PAIN MEDICINE BOARD REVIEW

PAIN MEDICINE BOARD REVIEW

EDITED BY

Marc A. Huntoon, MD

PROFESSOR OF ANESTHESIOLOGY

VIRGINIA COMMONWEALTH UNIVERSITY

RICHMOND VIRGINIA

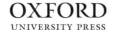
OXFORD

UNIVERSITY PRESS

OXFORD
UNIVERSITY PRESS

Oxford University Press is a department of the University of Oxford. It furthers
the University's objective of excellence in research, scholarship, and education
by publishing worldwide. Oxford is a registered trade mark of Oxford University
Press in the UK and certain other countries.

Published in the United States of America by Oxford University Press
198 Madison Avenue, New York, NY 10016, United States of America.

© Oxford University Press 2017

Library of Congress Cataloging-in-Publication Data
Names: Huntoon, Marc A., editor.
Title: Pain medicine board review / edited by Marc A. Huntoon.
Other titles: Pain medicine (Huntoon)
Description: Oxford ; New York : Oxford University Press, [2017] |
Includes bibliographical references and index.
Identifiers: LCCN 2016029256 (print) | LCCN 2016029915 (ebook) |
ISBN 9780190217518 (alk. paper) | ISBN 9780190217525 (e-book) |
ISBN 9780190217532 (e-book) | ISBN 9780190217549 (online)
Subjects: | MESH: Pain | Pain Management | Examination Questions
Classification: LCC RB127 (print) | LCC RB127 (ebook) | NLM WL 18.2 |
DDC 616/.0472076—dc23
LC record available at https://lccn.loc.gov/2016029256

This material is not intended to be, and should not be considered, a substitute for medical or other professional advice.
Treatment for the conditions described in this material is highly dependent on the individual circumstances. And, while
this material is designed to offer accurate information with respect to the subject matter covered and to be current as of
the time it was written, research and knowledge about medical and health issues is constantly evolving and dose schedules
for medications are being revised continually, with new side effects recognized and accounted for regularly. Readers must
therefore always check the product information and clinical procedures with the most up-to-date published product
information and data sheets provided by the manufacturers and the most recent codes of conduct and safety regulation.
The publisher and the authors make no representations or warranties to readers, express or implied, as to the accuracy or
completeness of this material. Without limiting the foregoing, the publisher and the authors make no representations
or warranties as to the accuracy or efficacy of the drug dosages mentioned in the material. The authors and the publisher
do not accept, and expressly disclaim, any responsibility for any liability, loss or risk that may be claimed or incurred as a
consequence of the use and/or application of any of the contents of this material.

1 3 5 7 9 8 6 4 2
Printed by WebCom, Inc., Canada

DISCLOSURES

The views expressed in Chapters 12 and 24 are those of the authors and do not necessarily reflect the official policy or position of the Department of the Navy, Department of Defense, or the United States Government.

CONTENTS

PREFACE

I undertook the writing of this book because of what I perceived as a gap in the available board review books at the time of my last recertification in pain medicine. There were a couple of books out then, but they seemed to be less focused on the actual key words and examination content outlines produced by the American Board of Anesthesiology (ABA) and other parent boards. As a former question writer for the ABA exam, I was well aware of the goals of those who develop those board exams. Despite the dearth of available review books, I (fortunately) did not find the exam to be too difficult. However, as someone who has led pain medicine programs at institutions such as the Mayo Clinic, Vanderbilt University, and now Virginia Commonwealth University, one should expect that academic faculty would stay abreast of the information relevant to a modern pain practice. The field of pain medicine has continued to evolve during the quarter century that I have been practicing, and the need for leadership in education has not lessened. Although no one book can be a sole source of study material for such an all-encompassing specialty area, it is my hope that this book will help medical students become interested in the field and that residents, fellows, or recertification candidates would become familiar enough with the material that they could pass the examination. I wish you the best, and hope that you find this field to be as fulfilling as I have, while remaining cognizant of the privilege it is to serve patients in pain. We must first be humble and strive to become knowledgeable to be the best we can.

Marc A. Huntoon, MD

CONTRIBUTORS

Ignacio Badiola, MD
Assistant Professor of Anesthesiology and Critical Care
University of Pennsylvania Perelman School of Medicine
Philadelphia, PA

William A. Beckman, MD, CAPT, MC, USN
Assistant Professor of Anesthesiology
Uniformed Services University of the Health Sciences
Staff Anesthesiologist and Pain Medicine Physician
Naval Medical Center Portsmouth, Virginia

Markus A. Bendel, MD
Department of Anesthesiology
Division of Pain Medicine
Mayo Clinic
Rochester, Minnesota

Gregory Carpenter, MD, MBA
Department of Anesthesiology
Vanderbilt University
Nashville, Tennessee

John Corey, MD
Assistant Professor of Clinical Anesthesiology
Division of Pain Medicine
Vanderbilt University
Nashville, Tennessee

Bryan Covert, MD
Pain Medicine Fellow
Department of Anesthesiology
Vanderbilt University
Nashville, Tennessee

Kurt F. Dittrich, MD
Assistant Professor of Clinical Anesthesiology
Division of Pain Medicine
Vanderbilt University
Nashville, Tennessee

David A. Edwards, MD, PhD
Assistant Professor of Anesthesiology
Vanderbilt University
Nashville, Tennessee

Ian M. Fowler, MD
Assistant Professor of Anesthesiology
Uniformed Services University of the Health Sciences
Staff Anesthesiologist and Pain Medicine Physician
Naval Medical Center San Diego
San Diego, California

Amitabh Gulati, MD
Director of Chronic Pain
Assistant Attending, Department of Anesthesiology
and Critical Care
Memorial Sloan Kettering Cancer Center
New York, New York

Robert J. Hackworth, MD
Division of Pain Medicine
Naval Medical Center
San Diego, California

M. Gabriel Hillegass, III, MD
Assistant Professor of Anesthesiology
Division of Pain Medicine
Department of Anesthesia and Perioperative Medicine
Medical University of South Carolina
Charleston, South Carolina

Joshua Horowitz, DO
Pain Medicine Fellow
Department of Anesthesiology
Vanderbilt University
Nashville, Tennessee

Joseph C. Hung, M.D.
Interventional Pain Management Physician
Tripler Army Medical Center
United States Department of Defense
New York, New York

Elizabeth Huntoon, MS, MD
Assistant Professor Physical Medicine and Rehabilitation
Assistant Professor Orthopedic Surgery and Rehabilitation
Director of Physical Medicine and Rehabilitation Medical
    Student Education
Vanderbilt Medical Group
Nashville, Tennessee

Adam K. Jacob, MD
Associate Professor of Anesthesiology
Mayo Clinic
Rochester, Minnesota

Usman Latif, MD, MBA
Assistant Professor of Anesthesiology
University of Kansas School of Medicine
Kansas City, Kansas

Daniel F. Lonergan, MD
Assistant Professor of Clinical Anesthesiology
Division of Pain Medicine
Vanderbilt University
Nashville, Tennessee

Maureen F. McClenahan, MD, CDR, MC, USN
Assistant Professor of Anesthesiology
Uniformed Services University of the Health Sciences
Director of Pain Medicine, Department of Anesthesiology and
Pain Medicine
Naval Medical Center
Portsmouth, Virginia

Kelly McQueen, MD, MPH
Professor of Anesthesiology
Division of Ambulatory Anesthesiology
Director, Vanderbilt Anesthesia Global Health &
    Development
Vanderbilt University
Nashville, Tennessee

Neel Mehta, MD
Medical Director, Pain Medicine
Department of Anesthesiology
Weill Cornell Medical College
New York-Presbyterian Hospital
New York, NY

Susan M. Moeschler, MD
Department of Anesthesiology
Division of Pain Medicine
Mayo Clinic
Rochester, Minnesota

Ramana K. Naidu, MD
Assistant Professor of Anesthesia & Perioperative Care
University of California, San Francisco
San Francisco, California

Andrea L. Nicol, MD, MS
Assistant Professor of Anesthesiology
University of Kansas School of Medicine
Kansas City, Kansas

Ryan Nobles, MD
Assistant Professor of Anesthesiology
Division of Pain Medicine
Department of Anesthesia and Perioperative Medicine
Medical University of South Carolina
Charleston, South Carolina

Daniel Pak, MD
Resident
Department of Anesthesiology
Weill Cornell Medical College
New York-Presbyterian Hospital
New York, NY

Meenal Patil, MD
Pain Management Center
Trenton, New Jersey

Julie R. Price, PsyD
Co-Interim Director for Health Psychology Services
Osher Center for Integrative Medicine at Vanderbilt
Assistant Professor of Clinical Psychiatry
Assistant Professor of Physical Medicine & Rehabilitation
Vanderbilt University School of Medicine
Nashville, Tennessee

Micah J. Price, PsyD
Director, Department of Psychology
Broward Health Medical Center
Assistant Clinical Professor of Psychology
Coordinator of Internship Training and
    Liaison Services
Nova Southeastern University
Fort Lauderdale, Florida

Antonio Quidgley-Nevares, MD
Associate Professor and Chairman of Physical Medicine &
    Rehabilitation
Staff Physiatrist and Pain Medicine Physician
Eastern Virginia Medical School
Norfolk, Virginia

Ellen W. K. Rosenquist, MD
Assistant Professor of Anesthesiology
Cleveland Clinic Lerner College of Medicine
Case Western Reserve University
Cleveland, Ohio

Martha J. Smith, MD
Assistant Professor of Anesthesiology
Division of Pain Medicine
Vanderbilt University
Nashville, Tennessee

Christopher Sobey, MD
Assistant Professor of Clinical
    Anesthesiology
Division of Pain Medicine
Vanderbilt University
Nashville, Tennessee

Natalie Strickland, MD
Assistant Professor of Anesthesiology
Emory University School of Medicine
Egleston Children's Hospital
Atlanta, Georgia

Hans P. Sviggum, MD
Medical Director, Obstetric Anesthesiology
Mayo Clinic
Rochester, Minnesota

Drew M. Trainor, DO
Denver Back Pain Specialists
Greenwood Village, CO

Anthony A. Tucker, MD
Assistant Professor of Anesthesiology
Uniformed Services University of the Health Sciences
Staff Anesthesiologist and Pain Medicine Physician
Naval Medical Center
Portsmouth, Virginia

Erik P. Voogd, MD
Division of Pain Medicine
Naval Medical Center
San Diego, California

Jenna L. Walters, MD
Assistant Professor of Clinical Anesthesiology
Division of Pain Medicine
Vanderbilt University
Nashville, Tennessee

Aaron Jay Yang, MD
Assistant Professor of Physical Medicine and Rehabilitation
Vanderbilt University
Nashville, Tennessee

Robert Yang, MD
Washington, DC

1.

PAIN ANATOMY AND PHYSIOLOGY

Daniel J. Pak and Neel Mehta

INTRODUCTION

This chapter focuses on pain anatomy and physiology to provide a comprehensive review of the mechanisms of nociception for preparation of the American Board of Anesthesiology Pain Medicine (PM) Examination. It reviews the anatomy of pain pathways (particularly the spinothalamic sensory tract) and the process of pain conduction from peripheral nociceptors to the cerebral cortex. It also reviews the different mechanisms of sensitization and inhibition at peripheral nociceptors (manifested as primary and secondary hyperalgesia), the spinal cord (wind-up and sensitization of second-order neurons), and supraspinal structures, which all affect the processing of nociceptive signals in the nervous system and, ultimately, the perception of pain.

QUESTIONS

1. Which of the following statements about nociceptors is false?

- A. Silent nociceptors respond to inflammation.
- B. Polymodal nociceptors are the most prevalent type.
- C. Mechanonociceptors respond to pinch and pinprick sensations.
- D. After repeated stimulation, nociceptors may demonstrate sensitization.
- E. Nociceptors have low thresholds for activation.

2. Arrange Aβ, Aδ, and C nerve fibers from the fastest to slowest conduction velocities.

- A. Aβ, C, Aδ
- B. Aβ, Aδ, C
- C. C, Aβ, Aδ
- D. C, Aδ, Aβ
- E. Aδ, Aβ, C

3. The following are true statements regarding abdominal visceral pain except:

- A. Nociceptive transmission occurs via C fibers.
- B. Distention of a hollow viscus has decreased intensity of pain compared to gut transection.
- C. Nociceptive transmission occurs with efferent sympathetic nerve fibers.
- D. Most gastrointestinal pain is characterized as a dull, aching sensation at the midline.
- E. Visceral pain is often associated with abnormal sympathetic activity.

4. Afferent pain fibers from most abdominal viscera nociceptors travel with sympathetic fibers in which of the following?

- A. Celiac plexus
- B. Superior hypogastric plexus
- C. Ganglion impar
- D. Stellate ganglion
- E. Hepatic plexus

5. All of the following statements are true regarding ascending pain pathways except:

- A. All first-order afferent nerve fibers enter the spinal cord via the dorsal spinal root.
- B. First-order neurons may synapse with sympathetic neurons.
- C. Second-order neurons in the dorsal horn mostly decussate to the contralateral side.

D. Wide dynamic range (WDR) neurons are second-order neurons.
E. Third-order neurons are located in the thalamus and send nerve fibers to the cortex.

6. Which of the following are excitatory neurotransmitters that modulate pain?

A. Substance P, glutamate, aspartate, γ-aminobutyric acid (GABA)
B. Substance P, glutamate, enkephalins, serotonin
C. Glutamate, aspartate, substance P, adenosine triphosphate (ATP)
D. Glutamate, serotonin, GABA, enkephalins
E. GABA, enkephalins, serotonin, ATP

7. Release of substance P may cause all of the following except:

A. Sensitization of nociceptors
B. Vasoconstriction
C. Enhanced chemotaxis
D. Mast cell degranulation
E. Increased neurokinin-1 activity

8. All of the following statements correctly characterize GABA activity except:

A. GABA is similar to glycine in that both are inhibitory neurotransmitters that inhibit ascending pain pathways.
B. Inhibition of pain signal transmission is facilitated by $GABA_B$ receptor activity.
C. GABA is an antagonist for *N*-methyl-D-aspartate (NMDA) receptors.
D. Benzodiazepines act on $GABA_A$ receptors.
E. All of the above statements are true.

9. Which of the following statements is true regarding WDR neurons compared to second-order nociceptive-specific neurons?

A. WDR neurons have smaller receptive fields compared to nociceptive-specific neurons.
B. WDR neurons are more prevalent than nociceptive-specific neurons.
C. WDR neurons decrease their firing rate with repeated stimulation.
D. WDR neurons only respond to noxious input.
E. Nociceptive-specific neurons can respond to non-noxious stimuli.

10. A 37-year-old otherwise healthy male experiences second-degree burns on the right forearm following a house fire. On physical exam, he has intense pain after application of mild heat at the site of injury. This is an example of:

A. Primary hyperalgesia
B. Secondary hyperalgesia
C. Allodynia
D. Paresthesia
E. Disinhibited pain

11. The same patient (from Question 10) returns 1 year later in clinic and says that after exposure to cold temperatures, he now experiences burning sensations in areas that were not injured during the house fire. Which of the following statements is incorrect regarding the patient's symptoms and central hypersensitivity?

A. WDR neurons exhibit a reduction in neural activation thresholds.
B. WDR. neurons have increased frequency of discharge with the same stimuli.
C. Substance P increases sensitization.
D. Nonsteroidal anti-inflammatory drugs (NSAIDs) do not have analgesic action on the spinal cord.
E. NMDA receptor activation increases sensitization.

12. A 71-year-old man who underwent an exploratory laparotomy for small bowel obstruction 2 weeks ago now experiences increased pain and allodynia at the surgical incision site. What direct role would NSAIDs have on relieving this patient's primary hyperalgesia?

A. Decrease prostacyclin and prostaglandin release
B. Decrease serotonin release
C. Decrease substance P release
D. Decrease calcitonin gene-related peptide (CGRP) release
E. Decrease all of the above substances

13. Which of the following statements is true regarding the spinothalamic tract?

A. The lateral spinothalamic tract projects mainly to the ventral posterolateral nucleus of the thalamus.
B. The lateral spinothalamic tract mediates emotional pain perception.
C. The medial spinothalamic tract carries information regarding intensity and location of pain.
D. The medial spinothalamic tract mediates perceptions of vibration and proprioception.
E. The spinothalamic tract mainly ascends in the gray matter of the spinal cord.

14. The periaqueductal gray (PAG) produces analgesia by all of the following mechanisms except:

A. Activation of interneurons in lamina II
B. Release of endogenous opioids
C. Inhibition of first-order neurons
D. Decreased release of substance P
E. All of the above statements are true

15. A 65-year-old male with intra-abdominal and retroperitoneal masses has persistent left-sided abdominal pain despite noninterventional treatments. His pain was refractory to oral medical therapy as well as intrathecal opioids. He underwent a unilateral percutaneous cervical cordotomy, an ablation procedure of the lateral spinothalamic (neospinothalamic) tract. However, he continues to complain of pain and severe distress following treatment. Which of the following statements is most likely true regarding this patient?

A. Cordotomies are more effective for relieving central pain rather than peripheral pain syndromes.
B. Ablation procedures such as cordotomies should not be recommended for patients with poor life expectancies.
C. A bilateral cordotomy would have been more effective for this patient.
D. Ablation of the medial spinothalamic (paleospinothalamic) tract could also be considered for this patient.
E. Cordotomies are not effective for reducing nociceptive pain.

16. Which of the following statements is most likely correct regarding the previous patient's pain (from Question 15)?

A. Inhibition of descending pain modulating pathways should decrease this patient's pain.
B. Spinothalamic fibers do not project to the PAG in the midbrain.
C. The PAG stimulates ascending pain fibers.
D. All pain fibers decussate to the contralateral spinal cord.
E. Other ascending pain pathways may contribute to this patient's pain.

17. A 58-year-old woman with recently diagnosed postherpetic neuralgia presents to the pain clinic after complaining of persistent hyperesthesia and allodynia. Which of the following best describes the most likely reason for her increased pain?

A. Decreased glutamate release
B. Activation of NMDA receptors
C. Lack of oral narcotic use

D. Decreased release of GABA
E. Lack of endogenous opiate release

18. The patient from Question 17 asks you about transcutaneous electrical nerve stimulation (TENS) as an additional modality of treatment for her pain. What is the most likely reason for the efficacy of TENS with relation to the gate control theory?

A. Inhibition of Aβ nerve fibers
B. Inhibition of the PAG
C. Inhibition of cutaneous nociceptors
D. Inhibition of C pain fibers
E. Inhibition of B fibers

19. A 49-year-old male with a history of poorly controlled type 2 diabetes mellitus presents to the pain clinic with bilateral lower extremity pain that is described as a constant burning sensation. He would like to avoid any opioid use due to gastrointestinal intolerances. He asks about the possible use of amitriptyline, a tricyclic antidepressant, as an analgesic option. Which of the following would be an appropriate response?

A. Tricyclic antidepressants would not be helpful because they do not have analgesic properties.
B. Tricyclic antidepressants would not be helpful because they are only effective for nociceptive pain syndromes.
C. Tricyclic antidepressants are adequate alternative analgesics because they predominantly act on μ-opiate receptors.
D. Tricyclic antidepressants are adequate alternative analgesics because they predominantly increase supraspinal inhibition.
E. Tricyclic antidepressants are adequate alternative analgesics because they predominantly act as glycine agonists.

20. Spinal cord gray matter is composed of 10 layers called Rexed laminae. Aδ fibers synapse predominantly on:

A. Lamina I and II
B. Lamina I and V
C. Lamina III and IV
D. Lamina VII
E. Lamina II and V

21. Neurons in Rexed lamina II (substantia gelatinosa) play an important role in modulating pain perception due to:

A. Inhibitory projections to ascending spinothalamic fibers
B. Increased release of substance P

C. Decreased release of GABA
D. High levels of WDR neurons that increase responsiveness to only noxious stimuli
E. Increased sensitization of cutaneous nociceptors

22. All of the following are true regarding the actions of endogenous opiates except:

A. Opioid receptors are distributed widely throughout the central nervous system, including the cerebral cortex, brainstem, dorsal horn, and dorsal root ganglion.
B. PAG stimulation decreases endogenous opiate release.
C. Presynaptic opiate receptor activation inhibits the release of glutamate and substance P.
D. Postsynaptic opiate receptor activation causes neuronal hyperpolarization.
E. Endogenous opiate peptides are antagonized by naloxone.

23. A 68-year-old male patient with a history of stage IVB hepatocellular carcinoma and diffuse bone metastases whom you have been treating for intractable pain has a pathologic femoral bone fracture. Which of the following systemic responses would you expect to see in this patient?

A. Tachycardia
B. Hyperglycemia
C. Increased oxygen consumption
D. Hypercoagulability
E. All of the above

ANSWERS

1. ANSWER: E

The vast majority of nociceptors are free nerve endings that respond to noxious stimuli, such as heat, mechanical, and chemical tissue injury. They have high activation thresholds and can increase neural firing rates depending on the intensity of the stimuli. Nociceptors also demonstrate functional plasticity, and with repeated stimulation they have sensitization. This can cause nerve transmission following a low-intensity noxious stimulus (hyperalgesia) or even after a non-noxious stimulus (allodynia). The three major nociceptor types are mechanonociceptors (responsive to pinch and pinprick sensations), silent nociceptors (responsive to inflammation), and polymodal mechano-heat nociceptors (the most common type; responsive to pressure, temperature, and neurochemical mediators such as histamine, capsaicin, and bradykinin).

FURTHER READING

Butterworth JF, Mackey DC, Wasnick JD. *Morgan and Mikhail's Clinical Anesthesiology*. 5th ed. New York, NY: McGraw-Hill; 2013.

2. ANSWER: B

Aβ afferent nerve fibers transmit non-noxious stimuli, whereas Aδ and C fibers transmit noxious stimuli (Table 1.1). In general, nerve conduction velocity is dependent on the diameter and degree of myelination of the nerve axon. Myelination increases the electrical insulation of the nerve and conducts the impulse at a higher velocity due to salutatory conduction along the axon. Larger nerves also have improved electrical conduction. As a result, conduction velocities are fastest for large, myelinated A fibers compared to smaller, nonmyelinated C fibers.

Table 1.1 **CHARACTERISTICS OF MAJOR AFFERENT NERVE FIBERS**

	C FIBERS	AΔ FIBERS	AB FIBERS
Function	Diffuse, dull pain	Sharp, localized pain	Light touch
Size (diameter; μm)	(0.3–1.6)	(1–4)	(6–22)
Myelination	–	+	++
Conduction velocity (m/s)	<2	5–25	>30

FURTHER READING

Barash PG, Cullen BF, Stoelting RK, et al. *Clinical Anesthesia*. 7th ed. Philadelphia, PA: Lippincott Williams & Wilkins; 2013.

3. ANSWER: B

Visceral nociceptors respond to chemical or mechanical stimuli, such as distention, ischemia, and inflammation. They do not respond as intensely to the localized transection or burning associated with surgery. These nerve fibers also synapse at several dermatomal levels and can cross the contralateral dorsal horn. As a result, pain is usually perceived at the midline and is characterized as a nonspecific dull and aching sensation. Visceral afferents travel via unmyelinated C fibers alongside efferent sympathetic nerve fibers. Consequently, afferent activity from these nociceptors is transmitted to the spinal cord between the levels of T1 and L2, and pain can be associated with abnormal sympathetic activity such as nausea, vomiting, and hemodynamic shifts.

FURTHER READING

Butterworth JF, Mackey DC, Wasnick JD. *Morgan and Mikhail's Clinical Anesthesiology*. 5th ed. New York, NY: McGraw-Hill; 2013.

4. ANSWER: A

The celiac plexus, which is anterior to the vertebral body of L1, carries afferent nociceptive and sympathetic innervation for most of the abdominal viscera. This includes innervation for the liver, pancreas, biliary tract, gallbladder, adrenal glands, spleen, kidneys, stomach, and small and large bowels. Therefore, celiac plexus blocks are effective for reducing chronic pain from upper abdominal visceral pathology (i.e., intractable pain from pancreatic cancer).

The superior hypogastric plexus, which is located anteriorly to the L5–S2 vertebral bodies, carries afferent and sympathetic innervation for the large bowel distal to the left colonic flexure and the pelvic viscera. The ganglion impar, which is located on the anterior surface of the coccyx, also provides afferent and sympathetic innervation for pelvic viscera. The stellate ganglion, located anteriorly to the C7 vertebral body, carries afferent and sympathetic innervation to portions of ipsilateral head, neck, and arm.

FURTHER READING

Kambadakone A, Thabet A, Gervais DA, et al. CT-guided celiac plexus neurolysis: A review of anatomy, indications, technique, and tips for successful treatment. *RadioGraphics*. 2011;31(6):1599–1621.

5. ANSWER: A

The transmission of pain signals starts with activation of first-order neurons, which mostly enter the dorsal horn of the spinal cord from the periphery via the dorsal spinal root. A minority of first-order neurons, however, may enter the spinal cord via the ventral nerve root, which is why some patients who undergo rhizotomies (transection of dorsal nerve roots in chronic pain patients for analgesia) can continue to feel pain following the procedure. First-order neurons may travel up or down several spinal segments in Lissauer's tract prior to synapsing with second-order neurons in the dorsal horn, which mostly decussate and cross the midline to the contralateral side of the spinal cord to ascend in the spinothalamic tract. Second-order neurons are either nociceptive-specific or WDR neurons. Both types receive noxious input from Aδ and C fibers, but WDR neurons receive non-noxious input as well. Second-order neurons then synapse with third-order neurons in the thalamus, which send fibers through the internal capsule to the cerebral cortex.

FURTHER READING

Butterworth JF, Mackey DC, Wasnick JD. *Morgan and Mikhail's Clinical Anesthesiology*. 5th ed. New York, NY: McGraw-Hill; 2013.
Hemmings HC, Egan TD. *Pharmacology and Physiology for Anesthesia: Foundations and Clinical Application*. Philadelphia, PA: Elsevier; 2013.

6. ANSWER: C

There are both excitatory and inhibitory neurotransmitters that act on afferent neurons transmitting pain information (Table 1.2). Substance P is an excitatory neuropeptide released by first-order neurons that acts on neurokinin-1

Table 1.2 NEUROTRANSMITTERS IN PAIN MODULATION

NEUROTRANSMITTER	MODULATING EFFECT
Glutamate	Excitatory
Aspartate	Excitatory
Substance P	Excitatory
Calcitonin gene-related peptide (CGRP)	Excitatory
Adenosine triphosphate (ATP)	Excitatory
γ-Aminobutyric acid (GABA)	Inhibitory
Acetylcholine	Inhibitory
Enkephalins	Inhibitory
β-Endorphins	Inhibitory
Serotonin	Inhibitory
Norepinephrine	Inhibitory

(NK-1) receptors to facilitate pain transmission. Other important excitatory neurotransmitters are glutamate and aspartate (both act on NMDA receptors), CGRP, and ATP.

FURTHER READING

Butterworth JF, Mackey DC, Wasnick JD. *Morgan and Mikhail's Clinical Anesthesiology*. 5th ed. New York, NY: McGraw-Hill; 2013.

7. ANSWER: B

Substance P is a neuropeptide that plays a major role as an excitatory neurotransmitter in nociception through its activation of NK-1 receptors. It is synthesized and released in response to painful stimuli from peripheral terminals of sensory nerve fibers and first-order neurons in the dorsal horn. In addition to its role as a facilitator of pain pathways, substance P sensitizes nociceptors, causes histamine degranulation from mast cells, and causes 5-HT release from platelets. Substance P is also a potent vasodilator via its activity on NK-1 receptors on the endothelium of blood vessels.

FURTHER READING

Butterworth JF, Mackey DC, Wasnick JD. *Morgan and Mikhail's Clinical Anesthesiology*. 5th ed. New York, NY: McGraw-Hill; 2013.

8. ANSWER: C

Both GABA and glycine are important neurotransmitters that are released by inhibitory interneurons in the dorsal horn and have an essential role for inhibiting other excitatory neural pathways. The major neurotransmitter for excitatory interneurons is glutamate. Through inhibition of WDR neurons and ascending pain fibers of the spinothalamic tract in the dorsal horn, G protein-coupled $GABA_B$ receptor activity plays an important role for analgesia. In fact, inhibition of $GABA_B$ receptors can lead to hyperesthesia and allodynia. $GABA_A$ receptors, on the other hand, are ligand-gated ion channels that increase Cl^- influx. Drugs such as benzodiazepines and barbiturates act on these receptors. GABA does not have any inherent NMDA receptor activity.

FURTHER READING

Butterworth JF, Mackey DC, Wasnick JD. *Morgan and Mikhail's Clinical Anesthesiology*. 5th ed. New York, NY: McGraw-Hill; 2013.

Hemmings HC, Egan TD. *Pharmacology and Physiology for Anesthesia: Foundations and Clinical Application.* Philadelphia, PA: Elsevier; 2013.

9. ANSWER: B

First-order neurons in the ascending pain pathway synapse with either second-order nociceptive-specific neurons or WDR neurons in the dorsal horn. WDR neurons are the most abundant in the dorsal horn. Both nociceptive-specific and WDR neurons receive noxious input from Aδ and C fibers, but WDR neurons receive non-noxious input as well. Therefore, WDR neurons are characterized by large receptive fields, whereas nociceptive-specific neurons have smaller, discrete receptive fields that are normally silent and responsive only to high-threshold noxious input. WDR neurons play a key role in central sensitization of pain. Repeated stimulation can exponentially increase the rate of firing of WDR neurons, causing a "wind-up" phenomenon that leads to increased second-order pain transduction for the same stimulus intensity.

FURTHER READING

Butterworth JF, Mackey DC, Wasnick JD. *Morgan and Mikhail's Clinical Anesthesiology.* 5th ed. New York, NY: McGraw-Hill; 2013.
Hemmings HC, Egan TD. *Pharmacology and Physiology for Anesthesia: Foundations and Clinical Application.* Philadelphia, PA: Elsevier; 2013.

10. ANSWER: A

This patient is experiencing hyperalgesia, which is an enhanced response to a noxious stimulant (Figure 1.1). Injury to the skin can cause two types: primary and secondary hyperalgesia. Primary hyperalgesia occurs at the site of injury and is due to release of various chemical modulators by the injured tissue (histamine, serotonin, bradykinin, and prostaglandins). This sensitizes nociceptors

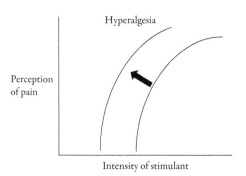

Figure 1.1 Hyperalgesia effect of pain perception.

and decreases the threshold for neural transmission. An enhanced response to the same stimulus intensity can be demonstrated, and continued transmission of pain signals following resolution of the stimulus is also common.

Secondary hyperalgesia develops in the region immediately surrounding the injured tissue and is a result of substance P release, which causes tissue edema, reddening or flaring of the skin around the site of injury, and sensitization to noxious stimuli. Unlike primary hyperalgesia, which occurs in response to both mechanical and heat stimuli, secondary hyperalgesia is triggered only by mechanical stimuli.

Allodynia refers to perception of pain following a nonnoxious stimulant, whereas paresthesia is an abnormal sensation (usually tingling or pricking) without an apparent stimulant.

FURTHER READING

Butterworth JF, Mackey DC, Wasnick JD. *Morgan and Mikhail's Clinical Anesthesiology.* 5th ed. New York, NY: McGraw-Hill; 2013.

11. ANSWER: D

Central sensitization refers to the enhancement and decreased inhibition of nociceptive pain pathways in the spinal cord to produce pain hypersensitivity. This can occur following an intense noxious stimuli or repeated exposure to stimuli.

Facilitation of central sensitization occurs primarily through one or more of the following mechanisms: (1) sensitization of second-order neurons where WDR neurons have increased response and frequency of discharge following stimulation, (2) a reduction in the neural activation threshold, and (3) an enlargement of the receptor fields such that adjacent neurons in the dorsal horn become responsive to both noxious (hyperalgesia) and innocuous (allodynia) stimuli. This patient is experiencing allodynia in areas beyond the original site of injury.

Substance P is one of the main mediators of central sensitization by facilitating increased neural membrane excitability through its interaction with G protein-coupled membrane receptors. Excitatory amino acids such as glutamate and aspartate also facilitate central sensitization through its activity on NMDA receptors. Prostaglandins help activate the release of these amino acids in the spinal cord; therefore, NSAIDs help reduce central sensitization.

FURTHER READING

Butterworth JF, Mackey DC, Wasnick JD. *Morgan and Mikhail's Clinical Anesthesiology.* 5th ed. New York, NY: McGraw-Hill; 2013.

Latremoliere A, Woolf CJ. Central sensitization: A generator of pain hypersensitivity by central neural plasticity. *J Pain*. 2009;10(9):895–926.

Hemmings HC, Egan TD. *Pharmacology and Physiology for Anesthesia: Foundations and Clinical Application*. Philadelphia, PA: Elsevier; 2013.

12. ANSWER: A

Tissue injury leads to the release of inflammatory mediators. This includes the production and release of prostaglandins, including prostaglandin E_2 (PGE_2), which activate and sensitize nociceptors. This leads to decreased nociceptor threshold for firing and an increased response to noxious stimuli as seen with primary hyperalgesia. NSAIDs counteract primary hyperalgesia through the decreased production of prostacyclin and prostaglandins via inhibition of the cyclooxygenase (COX) pathway. Recent studies have also indicated that COX inhibitors may decrease central sensitization of nociception in the spinal cord as well. Neurochemical mediators such as substance P, CGRP, and serotonin all have important excitatory effects on nociception but are not directly affected by NSAIDs.

FURTHER READING

Sinatra RS, Leon-Cassasola OA de, Viscusi ER. *Acute Pain Management*. New York, NY: Cambridge University Press; 2009.

13. ANSWER: A

The spinothalamic tract is the major ascending pain pathway that travels in the anterolateral portion of the spinal cord white matter. Axons of second-order neurons decussate via the anterior white commissure and ascend on the contralateral side to eventually project to supraspinal structures such as the thalamus, nucleus raphe magnus, and periaqueductal gray. Second-order neurons then synapse with third-order neurons in the thalamus to eventually project to the primary somatosensory cortex and the cingulate gyrus. It consists of two main pathways: the medial (paleospinothalamic) and lateral (neospinothalamic) tracts. The neospinothalamic tract transmits information regarding the location, duration, and intensity of pain and communicates to the ventral posterolateral nucleus (VPN) of the thalamus. The paleospinothalamic tract transmits emotional perceptions of pain and communicates to the medial thalamus.

FURTHER READING

Butterworth JF, Mackey DC, Wasnick JD. *Morgan and Mikhail's Clinical Anesthesiology*. 5th ed. New York, NY: McGraw-Hill; 2013.

14. ANSWER: E

The PAG of the midbrain plays an important role in supraspinal inhibition of ascending pain afferents. Stimulation of the PAG promotes excitatory connections with inhibitory interneurons in Rexed lamina II of the dorsal horn, which release endogenous opioids, such as enkephalin, that bind to μ-opiate receptors on axons of Aδ and C nerve fibers. Opiate receptor activation subsequently decreases substance P release from these primary afferent neurons, thereby inhibiting further activation of ascending second-order neurons and transmission of ascending pain signals. The PAG can also evoke antinociceptive action through adrenergic α_2 receptor activation in the dorsal horn. Deep brain stimulation of the PAG has been demonstrated to provide pain relief for some intractable pain syndromes, but it is not widely employed and remains "off-label" in the United States.

FURTHER READING

Boccard SGJ, Pereira EAC, Aziz TZ. Deep brain stimulation for chronic pain. *J Clin Neurosci*. 2015;22(10):1537–1543.

Budai D, Harasawa I, Fields HL. Midbrain periaqueductal gray (PAG) inhibits nociceptive inputs to sacral dorsal horn nociceptive neurons through α_2-adrenergic receptors. *J Neurophysiol*. 1998;80(5):2244–2254.

15. ANSWER: D

Patients with malignancies can experience severe pain that is refractory to opiates and intrathecal infusion therapies. Therefore, ablation procedures of the spinothalamic tract can be performed to relieve persistent nociceptive pain, with percutaneous cordotomy being an effective option for those with refractory unilateral nociceptive pain. Although effective at reducing pain, ablation procedures are usually recommended only in patients with limited life expectancies because the analgesic effects diminish over time. It is also more effective at relieving pain from peripheral nociceptor activation as seen with malignant pain syndromes in which tumors infiltrate bones or nerves. Neuropathic and central pain syndromes have less predictable results. Bilateral ablations are not commonly performed and are indicated only for bilateral or midline pain.

Cordotomies typically target ascending pathways in the lateral spinothalamic (neospinothalamic) tract, which transmits information regarding location, duration, and intensity of pain. Ablations of the medial spinothalamic (paleospinothalamic) tract do not provide analgesia by usual pain metrics, but they can provide relief of distress in malignancy pain syndromes and be helpful for managing the emotional perceptions of pain. Therefore, following an ablation of the paleospinothalamic tract, this patient may continue to perceive pain but not be distressed by it. Note that for this particular question, it is not necessary to know the specifics of what a cordotomy entails. However, one should know the differences between the two major spinothalamic pathways.

FURTHER READING

Frost EAM. *Clinical Anesthesia in Neurosurgery.* 2nd ed. Boston, MA: Butterworth-Heinemann; 1991.
Tollison CD, Satterthwaite JR, Tollison JW. *Practical Pain Management.* 3rd ed. Philadelphia, PA: Lippincott Williams & Wilkins; 2002.

16. ANSWER: E

Because there are multiple ascending pain pathways, some patients may continue to perceive pain following ablation procedures of the spinothalamic tract. Like the spinothalamic tract, the spinoreticular tract fibers decussate and ascend in the contralateral spinal cord to transmit signals to the thalamus and hypothalamus. These fibers mediate the emotional and autonomic aspects of pain. The spinocervical tract, another pathway for transmission of nociceptive pain, ascends ipsilaterally to the lateral cervical nucleus and projects to the contralateral thalamus. Dorsal column fibers that travel ipsilaterally and that were traditionally thought to transmit signals for proprioception have also been implicated to transmit visceral nociceptive information.

The PAG in the midbrain and the rostral ventromedial medulla are involved in regulating descending pathways that project to the dorsal horn to inhibit the ascending pain tracts. Therefore, stimulation of these areas with implants has been demonstrated to be potentially helpful in patients with chronic pain. It is important to know that fibers of the spinothalamic tract also project to the PAG and can modulate descending inhibitory pathways.

FURTHER READING

Butterworth JF, Mackey DC, Wasnick JD. *Morgan and Mikhail's Clinical Anesthesiology.* 5th ed. New York, NY: McGraw-Hill; 2013.
Frost EAM. *Clinical Anesthesia in Neurosurgery.* 2nd ed. Boston, MA: Butterworth-Heinemann; 1991.

Palecek J, Paleckova V, Willis WD. The roles of pathways in the spinal cord lateral and dorsal funiculi in signaling nociceptive somatic and visceral stimuli in rats. *Pain.* 2002;96(3):297–307.

17. ANSWER: B

This patient is experiencing wind-up, a mechanism of central pain sensitization. With repeated activation of C fibers, a progressive increase in the evoked response is seen such that WDR neurons increase their frequency of firing and also have prolonged firing after resolution of the stimulus. Glutamate and aspartate, both excitatory neurotransmitters, are important facilitators for wind-up through their activation of NMDA receptors, which can be found on WDR neurons. NMDA antagonists, such as ketamine, have been found to reduce wind-up pain in patients with postherpetic neuralgia and central neuropathic pain syndromes as well.

FURTHER READING

Eide PK. Wind-up and the NMDA receptor complex from a clinical perspective. *Eur J Pain.* 2000;4(1):5–15.

18. ANSWER: D

TENS is a noninvasive treatment that applies electrical current to the skin. This tactile, non-noxious stimulation activates Aβ fibers and modulates afferent information carried by ascending C pain fibers by inhibition within the substantia gelatinosa (or Rexed lamina II of the dorsal horn). This descending inhibition initiated by Aβ fibers is achieved via stimulation of the PAG. This has often been referred to as the gate control theory of pain. TENS has been associated with improving pain symptoms and decreasing opiate requirements in neuropathic pain syndromes, including postherpetic neuralgia, as well as in other acute pain syndromes.

FURTHER READING

Breivik H, Campbell WI, Nicholas MK. *Clinical Pain Management: Practice and Procedures.* 2nd ed. Boca Raton, FL: CRC Press; 2008.

19. ANSWER: D

Unlike nociceptive pain syndromes, chronic neuropathic pain syndromes are due to primary damage to nerve fibers of the peripheral or central nervous system. These conditions can be difficult to treat with conventional analgesics such as opiates and NSAIDs alone. Antidepressants such as tricyclic antidepressants (TCAs) and anticonvulsants such as gabapentin or pregabalin are typically considered first-line agents. TCAs inhibit serotonin and catecholamine reuptake in the synaptic nerve cleft, which increases monoamine-mediated inhibition of ascending pain pathways, thereby producing analgesia. This patient is experiencing diabetic neuropathic pain from his poorly controlled disease and would be considered an excellent candidate for antidepressant therapy.

FURTHER READING

Moore RA, Derry S, Aldington D, et al. Amitriptyline for neuropathic pain in adults. *Cochrane Database Syst Rev.* 2015;7:CD008242.

20. ANSWER: B

The spinal cord gray matter is divided into 10 Rexed laminae (Table 1.3), which follow a topographic organization and are organized based on different functions. Laminae I–VI comprise the dorsal horn and serve as the major area where both ascending and descending spinal pathways modulate pain. Some of the important layers are discussed here.

Table 1.3 REXED LAMINAE FUNCTIONS

REXED LAMINAE	FUNCTIONS
I	Somatic nociception, thermoreception
II	Somatic nociception, thermoreception, opiate responsive
III	Mechanoreception, proprioception
IV	Mechanoreception, proprioception
V	Visceral, somatic nociception, mechanoreception
VI	Mechanoreception, proprioception
VII	Preganglionic sympathies
VIII	Anterior motor horn
IX	Anterior motor horn
X	Central gray commissures

Lamina I contains second-order neurons that receive cutaneous and deep somatic nociceptive pain and temperature afferents. Lamina II (or substantia gelatinosa) contains second-order neurons that modulate cutaneous nociceptive information and are opiate responsive. Lamina III and IV second-order neurons receive non-nociceptive input and relay information regarding touch and proprioception. Lamina V processes visceral and somatic pain as well as non-noxious afferent information. Lamina VI relays proprioception information. Lamina VII contains preganglionic sympathetic neurons. Lamina VIII and IX comprise the anterior motor horn. Nociceptive C fibers synapse predominantly with second-order neurons in laminae I and II, whereas Aδ fibers terminate mainly on laminae I and V.

FURTHER READING

Butterworth JF, Mackey DC, Wasnick JD. *Morgan and Mikhail's Clinical Anesthesiology.* 5th ed. New York, NY: McGraw-Hill; 2013.
McMahon SB, Koltzenburg M, Tracey I, et al. *Wall and Melzack's Textbook of Pain.* 6th ed. Philadelphia, PA: Elsevier, 2013.

21. ANSWER: A

Rexed lamina II (substantia gelatinosa) neurons receive input from both Aδ and C fibers and play an essential role in modulating spinothalamic nerve fibers through their inhibitory interneurons. They do not release substance P. Lamina II interneurons also play an important role in analgesia through their expression of μ-opioid receptors. Although WDR neurons are common in the dorsal horn, they are most prevalent in lamina V. These second-order neurons have excitatory projections and respond to both non-noxious and noxious stimuli.

FURTHER READING

Trafton JA, Abbadie C, Marek K, et al. Postsynaptic signaling via the [mu] opioid receptor: Responses of dorsal horn neurons to exogenous opioids and noxious stimulation. *J Neurosci.* 2000;20(23):8578–8584.

22. ANSWER: B

The endogenous opiate system consists of three main peptides (β-endorphin, enkephalins, and dynorphins) and three main G protein-coupled receptors (μ, δ, and κ), which are widely expressed in the central nervous system, including the cerebral cortex, brainstem, limbic system, dorsal horn, and dorsal root ganglion. The release of endogenous opiates is triggered by activation of the PAG. Activation of opioid receptors leads to presynaptic inhibition of the release of excitatory chemical neurotransmitters, such as glutamate, substance P, and CGRP. Concurrently, opioid receptor activation also causes postsynaptic hyperpolarization for decreased neuronal excitability. Exogenous opioids have a predilection to act on second-order neurons in the substantia gelatinosa of the spinal cord. Both endogenous and exogenous opiates are antagonized by naloxone.

FURTHER READING

Benarroch EE. Endogenous opioid systems: Current concepts and clinical correlations. *Neurology*. 2012;79(8):807–814.

23. ANSWER: E

A neuroendocrine stress response is seen with acute pain syndromes that can be attributed to increased sympathetic activation and release of stress hormones. It can also be witnessed in chronic pain patients who experience prominent recurring nociceptive and central pain syndromes. Common cardiovascular effects include hypertension and tachycardia, which lead to increased cardiac output for patients with preserved cardiac function. This may also lead to increased oxygen consumption with increased work of breathing. An increase in the release of catecholamines and cortisol additionally leads to hyperglycemia as well as stress-related immunosuppression. Increased sympathetic activity can cause urinary retention or ileus. Hypercoagulability can also be seen with decreased fibrinolytic states. The patient described in this question is experiencing severe acute, superimposed on chronic pain, which places him at a high likelihood of developing the described systemic stress response.

FURTHER READING

Barash PG, Cullen BF, Stoelting RK, et al. *Clinical Anesthesia*. 7th ed. Philadelphia, PA: Lippincott Williams & Wilkins; 2013.
Butterworth JF, Mackey DC, Wasnick JD. *Morgan and Mikhail's Clinical Anesthesiology*. 5th ed. New York, NY: McGraw-Hill; 2013.
Hemmings HC, Egan TD. *Pharmacology and Physiology for Anesthesia: Foundations and Clinical Application*. Philadelphia, PA: Elsevier; 2013.

2.

LITERATURE REVIEW AND EVIDENCE

Andrea L. Nicol and Usman Latif

INTRODUCTION

This chapter reviews concepts underlying critical analysis of literature and evidence-based medicine because a thorough understanding of these topics is of utmost importance in the interpretation of medical literature and applicability of the results therein. Basic principles of valid clinical research and components of clinical trials are reviewed. The chapter explores specific topics pertaining to the designing, reporting, and interpreting of clinical studies about the treatment of pain. The effects of the analysis on the clinical applicability of study results are also discussed. Finally, the chapter identifies special features specific to the study of pain.

QUESTIONS

1. An investigator is performing a study in which there will be 100 separate independent comparisons in the analysis. At a significance level of 0.05, how many false-positive findings are possible on the average based on chance alone?

   A. 1
   B. 5
   C. 10
   D. 25
   E. 100

2. Which of the following is false regarding levels of evidence?

   A. Evidence meeting the highest standard is rated 1a.
   B. An individual randomized control trial (RCT) with a narrow confidence interval (CI) is rated as the highest level of evidence possible.
   C. An expert opinion is rated as a lower level of evidence than a case series.

   D. A common standard for levels of evidence allows for a uniform approach to comparison of different sources of data.
   E. Ratings are based on the design and quality of the study or paper.

3. Which of the following components of study design eliminates confounding by baseline variables, removes investigator bias, and guarantees that statistical tests will have valid false-positive error rates?

   A. Blinding
   B. Sample size calculation
   C. Informed consent
   D. Randomization
   E. Effect size

4. A researcher is interested in performing a randomized placebo-controlled trial for patients undergoing lumbar transforaminal steroid injections. Which of the following study parameters poses the greatest ethical challenge in the development and design of the proposed study?

   A. Placebo control
   B. Blinding
   C. Sample size
   D. Inclusion criteria
   E. Interim analysis

5. Which of the following is not an element of an informed consent?

   A. A statement that participation is voluntary
   B. A description of the benefits to the subject or others expected from the research
   C. Contact information for the US Department of Health and Human Services

D. A description of the foreseeable risks and discomforts to the subject

E. The expected duration of the subject's participation

6. Which of the following is true regarding grades of recommendation?

A. Grades of recommendation are used to describe the quality of the collection of evidence supporting an assertion using a range of 1 to 5.

B. Grades range from A to D.

C. 1a is the highest grade of recommendation.

D. Whether a recommendation is based on extrapolation is irrelevant to grading.

E. Grades of recommendation are ordered from lowest to highest levels of evidence strength.

7. Which of the following scales or questionnaires would be most beneficial to a pain researcher who is interested in measuring physical functioning as a marker of health-related quality of life in a study of patients with chronic low back pain?

A. Visual numerical pain score

B. Short Form (SF)-36

C. Visual analogue pain score

D. McGill Pain Questionnaire

E. Brief Pain Inventory

8. A study was performed to evaluate the efficacy of a new neuropathic drug in the treatment of postherpetic neuralgia. In the initial phase, all patients received the study drug, and outcome measures for changes in visual numerical pain scores were assessed before and after the study period. After the study period was complete, the researchers analyzed the data and selected only those patients who responded with a 30% or greater reduction in pain to continue the study in a randomized placebo-controlled trial. What specific type of study design is described here?

A. Crossover study design

B. Retrospective study design

C. Enrichment design

D. N-of-1 study design

E. Adaptive study design

9. An RCT study design is more likely to result in all of the following except:

A. Unbiased distribution of confounders

B. Facilitation of statistical analysis

C. Increased expense

D. Decreased volunteer bias

E. Attrition bias based on group allocation

10. Which of the following parameters provides clinicians with information on both the clinical significance and the statistical significance of an inferential statistical test?

A. p value

B. Effect size

C. Standard deviation

D. Confidence interval

E. Sample size

11. Which of the following is not a core outcome domain for chronic pain clinical trials as recommended by the Initiative on Methods, Measurement, and Pain Assessment in Clinical Trials (IMMPACT)?

A. Symptoms and adverse events

B. Physical functioning

C. Emotional functioning

D. Ratings of global improvement

E. Health care utilization

12. All the following are factors that should be considered when deciding whether you should use a parametric or nonparametric statistical analysis approach except:

A. The shape of the data distribution

B. The type of the data being analyzed

C. The assumption that samples are independent

D. The type of study design used

E. The assumption that variances are homogeneous

13. Match the following terms to the statements:
- **Case–control study**
- **Cross-sectional survey**
- **Crossover design**
- **Randomized controlled trial**
- **Cohort study**

A. What is a controlled trial in which each subject has both therapies at various points in time?

B. What design is best for studying the effect of an intervention?

C. What is a study design in which data are obtained from groups who have been exposed or not exposed to a variable of interest?

D. Which study design is best for the study of the effect of predictive risk factors on an outcome?

E. The prevalence of a disease or risk factor can be quantified best with which study design?

F. What is the only feasible study design for the study of very rare disorders?

14. A clinical trial is performed to evaluate the effectiveness of a new drug for fibromyalgia in a population sample of 120 patients. The mean decrease in pain scores after treatment in the active treatment group is 4.5. The mean decrease in average pain scores after treatment in the placebo group is 2.8. Assuming a normal distribution of the data, which statistical test is the best to utilize in comparing the mean change in average pain scores between the two groups?

A. Analysis of variance (ANOVA)
B. Student's *t*-test
C. Wilcoxon rank-sum test
D. Pearson coefficient of correlation
E. Chi-square test

15. Which of the following was developed as a tool to facilitate the complete and transparent reporting of trials and aid in their critical appraisal and interpretation in response to suboptimal and inadequate reporting of results from randomized controlled trials?

A. Cochrane database
B. PubMed
C. Consolidated Standards of Reporting Trials (CONSORT) Statement
D. Meta-analysis
E. EMBASE

16. What magnitude of change in visual analogue scale pain score is reported to be consistent with at least a moderately clinically meaningful reduction to chronic pain patients?

A. ≥20%
B. ≥30%
C. ≥40%
D. ≥50%
E. ≥60%

17. Which statistical principle is defined by the inclusion of all patients for analysis in the groups to which they were assigned, regardless of protocol adherence?

A. Intention-to-treat
B. Crossover
C. Per protocol
D. Bootstrapping
E. Subgroup analysis

18. Which of the following could be classified as an ordinal variable?

A. Color of eyes
B. Temperature (Celsius)

C. Satisfaction rating (very satisfied, moderately satisfied, etc.)
D. Height (cm)
E. Gender (male or female)

19. All of the following statements about research characteristics are true except:

A. In a double-blinded study, both patients and providers are unaware of the patients' group assignment.
B. Randomization is a process of selecting from a group in a manner that makes equal distribution of confounders likely.
C. If the patients who are likely to volunteer for a study are different than the general population, that is an example of confounding.
D. Stratification is a strategy in which patients are intentionally divided by an important characteristic prior to randomization.
E. In a triple-blinded study, patients, providers, and another group (e.g., data analyzers or support staff) are unaware of the patients' group assignment.

20. Which of the following is the probability of failing to reject the null hypothesis when there is an association between predictor and outcome?

A. Power
B. *p* value
C. Effect size
D. α
E. β

21. An investigator is researching the efficacy of two different drugs for painful diabetic polyneuropathy. In the study, there are two separate treatment periods separated by a period of time in which they are administered no medication. In the first treatment period, half of the group will be administered drug A and half will be administered drug B. In the second treatment period, the groups will receive the drug they did not receive in the first treatment period. What type of study design has this investigator employed for his research?

A. Crossover
B. Enrichment
C. Dose-finding
D. Randomized controlled trial
E. Adaptive

22. Which of the following groups of people are not considered to be vulnerable populations in research as

defined by the US Department of Health and Human Services?

A. Children and minors
B. Cognitively impaired persons
C. Cancer patients
D. Pregnant women
E. Prisoners

23. All of the following parameters are required to calculate sample size except:

A. Effect size
B. Variability (standard deviation)
C. α
D. β
E. p value

24. Which of the following components of clinical trial design specifies and defines the main characteristics of the sample population relevant to the research question?

A. Sample size
B. Inclusion criteria
C. Recruitment
D. Sampling error
E. Internal validity

25. Match the following terms to the statements:
- **Positive predictive value**
- **Number needed to treat (NNT)**
- **Power**
- **Specificity**
- **Sensitivity**

A. The inverse of the absolute risk reduction (ARR) is equal to which measure?
B. Which measure correlates with the proportion of negatives that are correctly identified as such?
C. The number of true positives divided by the sum of true positives and false positives is equal to?
D. Which measure quantifies the likelihood of identifying a significant effect when it exists?

ANSWERS

1. ANSWER: B

Many clinical trials have more than one measured outcome variable and several demographic variables of interest. Thus, a number of statistical comparisons will need to be made to analyze and interpret all of the data. The issue of multiple comparisons arises when enough significance tests are done, which leads to the increased likelihood that a test will be statistically significant based on chance alone. Multiple comparisons include repeated analyses of the same outcome variable and comparisons of multiple variables, including testing for differences in baseline characteristics and subgroup analyses. The significance level is also known as the type I error rate and is the probability of a false positive. It is denoted by the Greek letter α.

The implication of multiple comparisons is that the investigator should be cautious when interpreting the results. One way to counter the problem is to require a lower significance level; however, this will reduce the power of the trial. Another alternative is to increase the sample size so that a smaller significance level can be used while maintaining the power of the trial. This option may prove to be quite difficult for most investigators. Many adjustments can be used to approximate or control the significance level that should be used for interpretation of significant findings, including the Bonferroni correction, Holm procedure, and Hochberg procedure.

In the case of this investigator who is running 100 separate comparisons with a significance level of 0.05, 5 of them will be significant based on chance alone.

FURTHER READING

Cook TD, DeMets DL. Selected issues in the analysis. In: *Introduction to Statistical Methods for Clinical Trials*. Boca Raton, FL: Chapman & Hall/CRC Press; 2008: 333–370.

Friedman LM, Furberg CD, DeMets DL. Issues in data analysis. In: *Fundamentals of Clinical Trials*. 4th ed. New York, NY: Springer; 2010:345–390.

2. ANSWER: B

Utilizing a common framework for judging the strength of scientific work allows for a standard approach to comparing evidence and allows conflicting evidence to be weighted differentially. This systematic approach to levels of evidence is essential to the practice of evidence-based medicine. The Oxford Centre for Evidence-Based Medicine publishes and maintains a "Levels of Evidence" document.

Evidence is classified into one of five categories (Box 2.1). The evidence is then rated, in declining order of strength, as 1a, 1b, 1c, 2a, 2b, 2c, 3a, 3b, 4, or 5. The ratings are based on the design and quality of the study or paper. For example,

---

> *Box 2.1* EVIDENCE CATEGORIES
>
> Therapy/Prevention or Etiology/Harm
>
> Prognosis
>
> Diagnosis
>
> Differential Diagnosis or Symptom Prevalence Study
>
> Economic and Decision Analysis

for therapy studies, systematic reviews (with homogeneity) of RCTs receive the highest rating of 1a. Cohort studies and outcomes research generally receive a rating in the 2 category, whereas case–control studies are classified in the 3 category. A case series would be rated as 4, whereas an expert opinion paper would receive the lowest rating of 5.

FURTHER READING

Centre for Evidenced-Based Medicine (CEBM). Oxford Centre for Evidence-Based Medicine—Levels of evidence (March 2009). 2009. Available at http://www.cebm.net/oxford-centre-evidence-based-medicine-levels-evidence-march-2009. Accessed July 21, 2015.

3. ANSWER: D

Randomized control trials are comparative studies with an intervention group and a control group, in which the assignment of a subject to a group is determined by a formal process of randomization. In the simplest of terms, randomization is a procedure in which all participants are equally likely to be assigned to either the intervention group or the control group.

Randomization is an important concept and is advantageous for many reasons. First, randomization tends to produce comparable groups. This means that measured and unmeasured or unknown characteristics and prognostic factors of the participants will be, on average, evenly balanced between the intervention and control groups. Second, randomization removes the possibility of bias in the allocation of participants to the intervention group or to the control group, also known as selection bias. Selection bias can be conscious or subconscious and can easily invalidate comparisons, which is why randomization is so important. Finally, randomization provides a sound foundation for valid statistical inference and guarantees the validity of inferential tests of statistical significance. Thus, it ensures independence between assigned treatment and outcome and allows the researcher to state that observed differences between treatment groups are not attributable to chance.

Many different procedures can be employed to provide randomization for research studies, including blocked, stratified, adaptive, and play the winner.

FURTHER READING

Cook TD, DeMets DL. Randomization. In: *Introduction to Statistical Methods for Clinical Trials*. Boca Raton, FL: Taylor & Francis; 2008:141–170.

Friedman LM, Furberg CD, DeMets DL. Issues in data analysis. In: *Fundamentals of Clinical Trials*. 4th ed. New York, NY: Springer; 2010:345–390.

Piantadosi S. Treatment allocation. In: *Clinical Trials: A Methodologic Perspective*. 2nd ed. Hoboken, NJ: Wiley; 2005:331–353.

4. ANSWER: A

Although randomized, placebo-controlled trials are highly regarded to be the gold standard of clinical research, the use of a placebo in surgery and skill-dependent therapies, such as interventional pain management, is considered to be controversial due to the ethical considerations of performing a "sham" intervention. Sham interventions are apt to cause moral discomfort in clinician–investigators, who are trained to perform invasive interventions only for the medical benefit of patients.

Although sham interventions have the potential to harm subjects, research designs without a placebo or sham intervention are considered to be scientifically less vigorous. Horng and Miller contend that ethical objections—based on risk–benefit optimization and informed consent issues—do not support an absolute prohibition of the use of placebo/sham interventions when their use is methodologically necessary to answer clinically relevant questions. They suggest that each proposed trial involving sham procedures must be carefully evaluated in light of these ethical considerations. Furthermore, Miller and Kaptchuk purport that the use of sham interventions does not violate the rights of patient–subjects provided they have been adequately informed and fully understand that they will receive either a real or a sham intervention.

FURTHER READING

Horng S, Miller FG. Is placebo surgery unethical? *N Engl J Med*. 2002;347:137–139.

Miller FG, Kaptchuk TJ. Sham procedures and the ethics of clinical trials. *J R Soc Med*. 2004;97(12):576–578.

Piantadosi S. Contexts for clinical trials. In: *Clinical Trials: A Methodologic Perspective*. 2nd ed. Hoboken, NJ: Wiley; 2005:65–105.

5. ANSWER: C

Informed consent is an essential and important facet of clinical research. Instead of being viewed as a simple endpoint of a signature on a form, the consent document should be viewed as a basis for meaningful exchange of information between the investigator and the subject. Institutional review boards (IRBs), clinical investigators, and research sponsors all share responsibility to ensure that the informed consent process is adequate. The US Food and Drug Administration's *Code of Federal Regulations* Title 21 provides the required basic and optional additional elements of the informed consent document (Box 2.2).

Box 2.2 BASIC AND ADDITIONAL ELEMENTS OF INFORMED CONSENT

- Basic elements
  - A statement that the study involves research, including
    - Explanation of the purposes of the research
    - Expected duration of the subject's participation
    - Description of the procedures to be followed
    - Identification of experimental procedures
  - Description of reasonable foreseeable risks or discomforts to the subject
  - Description of any benefits to the subject or others that may be expected from the research
  - Disclosure of alternative procedures or treatment that may be advantageous to the subject
  - A statement describing how confidentiality of the records identifying the subject will be maintained
  - For research involving more than minimal risk
    - Explanation as to whether compensation and any medical treatments are available if injury occurs *and*
    - If so, what they consist of and where further information can be obtained
  - Contact information for answers to pertinent questions about the research and research subject's rights and whom to contact in the event of a research-related injury
  - A statement that participation is voluntary
    - Refusal to participate will involve no penalty or loss of benefits to which the subject is otherwise entitled
    - Subject may discontinue participation at any time without penalty
- Additional elements
  - A statement that there may be unforeseeable risks to the subject
  - Circumstances in which the subject's participation may be terminated by the investigator
  - Any additional costs to the subject that may result from participation in the research
  - Consequences of a subject's decision to withdraw from the research
    - Procedures for orderly termination of participation by the subject
  - A statement that significant new findings developed during the course of research that may relate to their willingness to continue participation will be provided
  - The approximate number of subjects involved in the study

FURTHER READING

US Department of Health and Human Services, Office for Human Research Protections. Informed consent checklist. Available at http://www.hhs.gov/ohrp/policy/consentckls.html. Accessed July 10, 2015.

US Food and Drug Administration. A guide to informed consent—Information sheet. Available at http://www.fda.gov/RegulatoryInformation/Guidances/ucm126431.htm. Accessed July 10, 2015.

US Food and Drug Administration. CFR—Code of Federal Regulations Title 21. Available at http://www.accessdata.fda.gov/scripts/cdrh/cfdocs/cfcfr/CFRSearch.cfm?fr=50.25. Accessed July 10, 2015.

6. ANSWER: B

When making an evidence-based recommendation, it is important to be able to summarize the quality of the underlying evidence. The Oxford Centre for Evidence-Based Medicine has designed a system for grading recommendations. Grades of recommendation range, in declining order of strength of underlying evidence, from A to D. The grading takes into account the levels of evidence assigned to the underlying studies. Also taken into account is whether extrapolation has occurred or whether the intended use situation has potential clinically important differences from the original study situation. This type of extrapolation generally results in a one category downgrade of the grade of recommendation. The Oxford Centre for Evidence-Based Medicine has summarized this grading scale (Table 2.1).

Table 2.1 GRADES OF RECOMMENDATION

GRADE	DESCRIPTION
A	Consistent level 1 studies
B	Consistent level 2 or 3 studies *or* extrapolations from level 1 studies
C	Level 4 studies *or* extrapolations from level 2 or 3 studies
D	Level 5 evidence *or* troublingly inconsistent/inconclusive studies of any level

FURTHER READING

Centre for Evidenced-Based Medicine (CEBM). Oxford Centre for Evidence-Based Medicine—Levels of evidence (March 2009). 2009. Available at http://www.cebm.net/oxford-centre-evidence-based-medicine-levels-evidence-march-2009. Accessed July 21, 2015.

7. ANSWER: E

In a clinical trial for chronic pain, pain reduction is a necessary outcome variable; however, it is important to consider other outcomes in clinical trials. In order to relieve clinical symptoms, the objectives of health care interventions include improvement of functioning and health-related quality of life. IMMPACT was formed with the mission to develop consensus reviews and recommendations for improving the design, execution, and interpretation of clinical trials for treatments of pain. IMMPACT recommendations and guidelines have been widely cited and have helped guide clinical trial design. Specific areas in which they have made recommendations include core outcome domains, core outcome measures, development of outcome measures, interpretation of clinical importance of treatment outcomes, core outcome and treatment measures for pediatric pain, clinical importance of group differences, analyzing multiple endpoints, research design for confirmatory clinical trials, research design for proof-of-concept studies, and design implications for chronic pain prevention studies.

With regard to the physical functioning domain of health-related quality of life, measures include the ability to carry out such daily activities as household chores, walking, work, travel, and self-care, in addition to strength and endurance measures. Based on the 2005 IMMPACT consensus publication, the group recommends use of either the Multidimensional Pain Inventory or the Brief Pain Inventory (BPI) for physical functioning measures. The BPI contains a Pain Interference Scale that provides reliable and valid measures of the interference of pain with physical functioning. The SF-36 Health Survey may be used as a more generic measure of health-related quality of life per IMMPACT's guidelines.

FURTHER READING

Dworkin RH, Turk DC, Farrar JT, et al. Core outcome measures for chronic pain clinical trials: IMMPACT recommendations. *Pain*. 2005;113:9–19.

Initiative on Methods, Measurement, and Pain Assessment in Clinical Trials (IMMPACT). IMMPACT website. http://www.immpact.org/index.html. Accessed July 13, 2015.

8. ANSWER: C

Treatment response is often highly variable among subjects in clinical trials for pain. Variability may be due to multiple factors, including different degrees of improvement due to placebo effects or other nonspecific factors, protocol adherence, difficulty in reliable and consistent pain reporting, difficulty tolerating the treatment, and treatments working better in some individuals than in others. The enrichment study design can be used in an attempt to decrease these various sources of variability in order to increase the chances of detecting an effect if it truly exists. An enrichment design uses run-in periods to identify and exclude subjects who have a prespecified level of treatment or placebo response, noncompliance, treatment intolerability, or variability in pain ratings. Thus, the enrichment design helps a researcher select subjects in whom a treatment effect may be more easily detected.

In the case of this study, by enriching the study with subjects based on a prespecified level of positive response to the investigational treatment, the second phase of the study will consist of a cohort of subjects for whom the treatment is likely to be efficacious. Limitations of enrichment study design include a limit on the generalizability of the results to a larger population of patients and the possibility of unblinding in the second phase as a patient who responds to a certain treatment may recognize the absence of pain relief or side effects if he or she is switched to placebo.

FURTHER READING

Dworkin RH, Turk DC, Peirce-Sandner S, et al. Research design considerations for confirmatory chronic pain clinical trials: IMMPACT recommendations. *Pain*. 2010;149:177–193.
Gewandter JS, Dworkin RH, Turk DC, et al. Research designs for proof-of-concept chronic pain clinical trials: IMMPACT recommendations. *Pain*. 2014;155:1683–1695.

9. ANSWER: D

Randomized controlled trials are experimental studies in which subjects are randomly assigned to treatment/intervention groups or control/placebo groups. RCTs are among the most rigorous study designs that can be employed. The advantages of such a design include increased likelihood of blinding (particularly in double-blinded studies), statistical analysis facilitated by randomization, and unbiased distribution of confounders.

The disadvantages include increased time to conduct the research; increased expense; and occasionally ethical ramifications having to do with randomizing patients to different treatment or nontreatment/placebo groups, especially if there is concern that one treatment option may be clearly superior. Attrition bias may occur when patients drop out of the study from one or the other of the study groups preferentially. For example, participants in the control group may be unhappy with a lack of progress and may drop out of the study to seek alternative treatment or participants in the treatment group may become lost to follow-up if treatment has been successful.

An additional disadvantage is volunteer bias. The goal of sampling is to obtain a representative sample of the larger population to be studied. Randomization is employed to improve the quality of the sample. However, patients are being randomized from a sample population consisting of volunteers willing to participate in the research. It may be possible that the individuals who are willing to volunteer for research are different in characteristics than the population as a whole. For example, it may be that more impoverished individuals volunteer for a paid drug trial, whereas affluent individuals do not.

FURTHER READING

Centre for Evidence-Based Medicine (CEBM). Study designs. 2014. Available at http://www.cebm.net/study-designs. Accessed July 21, 2015.
University of Texas at Austin. Common mistakes in using statistics: Biased sampling. 2015. Available at http://www.ma.utexas.edu/users/mks/statmistakes/biasedsampling.html. Accessed July 21, 2015.

10. ANSWER: D

The main purpose of clinical research is to perform a study in which the results obtained are applicable to a target population of people with a certain disease. Practically speaking, it is usually not possible to perform a study on "all" people in the target population. Instead, studies are performed on a sample of people drawn from the target population. The results of a clinical study are therefore used as estimates of what may happen if the treatment is given to the whole population of interest. Confidence intervals (CIs) provide a range of plausible values for a population parameter based on the study data results and give an indication of the precision of the measured treatment. The 95% CI is usually reported in the medical literature and represents the range in which there is 95% certainty that the true population parameter will lie. The width of a CI indicates the precision of the estimated parameter in that the wider the CI, the less the precision and higher amount of random error in the measurements.

CIs also provide useful information on the clinical importance of the results and, like p values, can be used to assess statistical significance. Clinical significance is represented by a difference in effect size between groups that could be considered important in clinical decision-making. If an effect size is known as being clinical important, CIs that contain that effect size values can indicate that the result of the test is likely of clinical significance. p values provide no information on the clinical importance of any observed differences between study groups. Whereas a p value indicates whether the results could or could not have arisen by chance, a statistically significant finding has little relation to clinical significance. CIs can provide information on statistical significance in that a p value will be less than 0.05 if the CI does not include whatever value is specified in the null hypothesis. For example, if a CI for a mean difference does not include 0, the data are not consistent with equal population means, and we can state that there is a statistically significant difference between the groups.

FURTHER READING

Akobeng AK. Confidence intervals and *p*-values in clinical decision making. *Acta Paediatr*. 2008;97:1004–1007.
Gardner MJ, Altman DG. Confidence intervals rather than *P* values: Estimation rather than hypothesis testing. *Br Med J (Clin Res Ed)*. 1986;292:746–750.

11. ANSWER: E

IMMPACT was formed with the mission to develop consensus reviews and recommendations for improving the design, execution, and interpretation of clinical trials for treatments of pain. IMMPACT recommendations and guidelines have been widely cited and have helped guide chronic pain clinical trial design. Specific areas in which it has made recommendations include core outcome domains, core outcome measures, development of outcome measures, interpretation of clinical importance of treatment outcomes, core outcome and treatment measures for pediatric pain, clinical importance of group differences, analyzing multiple endpoints, research design for confirmatory clinical trials, research design for proof-of-concept studies, and design implications for chronic pain prevention studies.

Turk et al. recommended that each of the six core outcome domains should be considered in all clinical trial designs for both efficacy and effectiveness of treatments for chronic pain. Furthermore, if one or more of the domains are not used as an outcome in a study, the reasons for excluding the outcome should be justified a priori. The six core outcome domains as recommended by IMMPACT are pain, physical functioning, emotional functioning, participant ratings of global improvement and satisfaction with treatment, symptoms and adverse events, and participant disposition. Additional or supplemental outcome domains that researchers may elect to use include role functioning, interpersonal functioning, pharmacoeconomic measures and health care utilization, biological markers, coping, clinician ratings of global improvement, neuropsychological assessments of cognitive and motor function, and suffering or other end-of-life issues.

FURTHER READING

Initiative on Methods, Measurement, and Pain Assessment in Clinical Trials. IMMPACT website. http://www.immpact.org/index.html. Accessed July 13, 2015.

Turk DC, Dworkin RH, Allen RR, et al. Core outcome domains for chronic pain clinical trials: IMMPACT recommendations. *Pain*. 2003;106(3):337–345.

12. ANSWER: D

Parametric and nonparametric are two broad classifications of statistical testing procedures. Parametric tests are based on assumptions about the distribution of the underlying population from which the sample was taken. The most common assumption is that the data are normally distributed, also known as a Gaussian distribution. Characteristics of normal distributions include the following : Data are symmetric about the mean, have bell-shaped density curves with a single peak, and are defined by mean (μ) and standard deviation (σ); and mean, median, and mode are the same. In normal distributions, 68% of the total area under the curve is within one standard deviation of the mean, 95% of the total area under the curve is within two standard deviations of the mean, and 99.7% of the total area under the curve is within three standard deviations of the mean. Other factors that determine whether or not a parametric test is suitable include the type of data being analyzed, homogeneity of variances, and whether or not the samples are independent. In contrast, nonparametric statistical procedures rely on few or no assumptions about the shape or parameters of the population distribution from which the sample was taken.

It is important to understand when to use a parametric versus a nonparametric statistical procedure. Nonparametric tests use less information and therefore are more conservative tests compared to their parametric alternatives. Thus, if a nonparametric test is used when you have parametric data, the power of the analysis can be decreased, meaning you are less likely to get a significant result when there truly is a significant result. However, if a parametric test is used wrongly when the data are actually nonparametric, the likelihood of incorrect conclusions increases. In addition to less power, results of nonparametric procedures are more difficult to interpret because many of the tests use rankings of the values in the data rather than using the actual data, which reduces the clinical understanding of the data and results.

FURTHER READING

Hoskin T. Parametric and nonparametric: Demystifying the terms. Available at http://www.mayo.edu/mayo-edu-docs/center-for-translational-science-activities-documents/berd-5-6.pdf. Accessed July 23, 2015.

13. ANSWERS:

A. A controlled trial in which each subject has both therapies at various points in time is a crossover design. Studies with a crossover design allow each subject to receive both therapies. They are randomized to treatment A or treatment B first and then switch to the other treatment at the crossover point. Subjects serve as their own controls, and all subjects receive treatment at least part of the time. This design can be problematic if the washout period for a treatment is lengthy or unknown. In addition, the treatment effect has to be reversible. In other words, if the treatment could lead to a permanent cure for a condition, then a crossover study design is not appropriate.

B. The design that is best for studying the effect of an intervention is the randomized controlled trial. See "randomized controlled trial" row in Table 2.2.

C. The study design in which data are obtained from groups that have been exposed or not exposed to a variable of interest is a cohort study. See "cohort study" row in Table 2.2.

D. The study design that is best for the study of the effect of predictive risk factors on an outcome is a cohort study. See "cohort study" row in Table 2.2.

E. The prevalence of a disease or risk factor can be quantified best with cross-sectional survey. See "cross-sectional survey" row in Table 2.2.

F. The only feasible study design for the study of very rare disorders is a case–control study. See "case–control study" row in Table 2.2.

FURTHER READING

Centre for Evidence-Based Medicine (CEBM). Study designs. 2014. Available at http://www.cebm.net/study-designs. Accessed July 21, 2015.

14. ANSWER: B

In this study, the analysis to be performed is to compare means between two independent groups. Given that the data are normally distributed, one can utilize a parametric test to compare the two groups. The appropriate parametric statistical procedure to compare the means of two independent groups is a Student's t-test. In Table 2.3, common analysis types and statistical procedures are categorized with corresponding parametric and nonparametric tests.

Table 2.2 **ATTRIBUTES OF RESEARCH STUDY DESIGNS**

STUDY DESIGN	DESCRIPTION	ADVANTAGES	DISADVANTAGES
Randomized controlled trial(RCT)	An experimental comparison study in which randomization is used to allocate participants into control/placebo or intervention/treatment groups. This is the best design to study the effect of an intervention.	• Unbiased distribution of confounders • Blinding • Statistical analysis facilitated by randomization	• Time-consuming and costly • Volunteer bias
Crossover design	Each study participant has both treatments or interventions. Subjects are randomized to which treatment they receive first. At the crossover point, the subjects switch treatments.	• Subjects serve as their own control, leading to reduced sample size requirements. • All subjects receive the treatment or intervention at some point. • Blinding	• Not a good design for nonreversible outcomes where treatment or intervention leads to a permanent change or cure • Not good for treatments with lengthy or unknown washout period
Cohort study	Subjects are identified who have already been exposed, or not exposed, to the factor. Data are then collected. The design is best for determining the effect of predictive risk factors on an outcome.	• Timing and directionality of events can be established. • It is more convenient and less expensive than an RCT.	• Difficult to identify controls and blind • Possibility of hidden confounder • No randomization • Not suited for rare diseases
Case–control study	A careful process is used to identify patients with or without a particular disease or outcome. Data are then collected on exposure to factors of interest.	• Fast and inexpensive • Feasible for rare disorders • Smaller sample size required in comparison to cross-sectional study	• Relies on historical data or recall to determine exposure • Possibility of confounders • Potential recall and selection bias
Cross-sectional survey	Exposure and outcome are measured at the same time in a defined population. This is best for determining the prevalence of a disease or risk factor.	• Inexpensive • Simple • No ethical implications	• Established association not causality • Possible recall bias • Neyman bias

Table 2.3 **PARAMETRIC AND NONPARAMETRIC STATISTICAL PROCEDURES BY TYPE OF ANALYSIS**

ANALYSIS TYPE	EXAMPLE	PARAMETRIC TEST	NONPARAMETRIC TEST
Compare means between two independent groups	Is the mean pain score at baseline for patients assigned to treatment group different from the mean pain score for patients assigned to the placebo group?	Student's *t*-test	Wilcoxon rank-sum test
Compare two numerical measurements taken from the same individuals	Was there a significant change in quality of life scores between baseline and the 3-month follow-up measurement in the treatment group?	Paired *t*-test	Wilcoxon signed-rank test
Compare means between three or more independent groups	Do baseline physical functioning scores differ at baseline in an experiment with three distinct groups (placebo, drug 1, and drug 2)?	Analysis of variance (ANOVA)	Kruskal–Wallis test
Compare multiple numerical measurements taken from the same individuals	Was there a significant change in pain scores in patients receiving treatment measured at baseline, 1 month, 3 months, and 6 months?	Repeated measures ANOVA	Friedman test

FURTHER READING

Hoskin T. Parametric and nonparametric: Demystifying the terms. Available at http://www.mayo.edu/mayo-edu-docs/center-for-translational-science-activities-documents/berd-5-6.pdf. Accessed July 23, 2015.

Sheskin DJ. *Handbook of Parametric and Nonparametric Statistical Procedures*. 5th ed. New York, NY: Chapman & Hall/CRC Press; 2011.

15. ANSWER: C

Comprehension of the results of an RCT entails that readers must have a complete understanding of its design, conduct, analysis, and interpretation. In order for this to occur, the authors of the study must provide complete transparency of all details. In the mid-1990s, CONSORT was developed by an international group of clinical trialists, statisticians, epidemiologists, and biomedical journal editors as a means of improving reporting of RCTs. The CONSORT Statement, most recently updated in 2010, is an evidence-based minimum set of recommendations including a checklist and flow diagram for reporting RCTs (Figure 2.1). It is meant to facilitate the complete and transparent reporting of trials and aid in their critical appraisal and interpretation.

Although use of the CONSORT Statement is not universal and not required by all medical journals and texts, a Cochrane review by Turner et al. concluded that journal endorsement of the CONSORT Statement may beneficially influence the comprehensiveness of RCT and trial reporting published in medical journals and texts.

FURTHER READING

Moher D, Schulz KF, Altman D. The CONSORT statement: Revised recommendations for improving the quality of reports of parallel-group randomized trials. *JAMA*. 2001;285(15):1987–1991.

Turner L, Shamseer L, Altman DG, et al. Consolidated Standards of Reporting Trials (CONSORT) and the completeness of reporting of randomised controlled trials (RCTs) published in medical journals. *Cochrane Database Syst Rev*. 2012; Issue 11:1–162.

16. ANSWER: B

In determining clinically important changes for outcome measures in the study of pain, interpretation of two separate aspects of the results must be distinguished. First, it must be established what change in the outcome measure represents a clinically meaningful difference for patients. Second, it must be established what difference in the magnitude of the response between the control and treatment groups is deemed to be large enough to ascertain the therapeutic significance of the results.

For clinical trials designed to evaluate the efficacy of chronic pain therapies, the primary outcome of interest commonly involves reduction in pain score intensity. Multiple studies have been performed to evaluate the magnitude of pain reduction that represents a clinically meaningful response to the pain treatment for patients, and an IMMPACT publication summarized the results with recommendations as noted in Box 2.3.

> *Box 2.3* CLINICALLY MEANINGFUL CHANGES IN VISUAL ANALOGUE SCALE PAIN SCORES
>
> - Minimal clinically meaningful change
>   - Raw pain score change of approximately 1 point
>   - 10–20% reduction in chronic pain intensity
> - Moderate clinically meaningful change
>   - Raw pain score change of approximately 2 points
>   - ≥30% reduction in chronic pain intensity
> - Substantial clinically meaningful change
>   - Raw pain score change of approximately 4 points
>   - ≥50% reduction in chronic pain intensity

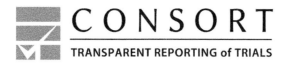

CONSORT
TRANSPARENT REPORTING of TRIALS

CONSORT 2010 Flow Diagram

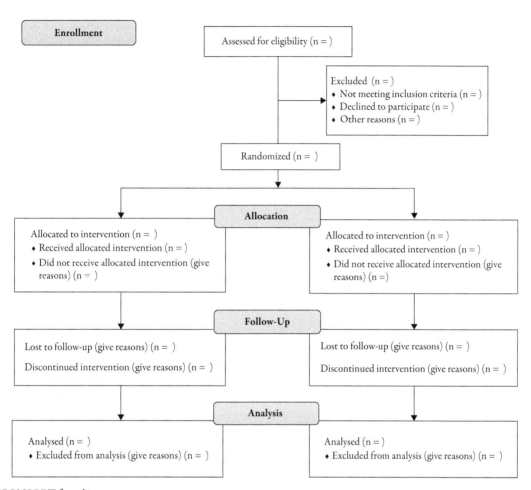

Figure 2.1 The CONSORT flow diagram.
SOURCE: CONSORT Group (http://www.consort-statement.org/consort-statement/flow-diagram).

FURTHER READING

Dworkin RH, Turk DC, Wyrwich KW, et al. Interpreting the clinical importance of treatment outcomes in chronic pain clinical trials: IMMPACT recommendations. *J Pain*. 2008;9(2): 105–121.

Farrar JT, Young JP Jr, LaMoreaux L, et al. Clinical Importance of changes in chronic pain intensity measured on an 11-point numerical pain rating scale. *Pain*. 2001;94:149–158.

Hanley MA, Jensen MP, Ehde DM, et al. Clinically significant changes in pain intensity ratings in persons with spinal cord injury or amputation. *Clin J Pain*. 2006;22:25–31.

Salaffi F, Stancati A, Silvestri CA, et al. Minimal clinically important changes in chronic musculoskeletal pain intensity measured on a numerical rating scale. *Eur J Pain*. 2004;8: 283–291.

17. ANSWER: A

The matter of which participants are to be included in a study's data analysis often arises during clinical research trials. Even the most carefully managed and well-designed trial cannot be perfectly executed. The protocol may not be exactly adhered to, outcome and response variable data may be missing, and some patients may not actually have been eligible for the study based on inclusion and exclusion criteria issues. This can lead to controversy when planning the statistical analyses for the data because these problems can introduce bias and potentially disrupt the validity of the results.

The intention-to-treat principle states that all participants randomized and all events should be accounted for in the primary analysis based on the group to which participants were randomized, regardless of whether or not they adhered to the assigned intervention. Following the intention-to-treat principle may underestimate the full effect of the treatment, but it guards against the more pressing issue of biased results. A per protocol analysis only includes participants who were fully adherent to the protocol with regard to the assigned study medication, follow-up visits and/or measurements, and had no other protocol violations. The main issue with per protocol analysis is that participants who adhere to study treatment and protocol may be different than those who drop out in ways that are related to the outcome of interest. If the results of intention-to-treat and per protocol analyses are different, then the intention-to-treat analysis results typically predominate for estimates of efficacy because they maintain the value of randomization. Unlike per protocol analysis, intention-to-treat analyses can only bias the estimated effect in the conservative direction by favoring the null hypothesis.

FURTHER READING

Friedman LM, Furberg CD, DeMets DL. Issues in data analysis. In: *Fundamentals of Clinical Trials*. 4th ed. New York, NY: Springer; 2010:345–390.

Grady D, Cummings SR, Hulley SB. Alternative trial designs and implementation issues. In: Hully SB, Cummings SR, Browner SR, et al. (Eds.), *Designing Clinical Research*. 3rd ed. Philadelphia, PA: Lippincott Williams & Wilkins; 2007:163–182.

Piantadosi S. Counting subjects and events. In: *Clinical Trials: A Methodologic Perspective*. 2nd Ed. Hoboken, NJ: Wiley; 2005:395–407.

18. ANSWER: C

Variables can be divided broadly into numerical and categorical categories with further subclassifications as outlined in Table 2.4.

Table 2.4 **CLASSIFICATION OF VARIABLES**

CLASS	SUBCLASS	DEFINITION
Categorical	Nominal	Variables that have two or more categories but lack any intrinsic order Example: Male or female
	Ordinal	Variables that have two or more categories that can be ordered or ranked Example: Strongly agree, moderately agree, etc.
Numerical	Interval	Numerical values that can be measured along a continuum Example: Temperature
	Ratio	Numerical values measured along a continuum where zero of that variable indicates that none of that variable is present Example: Weight

FURTHER READING

Laerd Statistics. Understanding the different types of variable in statistics. 2015. Available at https://statistics.laerd.com/statistical-guides/types-of-variable.php. Accessed July 27, 2015.

19. ANSWER: C

In a double-blinded study, both patients and providers are unaware of the patients' group assignment. In a triple-blinded study, another group, such as support staff or data analyzers, is also blinded. Randomization is a process of selecting from a group in a manner that makes equal distribution of confounders likely. Randomization will not work as well with small groups. Stratification is a strategy in which patients are intentionally divided by an important characteristic prior to randomization. Confounding occurs when study results are influenced by a factor other than that which is being studied. When a sample is skewed, it may be due to sampling error or related bias. For example, if diabetic patients are more likely than nondiabetics to volunteer for a study, that is a form of volunteer bias.

FURTHER READING

Stomp on Step 1. Confounding, randomization & blinding. 2015. Available at http://www.stomponstep1.com/confounding-placebo-stratification-randomization-blinding. Accessed July 27, 2015.

20. ANSWER: E

Four situations are possible when performing statistical tests to try to reject the null hypothesis in favor of the alternative hypothesis when interpreting the results of a study. In two of these situations, assuming the study is free from bias, the findings in the sample and what is reality in the population are concordant, and the inference by the investigator(s) will be correct. However, in the other two instances, a type I or type II error has been made, and the inference will not be correct.

Prior to beginning the study, the investigator(s) determines a priori what are the maximum chances he or she will accept in making type I or type II errors. The probability of committing a type I error is also known as α or the significance level. A type I error occurs when the null hypothesis is rejected when in reality there actually is no association between the predictor and outcome variable (a false-positive finding). The probability of a type II error is known as β. A type II error occurs when there is a failure to reject the null hypothesis when in reality an association does exist between predictor and outcome (a false-negative finding). Power is specified as $1 - \beta$ and is the probability of correctly rejecting the null hypothesis in the study sample if the actual effect in the population is greater than or equal to the effect size.

In an ideal world, both α and β would be set at zero, thus eliminating the possibility of false-positive or false-negative results. In real-life practice, these values are made as small as possible, with the caveat that the sample size will need to increase as these values decrease.

FURTHER READING

Browner WS, Newman TB, Hulley SB. Getting ready to estimate sample size: Hypotheses and underlying principles. In: Hully SB, Cummings SR, Browner SR, et al. (Eds.), *Designing Clinical Research*. 3rd ed. Philadelphia, PA: Lippincott Williams & Wilkins; 2007:51–63.

Friedman LM, Furberg CD, DeMets DL. Sample size. In: *Fundamentals of Clinical Trials*. 4th ed. New York, NY: Springer; 2010:133–167.

21. ANSWER: A

The crossover design is a special type of RCT in which each study treatment is administered at different times to every subject enrolled in the study. Participants in this type of design "cross over" or "switch" from one treatment to another by this strategy, with the intent to estimate differences between them. Typically, half of the participants are randomly assigned to start with one treatment (or control) and then switch to the other treatment (or control). In the case presented in this question, half would start with drug A and switch to drug B, and the other half would start with drug B and switch to drug A (Figure 2.2). This is the simplest type of crossover trial and is called the two-treatment,

two-period design. More complex crossover trial designs may be employed in various clinical circumstances.

The crossover design has multiple advantages for researchers. One advantage is that it minimizes variability because each participant serves as his or her own control and the subsequent paired analyses substantially increase the statistical power of the trial in that fewer participants are required. Thus, the crossover design takes advantage of making treatment comparisons based on within- rather than between-subject differences. This allows the treatment difference to be estimated with greater precision and less possibility for confounding. Recruitment may also be easier with this type of design because all subjects will receive all treatments under investigation, which may be an attractive attribute for some patients who are concerned about participating in clinical trials in which they may be randomized to a no-treatment or placebo arm.

Disadvantages of the crossover design are related to the issue of carryover effects and dropouts. Carryover effects are the residual influence of the intervention on the outcome during the period after which it has been discontinued. To reduce carryover effect, the investigator can use an untreated "washout" period between treatments with the hope that the outcome variable will return to its baseline before starting the next intervention. Another concern for carryover effects is if they lead to a permanent change or cure in the underlying condition of the patient. In this instance, the treatment during the second period could appear falsely or artificially superior. Finally, the patients' condition could change in the second treatment phase of the study, which possibly may affect how they respond to the second treatment.

The issue of dropouts is of concern for two reasons. First, the participant is exposed to more drugs or treatments

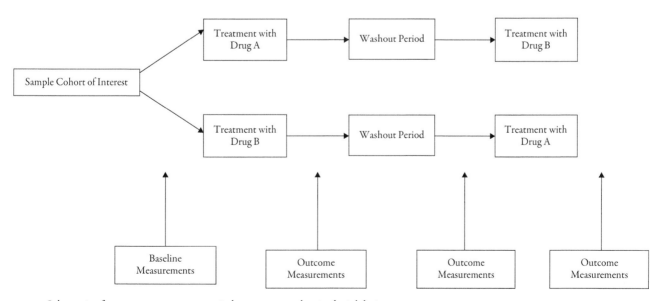

Figure 2.2 Schematic of a two-treatment, two-period, crossover randomized trial design.

in a crossover trial, increasing the chance of side effects that could contribute to dropping out. Second, the study is usually longer than a regular RCT, thus providing a longer period of opportunity to drop out. The consequences of dropouts are more impactful in a crossover design because the data loss is more significant; for example, if a participant drops out in the second treatment phase, the participant's data cannot be analyzed using only the first phase because that participant was acting as his or her own control and determining a treatment effect cannot occur.

FURTHER READING

Friedman LM, Furberg CD, DeMets DL. Basic study design. In: *Fundamentals of Clinical Trials.* 4th ed. New York, NY: Springer; 2010:67–96.

Grady D, Cummings SR, Hulley SB. Alternative trial designs and implementation issues. In: Hully SB, Cummings SR, Browner SR, et al. (Eds.), *Designing Clinical Research.* 3rd ed. Philadelphia, PA: Lippincott Williams & Wilkins; 2007:163–182.

Piantadosi S. Crossover designs. In: *Clinical Trials: A Methodologic Perspective.* 2nd ed. Hoboken, NJ: Wiley; 2005:515–527.

22. ANSWER: C

Certain groups of participants are considered to be particularly vulnerable to undue influence or coercion in a research setting. These groups, as outlined in 45 CFR 46, are children, wards of the state, prisoners, pregnant women and fetuses, persons who are mentally disabled or otherwise cognitively impaired, and economically or educationally disadvantaged persons. IRBs that review research studies involving all categories of vulnerable patients must determine that their use is adequately justified and that additional safeguards are implemented to minimize risks unique to each group.

FURTHER READING

US Department of Health & Human Services. CFR—Code of Federal Regulations Title 45, Part 46. Available at http://www.hhs.gov/ohrp/humansubjects/guidance/45cfr46.html. Accessed July 27, 2015.

US Department of Health and Human Services. IRB Guidebook: Chapter VI Special Classes of Subjects. Available at http://archive.hhs.gov/ohrp/irb/irb_chapter6.htm. Accessed July 27, 2015.

23. ANSWER: E

There are several variations on how sample sizes are estimated for a study or experiment, but there are common features and steps, including the following: stating the null hypothesis and either a one- or two-sided alternative hypothesis, the appropriate statistical test based on type of predictor and outcome variable in the hypotheses, a reasonable effect size between the two study groups, variability, and an a priori determination of α and β. Even if the exact value for one or more of these steps is uncertain or unknown, it is important to estimate the sample size prior to starting the study and early in the design phase. Many clinical trials are performed that lack the statistical power or ability to detect treatment effects of a magnitude that has some clinical importance. Conversely, some sample size estimations may assume an unrealistically large intervention effect, meaning the power for more realistic and smaller effects will be low. Finally, the danger in studies with low statistical power is that treatments that could be beneficial are discarded due to not finding statistical significance and may never be investigated again. Due to the approximate nature of sample size calculations, investigators should try to balance being realistic with being conservative in estimating the parameters discussed here.

FURTHER READING

Browner WS, Newman TB, Hulley SB. Estimating sample size and power: Applications and examples. In: Hully SB, Cummings SR, Browner SR, et al. (Eds.), *Designing Clinical Research.* 3rd ed. Philadelphia, PA: Lippincott Williams & Wilkins; 2007:65–94.

Friedman LM, Furberg CD, DeMets DL. Sample size. In: *Fundamentals of Clinical Trials.* 4th ed. New York, NY: Springer; 2010:133–167.

24. ANSWER: B

In designing a research study, one of the most important components is creating selection criteria that define the population to be studied. This is because of the possible effects of prognostic and selection factors on differences in outcome. The inclusion criteria define the main characteristics of the target population that pertain to the research question. Inclusion criteria typically include demographic characteristics (age, gender, and ethnicity), clinical characteristics (the disease being studied and its severity), geographic characteristics (patients from investigator's clinic or hospital or patients outside the investigator's practice), and time characteristics (study time frame from start to finish). Ultimately, inclusion criteria should be as specific as possible, sensible, used consistently throughout the study, and provide the basis for understanding to whom the published results and conclusions apply.

Exclusion criteria, on the other hand, indicate the subsets and characteristics of the population that might interfere with follow-up efforts, the quality of the data, or high risk of possible side effects. In clinical trials, exclusions tend to include specific causes of concern for the safety of the participants. As a good overall rule, having as few exclusion criteria as possible helps keep recruitment simple and preserves the number of potential study subjects.

FURTHER READING

Hulley SB, Newman TB, Cummings SR. Choosing the study subjects: Specification, sampling, and recruitment. In: Hully SB, Cummings SR, Browner SR, et al. (Eds.), *Designing Clinical Research*. 3rd ed. Philadelphia, PA: Lippincott Williams & Wilkins; 2007:27–36.

Piantadosi S. The study cohort. In: *Clinical Trials: A Methodologic Perspective*. 2nd ed. Hoboken, NJ: Wiley; 2005:309–330.

25. ANSWERS:

A. The inverse of ARR is equal to NNT). NNT represents how many people need to be treated or exposed to an intervention in order for one person to have an improved outcome. To calculate NNT, ARR must first be determined. ARR is defined as the difference between the control event rate and the experimental event rate. NNT is equal to the inverse of ARR.

FURTHER READING

Centre for Evidence-Based Medicine. Number needed to treat (NNT). 2014. Available at http://www.cebm.net/number-needed-to-treat-nnt. Accessed July 26, 2015.

B. Specificity correlates to the proportion of negatives that are correctly identified as such. Sensitivity is a measure of how likely a test will correctly identify a condition when it is present. Sensitivity is calculated as the number of true positives divided by the sum of true positives and false negatives. Specificity, on the other hand, is a measure of the likelihood that a person without a disease will have a negative test. It is calculated as the number of true negatives divided by the sum of the true negatives and false positives.

FURTHER READING

Williams M. Sensitivity and specificity: Precision of the clinical exam. 2015. Available at https://www.med.emory.edu/EMAC/curriculum/diagnosis/sensand.htm. Accessed July 26, 2015.

C. Positive predictive value is calculated as the number of true positives divided by the sum of true positives and false positives. It is the probability that a patient with a positive test actually has the disease. Negative predictive value, on the other hand, is the number of true negatives divided by the sum of the true negatives and false negatives.

FURTHER READING

Williams M. Sensitivity and specificity: Precision of the clinical exam. 2015. Available at https://www.med.emory.edu/EMAC/curriculum/diagnosis/sensand.htm. Accessed July 26, 2015.

D. Power quantifies the likelihood of identifying a significant effect when it exists. It can be calculated as $1 - \beta$.

FURTHER READING

Calkins K. Power and sample size: Applied statistics. 2015. Available at http://www.andrews.edu/~calkins/math/edrm611/edrm11.htm. Accessed July 26, 2015.

3.

PAIN RESEARCH
PLACEBO, ANIMAL MODELS, ETHICS, AND EPIDEMIOLOGY

David A. Edwards

INTRODUCTION

Research of pain requires not only that basic ethical standards for human studies research be followed but also that special consideration be given due to the potential for human suffering. The use of placebos as controls became widespread after World War II with the adoption of the randomized controlled trial. Other study designs have elucidated the risk factors for pain. The prevalence of pain in society is a measure of the burden of pain.

Experimentation using animals in pain research has provided considerable insight into the pathophysiology of pain in humans. Because the experience of pain is subjective, the study of pain in animals must be done in a way that limits potential suffering. Nociception and the response in animals must be considered to reflect pain, and so ethical principles to limit potential suffering in animals guide research in this area.

Historical abuses in human experimentation have driven the development of ethical guidelines for human subjects research. The *Belmont Report* serves as the modern standard of basic ethical principles on which institutional review boards (IRBs) judge human research studies.

QUESTIONS

1. In randomized controlled trials (RCTs), placebo response size is often difficult to quantify. Which of the following is not a confounder of positive placebo response in RCTs?

A. Response bias
B. Regression to the mean
C. Natural course of disease
D. An educated patient
E. Fluctuation in symptoms

2. A 50-year-old female is asked to rate her pain after receiving a placebo pill. She notices the research observer watching her and smiling; thus, she reports an improvement in her pain. This phenomenon is known as?

A. Response bias
B. Regression to the mean
C. Hawthorne effect
D. Mesmerism
E. Placebo response

3. Which of the following is true about the placebo effect?

A. It is a psychobiological event that can be attributed to the entire treatment experience.
B. Patient expectations negatively impact placebo response size.
C. Classical conditioning is the primary reason for the placebo response.
D. The Yale–Brown Compulsive Scale is used to rule out poor candidates in placebo-controlled trials.

4. Which of the following is a true definition of nocebo?

A. The paucity of effect from placebo
B. Negative side effects of a placebo
C. An active treatment not meant to cause the effect observed
D. A nonmedication placebo treatment
E. The observed effect of a placebo

5. A practitioner injects lidocaine into muscle trigger points and describes to the patient the triggering

muscles, saying, "When muscles twitch like this, I can tell it is really going to help you." This is an example of:

A. Social desirability
B. Nocebo
C. Conditioning
D. Placebo by instruction
E. Specific effects of treatment

6. A patient states, "My mother had epidural steroid injections and they were a lifesaver." A positive outcome in this patient after epidural steroid injection may partially be due to placebo as a result of which effect?

A. Nocebo effect
B. Conditioning effect
C. Instruction effect
D. Hawthorne effect
E. Social desirability effect

7. Which of the following is a true statement about the mechanism of placebo/nocebo?

A. Behavioral patterns influence response to placebo and are detectable by functional magnetic resonance imaging (fMRI) in the cerebellum.
B. Poor connectivity between glutamatergic spinal neurons is primarily responsible for nocebo responses.
C. fMRI of the spinal cord shows areas of overlap with nocebo and pain.
D. fMRI studies show that lower connectivity between frontal and midbrain structures is associated with poor response to placebo.
E. Placebo analgesia results in decreased conductivity between the prefrontal cortex and subcortical regions.

8. Janis is a study participant reporting the efficacy of a novel pain medication on peripheral neuropathic pain. Investigators observe that Janis reports improvement in her pain when it is injected by a person in a lab coat, and she reports no pain improvement when it is injected by a machine without her knowing. This scenario best describes which research model?

A. Double-blinded controlled
B. Open–hidden
C. Placebo controlled
D. Crossover
E. Positive–negative awareness

9. Ethical use of placebo assumes that:

A. The subject not be aware that he or she may receive a placebo.
B. There exists no effective treatment that can be used for comparison.
C. The side effects of the placebo are tolerable.
D. The study was designed by a physician.

10. Point Prevalence is:

A. The proportion of members of a population at risk of a disease who develop the disease over a specified time interval.
B. The total number of people in a population who are at risk for a disease.
C. A measure of how likely a disease will be acquired in a population.
D. The proportion of individuals at risk for a disease who have the disease.

11. Incidence is:

A. The proportion of members of a population at risk of a disease who develop the disease over a specified time interval.
B. The total number of people in a population who are at risk for a disease.
C. A measure of how likely a disease will be acquired in a population.
D. The proportion of individuals at risk for a disease who have the disease.

12. The most common pain conditions for which children and adolescents present are:

A. Headaches, bone fracture pain, stomach aches
B. Stomach aches, hip pain, back pain
C. Back pain, headaches, joint pain
D. Back aches, stomach aches, headaches
E. Joint pain, stomach aches, neck pain

13. The lifetime prevalence of low back pain is approximately:

A. <10%
B. 10–25%
C. 25–50%
D. 50–75%
E. >90%

14. The prevalence of migraine headaches in the United States is approximately:

    A. 10% in females and 5% in males
    B. 25% in females and 50% in males
    C. 10% in females and 20% in males
    D. 45% in females and 20% in males
    E. 60% in females and 10% in males

15. Which of the following statements is true?

    A. Workers with low back pain are most likely to return to work after a 3-year hiatus.
    B. For workers off work for 6 months with low back pain, the lifetime incidence of returning to work is 50%.
    C. The lifetime incidence of patients with acute-onset low back pain progressing to chronic low back pain is 50%.
    D. Lifetime incidence of low back pain and lifetime prevalence of low back pain are the same.

16. Observational studies:

    A. Include randomized controlled trials and case–control studies
    B. Provide level I evidence
    C. Are more difficult to perform due to ethical considerations
    D. Are analytical and help to identify risk factors
    E. Are better for investigating common exposures

17. Identify the true statement regarding risk factors for pain:

    A. Boys experience more pain than girls.
    B. Adult women report more severe levels of pain, but of shorter duration, than men.
    C. Chronic pain is as prevalent among adults before age 65 years as it is after age 65 years.
    D. There is little association between smoking and obesity and the development of chronic pain.
    E. There is strong evidence of a genetic influence on the development of chronic pain.

18. John underwent herniorrhaphy 6 months ago. At a follow-up visit in the clinic, he still reports achy pain despite a well-healed surgical site. Which of the following statements is true regarding risk factors for development of chronic postsurgical pain?

    A. Mental health has been a consistent predictor of development of chronic post-surgical pain.
    B. Preoperative pain intensity predicts postoperative acute pain but not development of chronic pain.

    C. Genetic profiles predict chronic pain in hernia surgery.
    D. Laparoscopic surgery has not been shown to decrease the risk of developing chronic pain after hernia repair.

19. Given the known risks of developing post-surgical pain, the most appropriate practice would be to:

    A. Increase a patient's opioid medication to reduce preoperative pain as low as possible
    B. Perform a paravertebral block for mastectomy
    C. Provide preoperative gabapentin 300 mg PO for below knee amputation
    D. Infuse lidocaine during lumbar spine surgery

20. What are the three basic ethical principles summarized in the *Belmont Report*?

    A. Respect for persons, beneficence, justice
    B. Respect, minimize suffering, replacement when possible
    C. Reduction in animal research, replacement when possible, fairness
    D. Fairness, equality, justice

21. What are the three R's of ethical animal research in pain?

    A. Replacement, refinement, and restoration
    B. Refinement, restoration, and reduction
    C. Reduction, refinement, and replacement
    D. Restoration, reduction, and replacement

22. Which of the following experimental models is a model for polyneuropathy pain?

    A. Implantation of osteosarcoma in the femur resulting in bone demineralization
    B. Distention of the bladder to induce a motor response (viscus distention)
    C. Use of streptozocin to ablate beta cells
    D. Partial ligation of the sciatic nerve

23. The hot-plate test involves placing an animal on a platform and gradually increasing the temperature until the threshold for heat pain is reached. The animal will react by lifting its feet off the surface. This is an example of which category of animal pain research?

    A. Category C—pain without relief
    B. Category D—distress relieved by analgesics
    C. Category E—minimal pain or distress

D. Category C—minimal pain or distress
E. Category D—pain distress relieved by analgesics

24. Select the true statement about using animal models as surrogates for pain in humans:

A. Animal models are valuable reflections of pain perception.
B. Rats are excellent animal models of pain because they show consistent response to pain tests across many different strains.
C. Physiologic mechanisms of pain are better determined in animal models given the lack of subjective bias.
D. Nociception-associated pain behaviors are assumed to be reflections of pain in animals.

25. Temperature, pressure, and electrical pain are modalities often tested in animal models. Which of the following is the best tool to measure pressure pain?

A. Calibrated von Frey filaments
B. The hot-plate test
C. The tail-flick test
D. Hargreaves model

26. A researcher wants to test whether tricyclic antidepressants affect thresholds of pressure pain sensation after mononeuropathy induced pain. Which model should the researcher choose?

A. Streptozocin-induced diabetic neuropathy model
B. Vincristine-induced neuropathy
C. Osteosarcoma cancer pain model
D. Viscous distention model
E. Common sciatic nerve ligature

27. A researcher receives funds from company X to attend a seminar. This same researcher carries out a study using a drug from company X. The study finds no benefit for pain treatment, so the company tells the researcher not to publish the results. The researcher should:

A. Publish the results despite the source of funding
B. Agree not to publish because funding was provided by a private company
C. Publish the results only if the study was partially funded by the National Institutes of Health
D. Inform the US Food and Drug Administration (FDA)

28. A researcher has proposed to study the effects of a new medication previously shown to have a 1% mortality. Which of the following standards lists among its

10 principles of ethical human experimentation that research must not include the possibility of death or disability?

A. Nuremberg Code
B. The National Research Act
C. Ethical principle of justice
D. The *Belmont Report*
E. The *Declaration of Helsinki*

29. Select the true statement about the history of ethical experimentation in humans:

A. The *Belmont Report* served as the blueprint for judgments delivered during the Nuremberg trials.
B. The National Commission for the Protection of Human Subjects of Biomedical and Behavioral Research produced the *Belmont Report.*
C. The *Belmont Report* lists three basic principles for ethical human experimentation: respect for persons, beneficence, and equality.
D. The Nuremberg Trial prosecuted the researchers responsible for the Tuskegee experiment.

30. In the *Belmont Report*, three basic ethical principles to protect human subjects during biomedical and behavioral research are outlined. These are:

A. Justice, refinement, replacement
B. Replacement, beneficence, respect for persons
C. Beneficence, respect for persons, justice
D. Restoration, refinement, replacement

31. A research study protocol is under review by the IRB. The IRB requests alterations to the protocol that proposed a trial of medication. The research is partially funded by the National Institutes of Health but sponsored by a company known to charge a high price for its nongeneric medications. The IRB plans to approve the study with assurance that the medication, if helpful to humans, be made available to all patients and not just to those who can afford it. This is an example of what basic ethical principle from the *Belmont Report?*

A. Respect for persons
B. Beneficence
C. Justice
D. Restoration
E. Refinement

32. A case–control study is recruiting subjects aged 50–90 years with Alzheimer's disease in order to observe the progression of disease and determine if social support impacts disease progression. Consent is done in the presence of another family member to ensure the

patient's rights are protected. This is an example of what ethical principle as defined in the *Belmont Report*?

    A. Respect for persons
    B. Beneficence
    C. Justice
    D. Restoration
    E. Refinement

33. An investigator has an obligation to make efforts to secure patient well-being. This is an example of what ethical principle as defined in the *Belmont Report*?

    A. Respect for persons
    B. Beneficence
    C. Justice
    D. Restoration
    E. Refinement

34. When designing a research study to test a new analgesic to be injected into the epidural space, a researcher delineates the risks of the procedure and the medication in her research design. She also outlines the potential benefits versus the potential risks. IRBs require this documentation based on what ethical principle from the *Belmont Report*?

    A. Respect for autonomy
    B. Nonmaleficence
    C. Beneficence
    D. Justice
    E. Refinement

35. From 1932 to 1972, the US Public Health Service conducted the Tuskegee study to research treatment and outcome of syphilis in African American men. During the study, effective treatment was withheld from hundreds of affected men in order to observe the progression of syphilis. In response to this, the *Belmont Report* was drafted. In the Tuskegee study, African American men were not treated even though an effective treatment for their disease was available. This would violate which basic principle from the *Belmont Report*?

    A. Restoration
    B. Justice
    C. Beneficence
    D. Maleficence
    E. Respect for persons

36. Janis is a 27-year-old female with cerebral palsy who experiences severe spasticity. A researcher would like to recruit subjects like Janis to investigate a new drug treatment for spasticity that has shown great promise in preclinical trials. Janis is mentally handicapped, so she will not be able to consent. Select the true statement relative to the *Belmont Report*:

    A. Respect for persons obligates the researcher to include Janis in the trial.
    B. Justice obligates the researcher to exclude Janis from the trial.
    C. Beneficence obligates the researcher to maximize the number of patients in the trial.
    D. Respect for persons obligates the researcher to obtain consent from Janis' health proxy.
    E. Justice obligates the researcher to ensure that the balance of benefits outweighs the risks.

37. In clinical research design, the requirement for scientific validity stipulates that risks cannot be incurred without:

    A. A functional research design
    B. Overriding benefits to subjects
    C. A plan to treat the potential harmful outcome
    D. Benefit to society

38. Although patients with chronic pain may be defined as a vulnerable population, they still deserve to benefit from potential treatments that medical science may discover. This is an example of:

    A. Justice
    B. Nonmaleficence
    C. Nonmalfeasance
    D. Balancing risk–benefit
    E. Respect for persons

39. The ethical use of placebos in pain research requires that:

    A. Subjects know when they receive the placebo
    B. No effective treatment exists that can be used as a comparison
    C. The placebo cause no harm
    D. The investigator be blinded to the placebo

ANSWERS

1. ANSWER: D

A placebo is an inactive treatment (or treatment experience), often a sugar pill, designed to seem like it is the real treatment. After World War II, the number of RCTs increased as a way to control for bias in clinical experimentation. However, up to 35% of patients in the treatment arm of an RCT will respond positively to placebo treatment, so it has become important to account for these effects. Furthermore, the effect size of placebo can be inflated by several confounding variables, making it less clear what part of the patient response is due to placebo.

Response bias can confound the true effect of placebo. When a patient who receives a placebo reports feeling better, it is difficult to determine if this is because the patient wants to please the clinician or provide a positive response when asked or if there is a true psychophysiological response that impacts the disease.

In some patients, disease may improve as a natural course of recovery or fluctuation in symptoms. An improvement in the disease may be misinterpreted as a positive response to placebo.

Patients may initially report extreme values but upon repeat measure report values closer to average. With enough measures, responses tend to average out. This is known as regression toward the mean and is considered a confounder when measuring the true influence of placebo.

The Hawthorne effect is a phenomenon in which patients alter their response as a result of being observed. Study patients may improve as a result of being studied, not directly as a result of receiving the placebo.

Co-intervention bias occurs when subjects receiving placebo alter their other concurrent treatment regimens due to a belief that they likely received the nonplacebo treatment. An example of this is when subjects treated with sham acupuncture reduce their opioids as a result of believing they received the true treatment and not as a result of reduced pain due to placebo response.

Social desirability is similar to response bias in that subjects respond in a particular way that avoids a negative stigma or implication. For example, it is more socially acceptable for a subject to underreport drug abuse (or overreport a placebo response) if there exists social pressure in a given direction.

Educated patients may demonstrate smaller placebo response. This is considered a way to reduce the effect size of placebo and not considered a bias of positive placebo response.

KEY FACTS: CONFOUNDING VARIABLES OF PLACEBO RESPONSE

- Natural course of disease
- Fluctuation of symptoms
- Regression to the mean
- Concurrent treatments (co-intervention)
- Social desirability
- Response bias
- Hawthorne effect

FURTHER READING

Finniss DG, Kaptchuk TJ, Miller F, et al. Biological, clinical, and ethical advances of placebo effects. *Lancet*. 2010;375:686–695.
Hróbjartsson A, Kaptchuk TJ, Miller FG. Placebo effect studies are susceptible to response bias and to other types of biases. *J Clin Epidemiol*. 2011;64:1223–1229.
van der Velden MG, Waisel DB. Ethics of research in patients with pain. In: Benzon HT, Rathmell JP, Wu CL, et al. (Eds.), *Practical Pain Management*. 5th ed. Philadelphia, PA: Mosby; 2014:1066–1070.

2. ANSWER: C

Determining the true effect of placebo is a challenge given several potential confounding variables. In the 1930s, at an electric company in Hawthorne, Illinois, research determined that productivity increased when employees were being studied. The Hawthorne effect is seen in clinical research as a result of subjects' tendency to perform better when they are being studied. This can result in a larger effect size, especially in the placebo response.

3. ANSWER: A

The word "placebo" originated from the mistranslation of Psalms 116 by St. Jerome. Hired mourners in the 13th century were known as "placebos" because of their fake behavior. Placebo controls were used in the 16th century by Catholics priests to identify those faking demon possession. In 1784, the Franklin Commission used placebo controls to debunk mesmerism. Following World War II and adoption of the RCT, placebo as a tool for medical research became widely used. Since then, understanding the mechanism of placebo has been the focus of great interest.

Modern research shows placebo to be the psychobiological response to not only the inert treatment but also including the entire therapeutic context. Expectation has an important psychological contribution to the placebo effect. Cues given to research subjects can influence the placebo effect positively (e.g., "This medication is really powerful") or negatively (e.g., "This substance is inert and you are unlikely to notice any change"). Conditioning can also influence the placebo response size, but it is not the primary contributor. Differentiating the effects of conditioning from expectation can be complex. The Yale–Brown

Obsessive Compulsive Scale is a psychological test unrelated to placebo.

FURTHER READING

Finniss DG, Kaptchuk TJ, Miller F, et al. Biological, clinical, and ethical advances of placebo effects. *Lancet*. 2010;375:686–695.

4. ANSWER: B

A nocebo response is a psychophysiological adverse effect or response that results following treatment with placebo. For example, worsened pain, advanced disease, or negative side effects after receiving an inert treatment are the result of nocebo response. Nocebo can be influenced, just as placebo is influenced, by several items.

Placebo response is enhanced in subjects who have observed others benefiting from a treatment (social observation). In conditioning, subjects exposed to improved conditions following treatment (e.g., reduced pain stimulus) have subsequent enhanced analgesic responses following reception of placebo (the opposite is true with nocebo response).

KEY FACTS: TRIGGERS THAT ENHANCE THE PLACEBO OR NOCEBO RESPONSE

- Social observation
- Conditioning
- Verbal instructions
- Interactions

FURTHER READING

Colloca L, Grillon C. Understanding placebo and nocebo responses for pain management. *Curr Pain Headache Rep*. 2014;18:1–7.

5. ANSWER: D

Placebo responses highly depend on subject expectations. If a positive outcome is expected, positive placebo response may be measured. If a negative outcome is expected, a nocebo response may occur. Because placebo response is the psychophysiological response to the entire treatment experience, a researcher/clinician can enhance a patient's expectation of a positive outcome by instructing the patient in the desired response and thereby directly influence the placebo effect.

FURTHER READING

Klinger R, Flor H. Clinical and ethical implications of placebo effects: Enhancing patients' benefits from pain treatment. *Handbook Exp Pharmacol*. 2014;225:217.

6. ANSWER: E

There are several triggers of enhanced placebo effects. Among these, a patient's observation of another's positive outcome with a treatment can make it more likely that the patient will benefit from a treatment him- or herself. Social observation can either positively (placebo) or negatively (nocebo) affect the response to treatment.

FURTHER READING

Colloca L, Grillon C. Understanding placebo and nocebo responses for pain management. *Curr Pain Headache Rep*. 2014;18:1–7.

7. ANSWER: C

Although the mechanism of placebo and nocebo effects are incompletely understood, certain aspects of the physiological response have consistently been measured in laboratory settings.

Placebo analgesia is associated with physiologic changes in the central nervous system. Specifically, connections between cortical structures (dorsolateral prefrontal cortex and anterior cingulate cortex) and midbrain structures (hypothalamus, amygdala, and periaqueductal gray) are enhanced, as measured by signal on fMRI. Pain sensation causes increased activity in the thalamus, insula, and somatosensory cortex, and placebo reduces this activity. fMRI of the spinal cord also shows a reduction in pain-induced activity with placebo. Both pain and nocebo effects are observed in overlapping areas in the spinal cord. These and other studies show the important central modulating effect of patient expectations.

At the biochemical level, placebo results in the release of endogenous opioids, cholecystokinin, oxytocin, and cannabinoids. The placebo response is also partially blocked by naloxone, confirming that endogenous opioids contribute. Genetic polymorphisms may make one group of patients more responsive to placebo (COMT and FAAH gene alleles regulating catecholamine and cannabinoid levels, respectively).

FURTHER READING

Benedetti F, Amanzio M. Mechanisms of the placebo response. *Pulm Pharmacol Ther* 2013;26:520–523.

8. ANSWER: B

Open–hidden models demonstrate that both active and inactive treatments can be enhanced by placebo effects. The placebo effect is positively reinforcing: There is a greater response when a treatment is given to a subject overtly than when given covertly. Likewise, the AD_{50} (dose required to reduce pain by 50%) of many analgesics is increased if given to patients covertly.

FURTHER READING

Colloca L, Grillon C. Understanding placebo and nocebo responses for pain management. *Curr Pain Headache Rep.* 2014;18:1–7.

9. ANSWER: B

Placebo use is critical for many study designs and a common feature of the RCT. In fact, placebo may be an essential requirement by the FDA for drug trials showing efficacy. The ethical use of placebos assumes the following:

- There is no effective treatment that can be used as a comparison.
- Risks of placebo use are acceptable.
- Validity of the study requires use of a placebo.
- Study subject is made aware that a placebo will be used as part of the informed consent.

FURTHER READING

van der Velden MG, Waisel DB. Ethics of research in patients with pain. In: Benzon HT, Rathmell JP, Wu CL, et al. (Eds.), *Practical Pain Management*. 5th ed. Philadelphia, PA: Mosby; 2014:1066–1070.

10. ANSWER: D

Prevalence and incidence are measures of disease proportion among populations and represent disease burden.

Prevalence is the proportion of members of a population at risk (e.g., females at risk of breast cancer or hospital nurses at risk of back pain) who are affected at a specific time or within an interval of time:

- Point prevalence: All persons affected with the disease at a specific time in a specific location
- Period prevalence: All incidences of the disease, new or old or recurring, counted over a time period (useful for recurring diseases such as the common cold)
- Lifetime prevalence: The proportion of members of the population who have ever had the disease (useful

in cohort studies in which populations are followed bvPrevalence is usually reported as a percentage of the population (e.g., 5%, or 5 in 100) or the proportion of a standardized population (e.g., 550 cases per 10,000).

Incidence is an expression of calculated risk of getting a disease. It is the proportion of members of a population at risk who *newly* develop the disease within a specified time frame.

FURTHER READING

Henschke N, Kamper SJ, Maher CG. The epidemiology and economic consequences of pain. *Mayo Clin Proc.* 2015;90:139–147.

11. ANSWER: A

Prevalence and incidence are measures of disease proportion among populations and represent disease burden.

Prevalence is the proportion of members of a population at risk (e.g., females at risk of breast cancer or hospital nurses at risk of back pain) who are affected at a specific time or within an interval of time:

- Point prevalence: All persons affected with the disease at a specific time in a specific location
- Period prevalence: All incidences of the disease, new or old or recurring, counted over a time period (useful for recurring diseases such as the common cold)
- Lifetime prevalence: The proportion of members of the population who have ever had the disease (useful in cohort studies in which populations are followed from birth)

Prevalence is usually reported as a percentage of the population (e.g., 5%, or 5 in 100) or the proportion of a standardized population (e.g., 550 cases per 10,000).

Incidence is an expression of calculated risk of getting a disease. It is the proportion of members of a population at risk who *newly* develop the disease within a specified time frame.

FURTHER READING

Henschke N, Kamper SJ, Maher CG. The epidemiology and economic consequences of pain. *Mayo Clin Proc.* 2015;90:139–147.

12. ANSWER: D

The most frequent pain conditions reported in pediatric patients are low back pain, headache, and abdominal pain

Table 3.1 **EPIDEMIOLOGY OF PAIN IN PEDIATRIC PATIENTS**

PAIN CONDITION	PREVALENCE
Back pain	9.8–49% (1-month prevalence), 11.8–33% (1-year incidence)
Headache	26–69% (1-month prevalence)
Abdominal pain	0.3–41.2% (1-month prevalence)

(Table 3.1). Measures of incidence (epidemiological measure of the development of new cases in an at-risk population over a defined interval) are not generally known because most studies report the period prevalence.

FURTHER READING

Henschke N, Kamper SJ, Maher CG. The epidemiology and economic consequences of pain. *Mayo Clin Proc.* 2015;90:139–147.

13. ANSWER: D

Although there are many different definitions of low back pain, most studies report a lifetime prevalence of between 51% and 84%. The 1-year incidence of first-time low back pain is between approximately 6% and 26%, and the incidence of recurrent low back pain is between approximately 24% and 80%.

KEY FACTS: EPIDEMIOLOGY OF PAIN IN ADULT PATIENTS

- Chronic low back pain (first time): 5.9–11.1% (1-month prevalence), 9% (lifetime prevalence)
- Low back pain: 14–90% (lifetime incidence)
- Sciatica: 0.4–16.4% (1-month prevalence), 9.3% (1-year incidence)
- Neuropathic pain (includes cancer): 0.9–39.1% (1-month prevalence)
- Fibromyalgia: 2–4% (point prevalence)
- Musculoskeletal: 14–28% (foot, ankle, and toe, pooled prevalence), 18–31% (shoulder, 1-month prevalence), 13–28% (knee, 1-month prevalence)

FURTHER READING

Henschke N, Kamper SJ, Maher CG. The epidemiology and economic consequences of pain. *Mayo Clin Proc.* 2015;90:139–147.

Malik KM, Jabri RS, Benzon HT. Overview of low back pain disorders. In: Benzon HT, Raja SN, Liu SS, et al. (Eds.), *Essentials of Pain Medicine.* 3rd ed. St. Louis, MO: Saunders; 2011:294–306.
Smith HS, Harris RE, Clauw DJ. –Fibromyalgia. In: Benzon HT, Raja SN, Liu SS, et al. (Eds.), *Essentials of Pain Medicine.* 3rd ed. St. Louis, MO: Saunders; 2011:345–350.

14. ANSWER: A

Migraine headaches are equally as common in males and females before puberty; however, after puberty the prevalence of migraines is 12–17.6% in females and 4–6% in males. Cluster headaches occur mostly in males (0.1–0.3% prevalence). Tension-type headaches are the most common; the lifetime prevalence approximates 90%.

KEY FACTS: EPIDEMIOLOGY OF HEADACHES

- Tension-type headache: 90% (lifetime prevalence)
- Migraine headache: ~15% in females, ~5% in males (prevalence)
- Cluster headache: ~0.2% (prevalence)

FURTHER READING

Henschke N, Kamper SJ, Maher CG. The epidemiology and economic consequences of pain. *Mayo Clin Proc.* 2015;90:139–147.
Rozental JM. Migraine headache and cluster In: Benzon HT, Raja SN, Liu SS, et al. (Eds.), *Essentials of Pain Medicine.* 3rd ed. St. Louis, MO: Saunders, 2011:261–267.

15. ANSWER: B

Spine pain is one of the most frequent reasons for lost workdays in the United States. Almost all individuals will experience low back pain in their lifetime. Depending on the definition and description of the problem, the lifetime incidence of low back pain ranges from 14% to 90%. Among working individuals who experience low back pain, 30% of these will develop chronic symptoms.

If a worker takes off work for 6 months due to low back pain, the likelihood of returning to work is 50% within that time frame. If the worker is off work for 1 year, the incidence of return to work is 25%, and if off for 2 years, the incidence of returning to work is less than 5%.

The terms *prevalence* and *incidence* are epidemiological terms used to describe proportions of populations affected by disease, and they represent a measure of societal burden:

- Prevalence is the proportion of a defined population that is at risk for a disease and that is also affected by the disease during a specified time period. The time period can be on a specific date (point prevalence) or over an interval of time (e.g., 1-year period—interval prevalence).
- Incidence is the proportion of members of a defined population who are at risk for a disease and who then *newly* become affected during a specified time interval.

The classic example is the Framingham Heart Study (Friedman et al., 1966), in which the population of Framingham, Massachusetts, was followed over 10 years to observe which persons developed coronary heart disease. Presumably all those in Framingham were at risk of developing heart disease, but certain individuals actually developed heart disease during the observation period. Those who developed heart disease were then compared to those who did not to identify potential risk factors such as cholesterol levels.

The prevalence of high cholesterol in those with coronary heart disease was 54%, whereas the prevalence of high cholesterol in those without coronary heart disease was 52%. In other words, at the end of 10 years, when cholesterol was measured, there was not a major difference in the prevalence of high cholesterol in either group. A major reason for this was that those with high cholesterol adjusted their diet so that by the end of the 10-year period, the two groups were nearly the same.

On the other hand, the 10-year incidence of high cholesterol was 75% in the group with coronary heart disease and 47% in the group without coronary heart disease. In other words, during the 10-year observation period, new cases of coronary heart disease were more often found in those with high cholesterol.

KEY FACTS: PREVALENCE VERSUS INCIDENCE

- Prevalence: The proportion of a population at risk affected by the disease at a specified point in time (a sum of all instances of a disease in a population at a certain time point)
  - Lifetime prevalence: The proportion of members of a population at risk who have been affected by the disease during any period of their lifetime
- Incidence: The proportion of members of a population at risk who become new cases of the disease during a time interval (a calculated risk of acquiring a disease in a certain time period)
  - Lifetime incidence: The proportion of members of a population at risk who become new cases (counting all recurrent events) of the disease during their lifetime (cumulative incidence)

FURTHER READING

Friedman GD, Kannel WB, Dawber TR, McNamara PM. Comparison of prevalence, case history and incidence data in assessing the potency of risk factors in coronary heart disease. *American Journal of Epidemiology*. 1966;83: 366–378.
Henschke N, Kamper SJ, Maher CG. The epidemiology and economic consequences of pain. *Mayo Clin Proc*. 2015;90:139–147.
Jewell NP. Measures of disease occurrence. In: Jewell NP (Ed.), *Statistics for Epidemiology*. Boca Raton, FL: Chapman & Hall/CRC Press; 2004:9–18.
Malik KM, Jabri RS, Benzon HT. Overview of low back pain disorders. In: Benzon HT, Raja SN, Liu SS, et al. (Eds.), *Essentials of Pain Medicine*. 3rd ed. St. Louis, MO: Saunders; 2011:294–306.

16. ANSWER: D

Analytic studies are used to determine what may be causing a disease to occur. These include the following:

- Experimental (control group and treatment group) studies
- Observational (no interventions) studies; there are three types of observational study designs:
  1. Cohort studies
  2. Case–control studies
  3. Cross-sectional studies

Cohort studies are either retrospective or prospective. In retrospective cohort studies, a cohort of subjects is selected based on an exposure, and an outcome of interest is measured among this cohort (e.g., failed back surgery syndrome among all patients who have undergone lumbar laminectomy). In prospective cohort studies (e.g., the Framingham Heart Study), a cohort of subjects at risk of a particular disease is identified and followed to observe occurrence of an outcome.

In case–control studies, cases of subjects with an outcome of interest are compared to those without the outcome from the same population.

What is the difference between a retrospective cohort study and a case–control study? In case–control studies, a researcher starts by knowing the disease/outcome (e.g., failed back surgery syndrome) and tries to determine the potential exposures or risk factors that are associated with the outcome (disability status, anxiety, etc.). In a retrospective cohort study, the researcher has identified the exposure/potential risk factor (e.g., anxiety) and tries to study the association of the exposure to the outcome (e.g., chronic pain).

The advantages and disadvantages of observational studies include the following:

- Cohort studies: Useful for rare *exposures* because individuals are chosen based on their exposure status; may need large sample size

- Retrospective: Inexpensive; data may be incomplete/inaccurate/insufficient
- Prospective: Expensive; better control over quality of data; potentially long follow-up needed
- Case–control studies: Useful for rare *outcomes* (diseases) because subjects are identified by already having the outcome and then compared to matched controls; quick; inexpensive; fewer subjects needed; can assess multiple potential risks
- Cross-sectional studies: Known as prevalence studies; not useful for cause–effect relationship of exposure to outcome because they examine disease and exposures at a specific time

KEY FACTS: LEVELS OF EVIDENCE

- Level I: RCT or systematic review of RCTs
- Level II: Low-quality RCT, prospective cohort, or systematic review of these
- Level III: Retrospective studies, case–control, or systematic review of these
- Level IV: Case series
- Level V: Expert opinion, case report

FURTHER READING

Henschke N, Kamper SJ, Maher CG. The epidemiology and economic consequences of pain. *Mayo Clin Proc*. 2015;90:139–147.
Song JW, Chung KC. Observational studies: Cohort and case–control studies. *Plast Reconstr Surg*. 2010;126:2234–2242.

17. ANSWER: C

Risk factors for the development of chronic pain are classified into the following general categories:

1. Age: The prevalence of many pain conditions increases or decreases with age, depending on the measure. Most recent studies show that the prevalence of chronic pain in adults younger than age 65 years can be as high as 76%, whereas that of adults older than age 65 years can be as high as 93%.
2. Sex: Among children, girls experience more pain than boys. Adult women report higher pain level, more frequent pain, and pain of longer duration than men.
3. Lifestyle choices: Smoking history, obesity, and comorbid conditions are associated with development of chronic pain.
4. Social: Socioeconomic factors influence development of chronic pain. Low education, low income, and higher unemployment are all associated with increased prevalence of chronic pain.
5. Occupation: High-demand jobs, job satisfaction, and occupational status all influence the development of chronic pain.
6. Psychosocial: The presence of anxiety, depression, stress, and chronic health problems may play a role in developing chronic pain.
7. Genetic: There is evidence of a genetic influence placing some patients at risk of developing chronic pain, but the strength of the influence is poorly understood.

FURTHER READING

Henschke N, Kamper SJ, Maher CG. The epidemiology and economic consequences of pain. *Mayo Clin Proc*. 2015;90:139–147.

18. ANSWER: A

Hernia repair is one of the most frequent surgeries performed in the United States. With improvement of surgical technique and introduction of laparoscopic approaches, complications of hernia repair surgery have decreased below 10%; however, the incidence of chronic pain after hernia repair has remained at approximately 10% so that it is the most frequent complication. Risk factors for development of chronic pain have thus garnered considerable attention.

KEY FACTS: RISK FACTORS FOR DEVELOPMENT OF CHRONIC PAIN AFTER SURGERY

- Type of surgery (e.g., limb amputation, thoracotomy, mastectomy, lumbar spine, abdominal hysterectomy, and hernia repair)
- Age (e.g., pediatric and elderly are less likely to develop chronic pain)
- Psychological factors (e.g., SF-12 mental summary, catastrophizing, and perceived control)
- Preexisting severity of acute pain and chronic pain

FURTHER READING

Edwards DA, Rathmell JP, Shah BJ. Post-herniorrhaphy pain. In: Hayek SM, Shah BJ, Desai MJ, et al. (Eds.), *Pain Medicine: An Interdisciplinary Case-Based Approach*. New York, NY: Oxford University Press; 2015:337–350.
Montes A, Roca G, Sabate S, et al. Genetic and clinical factors associated with chronic postsurgical pain after hernia repair, hysterectomy, and thoracotomy: A two-year multicenter cohort study. *Anesthesiology* 2015;122:1123–1141.

Perkins FM, Franklin JS. Prediction and prevention of persistent post-surgical pain. In: Benzon HT, Rathmell JP, Wu CL, et al. (Eds.), *Practical Pain Management*. 5th ed. Philadelphia, PA: Mosby; 2014:298–303.

19. ANSWER: B

It is appropriate practice to use evidence-based medicine whenever evidence exists. Although there remain many unknown contributors to the development of post-surgical chronic pain, a few risk factors have been shown to increase the odds of developing chronic pain. Best practice obligates the clinician to intervene, if possible, to mitigate the risks.

Although a patient may require surgery, the approach least likely to result in chronic pain may be considered, all else being equal. Reduction in opioid dose will make it easier to control perioperative pain, reduce opioid-related adverse events, and prevent opioid-induced hyperalgesia. There is evidence for the use of adjuvant medications, such as gabapentin and lidocaine, but there are no long-term studies to show efficacy in reducing the likelihood of chronic pain. Paravertebral blocks are an effective way of reducing the risk of persistent pain.

FURTHER READING

Perkins FM, Franklin JS. Prediction and prevention of persistent post-surgical pain. In: Benzon HT, Rathmell JP, Wu CL, et al. (Eds.), *Practical Pain Management*. 5th ed. Philadelphia, PA: Mosby; 2014:298–303.

20. ANSWER: A

The *Belmont Report* is the result of a meeting organized by the National Commission for the Protection of Human Subjects of Biomedical and Behavioral Research. The *Belmont Report* is a summary of the basic ethical principles identified by the Commission for human research. These are the following:

1. Respect for persons: Individuals should be treated as autonomous agents, or they should be protected if they have diminished autonomy.
2. Beneficence: This is the obligation to do no harm and to maximize possible benefits while minimizing possible harms.
3. Justice: Justice dictates who should benefit or who should shoulder the burden of research.

The first principle, *respect for persons*, applies when obtaining consent for study subjects. Persons involved should understand the research study and their role and be able to give consent based on their understanding. Furthermore, at any time they can withdraw from a study, being autonomous agents. Children, handicapped individuals, elderly, and all other persons with reduced capacity to understand and then give consent must be represented by surrogates who protect their rights and interests.

Beneficence means that a researcher has the obligation to maximize beneficial outcomes when designing research studies. Potential harm must not be significant. It is unethical to perform research on human subjects that may result in maiming individuals or causing their death.

The ethical principle of *justice* requires that persons not be excluded from potential benefits of research. Neither should classes of people shoulder the burden of research from which they may not benefit. For example, although it is necessary to protect the rights of children, it remains ethical to carry out studies on children who have diseases such as cancer. It is also unethical for a researcher to rely on a particular class of society that may never benefit from the results. For example, it is not ethical to study the effects of a drug on low-income individuals and then, if approved for human use, set the price point too high for anyone other than wealthy individuals to afford.

FURTHER READING

van der Velden MG, Waisel DB. Ethics of research in patients with pain. In: Benzon HT, Rathmell JP, Wu CL, et al. (Eds.), *Practical Pain Management*. 5th ed. Philadelphia, PA: Mosby; 2014:1066–1070.

21. ANSWER: C

Ethical animal research requires that studies are designed carefully so that there is a clear potential benefit to advance scientific understanding or health. Study design must therefore be *refined* to answer whether the outcomes sought require animals to be used at all. In many instances, animal studies can be *replaced* by in vitro or simulation models. If the study requires that animals be used, then the principle of *reduction* requires that the minimum number of animals necessary to answer the question be used.

KEY FACTS: THE THREE R'S OF ETHICAL ANIMAL RESEARCH

- Refine
- Reduce
- Replace

FURTHER READING

Russell WMS, Burch RL. *The Principles of Humane Experimental Technique*. London: Methuen; 1959.

22. ANSWER: C

Animal models used to study pain depend on objective observation of animal behaviors to quantify nociception. Pain models measure different pain modalities (Table 3.2): mechanical pain, thermal pain, chemical-induced pain, and inflammatory pain. To measure mechanical pain, calibrated von Frey filaments are used to determine the pressure threshold at which an animal will withdraw its foot. In models of allodynia and hyperalgesia (Table 3.2), the threshold for mechanical pain or heat/cold pain may change, and treatments may normalize pain thresholds.

In this question, streptozotocin is used to destroy pancreatic beta cells to cause chronic hyperglycemia and peripheral neuropathic pain. This is a model for what occurs in human diabetic neuropathy.

FURTHER READING

Chung JM. Animal models and experimental tests to study nociception and pain. In: Gebhart GF, Schmidt RF (Eds.), *Encyclopedia of Pain*. Berlin: Springer; 2013:154–157.

23. ANSWER: D

Animal experiments of pain are regulated by local institutional animal care and use committees. Animal experiments that cause pain are categorized by degree and duration of painful stimuli (Box 3.1).

Table 3.2 **ANIMAL MODELS OF ACUTE AND CHRONIC PAIN**

CATEGORY	PAIN MODALITY	MODEL	DESCRIPTION
Acute pain	Mechanical pressure	Paw pressure test	The *pressure threshold* to paw withdrawal is measured while a pressure pad is applied to the metacarpal of the toe.
		Withdrawal threshold	Calibrated von Frey filaments are applied to the hind foot and the smallest filament that elicits a withdrawal response is considered to be the *withdrawal threshold*.
	Temperature	Tail-flick test	Radiant heat is applied to the tail or the tail is placed in hot water that causes the animal to flick its tail out of the way. The time to withdrawal of the tail is measured as the *withdrawal latency*.
		Paw withdrawal test	Radiant heat is applied under the animal's foot. The *time to withdrawal* is measured. This test is more sensitive than the tail-flick test.
		Hot-plate test	An animal is placed on a hot plate of variable temperature. When the animal licks its feet or jumps off the plate, the *response latency* is recorded.
	Electrical	Electrical shock tail vocalization test	The *electrical threshold* to vocalization is measured with electrode-delivered current to the tail.
Subacute and chronic pain	Neuropathic (mononeuropathy)	Spared nerve injury	The peripheral nerve (tibial or common peroneal) is injured.
		Partial sciatic nerve ligation	The lateral third of the sciatic nerve is injured.
		Chronic constriction injury	The common sciatic is constricted.
		Spinal nerve ligation	L5 and L6 nerve roots are ligated (called Chung L5/L6 ligation).
	Neuropathic (polyneuropathy)	Diabetic neuropathy	Streptozocin causes hyperglycemia and results in peripheral neuropathy.
		Chemotherapy	Vincristine, paclitaxel, or cisplatin is given and results in neuropathy.
	Visceral	Chemical	Hypertonic saline, acetic acid, and capsaicin.
		Viscus distention	Distend hollow organs → visceromotor response.
	Cancer	Osteosarcoma	Implant osteosarcoma into femur → proliferates causing bone demineralization and pain.

Box 3.1 CATEGORIES OF ANIMAL PAIN
EXPERIMENTATION

- Category C
  - Minimal pain
  - Animal can escape the stimulus (i.e., von Frey filament—the animal can lift its foot away; hot plate—the animal can jump off the plate)
- Category D
  - Pain followed by treatment with analgesics (i.e., surgery that is treated with postoperative opioids)
- Category E
  - Pain that is not alleviated (i.e., models of neuropathic or cancer pain)

24. ANSWER: D

Nociception is the pathophysiological response to a harmful or potentially harmful stimulus. In humans, this results in the perception of pain. It is controversial whether or not animals perceive pain or if responses only reflect nociceptive behaviors. Despite this, ethical experimentation in pain on animals assumes that the observed behaviors represent pain and not just nociception.

Rat strains show different degrees of responses to pain modalities and different responses to treatments. This may reflect differential nociception as a result of genetic variation.

25. ANSWER: A

von Frey filaments are small wires calibrated to bend at specific pressure thresholds (Table 3.2). These wires are applied to the foot of an animal, and the wire that causes the animal to withdraw its foot indicates the pressure at which the animal pressure nociceptors are activated.

The hot-plate test, Hargreaves model, and tail-flick test are tools to measure heat temperature thresholds of nociception (Table 3.2). In the hot-plate test, the animal is placed on a heating platform and the temperature is gradually increased until the animal lifts its paws, licks its paws, or jumps off the surface. In the Hargreaves model, a small localized heat source is applied to the foot of the animal. In the tail-flick test, an animal's tail is placed in a heated water bath. The time to withdrawal is measured from the time the animal's tail is placed in the bath to the time it flicks its tail out.

FURTHER READING

Chung JM. Animal models and experimental tests to study nociception and pain. In: Gebhart GF, Schmidt RF (Eds.), *Encyclopedia of Pain*. Berlin: Springer; 2013:154–157.

26. ANSWER: E

Here, the only model of mononeuropathy is the common sciatic ligature model (Table 3.2). The others are models of polyneuropathy or cancer pain.

Tricyclic antidepressants (TCAs) have antinociceptive properties in rat models of electrical pain, formalin-induced pain, heat pain, and tissue injury/neuropathic pain. In 1992, Ardid and Guilbaud showed that in rats with ligatures tied around the common sciatic nerve, TCAs increased the threshold to vocalization of pain from the paw pressure test (phasic test) and reduced spontaneous pain-related behavior (tonic test).

FURTHER READING

Ardid D, Guilbaud G. Antinociceptive effects of acute and 'chronic' injections of tricyclic antidepressant drugs in a new model of mononeuropathy in rats. *Pain*. 1992;49:279–287.
Smith HS, Argoff CR, McCleane G. Antidepressants as analgesics. In: Benzon HT, Rathmell JP, Wu CL, et al. (Eds.), *Practical Pain Management*. 5th ed. Philadelphia, PA: Mosby; 2014:530–542.

27. ANSWER: A

For human subjects research to be ethical, the results must add to scientific understanding and be considered valuable to society. Unnecessarily repetitive research would thus be considered unethical to perform. Moreover, it is crucial to publish the results of studies with negative results to avoid repetitive research. There is considerable literature bias as a result of unpublished negative research. Indeed, level I data consisting of meta-analysis are limited by the non-inclusion of negative study results. It is considered unethical for a researcher to withhold human subjects research results.

FURTHER READING

van der Velden MG, Waisel DB. Ethics of research in patients with pain. In: Benzon HT, Rathmell JP, Wu CL, et al. (Eds.), *Practical Pain Management*. 5th ed. Philadelphia, PA: Mosby; 2014:1066–1070.

28. ANSWER: A

The Nuremberg Code (1947) outlined 10 standards for ethical human experimentation. Among these is the requirement that no experimentation be performed on human subjects that may result in death or disability.

KEY FACTS: NUREMBERG CODE—10 STANDARDS FOR ETHICAL HUMAN EXPERIMENTATION

- Voluntary informed consent is essential.
- Risks must be balanced against benefits.
- Avoid unnecessary physical and mental suffering.
- No experimentation is to be performed in which death or disability may result.
- Experiments must be designed to yield fruitful results for society.
- Experiments must be designed based on results of animal experiments and a knowledge of natural history of disease.
- Scientists must make preparations to protect subjects.
- The experiment should be conducted only by scientifically qualified persons.
- The subject should be at liberty to end the experiment at any time.
- The scientist in charge must be prepared to terminate the experiment at any stage.

FURTHER READING

van der Velden MG, Waisel DB. Ethics of research in patients with pain. In: Benzon HT, Rathmell JP, Wu CL, et al. (Eds.), *Practical Pain Management*. 5th ed. Philadelphia, PA: Mosby; 2014:1066–1070.

29. ANSWER: B

Following World War II and the atrocities by German researchers on human subjects, a series of trials collectively known as the Nuremberg Trials were conducted. This resulted in the conviction of 22 men and 1 woman; 7 were ultimately hanged, 9 were given prison terms, and 7 were determined not guilty. During the trials, the Nuremberg Code was drafted to designate what was considered ethical in human experimentation.

It was not until decades later, and partially in response to the unethical experimentation of African American men with syphilis during the Tuskegee experiments, that the United States government drafted the national Research Act (July 12, 1974), which created the National Commission for Protection of Human Subjects of Biomedical and Behavioral Research. The Commission was charged with outlining ethical principles for human experimentation.

The Commission published the *Belmont Report* on April 18, 1979, which summarized its recommendations. This report also serves as a reference for today's IRBs.

FURTHER READING

van der Velden MG, Waisel DB. Ethics of research in patients with pain. In: Benzon HT, Rathmell JP, Wu CL, et al. (Eds.), *Practical Pain Management*. 5th ed. Philadelphia, PA: Mosby; 2014:1066–1070.

30. ANSWER: C

The *Belmont Report* is the result of a meeting organized by the National Commission for the Protection of Human Subjects of Biomedical and Behavioral Research. The *Belmont Report* is a summary of the basic ethical principles identified by the Commission for human research. These principles are provided in Box 3.2.

FURTHER READING

van der Velden MG, Waisel DB. Ethics of research in patients with pain. In: Benzon HT, Rathmell JP, Wu CL, et al. (Eds.), *Practical Pain Management*. 5th ed. Philadelphia, PA: Mosby; 2014:1066–1070.

31. ANSWER: C

The principle of justice suggests that the benefits of research not be restricted to subpopulations (e.g., only the wealthy who can afford to pay for an approved medication) or that the burden of research not be placed unfairly on a vulnerable subpopulation (e.g., handicapped, prisoners, and the poor). See Box 3.2 for more information on the *Belmont Report*.

32. ANSWER: A

Respect for persons obligates a researcher to obtain informed consent from the research subject prior to including that person. If the person is unable to act as an autonomous agent (e.g., children and the mentally handicapped), then a health care proxy must act in his or her stead. The principle of respect for persons requires that those with diminished autonomy be protected. See Box 3.2 for more information on the *Belmont Report*.

33. ANSWER: B

The principle of beneficence includes the obligation to do no harm and so secure patient well-being. See Box 3.2 for more information on the *Belmont Report*.

34. ANSWER: C

The principle of beneficence requires that potential benefits should be maximized while potential risks are minimized. See Box 3.2 for more information on the *Belmont Report*.

35. ANSWER: E

Respect for persons requires that subjects of human studies research consent to participate and are allowed to withdraw from the study at any time. During the Tuskegee experiment, African American men were not informed that a treatment for their disease existed, violating this principle.

36. ANSWER: D

Respect for persons is an ethical principle outlined in the *Belmont Report* that stipulates that those with reduced capacity be represented by those who can consent on their behalf. The principle of justice, in this instance, might require that this study not be restricted and potentially deny benefit to this population.

37. ANSWER: A

Although all the answers given would be appropriate points to include when designing human subjects research, study design validity depends only on the ability of a study to answer the hypothesis and provide useful results. It is the responsibility of the researchers and the IRB to ensure it does this before any risks can be incurred or resources used.

FURTHER READING

van der Velden MG, Waisel DB. Ethics of research in patients with pain. In: Benzon HT, Rathmell JP, Wu CL, et al. (Eds.), *Practical Pain Management*. 5th ed. Philadelphia, PA: Mosby; 2014:1066–1070.

38. ANSWER: A

In pain research, individuals in pain are considered vulnerable given that they may be more inclined to consent to being experimented on in order to relieve their suffering. Despite this, it would be unethical in many instances to restrict research in this population and limited potential therapies that may be discovered to alleviate pain. The principle of justice thus requires that, in this case, potential benefits not be withheld.

FURTHER READING

van der Velden MG, Waisel DB. Ethics of research in patients with pain. In: Benzon HT, Rathmell JP, Wu CL, et al. (Eds.), *Practical Pain Management*. 5th ed. Philadelphia, PA: Mosby; 2014:1066–1070.

39. ANSWER: B

Placebo-controlled trials are often required by the FDA for drug trials. In pain research, the use of placebo is ethical only in the instance in which no effective treatment exists that can be used as a comparison.

FURTHER READING

van der Velden MG, Waisel DB. Ethics of research in patients with pain. In: Benzon HT, Rathmell JP, Wu CL, et al. (Eds.), *Practical Pain Management*. 5th ed. Philadelphia, PA: Mosby; 2014:1066–1070.

4.

PSYCHOLOGY OF PAIN
PSYCHOLOGICAL ASSESSMENT AND TREATMENT OF PAIN

Julie R. Price, Micah J. Price, and Marc A. Huntoon

INTRODUCTION

The role of psychosocial variables in the understanding, diagnosis, and treatment of pain has grown significantly in the past 30 years. Pain is no longer dichotomously thought of as either a purely psychological or physiological condition (mind–body dualism) but, rather, as a combination of biopsychosocial factors and experiences. The questions in this chapter consider the changing role of these psychosocial factors by exploring the fifth edition of the *Diagnostic and Statistical Manual of Mental Disorders* as well as other pain-related assessments and psychodiagnostics; cognitive behavioral, acceptance and commitment, behavioral, and other psychological interventions for pain management; the role of stages of change in selection of interventions; and biopsychosocial theoretical models for understanding pain. The questions in this chapter also provide detailed and empirically supported explanations of the biopsychosocial impact of pain, along with references to texts commonly utilized in the training of anesthesiologists, so as to promote a better understanding of the associated materials.

QUESTIONS

1. A "third-generation" psychotherapeutic treatment modality that views pain not as something that must be controlled or fought against but, rather, as a change in life that should be adapted to and experienced so that one can focus his or her energy on living life is most consistent with which therapy?

A. Hypnosis
B. Cognitive behavioral therapy
C. Guided imagery
D. Acceptance and commitment therapy

2. A patient recognizes that his or her current medication regimen is not providing sufficient pain management but struggles to engage in an active, nonpharmacological pain management approach/intervention at this time, despite inquiring about risks and benefits of nonpharmacological interventions. According to the transtheoretical model of behavioral change, the patient is in what stage of change?

A. Action
B. Precontemplation
C. Termination
D. Contemplation

3. Individuals with chronic and severe pain can often become fixed and unconsciously resistant to further gains. In order to overcome this rigidity in patients, clinicians have utilized approaches that directly address being "stuck" in the change process. This approach has demonstrated successful outcomes with substance abuse patients. Which of the following approaches has been shown to be effective with such patients?

A. Meditation
B. Motivational interviewing
C. Family systems therapy
D. Biofeedback

4. Which of the statements regarding cognitive behavioral therapy (CBT) for chronic pain is the most accurate?

A. CBT can be effective in a group therapy format.
B. CBT is often effective for acute pain but ineffective for chronic pain.
C. CBT is primarily useful for middle-aged adults with chronic pain, but it is often less effective for teens and older adults.

D.   CBT treatment for chronic pain focuses on psychological factors but ignores physiological factors.

5. Cognitive behavioral intervention as well as other psychotherapeutic strategies have been shown to exhibit what effects in pain patients?

A. Reduce the intensity of pain, but not improve the patient's reported pain symptomatology and psychosocial functioning
B. Improve both the patient's anxiety and depression symptomatology, but not improve reported pain intensity
C. Reduce pain intensity as well as improve activities of daily living and psychosocial functioning
D. Improve psychosocial functioning and reported pain behaviors, but not reduce pain intensity

6. You have been consulted to provide palliative care interventions for an elderly patient with terminal cancer. On your entering, the patient indicates experiencing significant pain and expresses fears of taking pain medication. As you start to explore the patient's fears, he begins to discuss his religion, indicates a need for "God's guidance," and requests prayer. In this instance, before addressing the medical needs of the consultation, what is the best approach for promoting psychological well-being and reducing physical distress?

A. Explore the patient's religious beliefs and, if not compromising your own beliefs, be willing to pray with or allow the patient to pray while you remain silent.
B. Tell the patient immediately you will consult the hospital chaplain because religion is outside of your scope of training.
C. Explore the patient's religious beliefs and, even if it would compromise your own beliefs, be willing to pray with the patient.
D. Utilize cognitive behavioral techniques to challenge the patient's fears and beliefs that he requires prayer to make appropriate decisions regarding his care.

7. A patient 6 months post joint replacement surgery reports that his pain has remained at a 9/10 since his 1-month follow-up visit. He reports that he does not like to take pain medication and discloses concerns about becoming "addicted to pain pills." The patient readily brings in his prescription bottle of hydromorphone, which has half of the pills remaining, but requests a refill. What area of exploration is not required to rule out/diagnosis an opioid use disorder?

A. Is the patient taking larger amounts of pain medication than intended and experiencing cravings?

B. Is the patient obtaining pain medication from other providers or spending excessive amounts of time seeking out pain medication?
C. Is the patient experiencing breakthrough pain due to insufficient use of pain medication?
D. Is the patient experiencing impairments in occupational and social functioning?

8. A significant predictor in the determination of successful physiological and psychological (mind–body) treatment interventions is the accurate assessment of pain. However, given that pain is a very individual and subjective experience, coupled with the existence of those who might be moved by secondary gains, thus potentially over-/underreporting pain, the ability to accurately measure pain intensity is a challenge at best. Given this, which of the following is not a valid measure of pain intensity?

A. Pain Catastrophizing Scale
B. Wong–Baker FACES Pain Scale
C. McGill Pain Questionnaire
D. West Haven–Yale Multidimensional Pain Inventory

9. A 38-year-old Caucasian American male presents with post-laminectomy syndrome and complaints of chronic back pain rated at 10/10 that developed after a motor vehicle collision 3 years ago. He is currently in legal litigation and has a history of arrests for narcotics distribution. Records reveal the patient has been seen by multiple pain providers and states hydrocodone is the only medication that "helps my pain." He is unusually guarded when discussing his pain medication, and recent urine drug screen results are negative for opioids. What diagnosis most likely fits this patient's presentation?

A. Somatic symptom disorder, with predominant pain
B. Conversion disorder
C. Factitious disorder
D. Malingering

10. You will be referring a 42-year-old patient with failed back syndrome for a presurgical psychological evaluation for an implantable device, specifically a spinal cord stimulator (SCS). You are aware that the patient has a long history of psychiatric instability, but currently the patient appears to be functioning quite well, other than what appear to be challenges relating to ineffective pain management. What psychological assessment instrument(s) would you like to see utilized, because it has demonstrated effectiveness for assessing psychopathology and personality, in order to fully evaluate your patient preoperatively?

A. Beck Depression and Anxiety Inventories (BDI/BAI)
B. Patient Health Questionnaire Screeners (PHQ)

C. Minnesota Multiphasic Personality Inventory-2 (MMPI-2)/Minnesota Multiphasic Personality Inventory-2–Restructured Form (MMPI-2-RF)
D. A structured clinical interview (SCI)

11. The multidisciplinary approach to rehabilitation, which often includes a combination of psychological, pharmacological, physical, occupational, and group-based interventions, is typically based on what model of health care?

A. Cognitive behavioral
B. Biological
C. Alternative
D. Biopsychosocial

12. What psychosocial factor has been found to be least predictive of poor treatment outcomes following lumbar and SCS surgery?

A. Presurgical pain intensity
B. Longer pain duration
C. Old age
D. Poor coping

13. What physiotherapy intervention has been shown to have a strong evidence base for its effectiveness in complex regional pain syndrome (CRPS) and uses a contralateral body part as a means of targeting cortical areas of the brain in order to reduce body perception disturbance and pain through reversal of abnormalities in the body map?

A. Guided imagery
B. Systematic desensitization
C. Biofeedback
D. Graded motor imagery

14. Which of the following descriptions best fits within the more modern integrated model of pain?

A. Pain is viewed as a physiological or somatic response to noxious stimulation of particular neuroreceptors within the body.
B. Pain is the conscious and sometimes unconscious experience of a noxious stimulus involving sensory, emotional, and cognitive processes within the brain.
C. Pain is viewed as a psychiatric response to childhood trauma, pain-prone personalities, or distorted thought processes.
D. Pain is a learned response to rewards and punishments that involves exposure to and/or removal of noxious stimuli as part of a reinforcement continuum.

15. A 48-year-old Hispanic female presents with low back pain and chronic left L5 radiculopathy status post lumbar fusion, which resulted from a motor vehicle collision 5 years earlier. Repeated imaging of the lumbar spine shows no new pathology. She has been adherent to her current medication regimen and physical therapy without effect. She endorsed trying "everything," but during her psychological evaluation for a spinal cord stimulator, she expressed expectation for either 100% pain relief or no pain relief at all. From a cognitive behavioral perspective, what type of cognitive distortion is she most likely exhibiting?

A. Overgeneralization
B. Catastrophizing
C. Jumping to conclusions
D. Dichotomous thinking

16. There is a vast body of research indicating the importance of cognitive and behavioral processes in how individuals adapt to chronic pain. Learning theory postulates that social and environmental variables have been shown to be associated with pain behaviors and disability levels. What has been consistently found to be associated with greater physical and psychosocial dysfunction, even after controlling for pain and depression levels?

A. Pain-related beliefs
B. Pain catastrophizing
C. Pain-related appraisals
D. Pain intensity

17. Research suggests the relationship between childhood trauma and chronic pain as an adult is which of the following?

A. Childhood trauma has a positive correlation with chronic pain in adulthood.
B. Childhood trauma has a negative correlation with chronic pain in adulthood.
C. Research suggests that children who experience trauma are often numb to all types of pain in adulthood.
D. Childhood trauma has no correlation with pain in adulthood.

18. After careful examination and medical history, a diagnosis of fibromyalgia was assigned, using the American College of Rheumatology (1990) criteria, to your 40-year-old female patient. If formulating an integrative approach to treatment, which of the following would likely have the greatest amount of benefit for your patient?

A. Nonsteroidal anti-inflammatory drugs (NSAIDs), vigorous aerobic exercise, procedural intervention, and cognitive behavioral or acceptance-based therapies

B. Cognitive behavioral or acceptance-based therapies, movement-based exercise (e.g., yoga), antidepressants, and an anti-inflammatory diet
C. Long-term psychodynamic therapies and procedural interventions
D. Cognitive behavioral or acceptance-based therapies, high-dose opioids, nutritional supplements, and vigorous aerobic exercise

19. A comprehensive psychological evaluation is a necessity when evaluating a patient presurgically for clearance for various surgical procedures (spinal cord stimulator, intrathecal pump, bariatric surgery, and organ transplantation). The use of either only a clinical interview or only psychological assessment instruments provides limited data and can miss how the psychological aspects of affective, behavioral, and cognitive dimensions interplay with sensory–physical ones. If a provider decides to conduct only a clinical interview, what will he or she be missing in this evaluation?

A. An objective norm-referenced measure to evaluate the validity of responses to assist in determination of whether the patient is over- or underreporting symptomatology
B. Opportunity to interact and collect information that may be relevant but not asked in questionnaires (e.g., ongoing fear resulting from the death of a close relative during surgery or unusual patient behaviors such as skin picking)
C. An opportunity to develop rapport with the patient
D. The patient's subjective view of his or her pain experiences and expectations/hopes for post-surgical outcomes

20. Biofeedback, a cognitive behavioral intervention, has been shown as successful for the treatment of peripheral neuropathy as a result of?

A. Relaxation and regulation of blood pressure
B. Reduction of HbA1c and increased blow flow to the extremities
C. Increased blood flow to the extremities
D. Improvement in pain management

21. A 65-year-old patient with a history of paroxysmal trigeminal pain that developed after fracture of the mandible following a motor vehicle collision returns 2 weeks after a surgical procedure with inadequate pain relief. The patient expressed complaints of facial tingling and difficulties in facial expression. The patient also expressed concerns that the surgery was a failure and is extremely unhappy with a wait-and-see approach. After medical examination, the surgery appears to have been successful. Of the following recommended interventions, which would likely lead to the most rapid increase in patient satisfaction?

A. Cognitive behavioral therapy to help the patient come to terms with unrealistic expectations
B. Schedule patient for follow-up surgery
C. Tell patient there is little more that can be done other than wait
D. Cognitive behavioral therapy with a focus on sensory retraining

22. A supportive relationship between the physician and the patient has been found to facilitate all of the following except?

A. Improved adherence/compliance
B. The flow of information
C. Patient avoidance of discussions regarding trauma/abuse history
D. Improved recovery

23. The view or formulation of pain as originating from psychological causes or "all in the patient's head" is termed?

A. Idiopathic view
B. Neuropathic view
C. Psychogenic view
D. Nociceptive view

24. A patient has shown improvement via a reduction in pain intensity but continues to struggle with acceptance issues regarding lifestyle changes as a result of his pain/medical condition. A cognitive behavioral group therapy intervention has been determined to be beneficial, but the physician is unsure if the patient would be a good fit for group therapy. What behavioral factor(s) would likely indicate the patient is a poor candidate for group therapy?

A. Inactivity or excessive dependence
B. Mild to moderate anxiety or depression
C. Anger and hostility
D. Negative self-talk or criticism

25. For the past 2 years, your patient has been on time to appointments, adhered to and taken medications as prescribed, and endorsed adequate pain control. However, the patient is experiencing increased difficulties with constipation and drowsiness. The patient reports no desire to change his treatment regimen at this time and refuses to consider active, nonpharmacological

interventions. According to the transtheoretical model of behavioral change, your patient is in the precontemplation stage. What intervention might be the most beneficial in promoting movement into the contemplation stage of change?

   A. Commend the patient for adherence to treatment recommendations. Then ask to briefly discuss the advantages and disadvantages of changing treatment interventions and provide personalized information on active, nonpharmacological interventions.
   B. Discuss a referral for ongoing care/termination as a means of creating a need for change.
   C. Continue same treatment, but shock the patient by providing only negative side effects/consequences.
   D. Discuss the consequences and offer inoculation by discussing that some patients fail at making change the first few times.

26. You are palliatively treating a recovering burn patient who is about to begin physical therapy. He enters the physical therapy room and becomes nervous and begins to complain of increased pain prior to beginning any treatment. The patient complains not only of increased pain in his arm, the current target of therapy, but also of unbearable pain in his back and legs, which were also burned. What intervention would primarily be utilized as an in vivo approach to focus on the anticipatory fear the patient is experiencing?

   A. Cognitive behavioral therapy
   B. Systematic desensitization
   C. Operant conditioning
   D. Eye movement desensitization and reprocessing (EMDR)

27. Coping refers to the use of a set of diverse techniques or methods by which an individual can deal with stressors including physical pain. Of the following, which is not a recognized coping technique/strategy?

   A. Coping self-statements
   B. Task persistence
   C. Self-actualization
   D. Medication use

28. A 78-year-old non-Caucasian male with terminal colorectal cancer is being evaluated as to his psychological readiness for a proposed intrathecal drug delivery device in the setting of inadequate pain control. Which of the following is a true statement(s) regarding cultural and racial disparities in pain expression and treatment?

   A. African and Hispanic Americans are more likely to report using prayer as a coping strategy than Caucasians.
   B. African Americans were found to have higher thresholds for pain in experimental thermal pain studies and also variation in certain pain transduction and opioid receptor gene polymorphisms.
   C. Barriers to effective pain care are almost entirely due to health care provider attitudes.
   D. All of the above.

29. For the optimal conduct of experiments in clinical pain, the following domain(s) is an important component of the research study:

   A. A validated measure of depression and/or emotional health
   B. A functional measure (e.g., the Oswestry Disability Scale)
   C. A scale representation of pain intensity such as a numeric rating scale
   D. All of the above
   E. Only B and C

30. A 13-year-old female is involved with her parents in a major motor vehicle collision that has left her with fractured ribs, sternum, left scapula, pelvis, and left femur. She is intubated and unable to respond when her nurse asks about pain. Which of the following is true about evaluation of pain in impaired patients?

   A. The Bieri faces scale is likely to be accurate even if she is intubated.
   B. Although verbal report of pain is best, this is not true for children her age.
   C. Vital sign changes are the most accurate pain indication in the critical care setting.
   D. The Critical-Care Pain Observation Tool (CPOT), Faces, Legs, Activity, Cry, and Consolability (FLACC), or Pain Behavioral Assessment Tool (PBAT) may all be appropriate to ascertain whether she may have pain.

31. Measuring pain in special populations such as the cognitively impaired elderly patient or young child can be challenging. Of the following, which is most true of pain assessment?

   A. In patients with severe dementia, the FLACC scale is always the most useful.

B. Children younger than age 6 years can routinely use the Faces scale revised version to rate their pain with high reliability.

C. When assessing pain in special populations, one should choose a scale and stick with it because applying multiple scales only confuses the picture.

D. When choosing a pain measurement, ensuring that most participants can utilize the scale and ensuring a large sample size and adequate power can overcome unreliability.

ANSWERS

1. ANSWER: D

Acceptance and commitment therapy (ACT) is a third-generation or third-wave treatment modality that utilizes six key principles or processes to promote healthy cognitive and behavioral coping and adaptation with the ultimate goal of gaining psychological flexibility. These principles are acceptance, cognitive fusion, being present or mindfulness, self as context, values, and committed action. The three with the greatest empirical support in pain management are acceptance, which involves an active and aware embrace of those thoughts/events once experienced without any attempt to change them in form or frequency; mindfulness or being in the present moment via nonjudgmental contact; and values, which are chosen qualities based on the patients' life directions that provide an underlying reason for purposeful movement. Research suggests acceptance shows the greatest benefit in pre- to post-treatment functioning, whereas values-based action dominates pretreatment to follow-up. Research also suggests changes in acceptance show benefit in reduction of pain-related fears. ACT, unlike CBT, avoids viewing a patient's struggle with pain as a maladaptive thought process. Guided imagery might be utilized as part of the mindfulness component of ACT treatment, and like hypnosis, it can be beneficial for pain intensity reduction, although both guided imagery and hypnosis are limited in that they fail to address more complex cognitive processes.

FURTHER READING

Cianfrini LR, Block C, Doleys DM. Psychological therapies. In: Deer TR, Leong MS, Buvanendran A, et al. (Eds.), *Comprehensive Treatment of Chronic Pain by Medical, Interventional, and Integrative Approaches*. New York, NY: Springer; 2013:827–844.
Hayes S. The psychological flexibility model. Available at https://contextualscience.org/the_six_core_processes_of_act. Accessed August 10, 2015.
Volwes K, Mccracken L. Acceptance and values-based action in chronic pain: A study of treatment effectiveness and process. *J Consult Clin Psychol*. 2008;76(3):397–407.

2. ANSWER: D

The transtheoretical model of behavioral change, developed by Prochaska and DiClemente in 1982, is a method of assessing an individual's readiness to change/engage in a new behavior. The model involves five stages: precontemplation, contemplation, preparation, action, and maintenance. It has been shown to be effective for understanding the level of engagement in treatment readiness for chronic pain patients because patients are unlikely to make a change in behaviors if they are not ready. The precontemplation stage involves individuals who are not intending to take action in the near future and who may even be unaware or even unwilling to see that their behavior is problematic. The contemplation stage involves individuals who are beginning to recognize a behavior as problematic and who begin to evaluate the advantages and disadvantages of their continued actions. The preparation stage involves individuals who intend to take action in the immediate future and may begin to make minor behavioral changes. In the action stage, individuals are making specific overt modifications toward modifying their problematic behaviors and/or engaging in new and healthier behaviors. The maintenance stage involves those who have sustained action for a period of 6 months or longer and are working to prevent relapse. Diagnostic tools are available to determine a patient's particular stage, and interventions can be utilized in each stage to provide motivation and support for progression to the next stage. After someone has progressed through the individual stages, he or she may regress to the beginning or prior stages or may reach a termination phase in which the change becomes accepted and a desire to return to the old behavior no longer exists. For this question, contemplation is the best choice because the patient recognizes and is weighing the advantages and disadvantages (or risks and benefits) of making a change.

FURTHER READING

Jensen MP. Enhancing motivation to change in pain treatment. In: Turk DC, Gatchel RJ (Eds.), *Psychological Approaches to Pain Management: A Practitioner's Handbook*. 2nd ed. New York, NY: Guilford; 2002:71–93.
Prochaska JO, DiClements CC. Transtheoretical therapy: Toward a more integrative model of change. *Psychother Theory Res Pract*. 1982;19:276–288.

3. ANSWER: B

Of the approaches listed in the answer choices, one that has been found effective in initiating change among patients with active substance abuse is motivational interviewing (MI). MI has been shown to be effective with the substance abuse population, and it has recently been adopted and is showing promise with the chronic pain population. MI has five principles or tasks that guide the provider: expressing empathy, developing discrepancy, avoiding argumentation, rolling with resistance, and supporting self-efficacy. MI utilizes strategies such as evaluating where the patient is in the change process via Prochaska's stage of change model and utilizing supportive challenges and encouragement to assist the patient in motivation for change. The clinician listens with empathy, asks open-ended questions, provides affirming feedback, and provides meaningful challenges to handle resistance to change. Although empathy is an innate characteristic, clinicians can demonstrate empathic listening through the use of body language (head nods and leaning in toward the patient) and verbal reflections of content. An open-ended question would be "How have you coped with your pain so far?" versus a closed question such as "What is your pain score out of 10?" Positive affirmations should focus on highlighting successes, such as "Even though you pain is an 8/10 today, you have made every appointment and are adherent to recommendations." All of these techniques would be approached from a tolerant and nonjudgmental standpoint. The other choices do not directly address patients who are fixed or "stuck" in the change processes.

FURTHER READING

Jensen MP. Enhancing motivation to change in pain treatment. In: Turk DC, Gatchel RJ (Eds.), *Psychological Approaches to Pain Management: A Practitioner's Handbook*. 2nd ed. New York, NY: Guilford; 2002:71–93.

Miller WR, Rollinick S. *Motivational Interviewing: Preparing People to Change Addictive Behavior*. New York, NY: Guilford; 1991.

Turk, DC. Psychological interventions. In: Benzon H, Rathmell J, Wu CL, et al. (Eds.), *Practical Management of Pain*. 5th ed. Philadelphia, PA: Mosby; 2014:615–628.

4. ANSWER: A

The goal of CBT is to modify maladaptive thoughts and behaviors. CBT teaches individual patients to identify and change maladaptive thought patterns that distort feelings and lead to unhealthy behaviors. By changing this maladaptive triad, psychological distress is reduced and the overall quality of life is improved. This reduction in psychological distress then results in a corresponding reduction in pain symptomatology and related chronic pain behaviors. Chronic pain-related impairments are exacerbated by the individual's maladaptive thoughts, feelings, and behaviors, which then lead to a downward spiraling decline in physical and emotional functioning. CBT has been empirically shown to be beneficial for patients with chronic neuropathic pain, which focuses on helping the patient develop an understanding of how pain consists of both physical and emotional experiences.

CBT utilizes individual and group therapeutic approaches to engage the patient in modification of maladaptive coping strategies that exacerbate pain-related impairments and losses to functioning via goal setting, cognitive restructuring, activity pacing, and relaxation training. CBT interventions can be delivered in brief 5-minute psychoeducational sessions in multiweek group rehabilitation programs. The effective patient population ranges from pediatrics to adults. CBT is effective for depression, anxiety, post-traumatic stress disorder, and substance abuse, as well as comorbid disorders.

FURTHER READING

Cianfrini LR, Block C, Doleys DM. Psychological therapies. In: Deer TR, Leong MS, Buvanendran A, et al. (Eds.), *Comprehensive Treatment of Chronic Pain by Medical, Interventional, and Integrative Approaches*. New York, NY: Springer; 2013:827–844.

Otis JD, Pincus DB, Murawski ME. Cognitive behavioral therapy in pain management. In: Ebert MH, Kerns RD (Eds.), *Behavioral and Psychopharmacologic Pain Management*. Cambridge, UK: Cambridge University Press; 2011:184–200.

Townsend CO, Rome JD, Bruce BK, et al. Interdisciplinary pain rehabilitation programs. In: Ebert MH, Kerns RD (Eds.), *Behavioral and Psychopharmacologic Pain Management*. Cambridge, UK: Cambridge University Press; 2011:114–128.

5. ANSWER: C

A literature review of psychotherapeutic treatment models for chronic pain investigated the outcomes of psychodynamic, cognitive behavioral, and behavioral therapies. Among other intervention types, insight oriented, motivational interviewing, relaxation, meditation, and guided imagery were explored. Turk et al. (2008) found specifically that CBT improved mood, coping, activities of daily living, and social functioning. They also found that CBT reduced pain intensity, along with substituting feelings of dependence, passivity, and avoidance with enhanced self-control and pain self-management. The authors expressed that all of the therapeutic interventions could lead to increased self-management of pain because they improved maladaptive pain beliefs, expectations, and attitudes. Other established pain intervention researchers also similarly support the potential benefits of CBT for reduction in pain-associated symptomatology. Answer C is the best choice because it is the only answer that incorporates improvements across the related areas.

FURTHER READING

Cianfrini LR, Block C, Doleys DM. Psychological therapies. In: Deer TR, Leong MS, Buvanendran A, et al. (Eds.), *Comprehensive Treatment of Chronic Pain by Medical, Interventional, and Integrative Approaches*. New York, NY: Springer; 2013:827–844.

Turk DC, Swanson KS, Tunks ER. Psychological approaches in the treatment of chronic pain patients—When pills, scalpels, and needles are not enough. *Can J Psychiatry*. 2008;53:213–223.

6. ANSWER: A

It is common for patients to experience existential issues when terminally ill or undergoing significant life changes. In an integrated approach to patient care, the provision of empathy, emotional comfort, and understanding has been shown to improve the doctor–patient relationship, increase adherence, and promote improvement in communication. For many patients, religious or spiritual needs can require being addressed during the provision of medical care. Although a clinician may not have specific training in religious practices, there are opportunities and strategies available that can help address these patient needs. A clinician should avoid imposing prayer or religious beliefs on the patient and only pray with the permission or at the request of the patient. The clinician should also be mindful of not compromising his or her own beliefs and not engage in religious practices that would do so. The clinician may, if comfortable and requested, lead a prayer or offer to stand silently while the patient prays. Clinicians can also take a "spiritual history," as discussed by Puchalski and Romer, by exploring "FICA." FICA is an acronym for exploring the patient's *faith* and beliefs, *importance* of those in the patient's life, the patient's spiritual *community*, and how the patient would desire those to be *addressed* in his or her care. The clinician can then, as comfortable, support the patient in meeting these needs as part of an integrative care approach. After exploring the FICA content areas, it is also appropriate to connect the patient with an appropriate spiritual mentor, such as a priest, minister, rabbi, or cleric.

FURTHER READING

Marchand LR. End-of-life care. In: Rakel D (Ed.), *Integrative Medicine*. 3rd ed. Philadelphia, PA: Saunders; 2012:732–743.
Puchalski C, Romer AL. Taking a spiritual history allows clinicians to understand patients more fully. *J Palliat Med*. 2003;3(1):129–137.

7. ANSWER: C

Data from the National Survey on Drug Use and Health (NSDUH) by the Substance Abuse and Mental Health Services Administration's Center for Behavioral Health Statistics and Quality indicate that in 2013, more than 4.5 million individuals were illicitly utilizing pain medications. Given that level of use, the chances of a patient presenting with a *Diagnostic and Statistical Manual of Mental Disorders*, fifth edition (DSM-5), diagnosable opioid use disorder are concerning. Patients who abuse substances can be creative and use various strategies in the attempt to demonstrate they are not misusing their medications, although not all aberrant drug-taking behaviors are associated with medication abuse/addiction. Proper diagnosis is a necessity in order to make proper treatment recommendations because a patient might just need psychomedical education on medication usage to overcome fears of addiction or might have significant dependency issues that need to be addressed via an inpatient substance treatment facility.

According to DSM-5 criteria, an opioid use disorder requires a patient to meet 2 of 11 diagnostic criteria occurring within a 12-month time frame. These criteria involving opioids include the following:

1. The use of larger amounts or taken over longer period of time than intended
2. Persistent or unsuccessful desire to reduce or control use
3. Significant effort/time spent obtaining, using, or recovering from opioids
4. A strong craving or desire to use
5. Failure to fulfill work, academic, or home obligations
6. Continued use despite social or interpersonal problems
7. Giving up or reducing social, occupational, or recreational activities
8. Recurrent use in physically hazardous situations
9. Continued use despite persistent or recurrent physical or psychological problems
10. Tolerance
11. Withdrawal

Note that patients who exhibit tolerance or withdrawal within prescribed and appropriate usage do not meet these criteria. Answer C, breakthrough pain, might be an important consideration in treatment but is not part of the diagnostic criteria, so it is the best answer.

FURTHER READING

American Psychiatric Association. *Diagnostic and Statistical Manual of Mental Disorders*. 5th ed. Arlington, VA: American Psychiatric Publishing; 2013.
Substance Abuse and Mental Health Services Administration, National Survey on Drug Use and Health. The NSDUH report. http://www.samhsa.gov/data/sites/default/files/NSDUH-SR200-RecoveryMonth-2014/NSDUH-SR200-RecoveryMonth-2014.htm. Accessed September 1, 2015.

8. ANSWER: A

Having a baseline score for measuring pain intensity can be invaluable in determining what effective biopsychosocial treatment intervention to utilize for pain management. Numerous measures for pain assessment measure various areas, such as intensity, quality, beliefs, acceptance, expectations, and psychosocial impact. The most commonly used measures for pain intensity are the numeric rating scale (NRS), verbal rating scale (VRS), and visual analogue scale (VAS). NRS and VAS typically utilize either a written or a verbal rating of pain on a ruler-type scale of 0–10 or 0–20, with 0 indicating no pain and 10 or 20 indicating the most severe or extreme pain possible. Some versions include numeric gradients, descriptive wording, or faces. The Wong–Baker FACES pain scale is a version of the VAS that includes faces and has been found to be highly useful with children and individuals who are nonverbal or non-English speaking. VRS utilizes verbal descriptors, which the patient verbally rates pain intensity on a Likert scale, including "none," "mild pain," "moderate pain," "severe pain," "very severe pain," and "worst possible pain."

Two other more commonly used pain assessment tools are the McGill Pain Questionnaire (MPQ) and the West Haven–Yale Multidimensional Pain Inventory (WHYMPI). The MPQ provides patients the ability to describe their quality of pain, as well as a measure of their pain intensity. Patients select words from various groups that have assigned numeric ratings, which are then scored with a minimum of 0 or no pain and a maximum of 78 being the highest possible pain. The MPQ also provides information regarding the location and exacerbating or ameliorating factors. The WHYMPI is a more complex 52-item measure that assesses multiple pain and physical domains with a 12-scale inventory that is divided into three parts. Part A, along with intensity, measures dimensions of the chronic pain experience. Part B assesses perceptions of responses of others to the patient's pain behaviors and complaints. Part C evaluates engagement in common everyday activities. The correct answer, the Pain Catastrophizing Scale, is a 13-item measure that assesses catastrophic thinking in relation to pain, which can impact severity and chronicity, but does not directly provide a measure of pain intensity.

FURTHER READING

Brunelli C, Zecca E, Martini C, et al. Comparison of numerical and verbal rating scales to measure pain exacerbations in patients with chronic cancer pain. *Health Qual Life Outcomes*. 2010;8:42.

Ferreira-Valenta MA, Pais-Ribeiro JL, Jensen MP. Validity of four pain intensity rating scales. *Pain*. 2011;152(10):2399–2404.

McGill Pain Questionnaire. Available at http://www.cebp.nl/vault_public/filesystem/?ID=1400. Accessed June 30, 2015.

Melzack R. The McGill Pain Questionnaire: Major properties and scoring methods. *Pain*. 1975;1:277–299.

Seng E, Kerns RD, Heapy A. Psychological and behavioral assessment. In: Gatchel H, Rathmell J, Wu CL, et al. (Eds.), *Practical Management of Pain*. 5th ed. Philadelphia, PA: Saunders; 2013:243–256.

West Haven–Yale Multidimensional Pain Inventory (WHYMPI/MPI). Available at http://www.va.gov/PAINMANAGEMENT/WHYMPI_MPI.asp. Accessed July 12, 2012.

9. ANSWER: D

Although in the DSM-5, malingering is not listed as a "mental disorder" but, rather, as "other conditions that may be a focus of clinical attention." The essential feature for malingering in the DSM-5 is intentional production of false or exaggerated symptomatology that is motivated by external gain or incentive. Patients rarely directly disclose external gains. Thus, careful consideration should be given to patients who have legal or criminal issues that relate to their current medical presentation, reported symptoms that are highly inconsistent with objective findings, antisocial personality disorder, and/or a high level of guardedness/lack of cooperation during evaluation and in adhering to prescribed treatment regimens. Toxicology results are also very useful in determining patient use or even non-use of medication and should be considered a standard of practice. In this case, the patient's negative toxicology report suggests he is non-adherent to his prescribed medication regimen, and given his prior arrest history for narcotics distribution and resulting financial gains, concerns are evident for both malingering and diversion. When considering pharmacological interventions for this patient, the associated street value of the prescribed medication should be considered to reduce the risk of diversion. Malingering differs from the psychiatric diagnosis of factitious disorder, in which the absence of external incentives/rewards must be present. It also differs from conversion and somatic disorders, whereby the patient is not intentionally feigning the symptoms. Note that although most would agree that some patients may feign symptoms for external gain, there are disagreements over methods of detection of feigned symptomatology and poor criteria for what it means to feign. However, external gain or even feigning symptoms does not preclude the patient experiencing pain or having a legitimate medical condition. Given such challenges, progress has been limited in objective detection of feigned physical or somatic symptoms.

FURTHER READING

American Psychiatric Association. *Diagnostic and Statistical Manual of Mental Disorders*. 5th ed. Arlington, VA: American Psychiatric Publishing; 2013.

Berry DTR, Nelson NW. DSM-5 and malingering: A modest proposal. *Psychol Inj Law*. 2010;3(4):295–303.

10. ANSWER: C

The MMPI-2, a 567-item, true–false questionnaire, and the MMPI-2-RF, a 338-item, true–false questionnaire, access personality traits and psychopathology. They have broad research support for people aged 18–80 years old with at least a fifth-grade reading level. They also have significant empirical support with norms specifically developed for chronic pain and spine surgery/spinal cord stimulator candidates (MMPI-2-RF). The MMPI-2 assesses numerous psychopathologies, including depression, anxiety, psychosis, mania, and somatic symptoms, as well as maladaptive personality patterns and treatment indicators. In addition, the MMPI-2 provides seven scales that assess validity, with three—the L, F, and K scales—being most relevant to the question asked. The L scale detects attempts to present in an overly favorable manner while denying the most common shortcomings. The F scale detects attempts at "faking good or bad" and is able to detect those who exhibit pathologies at a level beyond what would be expected even by severe psychiatric inpatients. The K scale measures defensiveness, which detects more subtle attempts to present in the best possible manner. All three scales, when used together, are beneficial in the assessment of patients who may be reporting a level of current symptoms that is inconsistent. The Beck Inventories and Patient Health Questionnaire Screeners are brief and optimal for rapid or repeat assessment of depression, anxiety, and somatic issues, but controversial factorial (construct) validity exists. These measures are highly "face valid," meaning that the content of the questions is obviously related to what is being assessed; thus, someone can easily under- or overreport symptomatology. A structured clinical interview can provide consistency across evaluations and allow for gathering patient-specific information, but it lacks the objective norms and validity indicators of more lengthy assessments.

FURTHER READING

Patient Health Questionnaire (PHQ) Screeners. Available at http://www.phqscreeners.com. Accessed May 12, 2015.
Richter P, Werner J, Heerlein A, et al. On the validity of the Beck Depression Inventory: A review. *Psychopathology*. 1998; 31(3):160–168.
Seng E, Kerns RD, Heapy A. Psychological and behavioral assessment. In: Benzon H, Rathmell J, Wu CL, et al. (Eds.), *Practical Management of Pain*. 5th ed. Philadelphia, PA: Mosby; 2014:243–256.

11. ANSWER: D

Multidisciplinary or interdisciplinary approaches to pain rehabilitation are based on the biopsychosocial model of health care. The biopsychosocial model for chronic pain suggests that the experience of pain is based on sensory phenomena, which are then influenced by behavioral, emotional, social, and environmental factors. Interventions are goal-directed with a focus on functional restoration, specifically improvements in both physical and psychosocial functioning. Emphasis is on specific activities, such as improvements in range of motion, pain management, activities of daily living, depressive and anxious symptomatology, social functioning, familial dynamics, resumption in pleasurable activities, and vocational-related function. The treatment team primarily consists of physicians, psychologists, physical and occupational therapists, and vocational specialists.

Although CBT is the primary psychological treatment modality, group therapy, movement (yoga, tai chi, and qigong), and mindfulness-based interventions are also indicated. Groups can focus on restructuring shared maladaptive cognitions or behaviors and/or provide psychoeducational support that encourages self-regulation, return of functioning, and relapse prevention.

Integrated multidisciplinary or interdisciplinary functional restoration programs have been found to be effective and are administered in the outpatient setting and time-limited in nature. Patients generally attend these programs 6–8 hours daily for 3 weeks. Many patients prescribed interdisciplinary approaches for pain management have received individual services from a variety of providers, with limited or incomplete relief in pain symptomatology.

FURTHER READING

Artner J, Kurz S, Cakir B, et al. Intensive interdisciplinary outpatient pain management program for chronic back pain: A pilot study. *J Pain Res*. 2012;5:209–216.
Hazard RG, Fenwick JW, Kalisch SM, et al. Functional restoration with behavioral support: A one-year prospective study of patients with chronic low-back pain. *Spine (Phila Pa 1976)*. 1989;14(2):157–161.
Townsend CO, Rome JD, Bruce BK, et al. Interdisciplinary pain rehabilitation programs. In: Ebert M, Kerns R (Eds.), *Behavioral and Psychopharmacologic Pain Management*. Cambridge, UK: Cambridge University Press; 2011:114–128.

12. ANSWER: A

Nelson et al. described patient selection for SCS implantation as a somewhat imprecise enterprise; however, there is evidence indicating a statistically significant link between psychosocial factors and poorer surgical outcomes. Psychological assessment has also repeatedly been shown to be successful in identifying these psychosocial factors. An analysis of 753 studies by Celestin et al. examined the relationship between presurgical predictor variables and treatment outcomes. Of those, only 25 studies and 4 SCS studies were identified that met their seven inclusion criteria. In 92% of the studies reviewed, a positive relationship was found between psychological factors and poor treatment outcomes. The psychosocial factors of presurgical somatization, depression, anxiety, and poor coping were found to have the greatest predictive validity of poorer outcomes for lumbar surgery and SCS. Some studies also found older age and longer pain duration to be predictive of poorer outcomes. The variables that were minimally predictive of poorer outcomes were pretreatment physical findings, activity interference, and presurgical pain intensity.

FURTHER READING

Celestin J, Edwards RR, Jamison RN. Pretreatment psychosocial variables as predictors of outcomes following lumbar surgery and spinal cord stimulation: A systematic review and literature synthesis. *Pain Med.* 2009;10(4);639–653.

Nelson DV, Kennington M, Novy DM, et al. Psychological selection criteria for implantable spinal cord stimulators. *Pain Forum.* 1996;5(2);93–103.

13. ANSWER: D

CRPS is a complex, disabling condition that consists of sensory, motor, and autonomic manifestations, including pain, allodynia, hyperalgesia, and potential loss of function. Treatment from an interdisciplinary team perspective is recommended because CRPS involves not only physiological issues with pain and muscle atrophy but also psychological issues such as disturbances in body perception, depression, and learned helplessness. Graded motor imagery (GMI) is a recommended treatment for CRPS that involves the patient placing the affected limb behind a mirror while purposely moving the contralateral body part. The patient attends to the reflection of the contralateral limb in the mirror, which provides visual feedback to aid the brain in configuration of a new body map. GMI treatment targets cortical areas of the brain and has been shown to reduce pain, perceptual disturbance, and limb guarding behaviors. The other treatments—guided imagery, systematic desensitization, and biofeedback—have potential to reduce psychological symptomatology (anxiety and depression) associated with CRPS, may aid in relaxation, and reduce limb guarding behaviors but do not use contralateral body parts in remapping of the brain.

FURTHER READING

Cossins L, Okel RW, Cameron H, et al. Treatment of complex regional pain syndrome in adults: A systematic review of randomized controlled trials published from June 2000 to February 2012. *Eur J Pain.* 2013;17:158–173.

Turk, DC. Psychological interventions. In: Benzon H, Rathmell J, Wu CL, et al. (Eds.), *Practical Management of Pain.* 5th ed. Philadelphia, PA: Mosby; 2014:615–628.

14. ANSWER: B

The experience of pain involves the conscious and sometimes unconscious experience of a noxious stimulus involving sensory, emotional, and cognitive processes of the brain. Nociception and the experience of pain are two different concepts. Nociception involves the ability to feel pain, caused by stimulation of a nociceptor, and occurs when a signal produced by a noxious stimulus is transmitted to the brain via the nervous system. The experience of pain involves a psychogenic component, which is cognitive–evaluative in nature, as well as sensory and emotional process components.

Modern, more integrative theories define pain as a reciprocal interaction between biological, psychological, and social variables that shape both the experience of and the response to pain. One's experience of pain can be triggered by cognitive learning processes or by actual or threatened noxious nerve stimulation or tissue damage. Central sensitization is an example of a non-associative learning process, in which repeat exposures to stimuli produce amplification of nerve cell responses. This type of learned response can be adaptive in that repeated exposure to minor stimulation can result in prevention. However, the perception of pain is also influenced by how one interprets sensations and injury. Individuals who attribute maladaptive or greater meaning to a painful stimulus tend to perceive pain with greater intensity. This interpretation can lead to guarding or avoidant behaviors and ultimately inactivity and physical deconditioning. Conditioning and psychosocial factors also either intensify or reduce persistence of pain-related behaviors, perception of pain intensity, and functional impairments. In addition, individuals with psychiatric conditions or who have a more pessimistic outlook tend to have greater pain sensitivity.

FURTHER READING

Otis JD, Pincus DB. Chronic pain. In: Boyer BA, Paharia MI (Eds.), *Comprehensive Handbook of Clinical Health Psychology.* Hoboken, NJ: Wiley; 2008:349–370.

Sperry L. Chronic pain. In: Sperry L (Ed.), *Treatment of Chronic Medical Conditions: Cognitive–Behavioral Therapy Strategies and Integrative Treatment Protocols.* Washington, DC: American Psychological Association; 2009:153–171.

15. ANSWER: D

According to Beck, cognitive distortions are individual thought processes that negatively skew the way in which one views the world, others, and oneself. These inaccurate thoughts are usually used to reinforce negative thinking or emotions; interfere with the patient's functioning; and are often based on biased, incomplete, or misinterpreted information. Common distortions often utilized by pain patients include overgeneralization, catastrophizing, jumping to conclusions (mind-reading/fortune-telling error), mental filter, and dichotomous thinking (all-or-nothing/black-and-white thinking). Overgeneralization is viewing a single negative event as a never-ending pattern of defeat. Catastrophization involves thinking the absolute worst about a situation or treatment outcome with exaggeration, rumination, and feelings of helplessness in regard to the symptoms. Jumping to conclusions (mind-reading/fortune-telling error) occurs when one makes a negative interpretation even though there are no definite facts that convincingly support one's conclusions. For example, you conclude that someone is reacting negatively to you, and you do not bother to check this out or you anticipate that things will turn out badly. You are convinced that your prediction is an already established fact. Mental filter involves picking out a single negative detail and dwelling on it exclusively. Of the possible choices, answer D is the best option because the patient is engaging in dichotomous thinking. She is viewing the outcome as either eliminating her pain presentation entirely or thinks she will get no pain relief.

FURTHER READING

Beck J. *Cognitive Behavior Therapy: Basics and Beyond.* 2nd ed. New York, NY: Guilford; 2011.
Benzon H, Turk DC. Psychological interventions. In: Benzon H, Rathmell J, Wu CL, et al. (Eds.), *Practical Management of Pain.* 5th ed. Philadelphia, PA: Mosby; 2014:615–628.
Burns DD. *Feeling Good.* New York, NY: Morrow, 1980.
Cianfrini LR, Block C, Doleys DM. Psychological therapies. In: Deer TR, Leong MS, Buvanendran A, et al. (Eds.), *Comprehensive Treatment of Chronic Pain by Medical, Interventional, and Integrative Approaches.* New York, NY: Springer; 2013:827–844.

16. ANSWER: B

Pain catastrophizing involves rumination about pain, the magnitude of threat of pain, and perceived inability to cope with pain and the resulting presentation. Pain catastrophizing has been consistently found to be associated with greater physical and psychosocial dysfunction, even after controlling for pain and depression levels. Fear avoidance has also been shown to be important in pain and physical and psychosocial function. Interventions often utilized for pain include cognitive restructuring, relaxation training, goal setting using a hierarchal structure, behavioral activation, activity pacing, and working to problem-solve barriers. Ehde et al. state, "The goals of CBT for pain are to reduce pain and psychological distress and to improve physical and role function by helping individuals decrease maladaptive beaviors, increase adaptive behaviors, identify and correct maladaptive thoughts and beliefs, and increase self-efficacy for pain management."

FURTHER READING

Edwards RR, Cahalan C, Mensing G, et al. Pain, catastrophizing, and depression in the rheumatic diseases. *Nature Rev Rheumatol.* 2011;7(4):216–224.

Ehde DM, Dillworth TM, Turner JA. Cognitive–behavioral therapy for individuals with chronic pain: Efficacy, innovations, and directions for research. *Am Psychol.* 2014;69(2):153–166.
Gatchel RJ, Peng YB, Peters ML, et al. The biopsychosocial approach to chronic pain: Scientific advances and future directions. *Psychol Bull.* 2007;133(4):581–624.

17. ANSWER: A

Meta-analytic studies have consistently found a relationship between chronic pain and childhood trauma when comparing those endorsing abuse with those not reporting childhood abuse or neglect. Depending on the type of childhood abuse considered (physical, sexual, or verbal), approximately 48% of chronic pain patients reported some type of abuse as a child. Multiple psychological traumas during childhood have been show to predispose individuals to chronic lower back pain. In studies specific to chronic back pain patients, those with minimal structural pathology were found to have three or more traumatic childhood psychological risk factors. Although there is a positive correlation between childhood abuse and reports of chronic pain, studies do not suggest that chronic pain patients are feigning their medical symptomatology/pain presentation. Research on childhood trauma and hypochondriasis found that only 32.1% of hypochondriacal patients reported a history of physical abuse, with the percentage reporting other types of childhood abuse being much lower. Given the significant difference between percentages of those reporting abuse and those found to be experiencing hypochondriasis, it is statistically likely that patients reporting chronic pain have experienced changes to underlying nervous system functioning and/or a component of central sensitization.

FURTHER READING

Barsky AJ, Wool C, Barnett MC, et al. Histories of childhood trauma in adult hypochondriacal patients. *Am J Psychiatry.* 1994;151:397–401.
Davis DA, Luecken LJ, Zautra AJ. Are reports of childhood abuse related to the experience of chronic pain in adulthood? A meta-analytic review of the literature. *Clin J Pain.* 2005;21(5):398–405.
Goldberg RT, Pachasoe WN, Keith D. Relationship between traumatic events in childhood and chronic pain. *Disabil Rehabil.* 1999;21(1):23–30.
Schofferman J, Anderson D, Mines R, et al. Childhood psychological trauma and chronic refractory low-back pain. *Clin J Pain.* 1993;9(4):227–310.

18. ANSWER: B

Fibromyalgia is a syndrome characterized by diffuse pain along with fatigue, emotional distress, and other associated features, such as headaches and irritable bowel syndrome.

Patients often believe they are dismissed or viewed from the psychosomatic lens. Therefore, one of the best initial interventions can be empathic listening, affirmation of patient experiences, and an explanation of current research regarding how physiological symptomatology is related to changes within the brain and how it processes sensory information. Beyond this initial interaction, much of the research into finding effective interventions for treating fibromyalgia has shown mixed outcomes. Currently, research suggests that 5–33% of patients may experience symptom improvement, with the overall goal of functional improvement and quality of life, not a cure. Some interventions have also demonstrated unclear, poor, little, or no efficacy, such as the use of NSAIDs and surgical interventions. Some studies have found omega-3 fatty acids, vitamin D, and anti-inflammatory diets beneficial, but little benefit from many other nutritional supplements has been found. Studies have also found benefits from aerobic exercise tailored to a patient's physical abilities, such as starting a patient with aqua therapy, tai chi, yoga, or stretching and progressing as the patient gains strength and mobility. However, starting with more vigorous exercise will result in many patients experiencing a significant increase in pain, which usually leads to resistance to and avoidance of physical activity. Medications have had mixed benefit: Antidepressants have been found to be beneficial for improvements in sleep and mood, and anticonvulsants (e.g., gabapentin and pregabalin) have been found to be beneficial for chronic and neuropathic pain, but significant controversy exists with regard to opioid use due to negative effects (e.g., constipation, addiction, and sedation). Psychotherapy and mind–body therapies, such as CBT, ACT, and mindfulness practices, have also been found to be beneficial.

FURTHER READING

Adams MCB, Clauw, D. Chronic widespread pain. In: Benzon H, Rathmell J, Wu CL, et al. (Eds.), *Practical Management of Pain*. 5th ed. Philadelphia, PA: Mosby; 2014:392–407.

Selfridge NJ, Muller D. Fibromyalgia. In: Rakel D (Ed.), *Integrative Medicine*. 3rd ed. Philadelphia, PA: Saunders; 2012:438–446.

19. ANSWER: A

The most up-to-date reporting outcomes on presurgical psychological evaluations recognize the incorporation of technology (SCSs and bariatric) within a multidisciplinary comprehensive evaluation and treatment process. Presurgical interventional pain interventions commonly include multiple assessment strategies, which consist of a clinical interview, standardized questionnaires, behavioral observations, formal mental status exam, psychophysiological pain assessments, objective psychological tests, and family member assessments. A clinical interview provides not only an opportunity to gather detailed subjective pain information but also the unique opportunity to interact and collect information that may be relevant but not asked in questionnaires, develop rapport with the patient, and obtain the patient's subjective view of his or her pain experiences and expectation for post-surgical outcomes. Objective assessment strategies, such as questionnaires, psychological tests, and various pain assessments, provide information as well as objective norm-referenced evaluation of factors that can assist in determining if the patient, in comparison to others, has a particular psychiatric condition, certain positive/negative treatment indications/factors, and/or is potentially over- or underreporting symptomatology. These measures can also assist in gathering large amounts of information through the use of hundreds of individual questions. Formal mental status examinations provide the ability to screen the patient's neurocognitive functioning, which can be useful in the determination of the patient's cognitive competency and ability to participate in a sufficiently informed manner. They can also be useful is evaluating the potential neurocognitive impact of pain medication or related medical conditions.

FURTHER READING

Doleys DM. Preparing patients for implantable technologies. In: Turk DC, Gatchel, RJ (Eds.), *Psychological Approaches to Pain Management: A Practitioner's Handbook*. 2nd ed. New York, NY: Guilford; 2002:334–348.

Nelson DV, Kennington M, Novy DM, et al. Psychological selection criteria for implantable spinal cord stimulators. *Pain Forum*. 1996;5(2);93–103.

Seng E, Kerns RD, Heapy A. Psychological and behavioral assessment. In: Benzon H, Rathmell J, Wu CL, et al. (Eds.), *Practical Management of Pain*. 5th ed. Philadelphia, PA: Mosby; 2014:243–256.

20. ANSWER: B

The peripheral nervous system is responsible for transmission of communications between the limbs and organs in the body to the central nervous system (brain and spinal cord). Peripheral neuropathy interferes with this communication and leads to sensory difficulties that cause pain, numbness, and/or motor difficulties, which can then result in challenges with movement and muscle control. Peripheral neuropathy commonly occurs in individuals with diabetes, alcoholism, patients who have undergone treatment with certain medications (e.g., chemotherapy agents), or patients who have been exposed to certain toxins.

Biofeedback is an intervention conducted by a psychologist or other trained medical professional that utilizes electronic equipment to help identify, monitor, and consciously manage physiological responses. Biofeedback helps individuals learn to control bodily functioning that is usually controlled by the autonomic nervous system. These functions include heart rate, blood pressure, oxygen saturation, temperature of/blood flow to the extremities, and muscle activity. Once these techniques are learned in the medical setting, they are then performed at home, usually without the use of electronic equipment. Biofeedback is also utilized to learn relaxation techniques for stress reduction and for the management of chronic pain, including headaches and chronic orofacial pain. In the treatment of peripheral neuropathy, biofeedback has been shown to directly reduce HbA1c and increase blood flow to the extremities. These changes lead to reductions in neuropathic pain and stress levels, as well as improvements in quality of life and psychological health.

FURTHER READING

Ehde DM, Dillworth TM, Turner JA. Cognitive–behavioral therapy for individuals with chronic pain: Efficacy, innovations, and directions for research. *Am Psychol.* 2014;69(2):153–166.

Haythornthwaite JA, Benrud-Larson LM. Psychological aspects of neuropathic pain. *Clin J Pain.* 2000;16(2):101–105.

Nahas R. Type 2 diabetes. In: Rakel D (Ed.), *Integrative Medicine.* 3rd ed. Philadelphia, PA: Saunders; 2012:297–311.

Sunil TP. Peripheral neuropathy. In: Rakel D (Ed.), *Integrative Medicine.* 3rd ed. Philadelphia, PA: Saunders; 2012:102–113.

21. ANSWER: D

Peripheral nerve injuries to the face typically involve stretching, inflammation, or compression of the trigeminal nerve. This condition is termed trigeminal neuralgia (TN) and is associated with extreme pain that can last minutes to hours and recur multiple times during the day. The pain may be associated with many areas of the face and can occur spontaneously or from stimulation involving touch, cold, or even wind.

CBT with a focus on sensory retraining (or sensory re-education) is a technique that can improve the patient's ability to interpret the altered sensory response from injured sensory nerves and also improve the patient's perception of function. Repetitive neural input (gentle touching or brushing with a makeup brush) from sensory retraining exercises also leads to changes in the somatosensory cortex. This neural reorganization through sensory retraining can, with varying levels of success, help compensate for impairments associated with nerve injury. Sensory retraining also helps the patient's perception of unpleasant orofacial sensations and strengthens weakened and damaged signal pathways.

Research on sensory retraining suggests that it is an inexpensive and noninvasive procedure that, if initiated soon after injury or surgery, can improve altered orofacial sensations. In a comparison of patients who have or have not received sensory retraining, those who received sensory retraining showed a much more rapid rate of recovery. These interventions have also been found to be highly effective at decreasing psychosocial challenges associated with altered hypoesthetic facial sensations. In addition, patients not receiving treatment for typical TN may see a transformation over time to an atypical TN presentation, with a change in the character of the pain to more constant and background pain with the development of sensory impairment. Therefore, early intervention to give the opportunity of pain relief without sensory deficits is recommended.

FURTHER READING

Dellon AL. Re-education of sensation. In: Dellon AL (Ed.), *Evaluation of Sensibility and Re-education of Sensation in the Hand.* Baltimore, MD: Lucas; 1988:203–246.

Phillips C, Blakey G, Essick GK. Sensory retraining: A cognitive behavioral therapy for altered sensation. *Atlas Oral Maxillofac Surg North Am.* 2011;19(1):109–118.

22. ANSWER: C

The relationship between the physician and the patient can be a significant social–environmental protective and/or risk factor. Protective factors reduce the probability of risk or harm, whereas risk factors increase the probability of risk or harm. When a physician is viewed as empathic and competent, as well as exhibits patience in asking open-ended questions, the patient is more likely to disclose issues with poor medication and treatment adherence. Improvements in flow of information can lead to disclosure of challenges in following prescribed treatment plans or even support the discussion of how prior traumatic events, family issues, and work challenges are impacting the patient's recovery. In contrast, a poor physician–patient relationship can result and lead to the patient withholding information, increase the risk of nonadherence, and delay recovery. Issues such as a history of a trauma/abuse or secondary gains from disability can significantly delay recovery, thus the importance of a supportive physician–patient relationship.

FURTHER READING

Cianfrini LR, Block C, Doleys DM. Psychological therapies. In: Deer TR, Leong MS, Buvanendran A, et al. (Eds.), *Comprehensive Treatment of Chronic Pain by Medical, Interventional, and Integrative Approaches.* New York, NY: Springer; 2013:827–844.

23. ANSWER: C

The psychogenic view of pain has existed since the development of psychodynamic theory; however, it was not more formally described until the 1960s. When physical explanations seem inadequate or disproportional to the painful stimuli or when treatment results are inconsistent and/or associated with psychological stressors, pain is attributed to psychological causes. This view suggests that chronic pain is based on psychopathological tendencies that are innate and maintain a patient's pain and will be resolved once the psychogenic mechanisms are resolved. The layperson's view is that the person's pain is "all in their head." Empirical support for this viewpoint is limited, and many people with chronic pain do not exhibit psychopathology. However, cases of secondary gain and malingering or substance abuse/addiction do exist and can be used to promote this viewpoint. In the past, the American Psychiatric Association has supported this view with the creation of a psychiatric disorder, somatoform pain disorder, but it has made some movement away from the psychogenic view of pain in the DSM-5), although it still maintains the diagnosis of somatic symptom disorder, with predominant pain.

FURTHER READING

American Psychiatric Association. *Diagnostic and Statistical Manual of Mental Disorders*. 4th ed. Washington, DC: American Psychiatric Association; 1994.

American Psychiatric Association. *Diagnostic and Statistical Manual of Mental Disorders*. 5th ed. Arlington, VA: American Psychiatric Publishing; 2013.

Turk, DC. Psychological interventions. In: Benzon H, Rathmell J, Wu CL, et al. (Eds.), *Practical Management of Pain*. 5th ed. Philadelphia, PA: Mosby; 2014:615–628.

Turk, DC. Psychosocial aspects of chronic pain. In: Benzon H, Rathmell J, Wu CL, et al. (Eds.), *Practical Management of Pain*. 5th ed. Philadelphia, PA: Mosby; 2014:139–148.

24. ANSWER: C

Group therapy has emerged as one of the major forms of psychological treatment for chronic pain. It has been shown to be effective at increasing social support and improving coping skills, acceptance, treatment maintenance/adherence, and overall psychiatric well-being. However, prior to referral/placement into group therapy, screening must occur to ensure that the patient is an appropriate fit for the group being offered. This screening can be conducted by the pain physician, but it is often completed by the clinician who is facilitating the group. Two highly important categories that should be examined for goodness of fit when referring patients to pain management groups are symptom/group match and behavioral, cognitive, and emotional variables.

A patient's symptoms or needs should match the type of group offered. Groups usually have a focus with specific goals, such as grief and loss, addiction, depression, general support, or adaptation to lifestyle changes, although some groups may be more process oriented and promote open discussion of thoughts and feelings. For a patient struggling to make acceptance-based lifestyle changes (pacing, etc.), being referred to an addictions group would likely result in poor attendance and dropout. For someone highly uncomfortable with lack of structure or sharing deep emotions, an open process group might be a poor fit.

A patient's behavioral, cognitive, and emotional variables should also be examined for goodness of fit. To benefit from group therapy, a patient must be motivated and willing to attend and participate in regular group meetings. Group therapy is indicated for those with deconditioning/inactivity, dependence on others, negative self-talk/criticism, and mild or moderate anxiety or depression. Group therapy is not indicated for those who are significantly angry and hostile, especially toward medical professionals, because they can monopolize time and use the group as an audience to vocalize their complaints. These individuals can also be a challenge to redirect and fail to respond to the group leader or member feedback. Patients with severe depression, anxiety, bipolar, or other psychiatric conditions may struggle to participate and have a higher potential to verbally monopolize group time.

FURTHER READING

Ehde DM, Dillworth TM, Turner JA. Cognitive–behavioral therapy for individuals with chronic pain: Efficacy, innovations, and directions for research. *Am Psychol*. 2014;69(2):153–166.

Keefe FJ, Beaupre PM, Gil KM, et al. Group therapy for patients with chronic pain. In: Turk DC, Gatchel, RJ (Eds.), *Psychological Approaches to Pain Management: A Practitioner's Handbook*. 2nd ed. New York, NY: Guilford; 2002:234–255.

25. ANSWER: A

The transtheoretical model of behavioral change, a method of assessing a patient's readiness to change, involves five stages: precontemplation, contemplation, preparation, action, and maintenance. The precontemplation stage involves individuals who are not intending to take action in the near future and may even be unaware or unwilling to accept that their behavior is problematic. During this stage, change can be best promoted by highlighting the patient's strengths, asking permission to discuss change, brief discussions of advantages and disadvantages of change (not the medication), and providing personalized information. The contemplation stage involves individuals who are beginning to recognize a behavior is problematic and who begin to evaluate the advantages and disadvantages of their continued actions. Promoting change at this stage involves helping the patient increase the advantages of changing and decrease the disadvantages, as well as exploration of fears and/or concerns. The preparation stage involves individuals who intend to take action in the immediate future and may begin to make small behavioral changes. Promoting change at this stage involves providing further education/information, discussions regarding support groups, highlighting strengths that will enable minor changes, and addressing any ambivalence that may arise. In the action stage, individuals are making specific overt modifications toward modifying their problematic behaviors and/or are engaging in new and healthier behaviors. To promote continued change while in this stage, it is important to encourage the patient's commitment, teach strategies supportive of change, connect the patient to someone who has been successful in the area the patient is currently pursuing for increased support, and review current medical recommendations/medications. Further discussion of support groups might also be warranted. The maintenance stage involves those who have sustained action for a period of 6 months or longer and are working to prevent relapse. In this stage, the clinician should review and support gains, inoculate against disappointment by discussing how people sometimes slip but recover, and promote the patient helping others enact change.

For patients who do not see a need to change, coercive and shock techniques have shown limited efficacy for long-term benefit and can result in the patient becoming more resistant to change. Premature termination of treatment can lead to the patient going elsewhere or even finding illicit means of acquiring treatments (medications or substitutes). Telling a patient that others fail at change prior to the patient beginning the process can encourage hopelessness and/or a reluctance to even consider making changes.

FURTHER READING

Jensen MP. Enhancing motivation to change in pain treatment. In: Turk DC, Gatchel RJ (Eds.), *Psychological Approaches to Pain Management: A Practitioner's Handbook.* 2nd ed. New York, NY: Guilford; 2002:71–93.

Prochaska JO, DiClements CC. Transtheoretical therapy: Toward a more integrative model of change. *Psychother Theory Res Pract.* 1982;19:276–288.

SAMSHA/CSAT Treatment Improvement Protocols (TIP). From precontemplation to contemplation: Building readiness. In: *TIP 35: Enhancing Motivation for Change in Substance Abuse Treatment.* Rockville, MD: Substance Abuse and Mental Health Services Administration; 1999.

26. ANSWER: B

Systematic desensitization is a form of behavioral therapy that is based on principles of classical conditioning. The goal is to utilize counterconditioning to remove a phobic or fear response and substitute a relaxation response to a conditional stimulus. There are three phases to the treatment: First, the patient breaks the event into progressive steps or a stepped hierarchy that invokes fear. Next, the patient is given training in relaxation techniques, such as deep breathing or guided imagery. Finally, the patient uses the relaxation techniques while progressing along the fear hierarchy in order to reduce the paired anxiety or phobic response. The patient can utilize imaginal (imaginary) or in vivo (in the situation) exposure techniques. When the patient feels comfortable at each progression, he or she moves on to the next stage in the hierarchy. Operant conditioning utilizes a system of positive or negative reinforcements and punishments to change behaviors or increase learning. Reinforcement increases a behavior, and punishment decreases a behavior. Positive means adding something pleasurable or unpleasurable, and negative means removing something pleasurable or unpleasurable. The question does not involve rewards or punishments; therefore, it is not a form of operant conditioning. CBT and EMDR are primarily talk therapies and might utilize systematic desensitization techniques, although their primary goals are to address the cognitions involved in the fear process.

FURTHER READING

McGlynn FD. Systematic desensitization. In: Weiner IB, Craighead WE (Eds.), *Corsini Encyclopedia of Psychology.* Hoboken, NJ: Wiley; 2010:1–3.

Turk DC. Psychosocial aspects of chronic pain. In: Benzon H, Rathmell J, Wu CL, et al. (Eds.), *Practical Management of Pain.* 5th ed. Philadelphia, PA: Mosby; 2014:139–148.

27. ANSWER: C

Coping styles can be either helpful or averse to outcomes for chronic pain patients. Of the choices, coping self-statements, task persistence, and medication use can all be strategies an individual might utilize to manage his or her painful experience. Self-actualization is part of Maslow's hierarchy of needs, a motivational needs progression whereby an individual feels fulfilled, having accomplished all of the things he or she is capable of achieving through personal growth and important experiences that are meaningful/emotional. In children and adolescents with chronic pain, distinct coping style differences have been noted. For example, whereas boys used behavioral distraction techniques, girls sought social support more often. Higher average pain intensity correlated negatively with coping efficacy. In girls, internalizing/catastrophizing also led to negative effects on coping efficacy. As opposed to children, adolescents tended to use affirmative coping self-statements.

FURTHER READING

Haythornwaite JA, Wegener ST, Heinberg LJ. Psychological evaluation and testing. In: Benzon H, Raja S, Liu S, et al. (Eds.), *Essentials of Pain Medicine*. 3rd ed. Philadelphia: Saunders; 2011:36.

Lynch AM, Kashikar-Zuck S, Goldschneider KR, et al. Sex and age differences in coping styles among children with chronic pain. *J Pain Symptom Manage*. 2007;33(2):208–216.

28. ANSWER: A

The influence of cultural and racial disparities in pain management has been underestimated. Barriers to effective pain treatment include patient factors such as beliefs and attitudes about pain, genetic differences in expression of transduction molecules such as transient receptor potential V-1, and opioid receptor genetic polymorphisms; health care provider barriers including inadequate pain training, beliefs about minority patients, or inadequate assessment of pain; and health care system barriers including poorer access to care, lack of insurance coverage, and lack of resource availability. Non-Caucasians are more likely to use prayer as a coping strategy, thus making answer A the most appropriate choice. In experimental testing of thermal pain thresholds, African American subjects had a lower threshold for pain than Caucasians, attributable in part to genetic differences.

FURTHER READING

Anderson KO, Green CR, Payne R. Racial and ethical disparities in pain: Causes and consequences of unequal care. *J Pain*. 2009;10(12):1187–1204.

29. ANSWER: D

The IMMPACT recommendations suggested that the following six core domains should be part of all rigorous clinical chronic pain trials: pain; physical functioning; emotional functioning; a patient rating of improvement and satisfaction; symptoms; and participant disposition, such as adherence to the treatment and dropout from the trial. The authors note that these are not intended to be absolute requirements because there may be cases in which one or more domains may not be indicated. However, because chronic pain is a biopsychosocial problem, inclusion of measures from all of these domains should set a standard by which comparison of various works can be accomplished.

FURTHER READING

Turk DC, Dworkin RH, Allen RR, et al. Core outcome domains for chronic pain clinical trials: IMMPACT recommendations. *Pain*. 2003;106:337–345.

30. ANSWER: D

Evaluation of impaired children and adults is difficult because they may be impaired by medication, their critical illness, intubation, or disorientation, or they may be pharmacologically paralyzed. The following is a suggested hierarchy for evaluating the presence of pain as suggested by the American Academy of Pain Medicine Nursing: (1) Attempt to elicit a self-report from the patient or document why self-report cannot be obtained, (2) identify pathologic conditions associated with potential for pain, (3) list patient behaviors indicative of pain (a behavioral assessment tool may be used), (4) identify behaviors that caregivers and others knowledgeable about the patient think may indicate pain, and (5) attempt an analgesic trial. Various behavioral tools have been developed for pediatric patients and nonverbal vulnerable individuals. In the intensive care unit, tools such as the CPOT, FLACC scale, and the PBAT have all been developed. These should be age and condition appropriate. In this case, the patient has multiple possible pain-causing conditions with the various fractures. Assuming she is intubated but not paralyzed by muscle relaxant agents, a behavioral tool may be useful. A faces scale would be expected to be appropriate for preverbal children up to approximately age 6 years, but it might also be affected by critical illness factors such as disorientation and intubation. Vital signs can be misleading, and although they can be factored into the complete picture, they should not be solely relied on.

FURTHER READING

Gelinas C, Johnston C. Pain assessment in the critically ill ventilated adult: Validation of the Critical-Care Pain Observation Tool and physiologic indicators. *Clin J Pain*. 2007;23(6):497–505.

Herr K, Coyne PJ, McCaffrey M, et al. Pain assessment in the patient unable to self-report: Position statement with clinical practice recommendations. Available at http://www.aspmn.org/documents/PainAssessmentinthePatientUnabletoSelfReport.pdf.

Hicks CL, von Baeyer CL, Spafford PA, et al. The Faces Pain Scale–Revised: Toward a common metric in pediatric pain measurement. *Pain*. 2001;83:173–183.

31. ANSWER: D

Measurement of pain in special populations such as children and patients with cognitive impairment or dementia can be difficult. Although scales such as the FLACC or the Faces Pain Scale revised version may work very well in some patients, this is not always the case. Thus, the best way to determine if a population's pain can be reliably measured is to try several methods to identify which scale works best. Although the Faces Pain Scale revised version has been validated in children, for example, there is evidence from one study that in children younger than age 6 years, more than half had problems understanding the scale. Thus, for most trials, the best approach is to ensure a large study population and adequate power (answer D) to overcome unreliability in measuring pain intensity and, in some cases, to add a behavioral measure of pain.

SUGGESTED READING

Hicks CL, von Baeyer CL, Spafford PA, et al. The Faces Pain Scale–Revised: Toward a common metric in pediatric pain measurement. *Pain*. 2001;83:173–183.

Jensen MP. Measurement of pain. In Fishman S, Ballentyne J, Rathmell J (Eds.), *Bonica's Management of Pain*. 4th ed. Philadelphia, PA: Lippincott Williams & Wilkins; 2010.

GENDER DIFFERENCES IN PAIN

Gregory Carpenter and Meenal Patil

INTRODUCTION

Research regarding sex, gender, and pain has proliferated in recent decades. Epidemiologic and clinical findings strongly demonstrate that women are at an increased risk for chronic pain, experience greater pain-related distress, and in experiments show heightened sensitivity for pain compared to men. Research on sex-based differences in the experience of pain and its treatment is beginning to uncover patterns that may allow for more precise tailoring of treatments.

There are differences in analgesic responses to pain and to both opioid and non-opioid medications, as well as for endogenous analgesic processes. Many stress-related disorders, such as fibromyalgia and chronic pain, are more prevalent in women. Studies of experimentally induced pain have produced a very consistent pattern of results, with women exhibiting greater pain sensitivity, enhanced pain facilitation, and reduced pain inhibition compared to men.

Several mechanisms have been implicated in the underlying sex differences, including biological involvement of estrogen and progesterone versus testosterone. Most of the research to support sex hormone effects on pain stems from studies demonstrating exacerbation of clinical pain across the menstrual cycle. Sex-related differences in pain may also reflect differences in the endogenous opioid system.

Other mechanisms include steroid action differences in adulthood; modulation of various biological systems such as the cardiovascular and inflammatory pathways; and sociocultural differences, including disparities in gender roles and gender role expectations. Most studies suggest that additional investigational research is necessary to further elucidate these differences in order to target therapy appropriately.

QUESTIONS

1. Prior to puberty, the gender gap in pain reporting shows:

A. Increased pain severity for girls
B. Decreased pain threshold for girls
C. No differences between boys and girls
D. Increased chronic pain syndromes for girls

2. Which phase of the menstrual cycle is most associated with a higher incidence of pain and a lower pain threshold?

A. Follicular
B. Luteal
C. Perimenstrual
D. All phases of the menstrual cycle appear to be equal

3. Women are more likely than men to have all of the following except:

A. Fibromyalgia
B. Migraines
C. Cluster headaches
D. Irritable bowel syndrome

4. Reference values for the pain threshold in a normal population demonstrate:

A. Decreased pain threshold in women compared to men
B. Increased pain threshold in women compared to men

C. A difference in thresholds between genders that persists with age

D. A difference in thresholds between genders that increases with age

5. In studies of the use of opioid patient-controlled analgesia (PCA) in men and women, women demonstrate:

A. Lower opioid consumption postoperatively

B. Higher opioid consumption postoperatively

C. Lower patient satisfaction with PCA

D. No differences compared to men

6. What are potential biases in the identification and treatment of pain between the sexes?

A. There is an increased likelihood to undertreat pain in women compared to men.

B. In the postoperative setting, women are more likely to receive sedatives than opioids compared to men.

C. Medical providers are more likely to identify pain and prescribe opioids to patients of the same sex.

D. All of the above are correct.

7. Which of the following is true about individuals who self-identify as more masculine, in terms of gender roles and personality traits?

A. More masculinity directly correlates with higher pain threshold.

B. More masculinity inversely correlates with pain threshold.

C. More masculinity does not correlate with pain threshold at all.

D. More masculinity only correlates with higher pain thresholds in men and not in women.

8. In experimental testing of pain thresholds, with all other factors being equal, which individual is most likely to show the highest pain threshold?

A. A female participant with a female examiner

B. A male participant with a male examiner

C. A female participant with a male examiner

D. A male participant with a female examiner

9. Which of the following statements is true regarding sex hormones and their relationship to pain?

A. One-third of patients being treated with anti-androgen therapy will develop chronic pain.

B. Average female estrogen levels are associated with a heightened inflammatory response compared to average male levels.

C. Postmenopausal women taking hormone replacement therapy (HRT) display lower pain thresholds than women not on HRT.

D. All of the above are true.

10. In biopsychosocial models that deal with pain, women are more likely than men to utilize which mechanism?

A. Catastrophizing

B. Denial

C. Behavioral distraction

D. Isolation

11. Low estradiol states are associated with what pattern of pain sensitivity in women?

A. Increased pain sensitivity and decreased endogenous opioid neurotransmission

B. Decreased pain sensitivity and increased endogenous opioid neurotransmission

C. Increased pain sensitivity and increased endogenous opioid neurotransmission

D. Decreased pain sensitivity and decreased endogenous opioid neurotransmission

12. Research has shown that functional magnetic resonance imaging illuminates significant differences in the central nervous system between men and women. Regarding painful stimulation in patients with irritable bowel syndrome, which area(s) is activated in men compared to women?

A. Insula

B. Amygdala

C. Mid-cingulate

D. Left thalamus and ventral striatum

13. When two groups of mice (those in pain/affected vs. unaffected) were studied, which correlation was noted regarding the theory of social interaction modulating pain?

A. Female unaffected mice spent more time with their affected cagemates, which subsequently had lower rates of pain behavior.

B. Male unaffected mice spent more time with their affected cagemates, which subsequently had lower rates of pain behavior.

C. There was no difference in pain behavior when unaffected mice approached affected cagemates.

D. Female unaffected mice spent less time with their affected cagemates, which subsequently had lower rates of pain behavior.

14. **Which of the following mechanisms have been proposed as explanations for sexual differences in pain and analgesia?**

   A. Experiential: Sex difference is due to differential painful experiences either by sex or experiences that can affect pain, such as labor pain.
   B. Genetic: Sex difference is due to sex chromosome effects.
   C. Organizational: Sex difference is due to steroid action of development.
   D. All of the above.

15. **As studies continue to evaluate the pain experience and variables, what factors have been implicated regarding health care provider practices?**

   A. Both male and female physicians prescribed more pain medications for female neck pain patients compared to males in one study.
   B. Both male and female physicians prescribed higher opiates for same-sex low back pain patients in one study.
   C. No gender disparities were found in physician prescription of opioid analgesics in one study.
   D. All of the above.

ANSWERS

1. ANSWER: C

Several studies have shown no or only minor differences in pain reporting in young children (<12 years old). As children age, there is an increasing prevalence of chronic pain issues in girls compared to boys. The most common differences in girls that emerge during puberty include higher prevalence of any pain, more common pain at multiple sites, and more likely to experience recurrent headaches. This evidence suggests that sex hormones play a role in the development of gender differences in pain.

FURTHER READING

Fillingim RB, King CD, Ribeiro-Dasilva MC, et al. Sex, gender, and pain: A review of recent clinical and experimental findings. *J Pain*. 2009;10(5):447–485.

2. ANSWER: B

A number of experimental studies suggest that pain sensitivity varies across the menstrual cycle, with the luteal phase being most sensitive. A meta-analysis of 16 studies found that pain thresholds were higher during the follicular phase (lower levels of estradiol and progesterone), with several experimental studies showing the largest decrease in threshold during the luteal phase. This effect has been shown across multiple pain modalities, including mechanical, thermal, and ischemic, but not for electrical stimuli. This evidence highlights the likely role of sex hormones in the modulation of pain.

FURTHER READING

Bartley EJ, Fillingim RB. Sex differences in pain: A brief review of clinical and experimental findings. *Br J Anaesth*. 2013;111:52–58.
Fillingim RB, King CD, Ribeiro-Dasilva MC, et al. Sex, gender, and pain: A review of recent clinical and experimental findings. *J Pain*. 2009;10(5): 447–485.
Riley JL, Robinson ME, Wise EA, et al. A meta-analytic review of pain perception across the menstrual cycle. *Pain*. 1999;81(3): 225–235.

3. ANSWER: C

Chronic pain, in general, is more likely to occur in women, which translates to the vast majority of chronic pain conditions having a strong female predominance. For conditions that are found in both genders, female-predominate conditions include chronic fatigue syndrome,

fibromyalgia, interstitial cystitis, temporomandibular disorder, headache, migraine, and osteoarthritis (back, neck, and knee). Male-predominate, or male-only, disorders include chronic prostatitis, gout, and cluster headache. There are additional chronic pain disorders that affect only females, such as endometriosis, vulvodynia, and menstrual pain.

FURTHER READING

Mogil JS. Sex differences in pain and pain inhibition: Multiple explanations of a controversial phenomenon. *Nat Rev Neurosci*. 2012;13(12):859–866.

4. ANSWER: A

In an experimental study by Neziri and colleagues to determine reference values for pain thresholds to mechanical and thermal pain, several demographic variables were found to be important. Gender, age, and interaction of gender and age appear to have an influence on an individual's ability to tolerate painful stimuli. Women were found to have lower pain thresholds, which is consistent with results from multiple other studies. There are conflicting data for age, with no clear consensus regarding whether older individuals have increased, decreased, or unchanged pain thresholds. The gender discrepancies between men and women with regard to pain thresholds appear to decrease with age. Interestingly, the postmenopausal state is characterized by low serum concentrations of estrogen and progesterone, which may provide additional evidence correlating pain and sex hormones.

FURTHER READING

Neziri AY, Scaramozzino P, Andersen OK, et al. Reference values of mechanical and thermal pain tests in a pain-free population. *Eur J Pain*. 2011;15(4):376–383.

5. ANSWER: A

A recent meta-analysis of opioid analgesia in men and women postoperatively appeared to show a greater analgesic response to opioids (especially morphine) in women compared to men. This effect was greatest in PCAs, leading to women consuming a statistically significant lesser amount of opioid in both total milligrams and milligrams per kilogram. Although side effects (nausea, pruritus, and sedation) potentially may have driven the decreased amount of opioid usage, there was no difference in reported pain scores between the genders. This seems to support an increased analgesic response to opioids in women.

FURTHER READING

Bartley EJ, Fillingim RB. Sex differences in pain: A brief review of clinical and experimental findings. *Br J Anaesth*. 2013;111:52–58.
Niesters M, Dahan A, Kest B, et al. Do sex differences exist in opioid analgesia? A systematic review and meta-analysis of human experimental and clinical studies. *Pain*. 2010;151:61–68.

6. ANSWER: D

Gender bias in the provision of pain management is a well-documented phenomenon. In multiple studies, women have been shown to be less likely to receive analgesics compared to men. When presented with the same standardized vignette, medical students were more likely to give nonspecific somatic diagnoses, address psychosocial factors, and prescribe psychoactive medications when the patient was given a female gender compared to a male gender. In addition, medical providers of the same sex as the patient (both male–male and female–female combinations) were more likely to prescribe opioid medication for low back pain.

FURTHER READING

Fillingim RB, King CD, Ribeiro-Dasilva MC, et al. Sex, gender, and pain: A review of recent clinical and experimental findings. *J Pain*. 2009;10(5):447–485.

7. ANSWER: D

Numerous studies have been performed in which individuals complete a self-assessment on their masculine or feminine characteristics (questionnaires include the Personal attributes questionnaire, Bem Sex Role Inventory, or the Hypermaculinity inventory assessments). Consensus from these studies appears to show a direct correlation between the gender role and the pain threshold. Interestingly, the correlation appears to affect only males, whereas the connection in females seems to be insignificant. These studies suggest that societal norms and expectations play a role in how pain is perceived and expressed by individuals.

FURTHER READING

Alabas OA, Tashani OA, Tabasam G, et al. Gender role affects experimental pain responses: A systematic review with meta-analysis. *Eur J Pain*. 2012;16(9):1211–1223.

8. ANSWER: D

Meta-analysis of gender role and pain responses seems to suggest that the sex of the investigator may influence the reporting of pain by a study participant. The greatest effect was on men, with their threshold being much higher when in the presence of a female investigator compared to a male investigator. Females were not reported to consistently show a change in thresholds in the presence of a female or male investigator, although they possibly also showed increased tolerance in the presence of the opposite sex. Although the extent of the effect is known, it may play a factor in clinical medicine when trying to assess the pain of a patient who is of the opposite sex.

FURTHER READING

Alabas OA, Tashani OA, Tabasam G, et al. Gender role affects experimental pain responses: A systematic review with meta-analysis. *Eur J Pain*. 2012;16(9):1211–1223.

9. ANSWER: D

Fillinghim et al. reviewed relatively recent clinical and experimental findings and found that a number of differences in pain sensitivity can be ascribed to sex hormone effects. Supplemental estrogen (hormone replacement therapy (HRT)) has been shown to increase pain in both postmenopausal women and transsexual patients undergoing hormone therapy transition. Conversely, postmenopausal women with no HRT show pain sensitivity similar to men, and female-to-male transsexuals have improved pain after beginning testosterone therapy. Women show an increased inflammatory response compared to men, which may be affected by estrogen levels.

FURTHER READING

Fillingim RB, King CD, Ribeiro-Dasilva MC, et al. Sex, gender, and pain: A review of recent clinical and experimental findings. *J Pain*. 2009;10(5):447–485.

10. ANSWER: A

Coping mechanisms are the cognitive and behavioral adaptations used by individuals to deal with stressors. With regard to pain, it appears that women are more likely to utilize catastrophizing (believing something is worse than it really is), support seeking, and positive statements, whereas men are more likely to use behavioral distraction. The higher levels of catastrophizing have been shown to be a mediator in the gender differences in pain between the sexes, with higher levels being associated with higher reports of pain.

FURTHER READING

Fillingim RB, King CD, Ribeiro-Dasilva MC, et al. Sex, gender, and pain: A review of recent clinical and experimental findings. *J Pain.* 2009;10(5):447–485.

11. ANSWER: A

Sex-related differences in pain may also reflect differences in the endogenous opioid system. There are differences in pain-related activation of brain mu opioid receptors. Smith and colleagues found that women in high estradiol/low progesterone states exhibit decreased pain sensitivity compared to women in low estradiol states, whereas decreased endogenous opioid neurotransmission is associated with low estradiol.

FURTHER READING

Bartley EJ, Fillingim RB. Sex differences in pain: A brief review of clinical and experimental findings. *Br J Anaesth.* 2013;111:52–58.
Smith YR, Stahler CS, Nichols TE, et al. Pronociceptive and antinociceptive effects of estradiol through endogenous opioid neurotransmission in women. *J Neurosci.* 2006;26:5777–5785.
Zubieta J-K, Smith YR, Bueller JA, et al. Mu-opioid receptor-mediated antinociceptive responses differ in men and women. *J Neurosci.* 2002;22:5100–5107.

12. ANSWER: D

Positron emission tomography and magnetic resonance imaging techniques have been used to investigate processing differences between the sexes in the central nervous system. Mildly painful rectal distension in patients with irritable bowel syndrome produced activation of the left thalamus and ventral striatum only in men. In women, areas of the amygdala and mid-cingulate were deactivated during uncomfortable and mild pain stimuli, respectively. During anticipation and uncomfortable (nonpainful) distension, men showed greater activation in areas of the insula.

FURTHER READING

Paller CJ, Campbell C, Edward R, et al. Sex-based differences in pain perception and treatment. *Pain Med.* 2009;10(2):289–299.

13. ANSWER: A

Animal studies show robust interactions between sex and other factors in relation to pain sensitivity. Recent studies also reveal that social interaction modulates pain in mice. In studies in which affected (pain stimulus applied) and unaffected (no pain stimulus) mice were placed in cages together, female mice, but not male mice, approached cagemates (but not strangers) that were in pain and spent excess time in physical proximity to their hurting familiar. A negative correlation was obtained between contact time and pain behavior. In other studies of male mice, after only one in a dyad was injected with acetic acid, either stress-induced analgesia or stress-induced hyperalgesia was observed, depending on the threat level dictated by facets of the testing situation.

FURTHER READING

Langford DL, Tuttle AH, Brown K, et al. Social approach to pain in laboratory mice. *Social Neurosi.* 2009;5:163–170.
Langford DL, Tuttle AH, Briscoe C, et al. Varying perceived social threat modulates pain behavior in male mice. *J Pain.* 2011;12:125–132.

14. ANSWER: D

Explanations for sexual differences in pain and analgesia have been divided into two groups: the ultimate causes, which aim to explain why there is a sex difference, and the proximate causes, which aim to explain how the sex difference is instantiated. Proximate causes include experiential (due to painful experiences such as abuse, labor pain, and clinical pain frequency), psychological (anger, negative affect, and anxiety), genetic (buffering from allelic mosaicism and X chromosome gene imprinting), neurochemical (sex-dependent levels of pain-related neurochemicals and/or their receptors such as cytokine expression, monoamine receptors, and NMDA receptors), organizational (steroid activation on development), activational (steroid action in adulthood, androgens, estrogens, and progesterone), systems level (cardiovascular system modulation, inflammation, and vagal nerve modulation), and sociocultural (differences in gender roles and gender role expectations).

FURTHER READING

Mogil J. Sex differences in pain and pain inhibition: Multiple explanations of a controversial phenomenon. *Nat Rev Neurosci.* 2012;13:859–866.

15. ANSWER: D

Psychological factors, including anxiety, depression, use of specific pain-coping strategies, and catastrophizing, are associated with the experience of pain. Health care provider characteristics have also been implicated in the experience because various studies have suggested biases between male and female providers.

FURTHER READING

Heins JK, Heins A, Grammas M, et al. Disparities in analgesia and opioid prescribing practices for patients with musculoskeletal pain in the emergency department. *J Emerg Nurs*. 2006;32(3):219–224.

Paller CJ, Campbell C, Edward R, et al. Sex-based differences in pain perception and treatment. *Pain Med*. 2009;10(2):289–299.

Weisse CS, Sorum PC, Sanders KN, et al. Do gender and race affect decisions about pain management? *J Gen Intern Med*. 2001:16(4):211–217.

6.

IMAGING

Markus A. Bendel, Drew M. Trainor, and Susan M. Moeschler

INTRODUCTION

This chapter focuses on diagnostic and procedural imaging techniques that are essential for the pain medicine practitioner. Attention is given to most modern imaging modalities, including ultrasonography, fluoroscopy, computed tomography (CT), and magnetic resonance imaging (MRI). It includes a review of many advanced pain medicine procedures, such as celiac plexus and stellate ganglion blocks. A discussion regarding the use of imaging to elucidate a problem with an implanted intrathecal drug delivery system is included as well. In addition to the procedure suite, this chapter provides a review of common radiological findings that are critical for the proper diagnosis and management of pain patients including spondylolysis and a review of Modic changes. Special attention is paid to the use of ultrasound in pain medicine, including diagnostic techniques in musculoskeletal disorders. Many questions contain a review of the significant anatomic considerations with each procedural technique.

QUESTIONS

1. A patient with an opioid and baclofen intrathecal drug delivery system in place begins to have symptoms of pruritus, agitation, and increased lower extremity spasticity 1 week after a routine reservoir refill. A complete workup is started, including an urgent catheter dye study (Figure 6.1). What is the most likely etiology of the patient's symptoms?

A. Intrathecal drug delivery system infection
B. Empty pump reservoir
C. Mechanical disruption of the pump circuit
D. Failure of the pump mechanism
E. Granuloma formation

2. A patient undergoes spinal cord stimulator trial lead placement. The leads are positioned as shown in

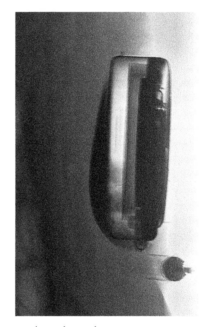

Figure 6.1 Urgent catheter dye study.

Figure 6.2. Classic stimulation-induced paresthesia would be located in:

A. Feet
B. Axial lumbar spine
C. Groin
D. Abdomen
E. Thorax

3. A patient with a history of ongoing pseudoclaudication after lumbar decompression undergoes the procedure shown in Figure 6.3. Which of the following is successfully traversed for proper needle placement?

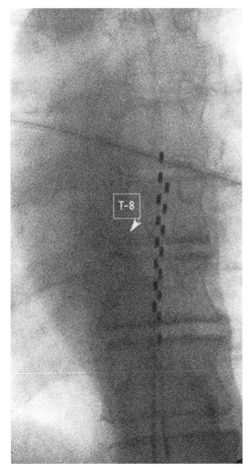

Figure 6.2 A representation of spinal cord stimulator trial lead placement.

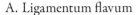

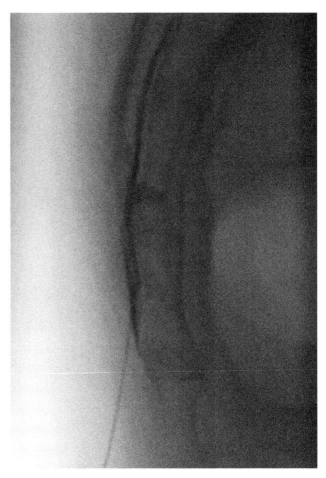

Figure 6.3 Lateral view contrast spread in a caudal epidural steroid injection.

A. Ligamentum flavum
B. S3 foramen
C. Retrodural space of Okada
D. Sacrococcygeal ligament
E. Sacrococcygeal disc space

4. A patient is clinically diagnosed with facetogenic axial lumbar pain. He undergoes successful differential medial branch block procedures and proceeds to radiofrequency denervation. Shown in Figure 6.4 are the final needle positions from that procedure. Which medial branch nerve is being ablated with the top needle placement?

A. L1
B. L2
C. L3
D. L4
E. L5

5. A 67-year-old male has a history of axial cervical spine pain and daily headache. A neurologic examination is unrevealing, and a head MRI is normal. A sagittal slice of his cervical CT is shown in Figure 6.5. Which intervention is most likely to benefit his spine pain?

A. Interlaminar epidural steroid injection
B. Transforaminal epidural injection
C. Cervical facet medial branch block and radiofrequency ablation
D. Cervical discography
E. Cervical vertebroplasty

6. A 75-year-old female presents to the pain clinic for midline thoracic spine pain. There is no radicular component. Initial workup yields the lateral X-ray findings as shown in Figure 6.6. Initial consideration should be given to which intervention?

A. Discography
B. Spinal cord stimulation
C. High-dose opioids
D. Capsaicin treatment
E. Vertebroplasty/kyphoplasty

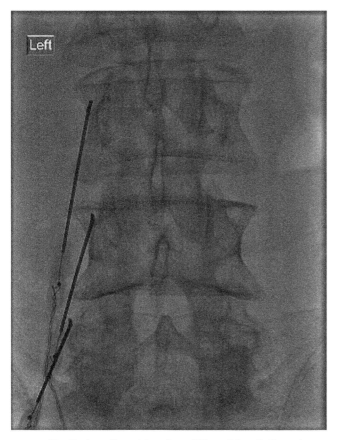

Figure 6.4 The final needle positions from differential medial branch block procedures and radiofrequency denervation.

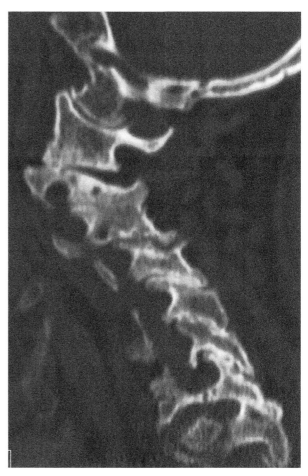

Figure 6.5 A sagittal slice of cervical CT from a 67-year-old male with a history of axial cervical spine pain and daily headache.

7. The National Council on Radiation Protection and Measurements recommends a maximum whole body yearly radiation exposure limit of:

A. 0.005 mSv
B. 0.05 mSv
C. 0.5 mSv
D. 5 mSv
E. 50 mSv

8. A patient is sent to the pain clinic for continued low back and groin pain. Symptoms are worse with ambulation and entering/exiting a car. Exam is significant for a positive Stinchfield test. An X-ray (Figure 6.7) is reviewed which demonstrates that the initial clinical efforts should be directed toward:

A. Treatment of hip osteoarthritis
B. Sacroiliac joints
C. Coccyx
D. Oncologic treatment
E. Trochanteric bursas

9. When performing the injection as seen in Figure 6.8, it is of paramount importance to avoid the lateral portion of the target joint due to:

A. Nerve root irritation
B. Intrathecal spread
C. Vascular uptake
D. Ineffective pain relief
E. Increased pain from injection

10. When working with an ultrasound to complete a piriformis injection on a patient with an elevated body mass index (BMI), altering which of the following will allow for greater depth of penetration of the tissue?

A. Increase frequency
B. Gain
C. M-mode
D. Dynamic range
E. Decrease frequency

11. A 28-year-old male is scheduled to undergo an outpatient arthroscopic repair of a recently diagnosed glenoid labral tear. An ultrasound-guided interscalene block is the preferred anesthesia by the surgical team.

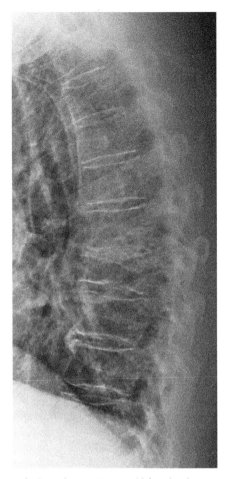

Figure 6.6 X-ray findings from a 75-year-old female who presents with midline thoracic spine pain.

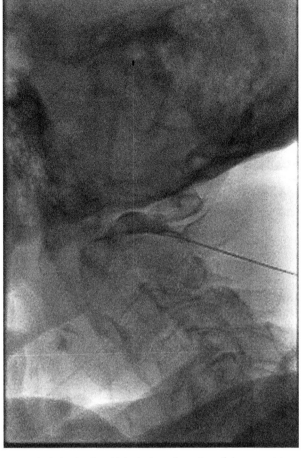

Figure 6.8 An injection in which the lateral portion of the target joint must be avoided.

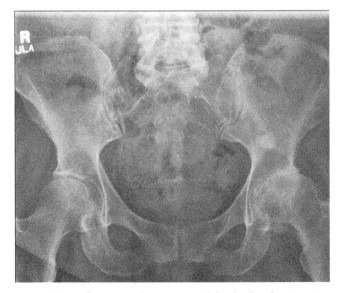

Figure 6.7 X-ray of a patient who presents with low back and groin pain.

What are the correct needle placement and targeted structures for this block?

A. Sternocleidomastoid and the anterior scalene—middle and lower trunks of brachial plexus
B. Middle and posterior scalenes—posterior chord of the brachial plexus
C. Middle and anterior scalenes—superior and middle trunks of the brachial plexus
D. Middle and anterior scalenes—lower trunk of the brachial plexus and axillary nerve
E. Middle and posterior scalenes—middle and lower trunks of the brachial plexus

12. Which of the following patients would be most likely to have a positive response to the ultrasound-guided injection in Figure 6.9?

A. 76-year-old female with burning dysesthesias over the anterolateral thigh and a positive reverse straight leg raise
B. 68-year-old female with chronic hip pain and significant tenderness to palpation over the greater trochanter
C. 29-year-old female who is 34 weeks pregnant and has severe low back pain with radiation into the buttock

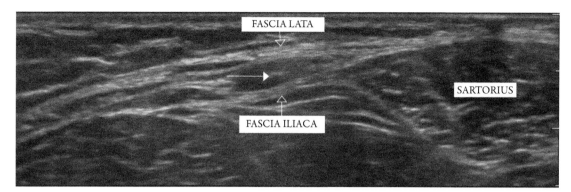

Figure 6.9 An ultrasound-guided injection.

D. 37-year-old obese male with burning dysesthesias over the anterolateral thigh

E. 71-year-old male with burning dysesthesias along the anterolateral thigh and weakness with hip flexion

13. A 46-year-old female with chronic low back, buttock, and posterior thigh pain presents to your office for evaluation. On examination, she has a positive PACE sign. You elect to perform an ultrasound-guided piriformis injection. Inadvertent block of the neural structure that is in the region of the piriformis would produce which of the following symptoms in the right lower limb?

A. Weakness in dorsiflexion at the ankle
B. Weakness in hip flexion and adduction
C. Paresthesias over the medial lower leg
D. Weakness in abduction of the hip
E. Paresthesias over the medial thigh just above the knee

14. A 56-year-old male with chronic axial low back pain undergoes an MRI of the lumbar spine. What image finding of the vertebral subchondral bone marrow would suggest an acute inflammatory process that is strongly associated with degenerative disc disease?

A. Increased signal intensity on both T_1- and T_2-weighted images
B. Decreased signal intensity on T_1- and T_2-weighted images
C. Increased signal intensity on T_1- and decreased signal intensity on T_2-weighted images
D. Decreased signal intensity on T_1- and increased signal intensity on T_2-weighted images
E. Decreased signal intensity on T_2-weighted images post contrast

15. A 62-year-old female with a past medical history significant for a right total hip arthroplasty 2 years ago presents with deep right buttock pain for the last 2 months. On physical examination, she has reproduction of her symptoms when the hip is passively extended, adducted, and externally rotated. What on an MRI of the pelvis would suggest ischiofemoral impingement as her source of pain?

A. Edema within the piriformis muscle
B. Narrowing between the lateral angle of the sacrum and the greater trochanter
C. Increased T_2 signal intensity at the proximal origin of the hamstring complex
D. Enlargement of the sciatic nerve just proximal to the piriformis
E. Narrowing between the ischial tuberosity and the lesser trochanter

16. Which muscle becomes impinged in ischiofemoral impingement?

A. Quadratus femoris
B. Gluteus medius
C. Iliopsoas
D. Piriformis
E. Semimembranosus

17. The most appropriate indication for the procedure being performed in Figure 6.10 would be?

A. Cancer-related pain secondary to pancreatic cancer
B. Cancer-related pain secondary to uterine cancer
C. Complex regional pain syndrome (CRPS) of the lower extremity
D. Chronic abdominal pain related to Crohn's disease
E. Pain related to degenerative disc disease

18. An indication of a successful block in the procedure being performed in Figure 6.10 would include?

A. An increase in systolic blood pressure of 10 mm Hg
B. An increase in the temperature of the affected limb by 1°C
C. Visible hidrosis of the affected limb

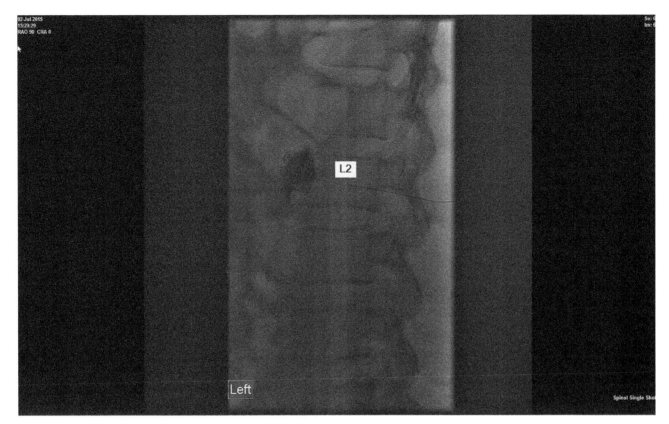

Figure 6.10 Lumbar sympathetic block.

D. Reduction in edema of the affected limb

E. Anesthesia in the area of pain in the affected limb

19. Inadvertent motor blockade in the procedure being performed in Figure 6.10 would result in weakness of?

A. Hip flexion

B. Ankle dorsiflexion

C. Hip abduction

D. Ankle inversion

E. Knee flexion

20. A patient with the MRI findings in Figure 6.11 could present with all of the following except:

A. Pain in the buttock and leg with standing and walking

B. Worsening of back pain with lumbar extension

C. Paresthesias or weakness in the lower limb

D. Worsening of back pain with prolonged sitting

E. Reduced reflexes in the lower limb

21. When scanning and performing a transversus abdominis plane block (TAP) (Figure 6.12), the layers can be identified in the following order (from superficial to deep):

A. External oblique, transversus abdominis, internal oblique

B. Internal oblique, transversus abdominis, external oblique

C. Transversus abdominis, internal oblique, external oblique

D. External oblique, internal oblique, transversus abdominis

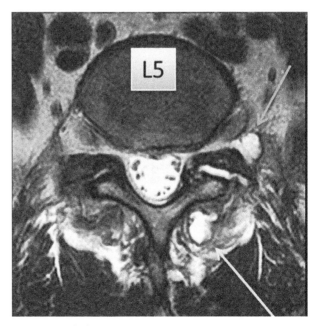

Figure 6.11 MRI findings.

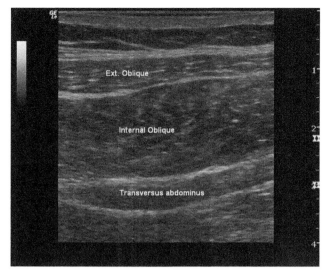

Figure 6.12 The fascial plane between the internal oblique and the transversus abdominis muscle.

22. Transversus plane blocks are an indication for acute perioperative pain for all of the following except:

A. C-section pain
B. appendectomy
C. hemorrhoidectomy
D. cholecystectomy

23. A needle placed for a stellate ganglion block is advanced to target the stellate and cervical chain that lies just anterior to the _____ muscle (Figure 6.13):

A. Longus colli
B. Sternocleidomastoid
C. Anterior scalene
D. Middle scalene

24. What is the structure with the star in the ultrasound image in Figure 6.14?

A. Internal jugular vein
B. External jugular vein
C. Internal carotid artery
D. Inferior thyroid artery

25. Pain from which of the following sites would not improve with this procedure (Figure 6.15):

A. Ureter
B. Stomach
C. Liver
D. Ascending colon

26. After placement of the right needle, it is aspirated and blood returns via the connection tubing

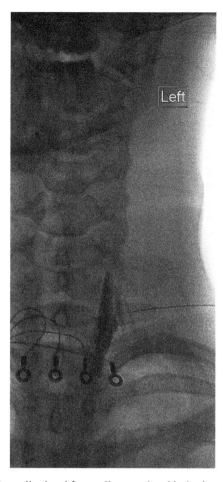

Figure 6.13 A needle placed for a stellate ganglion block advanced to target the stellate and cervical chain.

(Figure 6.15). The needle is most likely within the following vessel:

A. Superior vena cava
B. Inferior vena cava
C. Aorta
D. Iliac artery

27. The most frequent complication from this procedure is:

A. Incontinence
B. Hypotension
C. Diarrhea
D. Hematoma

28. This procedure is indicated in patients with (Figure 6.16):

A. Perineal pain
B. Urinary incontinence
C. Interstitial cystitis
D. Piriformis syndrome

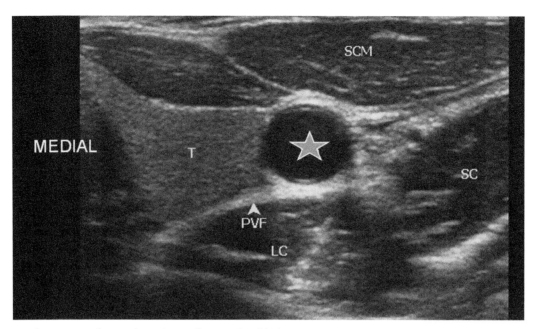

Figure 6.14 Ultrasound image providing guidance for a stellate ganglion block.

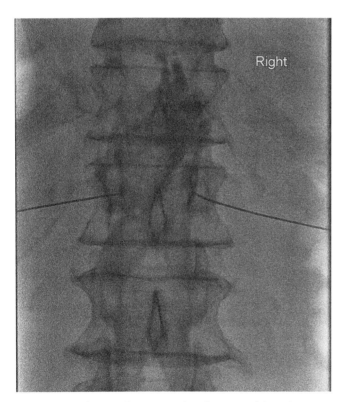

Figure 6.15 Procedure to relieve pain. After placement of the right needle, it is aspirated and blood returns via the connection tubing.

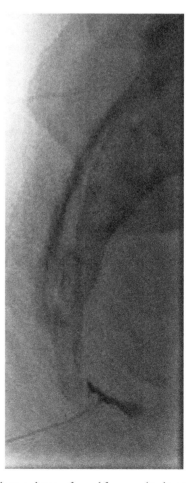

Figure 6.16 Block procedure performed for several indications.

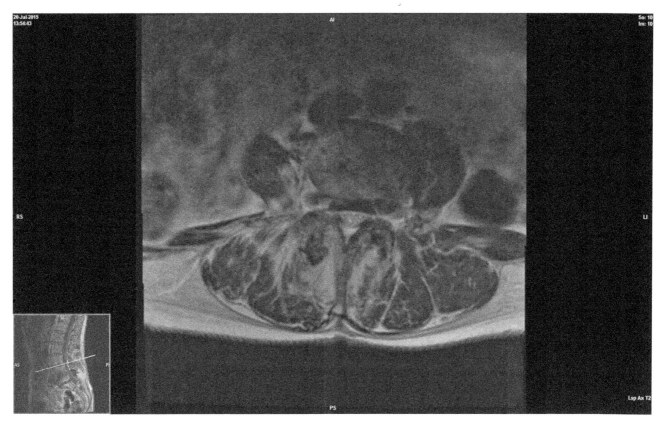

Figure 6.17 MRI of a 78-year-old patient who presents with pain.

29. A 78-year-old patient presents to clinic for pain. An MRI (Figure 6.17) is ordered to ascertain if the pathology in his spine is contributing to his pain complaint. Which is most likely?

A. Left leg pain in an L5 distribution with ambulation
B. Right Leg pain in an L5 distribution with ambulation
C. Bilateral groin pain with ambulation
D. Bilateral calf pain with ambulation

30. The definitive treatment for spinal stenosis is:

A. Nonsteroidal anti-inflammatory drug (NSAID) therapy
B. Gabapentin trial
C. Lumbar facet injections
D. Surgical decompression

ANSWERS

1. ANSWER: C

Figure 6.1 clearly shows contrast extravasation posterior to the intrathecal reservoir in the lateral view. This would be most consistent with a disruption in the circuit between the intrathecal reservoir and the tip of the catheter. In this case, the hub connecting the end of the catheter to the reservoir outlet had come dislodged.

Baclofen withdrawal is a syndrome that consists of classic symptoms that must be quickly recognized and treated because untreated baclofen withdrawal could be fatal. Seizures, myoclonus, rigidity, and death are possible results of acute baclofen withdrawal. Patients utilizing intrathecal baclofen therapy must be educated on the symptoms of baclofen withdrawal. Treatment with oral baclofen, monitoring, and close follow-up by a team of experts are essential in a severe case of baclofen withdrawal.

KEY FACTS

- Intrathecal baclofen withdrawal can be consistent with a medical emergency. Close observation and treatment by trained personnel are imperative.
- An intrathecal dye study can be helpful in assessing an intrathecal drug delivery system for a possible mechanical interruption.

FURTHER READING

Kari M, Jaycox M. Complications associated with intrathecal drug delivery systems. In: Buvanendran A, Diwan S, Deer T (Eds.), *Intrathecal Drug Delivery for Pain and Spasticity*. Philadelphia, PA: Saunders; 2011:102–112.

2. ANSWER: B

Figure 6.2 is a representation of a spinal cord stimulator trial. The leads are spanning the T8 vertebral body to the T7–T8 junction. Both leads are positioned close to the midline. This would classically be thought to give paresthesia coverage for axial spine pain. For lower extremity paresthesias, one would expect the leads to be placed between T9 and T12. Upper extremity paresthesia coverage is routinely obtained between C2 and C7. There is wide interpatient variability. This makes the trialing of the stimulation pattern essential to obtain proper paresthesia coverage for traditional stimulator programming.

KEY FACT

- Spinal cord stimulation paresthesia patterns have a significant degree of interpatient variability.

FURTHER READING

Rauck RL, Nagel S, North JL, et al. Spinal cord stimulation implantation techniques. In: Hayek SH, Levy R, Deer T (Eds.), *Neurostimulation for the Treatment of Chronic Pain*. Philadelphia, PA: Saunders; 2011:54–64.

3. ANSWER: D

Figure 6.3 shows classic lateral view contrast spread in a caudal epidural steroid injection. This technique can be employed in patients who have continued lumbosacral radicular symptoms after a surgical intervention. Occasionally, the caudal epidural space is the only means to safely access the epidural space in a postsurgical patient with altered anatomy.

A caudal injection is performed by palpating the sacral cornu that mark the entrance to the sacral hiatus. Utilizing fluoroscopy, anteroposterior (AP) and lateral views are obtained to ensure midline needle placement in the AP orientation and placement in the sacral hiatus on the lateral view. Contrast is injected to confirm appropriate spread in both AP and lateral views. The ligament overlying the sacral hiatus is the sacrococcygeal ligament. As the needle passes through this ligament, often a "pop" is palpable, signifying the entrance into the caudal epidural space.

The S3 foramen is certainly not traversed in a caudal injection, although it can serve as a marker for the most cephalad positioning of the needle in the caudal space. Any more cephalad positioning could result in the needle being positioned in the intrathecal space.

The ligamentum flavum is associated with the interlaminar epidural steroid injection. Sacrococcygeal disc space is encountered with a ganglion impar injection, and the retrodural space of Okada is a potential space posterior to the ligamentum flavum.

KEY FACT

- Caudal epidural steroid injection can be a route of access for patients with impediment to interlaminar or transforaminal access.

FURTHER READING

Petrolla JJ, Furman MB. Caudal epidural steroid injection. In: Furman MB (Ed.), *Atlas of Image-Guided Spinal Injections*. 2nd ed. Philadelphia, PA: Saunders; 2012:57–62.

4. ANSWER: B

The L2 medial branch is ablated at the junction point of the L3 superior article process (SAP) and L3 transverse process

(TP). This can create confusion when discussing (or ordering) procedures between providers. Discussing ablation of the L2 and L3 medial branch nerves is different than discussing the denervation of the L2–L3 facet joint. This would result in different needle placement in the procedure suite. In order to denervate the L2–L3 facet joint, one would place a needle at the L2 SAP–TP junction and L3 SAP–TP junction. Doing this would actually ablate the L1 and L2 medial branch nerves. The L1 medial branch nerve branches from the L1 spinal nerve root after it exits the spinal foramen (below the L1 TP). It then crosses the L2 SAP–TP junction and innervates the L1–L2 facet and the L2–L3 facet via articular branches. The L2 branch follows a similar path and innervates the L2–L3 facet and the L3–L4 facet. Thereby, abating the L1 and L2 medial branch nerves will successfully denervate the L2–L3 facet. Knowing the difference between the numbering of the medial branches and the facet joints will prevent any wrong level procedures and subsequent patient dissatisfaction.

KEY FACTS

- Anatomy of medial branch nerves is important to ensure that the ordering provider and proceduralist are in sync.
- Each facet joint receives innervation from the medial branch located one vertebral level above and from the exiting root at the level in question.

FURTHER READING

Waldman SD. *Atlas of Interventional Pain Management.* 4th ed. Toronto: Elsevier; 2015:463–472.

5. ANSWER: C

Figure 6.5 is significant for advanced cervical facet disease. The intervention most likely to succeed would be aimed at decreasing pain or pain transmission from these structures. A cervical radiofrequency ablation procedure would accomplish this goal.

The pain literature lacks strong evidence for many procedures that are commonly performed. Reasonable evidence exists for the use of radiofrequency ablation in the cervical and lumbar spine to alleviate facetogenic discomfort.

KEY FACTS

- Cervical facet arthritis is a common cause of axial neck pain and can be treated with medial branch radiofrequency ablation.
- Identification of spondylosis is essential for the pain physician.

FURTHER READING

Manchikanti L, Kaye AD, Boswell MV, et al. A systematic review and best evidence synthesis of the effectiveness of therapeutic facet joint interventions in managing chronic spinal pain. *Pain Physician.* 2015;18;E535–E582.

6. ANSWER: E

The included lateral chest X-ray is significant for the presence of a midthoracic vertebral compression fracture. Depending on several factors (age of fracture, degree of vertebral body height loss, and symptoms), the patient may be a good candidate for a vertebroplasty or kyphoplasty. There remains debate in the literature regarding the effectiveness of percutaneous vertebroplasty/kyphoplasty, but a pain physician should recognize a vertebral compression fracture as the likely source of discomfort in this patient.

KEY FACTS

- Vertebral body compression fractures can be a cause of significant discomfort.
- This diagnosis should be explored in elderly patients with risk factors for osteoporosis.

FURTHER READING

Buchbinder R, Golmohammadi K, Johnston RV, et al. Percutaneous vertebroplasty for osteoporotic vertebral compression fracture. *Cochrane Database Syst Rev.* 2015 Apr 30;4:CD006349.
McGirt MJ, Parker SL, Wolinsky JP, et al. Vertebroplasty and kyphoplasty for the treatment of vertebral compression fractures: An evidenced-based review of the literature. *Spine J.* 2009;9(6):501–508.

7. ANSWER: B

The maximum whole body radiation dose has been set at 0.05 mSv (5 rem). A pregnant woman has a 10-fold lower maximum of 0.005 mSv (0.5 rem). The thyroid, extremities, and gonads have yearly limits individually of 0.5 mSv (50 rem). This is important information to know given the well-documented effects of radiation overexposure. The amount of radiation that will result in pathologic effects to certain organs has also been established. The lens of the eye, for example, will begin to develop cataracts at a total radiation dose of 200 rad. The skin will exhibit erythema at 500 rad and permanent alopecia at 700 rad.

KEY FACTS

- The maximum whole body radiation dose is 0.05 mSv.
- Special precaution and monitoring should be provided for pregnant practitioners.

FURTHER READING

Benzon H, Rathmell JP, Wu CL, et al. Radiation safety and the use of radiographic contrast agents in pain medicine. In: Benzon H, Rathmell JP, Wu CL, et al. (Eds.), *Practical Management of Pain*. Philadelphia: Mosby; 2014:981–998.

8. ANSWER: A

Figure 6.7 is most significant for advanced osteoarthritis of the left hip. This is very likely the reason for the patient's groin and low back pain. Conservative measures for osteoarthritis include physical therapy, medications, and injections. Degenerative arthritis of this degree may require surgery in an otherwise appropriate candidate.

KEY FACTS

- Hip pathology can present as low back pain.
- A hip examination and investigation should be performed because the hip may be a a cause of low back in many patients.

FURTHER READING

Waldman SD. Arthritis pain of the hip. In: Waldman SD (Ed.), *Atlas of Common Pain Syndromes*. 3rd ed. Philadelphia, PA: Saunders; 2011:279–281.

9. ANSWER: C

Figure 6.8 demonstrates a fluoroscopically guided C1–C2 (atlanto-axial) joint injection. The technique involves dividing the joint space into thirds. Between the lateral and middle third is the intended injection target. This will allow for safe entry into the joint with the least possible risk of nerve injury or vascular uptake in the vertebral artery. Medial placement of the needle may lead to inadvertent intrathecal uptake or nerve root injury. Lateral placement of the needle may lead to intravascular needle placement in the vertebral artery at this level.

KEY FACTS

- Lateral placement of a C1–C2 joint injection places the patient at risk of vertebral artery injury or vascular injection.
- Medial placement of the C1–C2 injection increases the risk of nerve root injury or intrathecal injection.

FURTHER READING

Rolle W. Atlantoaxial joint intraarticular injection. In: Furman, ed. *Atlas of Image Guided Spinal Procedures*. Elsivier, Philadelphia, 2013.

10. ANSWER: E

A commonly tested relationship is that between frequency, resolution, and tissue penetration. High-frequency probes will provide the best resolution but have low tissue penetration. Lower frequency probes, on the other hand, will penetrate deeper tissues better but will have less resolution than higher frequency probes.

KEY FACTS

- Increased frequency will allow for better resolution of an ultrasound probe but less tissue penetration.
- Lowered frequency will allow for better tissue penetration but decreases resolution.

FURTHER READING

Gray A. Ultrasound. In: *Atlas of Ultrasound Guided Regional Anesthesia*. 2nd ed. Toronto: Elsevier; 2013.

11. ANSWER: C

The proper needle placement for regional anesthesia of the proximal upper extremity using an ultrasound-guided interscalene block is the tissue between the anterior and middle scalenes with injection of local anesthetic around the superior and middle trunks of the brachial plexus.

The technique is commonly performed with the patient in the supine position with his or her head rotated in the opposite direction. Then, using a linear transducer oriented on the transverse plane, the carotid artery is identified. The transducer is then moved laterally until the anterior and middle scalenes come into view with the trunks of the brachial plexus sandwiched between them. After proper identification of the structures, a 22-gauge needle is advanced 1–3 cm, and 15–25 ml of local anesthetic is injected, displacing the neural structures. For distal upper limb anesthesia, the lower trunk of the brachial plexus can be blocked in a similar manner.

Other methods of interscalene blockade include the landmark-based and neurostimulation techniques. The ultrasound-guided technique may be superior to other techniques, providing more rapid block onset times, fewer needle sticks, higher block success rates, lower effective doses of local anesthetic, reduced procedure times, and less procedure-related discomfort. Given the more rapid onset of anesthesia, care must be taken to avoid injecting under high resistance, which could indicate intraneural injection and related nerve damage.

KEY FACTS

- Proper needle placement for regional anesthesia of the proximal upper limb using the ultrasound-guided

interscalene approach is between the anterior and middle scalenes, with blockade of the superior and middle trunks of the brachial plexus.
• Potential benefits of using the ultrasound-guided approach compared to other techniques are more rapid onset of blockade with lower effective dose of local anesthetic and lower procedure-related discomfort of the patient.

FURTHER READING

Liu SS, YaDeau JT, Shaw PM, et al. Incidence of unintentional intraneural injection and postoperative neurological complications with ultrasound-guided interscalene and supraclavicular nerve blocks. *Anaesthesia* 2011;66(3):168–174.
Singh A, Kelly C, O'Brien T, et al. Ultrasound-guided interscalene block anesthesia for shoulder arthroscopy: A prospective study of 1319 patients. *J Bone Joint Surg.* 2012;94(22):2040–2046.

12. ANSWER: D

The lateral femoral cutaneous nerve (LFCN) is a primary sensory nerve that originates from the lumbar plexus with varying contributions of L1–L3. It emerges from the lateral border of the psoas, courses over the iliacus, medial to the anterior superior iliac spine (ASIS), deep to the inguinal ligament, and superficial to the sartorius, where it divides into an anterior and a posterior branch and provides sensation to the anterolateral thigh.

Meralgia paresthetica is a nerve entrapment of the LFCN and produces symptoms of dysesthesias, paresthesias, and sensory loss over the distribution of the LFCN. It tends to affect males in their 30s and 40s, and risk factors include obesity (BMI >30), tight-fitting jeans, pregnancy, seat belts, and direct trauma. The differential diagnosis of meralgia paresthetica includes upper lumbar radiculopathy, trochanteric bursitis, lumbar plexopathy, and retroperitoneal hemorrhage.

The diagnosis of meralgia paresthetica can be challenging because it often mimics other more common diagnoses, such as spine pathology. Ultrasound-guided injection of the LFCN can be both diagnostic and therapeutic in nature. The procedure involves the use of a high-frequency linear probe with the lateral border on the hyperechoic ASIS in the transverse plane. The medial border of the probe is then directed caudally, and the entire probe is translated in a medial–caudal direction until the oval hyperechoic structure of the LFCN is appreciated in the fascial plane superficial to the fascia lata and deep to the fascia iliaca. Then, under image guidance, a 25-guage needle is advanced into the fascial plane, and local anesthetic and corticosteroid are injected.

KEY FACTS

• Meralgia paresthetica is a compressive neuropathy of the lateral femoral cutaneous nerve and presents with dysesthesias, paresthesias, and sensory loss in the anterior and lateral thigh.
• Risk factors for the development of meralgia paresthetica include male gender, age 30–40 years, obesity (BMI >30), tight garments, pregnancy, seat belts, and direct nerve trauma.
• The differential diagnosis of meralgia paresthetica includes upper lumbar radiculopathy, trochanteric bursitis, lumbar plexopathy, and retroperitoneal hemorrhage.
• Ultrasound-guided injection of the LFCN can be both diagnostic and therapeutic in the management of meralgia paresthetica.

FURTHER READING

Cheatham SW, Kolber MJ, Salamh PA. Meralgia paresthetica: A review of the literature. *Int J Sports Phys Ther.* 2013;8(6);883–893.
Hurdle MF, et al. Ultrasound-guided blockade of the lateral femoral cutaneous nerve: Technical description and review of 10 cases. *Arch Phys Med Rehabil.* 2007;88(10):1362–1364.

13. ANSWER: A

Piriformis syndrome is often an overlooked cause of chronic low back and buttock pain. According to Kean Chen and Nizar, the prevalence of piriformis syndrome in the low back pain population is 17.2%. The most common presentation of piriformis syndrome is pain in the gluteal region with radiation down to posterior thigh, and it is thought to be secondary to myofascial trigger points. A less common presentation of piriformis syndrome is pain radiating into the lower extremity in the distribution of the L5 and S1 nerve roots. This is thought to be secondary to compression of the sciatic nerve as it courses under (and sometimes through) the piriformis. Patients with piriformis syndrome will often have reproduction of their pain with resisted abduction and external rotation, which is known as Pace test or sign.

It is reasonable to pursue ultrasound-guided injection in patients who have pain clinically consistent with piriformis syndrome. Some studies have shown the accuracy of injection to be 95% using ultrasound guidance compared to only 30% when using fluoroscopic guidance. One potential complication of injecting the piriformis with either imaging modality is inadvertent blockade of the sciatic nerve. This results in weakness of the muscles supplied by the sciatic nerve, and it presents clinically by weakness in dorsi/plantar flexion and eversion/inversion of the ankle. Sensory disturbances may also be present, including paresthesias over the posterolateral leg and dorsal/plantar surfaces of the foot.

KEY FACTS

• Piriformis syndrome is a underrecognized cause of low back and buttock pain in the low back pain population.

- Patients with piriformis syndrome often have pain with resisted abduction and external rotation of the hip (Pace test or sign).
- One complication of injecting the piriformis using either ultrasound or fluoroscopy is inadvertent block of the sciatic nerve. This presents clinically with motor and sensory disturbances in the distribution of the sciatic nerve.

FURTHER READING

Finnoff JT, Hurdle MF, Smith J. Accuracy of ultrasound-guided versus fluoroscopically guided contrast-controlled piriformis injections: A cadaveric study. *J Ultrasound Med.* 2008;27(8):1157–1163.

Jankovic D, Peng P, van Zundert A. Brief review: Piriformis syndrome—Etiology, diagnosis, and management. *Can J Anaesth.* 2013;60(10):1003–1012.

Kean Chen C, Nizar AJ. Prevalence of piriformis syndrome in chronic low back pain patients: A clinical diagnosis with modified FAIR test. *Pain Pract.* 2013;13(4):276–281.

14. ANSWER: D

Modic changes are seen in the vertebral subchondral bone marrow of patients with degenerative disc disease. There are three main types of Modic changes seen on MRI. Type I shows decreased signal intensity on T_1-weighted images and increased signal intensity on T_2-weighted images. It is thought to represent an acute inflammatory process in the setting of degenerative disc disease and is strongly correlated with pain. Type II Modic changes represent a more stable phase of degenerative disc disease and are associated with increased signal intensity on both T_1- and T_2-weighted images. Type III Modic changes are represented by decreased signal intensity on both T_1- and T_2-weighted images and represent the most chronic change associated with subchondral sclerosis.

KEY FACTS

- Modic type I changes on MRI are represented by decreased signal intensity on T_1-weighted images and increased signal intensity on T_2-weighted images.
- Modic type I changes are associated with an acute inflammatory process and are strongly correlated with pain.

FURTHER READING

Jarvinen J, Karppinen J, Niinimäki J, et al. Association between changes in lumbar Modic changes and low back symptoms over a two-year period. *BMC Musculoskel Disord.* 2015;16:98.

Maatta J, Karppinen J, Luk KD, et al. Phenotype profiling of Modic changes of the lumbar spine and its association with other MRI phenotypes: A large-scale, population-based study. *Spine J.* 2015;15(9):1933–1942.

15. ANSWER: E

Ischiofemoral impingement is one of the two impingement syndromes of the hip. It is more common in middle-aged females and those who have had a total hip arthroplasty. It typically manifests as buttock, groin, or medial thigh pain that is reproduced with extension, adduction, and external rotation of the hip.

16. ANSWER: A

The pain from ischiofemoral impingement is caused by the impingement of the quadratus femoris muscle between the ischial tuberosity and the lesser trochanter of the femur. An MRI of the pelvis will show narrowing of the ischiofemoral space, which is defined as the narrowest distance between the ischial tuberosity and the lesser trochanter. Other imaging criteria include edema within the quadratus femoris muscle or narrowing of the quadratus femoris space (space between the hamstring tendons and the iliopsoas tendon or lesser trochanter).

KEY FACTS

- Ischiofemoral impingement is a potential cause of buttock, groin, or medial thigh pain.
- Ischiofemoral impingement is caused by narrowing of the ischiofemoral space, which can be appreciated on an MRI of the pelvis.
- The quadratus femoris muscle is the implicated structure in ischiofemoral impingement.
- The pain associated with ischiofemoral impingement can be reproduced with passive extension, adduction, and external rotation of the hip.

FURTHER READING

Finnoff JT, Bond JR, Collins MS, et al. Variability of the ischiofemoral space relative to femur position: An ultrasound study. *PM R* 2015;7(9):930–937.

Lopez-Sanchez MC, Péreza VA, Montero Furelosb LA, et al. Ischiofemoral impingement: Hip pain of infrequent cause. *Reumatol Clin.* 2013;9(3):186–187.

Singer AD, Subhawong TK, Jose J, et al. Ischiofemoral impingement syndrome: A meta-analysis. *Skeletal Radiol.* 2015;44(6): 831–837.

17. ANSWER: C

The procedure being performed in Figure 6.10 is for CRPS of the lower extremity. Lumbar sympathetic blocks have been used to treat a number of pain syndromes involving the lower limbs, including CRPS, postherpetic neuralgia, phantom limb pain, and ischemic pain secondary to vascular insufficiency.

18. ANSWER: B

Although studies have demonstrated variability in both the location and the number of lumbar sympathetic ganglia, there are typically three ganglia that lie anterior and lateral to the lower lumbar vertebral bodies and discs (most commonly at the L2–L3 disc). The lumbar sympathetic ganglia are commonly blocked at the vertebral bodies of L2–L4 using either a 22-gauge or a 25-gauge 5½-in. needle that is advanced in an oblique manner under fluoroscopic guidance until the tip lies immediately anterior to the vertebral body. After satisfactory spread of contrast, 10–15 cc of long-acting local anesthetic is injected. Ropivacaine is the preferred local anesthetic because it is less cardiotoxic than bupivacaine. With appropriate sympathetic blockade, there should be an observed temperature rise in the affected limb.

19. ANSWER: A

One of the more common complications of performing a lumbar sympathetic block is inadvertent blockade of the L2 nerve root, which can result in weakness of the hip flexors.

KEY FACTS

- Lumbar sympathetic blocks are commonly used to treat CRPS affecting the lower limb.
- A temperature rise in the affected limb is an indication of a successful sympathetic block.
- Hip weakness may be observed after a lumbar sympathetic block due to inadvertent blockade of the L2 nerve root.

FURTHER READING

Abramov R. Lumbar sympathetic treatment in the management of lower limb pain. *Curr Pain Headache Rep*. 2014;18(4):403.
Hong JH, Oh MJ. Comparison of multilevel with single level injection during lumbar sympathetic ganglion block: Efficacy of sympatholysis and incidence of psoas muscle injection. *Korean J Pain*. 2010;23(2):131–136.

Tang YZ, Ni JX, An JX. Complex regional pain syndrome type I following discTRODE radiofrequency treated with continuous lumbar sympathetic trunk block using patient-controlled analgesia. *Pain Med*. 2013;14(2):309–310.

20. ANSWER: D

The MRI of the lumbar spine is demonstrating a facet synovial cyst. Although the exact cause of these cysts is unknown, it is likely related to advanced degenerative changes within the facet joint. Facetogenic pain is often worse with extension of the spine. When these cysts are large in size, they can cause neuroforaminal stenosis and a resulting radiculopathy. A radiculopathy can present with paresthesias, weakness, and reflex changes in the lower limb. Less commonly, they can cause lateral recess stenosis, which can present as neurogenic claudication, including pain in the buttock or leg with prolonged standing or walking. Back pain with prolonged sitting is a more common presentation for discogenic pain.

KEY FACTS

- Facet synovial cysts are often associated with degenerative changes within the facet joint.
- These cysts can be associated with facetogenic pain.
- Facet synovial cysts can cause neuroforaminal stenosis and radiculopathy.
- Facet synovial cysts can cause lateral recess stenosis and present as neurogenic claudication.

FURTHER READING

Kalevski SK, Haritonov DG, Peev NA. Lumbar intraforaminal synovial cyst in young adulthood: Case report and review of the literature. *Global Spine J*. 2014;4(3):191–196.
Mavrogenis AF, et al. Lumbar synovial cysts. *J Surg Orthop Adv*. 2012;21(4):232–236.
Pindrik J, Macki M, Bydon M, et al. Midline synovial and ganglion cysts causing neurogenic claudication. *World J Clin Cases*. 2013;1(9):285–289.

21. ANSWER: D

The TAP block is defined as the fascial plane between the internal oblique and the transversus abdominis muscle (Figure 6.12). It has been described as the "triangle of petit" and is anatomically defined by the latissimus dorsi, the external oblique, and the iliac crest. This can be identified by placing the ultrasound transducer between the subcostal margin and the iliac crest at the mid-axillary line and scanning posterior to anterior. The somatic fibers traverse within the TAP plane; thus, an injection at this plane will cause anesthesia of the unilateral abdominal wall.

KEY FACTS

- The anatomy of the abdominal wall is important in the safe performance of a TAP block.
- The TAP block is performed between the internal oblique and transversus abdominus layers.

FURTHER READING

Jankovic ZB, du Feu FM, McConnell P. An anatomical study of the transversus abdominis plane block: Location of the lumbar triangle of Petit and adjacent nerves. *Anesth Analg.* 2009;109(3):981–985.

22. ANSWER: C

TAP blocks have been described in the literature for opioid-sparing postoperative pain control for multiple surgical procedures, including hernia repairs, cholecystectomies, and renal transplants, as well as post-cesarean section pain. Surgery that involves the abdominal wall is amenable to such a regional technique. However, the sacral innervation to the rectal region would not be anesthetized via a TAP block and thus it is not an indication for this procedure.

KEY FACT

- Abdominal wall pain is an indication for TAP blockade.

FURTHER READING

Abdallah FW, Halpern SH, Margarido CB. Transversus abdominis plane block for postoperative analgesia after Caesarean delivery performed under spinal anaesthesia? A systematic review and meta-analysis. *Br J Anaesth.* 2012;109(5):679–687.
Jankovic ZB, du Feu FM, McConnell P. An anatomical study of the transversus abdominis plane block: Location of the lumbar triangle of Petit and adjacent nerves. *Anesth Analg.* 2009;109(3):981–985.
Takebayashi K, Matsumura M, Kawai Y, et al. Efficacy of transversus abdominis plane block and rectus sheath block in laparoscopic inguinal hernia surgery. *Int Surg.* 2015;100(4):666–671.

23. ANSWER: A

The sympathetic fibers that course from the head, neck, and upper extremities coalesce into the upper cervical and thoracic sympathetic chain, of which the stellate ganglion is the formation of the inferior cervical chain with the thoracic sympathetic chain. The cervical chain runs just superficial to the surface to the longus colli muscle belly and is one of the landmarks and targets of an ultrasound-guided stellate ganglion block. The brachial plexus passes between the anterior and middle scalene muscles and is the intended target of interscalene blocks.

KEY FACT

- The stellate ganglion block is performed just anterior to the longus colli muscle at the C6 or C7 vertebral level.

FURTHER READING

Narouze S. Ultrasound-guided stellate ganglion block: Safety and efficacy. *Curr Pain Headache Rep.* 2014;18(6):424.

24. ANSWER: C

A stellate ganglion block is most commonly performed at the level of C6 or C7. Under ultrasound guidance, the internal jugular vein can be viewed lateral from the internal carotid and is easily collapsible under the ultrasound probe. The internal carotid artery, in contrast, is not easily collapsible, is pulsatile under color Doppler, and is superficial to the longus colli muscle. The inferior thyroid artery has been described as coursing through the intended pathway in some patients when performing a stellate ganglion block, although it is not as reliably imaged as the internal carotid. Vigilance is required when planning the needle trajectory for this procedure as well as throughout needle placement and injection of the medication to avoid intravascular injection.

KEY FACT

- Several important vascular structures can lie within the intended path for stellate blockade, and vigilance is of paramount importance.

FURTHER READING

Narouze S. Beware of the "serpentine" inferior thyroid artery while performing stellate ganglion block. *Anesth Analg.* 2009;109(1): 289–290.

25. ANSWER: A

The celiac plexus is a network of sympathetic and parasympathetic fibers located in the retroperitoneal space at the level of the T12 and L1 vertebrae. The celiac plexus receives sympathetic fibers from greater, lesser, and least splanchnic nerves, which are variable in number. These nerve fibers surround the celiac trunk, continuing inferiorly to the level of the superior and inferior mesenteric plexus. The celiac plexus innervates most of the abdominal viscera, including the stomach, liver, biliary tract, pancreas, spleen, kidneys, adrenals, omentum, small bowel, and colon to the splenic flexure.

Neurolytic celiac plexus and splanchnic nerve blocks are commonly performed to control pain in the epigastric viscera, especially due to either primary or metastatic upper abdominal cancers.

KEY FACT

• The ureter is not innervated by the celiac plexus.

FURTHER READING

Moeschler SM, Rosenberg C, Trainor D, et al. Interventional modalities to treat cancer-related pain. *Hosp Pract.* (1995) 2014;42(5):14–23.
Nagels W, Pease N, Bekkering G, et al. Celiac plexus neurolysis for abdominal cancer pain: A systematic review. *Pain Med.* 2013;14(8):1140–1163.

26. ANSWER: B

At the level of needle placement to the T12–L1 vertebral bodies, the inferior vena cava resides lateral and deep from the anterior border of the vertebral body. In contrast, the aorta is anterior and slightly to the left of the vertebral body. A transaortic approach to the celiac plexus may be performed in which the leftward needle is advanced through the aorta.

KEY FACT

• Major vessels are at risk of puncture during a celiac plexus blockade.

FURTHER READING

Nagels W, Pease N, Bekkering G, et al. Celiac plexus neurolysis for abdominal cancer pain: A systematic review. *Pain Med.* 2013;14(8):1140–1163.

27. ANSWER: B

Neurolysis of the splanchnic nerves, often referred to as a celiac plexus block, is performed for analgesia related to

cancer or pathology of the midgut organs. Thus, visceral pain originating in the distal esophagus, intestines, pancreas, stomach, and colon may be alleviated with such a procedure. There are several described approaches to this procedure, including retrocrural, transaortic, as well as endoscopically guided via the stomach. These procedures can decrease the need for opioid medications and their side effects. Risks related to this procedure include nerve injury, bleeding, pneumothorax, diarrhea, and hypotension. Most patients experience a decrease in blood pressure following the procedure secondary to vasodilatation. It is important to provide a fluid bolus prior to the procedure because these patients often have poor nutritional and fluid status secondary to their disease.

KEY FACTS

• Transient hypotension should be expected after a celiac plexus block.
• A fluid bolus is often sufficient to prevent or treat symptomology.

FURTHER READING

Wong GY, Schroeder DR, Carns PE, et al. Effect of neurolytic celiac plexus block on pain relief, quality of life, and survival in patients with unresectable pancreatic cancer: A randomized controlled trial. *JAMA* 2004;291(9):1092–1099.

28. ANSWER: A

The ganglion impar is a sympathetic ganglia located just anterior to the sacrum. Ganglion impar blocks are performed for several indications, including perineal pain and coccydynia. The ganglion impar is often targeted via a transsacrococcygeal approach with fluoroscopic guidance.

KEY FACT

• Ganglion impar blockade is traditionally performed for perineal pain.

FURTHER READING

Bogduk N. Ganglion impar blocks for coccydynia: A case series prerequisite for efficacy trial. *Pain Med.* 2015;16(7):1245.
Toshniwal GR, Dureja GP, Prashanth SM. Transsacrococcygeal approach to ganglion impar block for management of chronic perineal pain: A prospective observational study. *Pain Phys.* 2007;10(5):661–666.

29. ANSWER D

Lumbar spinal stenosis is caused by narrowing of the central canal related to ligamentum flavum hypertrophy, disc bulge, and/or facet arthropathy, with the latter being the most common contributor. Patients may experience bilateral leg pain with walking, often referred to as neurogenic claudication. Figure 6.17 demonstrates a narrowed central canal at the L4–L5 level that is the likely cause of this patient's pain. Often, patients describe a "shopping cart" sign in which their pain improves when they flex forward by leaning on a shopping cart when walking.

KEY FACT

- Spinal stenosis can often present with neuroclaudicatory symptoms (i.e., increased pain with ambulation).

FURTHER READING

Zaina F, Tomkins-Lane C, Carragee E, et al. Surgical versus nonsurgical treatment for lumbar spinal stenosis. *Spine*. 2016;41(14): E857–E868.

30. ANSWER: D

Spinal stenosis is often associated with pain when patients are standing and walking, and it is relieved when patients are sitting or flexed forward, such as when walking behind a shopping cart or gait aid. Thus, NSAIDs are unlikely to be beneficial in these patients. Although epidural steroid injections may provide some relief in these patients and are often trialed before surgery, facet injections are not indicated in patients with neurogenic symptoms. Surgical decompression of the level(s) of the stenosis will likely provide relief from lower extremity symptoms, although any back pain symptoms may not be improved.

KEY FACT

- Surgical intervention may be necessary for patients with significant stenosis, neurologic compromise, or failure of conservative care.

FURTHER READING

Katz JN, Harris MB. Clinical practice: Lumbar spinal stenosis. *N Engl J Med*. 2008;358(8):818–825.

7.

ADDICTION AND PAIN

Daniel F. Lonergan

INTRODUCTION

Patients who struggle with both pain and addiction present with some of the most challenging scenarios in clinical medicine. An understanding of the neurophysiologic basis of addiction is a key element in the proper management of acute and chronic pain. Physicians should appropriately screen for addiction and employ a comprehensive and safe approach to pain management, especially for patients with risk factors or a history significant for opioid addiction. Physicians should also understand the legal and regulatory issues governing the prescribing and dispensing of controlled substances in the course of treatment for acute pain, chronic pain, and addiction.

QUESTIONS

1. Approximately what percentage of addiction vulnerability is attributable to genetic factors?

    A. 10%
    B. 25%
    C. 50%
    D. 75%

2. A patient is genotyped for the CYP2D6 gene, which expresses the cytochrome P450 2D6 enzyme, and determined to be an ultrarapid metabolizer. What will likely be the resulting clinical effect when codeine is administered to this patient?

    A. A blunted analgesic response
    B. An exaggerated analgesic response
    C. An improved side effect profile
    D. No change in effect because codeine is not metabolized by this enzyme

3. Which basal ganglia structure plays a critical role in drug reward and the development of addiction by initiating the drug reward pathway and stimulating downstream dopamine release in the nucleus accumbens?

    A. Ventral tegmental area
    B. Substantia nigra
    C. Striatum
    D. Superior colliculus

4. Which opioid receptor is thought to have reduced abuse risk and is less associated with reward pathways?

    A. Delta
    B. Kappa
    C. Mu
    D. Sigma

5. Which protein is uncoupled from the opioid receptor by repeated or constant opioid activation and initiates a cascade of intracellular processes that leads to pharmacodynamic opioid tolerance?

    A. Protein kinase
    B. Delta FosB
    C. cAMP response element binding protein
    D. G protein

6. Patients with drug addiction show increased compulsivity and impulsivity, which is associated with decreased baseline activity in which brain region?

    A. Ventral tegmental area
    B. Anterior cingulate gyrus
    C. Nucleus accumbens
    D. Cerebellum

7. Many patients who suffer from persistent, chronic pain take prescription opioids on a daily basis. Based on current research, the majority of such patients take these medications primarily for what reason?

A. For the euphoric effects of the medication
B. For the analgesic effects of the medication
C. For the sedative effects of the medication
D. Because they are addicted to the medication

8. According to current research, approximately what percentage of chronic pain patients abuse substances, including prescription opioids and alcohol?

A. 1–2%
B. 10–20%
C. 40–50%
D. 60–80%

9. What is a key factor in identifying addiction among patients with chronic pain?

A. Physical dependence
B. Development of tolerance
C. Continued daily use of a substance
D. Impaired control over drug use

10. Which clinical screening tool, administered prior to initiation of opioid therapy, utilizes the following five assessment categories?
- Family history of substance abuse (alcohol, illegal drugs, prescription drugs)
- Personal history of substance abuse (alcohol, illegal drugs, prescription drugs)
- Age
- History of preadolescent sexual abuse
- Psychologic disease (attention deficit disorder, obsessive-compulsive disorder, bipolar, schizophrenia, depression)

A. Screener and Opioid Assessment for Patients with Pain (SOAPP)
B. Pain Medication Questionnaire (PMQ)
C. Opioid Risk Tool (ORT)
D. Diagnosis, Intractability, Risk and Efficacy Score (DIRE)

11. A 50-year-old female presents for a routine follow-up visit to a pain management clinic. A urine sample is collected and is positive for her regularly prescribed opioid medication as well as nordiazepam, temazepam, and oxazepam. This is most consistent with use of which benzodiazepine(s)?

A. Clonazepam
B. Oxazepam
C. Diazepam
D. The patient is using multiple benzodiazepines.

12. Urine screening for marijuana in frequent users may show positive results for up to how many days after the last use?

A. 2
B. 7
C. 27
D. 47

13. Which class of illicit drugs commonly tested in urine drug screens is most likely to yield a false-positive result?

A. Opioids
B. Benzodiazepines
C. Methamphetamines
D. Cannabinoids

14. A 21-year-old male patient presents for consultation at an outpatient pain practice seeking a prescription for extended-release oxymorphone for the treatment of chronic pain. Urine drug screening is positive for morphine, hydromorphone, oxymorphone, and methadone. The most appropriate descriptor for this patient is which one of the following?

A. "Strung out"
B. "A patient with opioid addiction"
C. "Junkie"
D. "Drug seeker"

15. What is the mechanism of action of naloxone?

A. $GABA_A$ receptor agonist
B. Mu opioid agonist
C. Mu opioid antagonist
D. Partial mu opioid agonist

16. What is the mechanism of action of buprenorphine?

A. $GABA_A$ receptor agonist
B. Mu opioid agonist
C. Mu opioid antagonist
D. Partial mu opioid agonist

17. What is the mechanism of action of methadone?

A. $GABA_A$ receptor agonist
B. Mu opioid agonist

C. Mu opioid antagonist
D. Partial mu opioid agonist

18. A 30-year-old uninsured male patient presents to an addiction specialist in an outpatient medical office seeking assistance for treatment of opioid addiction. He discloses a 2-year history of daily opioid use, which has recently escalated to occasional intravenous (IV) heroin use. He also has been using oral alprazolam 2-mg tablets, three or four times daily for several years, that he obtains from various sources. His last dose of either drug was 24 hours prior. The Clinical Opiate Withdrawal Scale (COWS) is 20, indicative of moderate withdrawal. What is the best course of action?

A. Induce the patient with buprenorphine/naloxone as part of a comprehensive outpatient treatment strategy. Instruct the patient to stop benzodiazepines and that they are absolutely not to be used in combination with this therapy.
B. Prescribe clonidine 0.1 mg twice daily and recommend complete abstinence from further illicit drug use.
C. Formulate a comprehensive treatment strategy to include induction of buprenorphine/naloxone under close supervision, as well as recommendation of a slow benzodiazepine taper.
D. Refer the patient to a local Narcotics Anonymous program and recommend complete abstinence from further illicit drug use.

19. A 23-year-old intubated male arrives in the trauma intensive care unit (ICU) with multiple traumatic injuries following a motorcycle accident. A family member discloses that he struggles with an active heroin addiction. What is the best approach in treating this patient's pain during his stay in the ICU?

A. Avoid treatment with any opioid medications to prevent enabling and furthering his addiction.
B. Initiate a methadone titration for the treatment of pain as well as addiction maintenance.
C. Treat heroin withdrawal with intramuscular (IM) buprenorphine and IV clonidine according to the COWS protocol.
D. Implement a multimodal treatment strategy, including treatment with adequate opioid analgesics as needed, with the understanding that this patient's opioid requirement may be increased due to chronic heroin use and opioid tolerance.

20. A 23-year-old male with a medical history of opioid addiction is recovering in the hospital 2 weeks after sustaining multiple traumatic injuries in a motorcycle accident. The primary service requests a consultation from the inpatient pain service. On initial evaluation, he is agitated and complains of uncontrolled pain. His medication regimen includes extended-release morphine 60 mg twice daily, immediate-release oxycodone 20 mg every 6 hours as needed for pain, and multiple adjunctive non-opioid agents. The patient's nurse notes that he is sedated for 1 or 2 hours following oxycodone administration, but the patient becomes agitated and requests more pain medication immediately upon awakening. His vital signs are regularly monitored and have been stable. The primary service would like to discharge the patient as soon as his pain is adequately controlled. What is the best course of action?

A. Discharge the patient on the current regimen because the optimal dose has been achieved.
B. Increase the dosage of extended-release morphine to achieve more stable pain control.
C. Coordinate with the psychiatry service to formulate a plan to address the patient's opioid addiction.
D. Stop oxycodone due to concern for excessive sedation and respiratory depression.

21. Naloxone distribution for patients at risk of opioid overdose is an example of a harm reduction approach to prevent overdose fatalities. Which one of the following statements is true about harm reduction?

A. This approach encourages users to continue risky drug-related behaviors.
B. Published research has shown this approach to be ineffective in reducing mortality.
C. Physicians who do not supply injectable naloxone to addicted patients are at risk of sanction by the medical board.
D. Opioid overdose prevention programs (OOPPs) train nonmedical bystanders to identify the symptoms of overdose and then administer naloxone prior to the arrival of emergency and medical personnel.

22. According to the 2013 Substance Abuse and Mental Health Services Administration's National Survey on Drug Use and Health (NSDUH), the majority of persons who use opioids for nonmedical purposes obtain them from what source?

A. Family or friends
B. The Internet
C. A drug dealer
D. Multiple doctors

23. A woman with a history of IV heroin use has been successfully managed by a methadone maintenance treatment center at 30 mg methadone daily. A pregnancy test is positive. She should be advised to:

A. Stop methadone immediately and be abstinent from all opioids throughout the pregnancy
B. Completely wean off of methadone by the third trimester to prevent neonatal abstinence syndrome (NAS)
C. Stop methadone and start sublingual buprenorphine 16 mg daily
D. Continue methadone treatment and that her dose may need to be increased in the third trimester of pregnancy

24. A woman with a history of IV heroin abuse delivers a newborn infant at 39 weeks of gestation. She has been maintained on 80 mg methadone daily throughout the pregnancy. The infant is most at risk for having which of the following physical characteristics?

A. Smooth philtrum
B. Short palpebral fissures
C. Small for gestational age
D. Congenital heart disease

25. What is an appropriate conclusion from the Maternal Opioid Treatment: Human Experimental Research (MOTHER) trial?

A. Buprenorphine is superior to methadone for use during pregnancy and is the new gold standard.
B. Methadone is superior to buprenorphine for use during pregnancy and remains the gold standard.
C. Buprenorphine is as safe as methadone for use during pregnancy and may lead to less neonatal withdrawal.
D. Buprenorphine/naloxone combinations should not be used in pregnancy.

26. According to the "Public Policy Statement on the Rights and Responsibilities of Healthcare Professionals in the Use of Opioids for the Treatment of Pain," a consensus document issued by the American Academy of Pain Medicine, the American Pain Society, and the American Society of Addiction Medicine, health care professionals should be held responsible for which one of the following?

A. To prevent and recognize willful and deceptive behavior of patients who are seeking out opioids for nonmedical purposes
B. To follow patients at reasonable intervals to confirm medications are being used as prescribed and that the goals of treatment are being met
C. To only prescribe opioid medications for patients with objective findings that correlate with their complaints of pain

D. To refuse to prescribe opioid medications for patients with a history of addiction or high-risk factors for the development of addiction

27. In the United States, the enactment of the Drug Addiction Treatment Act of 2000 (DATA 2000) allowed for which one of the following?

A. Opioid treatment programs (OTPs) to dispense Schedule II opioid medications, such as methadone, for the treatment of both pain and addiction
B. Physicians in a medical office, outside of an OTP, to prescribe Schedule III, IV, and V opioid medications approved by the US Food and Drug Administration (FDA) (e.g., buprenorphine/naloxone) for the treatment of addiction
C. OTPs to prescribe Schedule II opioid medications, such as methadone, to be dispensed by pharmacies in 30-day quantities
D. Physicians in a medical office or hospital to prescribe opioid medications to patients with documented pain, despite a personal history of addiction, without threat of legal sanction

28. A 44-year-old male with a remote history of heroin addiction presents to an outpatient pain practice for an initial consultation. He has been treated for the past 5 years with maintenance methadone therapy through a local OTP, with a current daily dose of 60 mg methadone per day. He also has debilitating low back pain, and the methadone has been very effective in managing his chronic pain. Due to the expense of frequent visits to the OTP, he requests transfer of his methadone management to the pain practice. What is the most appropriate action?

A. Assume the methadone prescription but slowly wean the dose while implementing a multidisciplinary plan to address chronic low back pain.
B. Convert the current methadone dose to an equivalent dose of extended-release opioid such as morphine or oxycodone for improved safety profile.
C. Do not write a methadone prescription and direct the patient back to an appropriate facility for ongoing treatment of opioid addiction.
D. Assume the methadone prescription at 60 mg daily and implement appropriate screening measures for substance abuse.

29. Which US legislation mandated that opioid medications are not to be prescribed for the treatment of opioid addiction?

A. Harrison Act of 1914
B. Narcotic Addict Treatment Act of 1974

C. Anti-Drug Abuse Act of 1986
D. Drug Addiction Treatment Act of 2000

30. A 53-year-old male presents to an outpatient pain clinic for initial evaluation of chronic low back pain. He is employed as a bus driver for the local school district. As a part of routine evaluation, a urine drug screen is positive for heroin, which is then confirmed with mass spectroscopy. What is the best course of action?

A. Notify the local school district immediately of this finding because children may be at risk.
B. Discharge the patient from the practice.
C. Meet with the patient to discuss the findings and encourage referral to an addiction treatment program.
D. Initiate treatment for chronic pain with an extended-release opioid because this will have a safer profile than heroin use.

31. In general, patients with active opioid addiction will have preference for what type of opioid formulations and delivery systems?

A. Long-acting, extended-release oral formulations
B. Long-acting sublingual formulations (i.e., buprenorphine products)
C. Short-acting oral formulations
D. Short-acting IV formulations

ANSWERS

1. ANSWER: C

Several gene polymorphisms have been identified in both human and animal studies to be involved in altered drug responses and the development of addiction. It is estimated that approximately 40–60% of addiction vulnerability may be attributable to genetic factors.

FURTHER READING

Herron A, Brennan T (Eds.). *The ASAM Essentials of Addiction Medicine*. 2nd ed. Chevy Chase, MD: American Society of Addiction Medicine; 2015:Chap. 1.

Ries R, Fiellin D, Miller S, et al. (Eds.). *The ASAM Principles of Addiction Medicine*. 5th ed. Chevy Chase, MD: American Society of Addiction Medicine; 2014:Chap. 1.

2. ANSWER: B

Cytochrome P450 2D6 metabolizes codeine to morphine. An ultrarapid metabolizer will experience a rapid elevation in morphine levels after codeine administration. This would yield an exaggerated analgesic response and potential for morphine intoxication.

FURTHER READING

Herron A, Brennan T (Eds.). *The ASAM Essentials of Addiction Medicine*. 2nd ed. Chevy Chase, MD: American Society of Addiction Medicine; 2015:Chap. 6.

Ries R, Fiellin D, Miller S, et al. (Eds.). *The ASAM Principles of Addiction Medicine*. 5th ed. Chevy Chase, MD: American Society of Addiction Medicine; 2014:Chap. 6.

3. ANSWER: A

The VTA of the basal ganglia initiates a complex firing of interconnecting neurons involved in reward pathways. This is initiated by inhibition of GABA at the VTA, which ultimately causes a flood of glutamate and dopamine release downstream at the nucleus accumbens (Figure 7.1). These basal ganglia reward pathways are thought to be more controlled by instinctual drive and pleasure and less mediated by rational thought (which is moderated by the prefrontal cortex). The substantia nigra is involved in dopamine production and has been linked with reward and addiction through more indirect and complex interactions. Dopaminergic loss in the substantia nigra is associated with Parkinson's disease. The striatum is an inhibitory nucleus

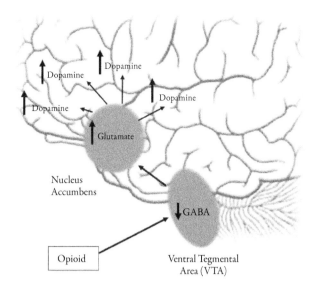

Figure 7.1 Opioid administration inhibits GABA at the ventral tegmental area of the basal ganglia, which then activates glutamate release downstream at the nucleus accumbens and leads to a surge in central dopamine levels and activation of reward pathways.

with complex involvement in a number of functions, including motor control. Atrophy of the striatum medium spiny neurons is associated with Huntington's disease and choreas. The superior colliculus is primarily involved in controlling eye movements.

FURTHER READING

Passik S, Smith H (Eds.). *Pain and Chemical Dependency*. New York, NY: Oxford University Press; 2008:Chap. 6.

Webster L, Dove B. *Avoiding Opioid Abuse While Managing Pain*. Forest Lake, MN: Sunrise River Press; 2007:Chap. 2.

4. ANSWER: B

Kappa opioid agonists do not cause self-administration or conditioned place preference (CPP) in animal models; therefore, they may have less abuse potential than the other receptors listed. Mu opioids do cause both self-administration and CPP in animal models. Delta opioids are associated with reduced respiratory depression and fewer gastrointestinal side effects, but like mu receptors, they are also involved in reward pathways. Although sigma receptors were once thought to be an opioid receptor subtype, it was later learned that these receptors have no structural similarity with opioid receptors and are not activated by opioid ligands. Sigma activation can produce euphoric or hallucinogenic effects in some subjects and therefore does have some abuse liability.

FURTHER READING

Guitart X, Codony X, Monroy X. Sigma receptors: Biology and therapeutic potential. *Psychopharmacology*. 2004;174(3):301–319.

Passik S, Smith H (Eds.). *Pain and Chemical Dependency*. New York, NY: Oxford University Press; 2008:Chap. 8.

Ries R, Fiellin D, Miller S, et al. (Eds.). *The ASAM Principles of Addiction Medicine*. 5th ed. Chevy Chase, MD: American Society of Addiction Medicine; 2014:Chap. 97.

Webster L, Dove B. *Avoiding Opioid Abuse While Managing Pain*. Forest Lake, MN: Sunrise River Press; 2007:Chap. 2.

5. ANSWER: D

Opioid receptors are G protein-coupled receptors. Repeated exposure to opioid ligands can cause uncoupling of the G protein, which renders receptors less functional and initiates a cascade of intracellular events that can lead to tolerance. The other proteins listed are also involved downstream in this cascade but are not coupled with opioid receptors.

FURTHER READING

Ries R, Fiellin D, Miller S, et al. (Eds.). *The ASAM Principles of Addiction Medicine*. 5th ed. Chevy Chase, MD: American Society of Addiction Medicine; 2014:Chap. 93.

Webster L, Dove B. *Avoiding Opioid Abuse While Managing Pain*. Forest Lake, MN: Sunrise River Press; 2007:Chap. 2.

6. ANSWER: B

Addicted patients show decreases in baseline functional magnetic resonance imaging (fMRI) activity of the prefrontal cortex, which is the "hub" of executive functioning in the brain. This includes the anterior cingulate gyrus, which is involved with inhibitory control, and the orbitofrontal cortex, which is involved in rational decision-making in relation to reward or punishment. These patients will subsequently be influenced more by limbic reward pathways, which include the ventral tegmental area and the nucleus accumbens, and will demonstrate increased baseline activity in these structures on fMRI. The cerebellum, a component of the hindbrain, is involved primarily in motor control.

FURTHER READING

Herron A, Brennan T (Eds.). *The ASAM Essentials of Addiction Medicine*. 2nd ed. Chevy Chase, MD: American Society of Addiction Medicine; 2015:Chaps. 1 and 3.

Ries R, Fiellin D, Miller S, et al. (Eds.). *The ASAM Principles of Addiction Medicine*. 5th ed. Chevy Chase, MD: American Society of Addiction Medicine; 2014:Chaps. 1 and 3.

7. ANSWER: B

The majority of patients with chronic pain likely take their medication for the appropriate reason: because of the analgesic, pain-relieving properties of the medication. If the goals of administration are met, they should also have a functional improvement related to medication use. Some patients may misuse their medication for a euphoric effect, or to "get high," but most patients on chronic opioid therapy do not experience significant cognitive dysfunction or sedating side effects from the medication; this may be more common when initiating opioid therapy but typically resolves with chronic use. The term "addiction" implies a pattern of aberrant or unhealthy behavior and should not be applied to the majority of patients who use opioids for the treatment of persistent pain. Professional attitudes regarding the risk and efficacy of opioid therapy for chronic nonmalignant pain continue to evolve, and this remains a controversial area in pain-related research and clinical practice.

FURTHER READING

Webster L, Dove B. *Avoiding Opioid Abuse While Managing Pain*. Forest Lake, MN: Sunrise River Press; 2007:Chap. 1.

8. ANSWER: B

Research in this area is somewhat limited, but studies indicate that patients with chronic pain have a tendency to abuse substances, including alcohol, at a rate of 10–18%, which is slightly higher than the rate in the general population. Approximately 2–5% of the chronic pain population manifest addiction to opioids, which is also a higher rate than that of the general population. Importantly, addiction and substance abuse are not interchangeable terms. The term addiction implies a chronic, maladaptive, relapsing disease of uncontrolled drug use despite ongoing negative consequences and self-harm. Substance abuse refers to the inappropriate use of an illegal substance or use of a legal substance excessively or for purposes other than that which it was prescribed. The term physical dependence also is not interchangeable with addiction. Physical dependence is characterized by a withdrawal syndrome if an opioid is stopped or decreased abruptly, but it is a physiological result of ongoing use and does not by itself indicate a pattern of aberrant behavior or addiction.

FURTHER READING

Savage S, Covington E, Gilson A, et al. Public policy statement on the rights and responsibilities of healthcare professionals in the use of opioids for the treatment of pain. A consensus document from the

American Academy of Pain Medicine, the American Pain Society, and the American Society of Addiction Medicine; 2004.

Webster L, Dove B. *Avoiding Opioid Abuse While Managing Pain.* Forest Lake, MN: Sunrise River Press; 2007. Chapter 1.

Webster L, Webster R. Predicting aberrant behaviors in opioid-treated patients: Preliminary validation of the Opioid Risk Tool. *Pain Med.* 2005;6(6):432–442.

9. ANSWER: D

The fifth edition of the *Diagnostic and Statistical Manual of Mental Disorders* (DSM-5) criteria for substance use disorder (Box 7.1) must be utilized cautiously in patients using opioids for pain, especially in relation to tolerance and physical dependence. Continued use of a substance, tolerance,

---

Box 7.1 DSM-5 CRITERIA FOR SUBSTANCE USE DISORDER

Definition: A problematic pattern of substance use leading to clinically significant impairment or distress as manifested by at least two of the following occurring in a 12-month period:

1. The substance is often taken in larger amounts or over a longer period of time than intended.
2. There is a persistent desire or unsuccessful efforts to cut down or control substance use.
3. A great deal of time is spent in activities necessary to obtain the substance, use, or recover from its effects.
4. Craving, or a strong desire to use the substance.
5. Recurrent substance use resulting in failure to fulfill major role obligations at work, school, or home.
6. Continued substance use despite having persistent or recurrent social or interpersonal problems caused or exacerbated by the effects of the substance.
7. Important social, occupational, or recreational activities are given up or reduced because of substance use.
8. Recurrent substance use in situations in which it is physically hazardous.
9. Continued use despite knowledge of having a persistent or recurrent physical or psychological problem that is likely to have been caused or exacerbated by the substance.
10. Tolerance, as defined by either of the following:
    (a) A need for markedly increased amounts of the substance to achieve intoxication or desired effect.
    (b) Markedly diminished effect with continued use of the same amount of the substance.
11. Withdrawal, as manifested by either of the following:
    (a) The characteristic withdrawal syndrome for the substance.
    (b) The substance is taken to relieve or avoid withdrawal symptoms.

---

physical dependence, and withdrawal may apply to a patient using opioids appropriately for pain without a diagnosis of addiction.

FURTHER READING

American Psychiatric Association. *Diagnostic and Statistical Manual of Mental Disorders* 5th ed. Arlington, VA: American Psychiatric Publishing; 2013.

Passik S, Smith H (Eds.). *Pain and Chemical Dependency.* New York, NY: Oxford University Press; 2008:Chap. 1.

10. ANSWER: C

The ORT assesses risk through a scoring system based on the five categories listed in Question 10. A score of 0–3 is considered low risk, a score of 4–7 is considered moderate risk, and a score of 8 or greater is high risk for opioid addiction.

FURTHER READING

Webster L, Webster R. Predicting aberrant behaviors in opioid-treated patients: Preliminary validation of the Opioid Risk Tool. *Pain Med.* 2005;6(6):432–442.

11. ANSWER: C

The interpretation of urine drug screens is complicated by the variety of drugs available and their various metabolites. Diazepam is rapidly metabolized into three active metabolites: nordiazepam, temazepam, and oxazepam. The parent drug will often not test positive because of relatively rapid metabolism. The use of oxazepam alone would not be associated with the presence of the other two metabolites. Importantly, oxazepam is the end product of diazepam metabolism and may be the sole metabolite remaining several days after infrequent diazepam use. Clonazepam is metabolized to 7-aminoclonazepam and may not be detected on many standard urine drug screens.

FURTHER READING

Herron A, Brennan T (Eds.). *The ASAM Essentials of Addiction Medicine.* 2nd ed. Chevy Chase, MD: American Society of Addiction Medicine; 2015:Chap. 19.

Practical Pain Management. Understanding the toxicology of diazepam, 2012. Available at http://www.practicalpainmanagement.com.

12. ANSWER: C

Tetrahydrocannabinol (THC) is the primary active component of the marijuana plant. Although the half-life is

20–30 hours, THC is highly lipophilic and absorbed into fat tissues and then is slowly released over time. The detection time for marijuana varies depending on frequency and chronicity of use and the sensitivity of the assay. In frequent users, urine specimens have been shown to be positive for up to 27 days after last use.

FURTHER READING

Herron A, Brennan T (Eds.). *The ASAM Essentials of Addiction Medicine*. 2nd ed. Chevy Chase, MD: American Society of Addiction Medicine; 2015:Chap. 19.

13. ANSWER: C

Urine toxicology results should be interpreted with caution. False-positive results for amphetamines and methamphetamines are more commonly reported than for opioids, benzodiazepines, and cannabinoids. Results from rapid-screening immunoassays should be confirmed using additional analytical methods, such as gas chromatography–mass spectrometry, and findings should be utilized in conjunction with consideration of clinical trends, risk assessment, and a complete patient assessment.

FURTHER READING

Brahm N, Yeager L, Fox M, et al. Commonly prescribed medications and potential false-positive urine drug screens. *Am J Health Syst Pharm*. 2010;67(16):1344–1350.

14. ANSWER: B

Addiction is now recognized as a disease that necessitates appropriate screening, prevention, and intervention, which requires full participation of the medical community. Medical professionals should avoid using slang terms and should treat patients with dignity and respect regardless of the disease process involved, including the disease of addiction.

FURTHER READING

Ries R, Fiellin D, Miller S, et al. (Eds.). *The ASAM Principles of Addiction Medicine*. 5th ed. Chevy Chase, MD: American Society of Addiction Medicine; 2014:Chap. 1.

15. ANSWER: C

Naloxone is a semisynthetic mu opioid antagonist typically available in IV, IM, or intranasal formulations and is primarily utilized for reversal of opioid overdose. The duration of action is 30–60 minutes. It is also used as an abuse deterrent in some oral drug formulations, such as buprenorphine/naloxone combination products to prevent IV drug abuse.

FURTHER READING

Herron A, Brennan T (Eds.). *The ASAM Essentials of Addiction Medicine*. 2nd ed. Chevy Chase, MD: American Society of Addiction Medicine; 2015:Chap. 9.
Ries R, Fiellin D, Miller S, et al. (Eds.). *The ASAM Principles of Addiction Medicine*. 5th ed. Chevy Chase, MD: American Society of Addiction Medicine; 2014:Chap. 9.

16. ANSWER: D

The pharmacology of buprenorphine is complex. It is a partial mu opioid agonist and a partial kappa agonist. It has high affinity for the opioid receptor, thus the risk for precipitated withdrawal if given following recent use of a full opioid agonist. The drug has a ceiling effect and thus decreased risk for respiratory depression compared with full opioid agonists. The sublingual formulation of buprenorphine is typically used for the treatment of opioid addiction. There is also a transdermal formulation that is FDA approved for the treatment of pain.

FURTHER READING

Ries R, Fiellin D, Miller S, et al. (Eds.). *The ASAM Principles of Addiction Medicine*. 5th ed. Chevy Chase, MD: American Society of Addiction Medicine; 2014:Chap. 97.

17. ANSWER: B

Methadone is a synthetic, full mu opioid agonist. It also has NMDA antagonist properties, which may make it more effective for neuropathic pain and less likely to contribute to hyperalgesia and tolerance. The half-life of racemic methadone is long and unpredictable (5–130 hours) but averages approximately 24 hours. The analgesic effects of methadone are short-lived in comparison to the respiratory depressant effects. Incomplete cross-tolerance with other opioid agonists is common, and conversion to methadone from other opioids is very complex with wide dose variability. These factors necessitate very slow, cautious titration when implementing methadone treatment. Methadone is metabolized by cytochrome P450 and has multiple drug interactions. At higher doses, it can cause significant QTc prolongation, which can progress to torsades de pointes. Methadone is highly lipophilic and has a prolonged elimination phase. Methadone and its metabolites are eliminated by both renal and fecal routes. Interestingly, methadone was developed by Germany prior to the start of World War II because of the need by the Nazi regime for a reliable internal source of opioids.

FURTHER READING

Passik S, Smith H (Eds.). *Pain and Chemical Dependency*. New York, NY: Oxford University Press; 2008:Chap. 16.
Ries R, Fiellin D, Miller S, et al. (Eds.). *The ASAM Principles of Addiction Medicine*. 5th ed. Chevy Chase, MD: American Society of Addiction Medicine; 2014:Chap. 97.

18. ANSWER: C

Although opioid withdrawal is rarely fatal in healthy subjects, abrupt benzodiazepine withdrawal may be life threatening. A closely supervised comprehensive strategy should be formulated, whether inpatient or outpatient, that also takes into consideration the medical dangers of benzodiazepine withdrawal. Although combining buprenorphine or any opioid with benzodiazepines increases the risk for respiratory depression and death, abrupt benzodiazepine withdrawal is not a safe option in this situation. Clonidine is a useful adjunct to treat the sympathetic effects during withdrawal. Recommending immediate complete abstinence is not likely to be effective. Narcotics Anonymous programs have been shown to be useful in the long-term treatment of addiction, but these will not address the immediate effects of withdrawal and are generally more effective at preventing relapse when combined with a comprehensive strategy that includes some form of medical maintenance, especially in the initial treatment phase.

FURTHER READING

Herron A, Brennan T (Eds.). *The ASAM Essentials of Addiction Medicine*. 2nd ed. Chevy Chase, MD: American Society of Addiction Medicine; 2015:Chap. 9.
Ries R, Fiellin D, Miller S, et al. (Eds.). *The ASAM Principles of Addiction Medicine*. 5th ed. Chevy Chase, MD: American Society of Addiction Medicine; 2014:Chap. 9.

19. ANSWER: D

In an acute setting, patients with opioid addiction should be managed in a similar manner as any other patient. Opioid analgesics, multimodal therapies, and regional anesthetics should be implemented where appropriate. Understanding that a patient struggles with opioid addiction may help in titrating opioid analgesics to appropriate dosages to adequately manage acute and subacute pain. Throughout the rehabilitation process, a plan for opioid optimization or discontinuation and addiction treatment should be openly implemented in coordination with the patient and other caregivers. The ICU is generally not an appropriate setting to initiate methadone maintenance for the treatment of addiction, although methadone may be a useful adjunctive agent in the treatment of pain if the medical providers are experienced with its use and understand its unique pharmacology. Although the COWS and a corresponding treatment protocol with clonidine and buprenorphine would be an appropriate avenue for a hospitalized patient seeking treatment for addiction, it would not be initiated in an acute setting of trauma.

FURTHER READING

Ries R, Fiellin D, Miller S, et al. (Eds.). *The ASAM Principles of Addiction Medicine*. 5th ed. Chevy Chase, MD: American Society of Addiction Medicine; 2014:Chap. 97.

20. ANSWER: C

Patients with both pain and addiction often present under very challenging clinical circumstances. Even with attentive care in a hospital setting, it can be very difficult to safely and effectively achieve appropriate analgesia. Patients who are highly tolerant to opioids may have more postoperative or post-traumatic pain despite escalating doses, and they may be more prone to developing opioid-induced sedation and respiratory depression. Opioid-induced hyperalgesia may also contribute to increases in pain as opioids are titrated upward. In addition, addicted patients seeking the euphoric effects of opioids may not reliably report their analgesic response. Non-opioid interventions should be maximized as much as possible. A multidisciplinary approach to the treatment of both pain and addiction should be implemented, and addiction specialists should be utilized where possible to assist with both immediate and long-term planning.

FURTHER READING

Ries R, Fiellin D, Miller S, et al. (Eds.). *The ASAM Principles of Addiction Medicine*. 5th ed. Chevy Chase, MD: American Society of Addiction Medicine; 2014:Chap. 98.

21. ANSWER: D

OOPPs train family members and bystanders to recognize the signs of opioid overdose and then properly administer treatment with injectable naloxone. Although harm reduction programs are not specifically focused on reducing the prevalence of drug use, there may be motivation for some users involved in these programs to seek help in reducing or discontinuing drug use. Although the benefits of naloxone distribution programs have not been definitively established, the evidence is encouraging that such programs may reduce mortality at the population level. More research is needed to determine the benefits of these programs and the most appropriate methods for implementation. Currently, there is no established standard of care or evidence-based guideline that would mandate naloxone distribution to patients at risk for opioid overdose.

FURTHER READING

Herron A, Brennan T (Eds.). *The ASAM Essentials of Addiction Medicine*. 2nd ed. Chevy Chase, MD: American Society of Addiction Medicine; 2015:Chap. 30.
Ries R, Fiellin D, Miller S, et al. (Eds.). *The ASAM Principles of Addiction Medicine*. 5th ed. Chevy Chase, MD: American Society of Addiction Medicine; 2014:Chap. 30.

22. ANSWER: A

The 2012–2013 NSDUH reported the following statistics for persons who used opioids for nonmedical purposes:

- 53% received them from a friend or relative for free. 84% of these persons reported that their friend or relative obtained the drugs from just a single doctor.
- 21% received them through a prescription from one doctor.
- 15% bought or took them from a friend or relative.
- 4% got them from a drug dealer or other stranger.
- 2.6% got them from more than one doctor.
- 0.1% bought pain relievers on the Internet.
- 0.7% stole them from a doctor's office, clinic, hospital, or pharmacy.

FURTHER READING

Substance Abuse and Mental Health Services Administration (SAMHSA). Results from the 2013 National Survey on Drug Use and Health: Summary of national findings. NSDUH Series H-48, HHS Publication No. (SMA) 14–4863. Rockville, MD: SAMHSA; 2014.

23. ANSWER: D

There is no FDA-approved treatment for opioid addiction in pregnant patients, although methadone maintenance therapy has been considered the gold standard for decades. Medical withdrawal of the pregnant patient from opioids is not recommended because of the high rate of relapse, which exposes the mother to increased risk and also increases the likelihood of fetal intrauterine death. Maintaining a stable methadone dose reduces the stress on the fetus and prevents maternal relapse and harm from exposure to illicit substances. Larger plasma volume, increased methadone metabolism and clearance, decreased plasma protein binding, and increased tissue binding may necessitate increased methadone doses in the third trimester of pregnancy.

FURTHER READING

Herron A, Brennan T (Eds.). *The ASAM Essentials of Addiction Medicine*. 2nd ed. Chevy Chase, MD: American Society of Addiction Medicine; 2015:Chap. 83.
Ries R, Fiellin D, Miller S, et al. (Eds.). *The ASAM Principles of Addiction Medicine*. 5th ed. Chevy Chase, MD: American Society of Addiction Medicine; 2014:Chap. 83.

24. ANSWER: C

Both methadone and buprenorphine maintenance during pregnancy are most likely to be complicated by low birth weight and NAS. The other choices are physical characteristics commonly found in children with fetal alcohol syndrome.

FURTHER READING

Herron A, Brennan T (Eds.). *The ASAM Essentials of Addiction Medicine*. 2nd ed. Chevy Chase, MD: American Society of Addiction Medicine; 2015:Chap. 83.
Ries R, Fiellin D, Miller S, et al. (Eds.). *The ASAM Principles of Addiction Medicine*. 5th ed. Chevy Chase, MD: American Society of Addiction Medicine; 2014:Chap. 83.

25. ANSWER: C

The MOTHER trial compared buprenorphine maintenance with methadone maintenance for opioid-dependent women during pregnancy. Buprenorphine was shown to be just as safe as methadone for use during pregnancy and likely leads to less severe NAS. Buprenorphine/naloxone combinations were not studied in this trial. Generally, it is accepted that naloxone should not be administered to a pregnant woman because abrupt, precipitated withdrawal can lead to severe fetal distress, premature labor, or spontaneous abortion.

FURTHER READING

Jones H, Kaltenback K, Heil S, et al. Neonatal abstinence syndrome after methadone or buprenorphine exposure. *N Engl J Med.* 2010;363(24):2320–2331.

26. ANSWER: B

Health care professionals (HCPs) should "use clear and reasonable medical judgment to establish that a pain state exists and to determine whether opioids are an indicated component of treatment." Patients should be followed at reasonable intervals to confirm that the medications are being used as prescribed and that the goals of treatment are being met. HCPs who use reasonable medical judgment "should not be held responsible for the willful and deceptive behavior of patients who successfully obtain opioids for nonmedical purposes." Medical judgment regarding the appropriateness of the use of opioids for pain is made by examining multiple factors in the context of the provider–patient relationship and will vary depending on the clinical situation. It is the HCPs responsibility to make an informed clinical decision using sound medical judgment; this may include prescribing opioids for patients without objective physical exam findings or for patients with risk factors for addiction.

FURTHER READING

Savage S, Covington E, Gilson A, et al. Public policy statement on the rights and responsibilities of healthcare professionals in the use of opioids for the treatment of pain. A consensus document from the American Academy of Pain Medicine, the American Pain Society, and the American Society of Addiction Medicine; 2004.

27. ANSWER: B

DATA 2000 was implemented to provide greater access to treatment for patients with opioid addiction. Prior to its enactment, this was essentially limited to the use of methadone, a Schedule II substance, which was only to be dispensed in federally approved OTPs. DATA 2000 allows for physicians in a regular medical office to dispense or prescribe Schedule III, IV, and V opioid medications that have been approved by the FDA for the treatment of addiction (i.e., buprenorphine/naloxone), although with some restrictions. Treating physicians must obtain a "DATA waiver" by completing a basic training course and applying for a special DEA number—an "X-number." Physicians are given a waiver to prescribe for a total of 30 patients per month for the first year, and they can apply for a waiver to treat 100 patients per month thereafter. Some states have passed provisions that further regulate treatment protocols beyond DATA 2000, such as restricting the use of buprenorphine monoproduct (Subutex) except for pregnant women and nursing mothers and patients with documented naloxone allergy and prohibiting the off-label use of sublingual buprenorphine products for the treatment of pain. Physicians prescribing buprenorphine products should become familiar with the specific regulations of that state. Transdermal buprenorphine products (butrans) are FDA approved for the treatment of pain and therefore do not require a special waiver.

FURTHER READING

Center for Substance Abuse Treatment (CSAT). *Clinical Guidelines for the Use of Buprenorphine in the Treatment of Opioid Addiction.* Treatment Improvement Protocol (TIP) Series 40, Executive Summary. Rockville, MD: CSAT; 2004.

28. ANSWER: C

There is no legal avenue, outside of an OTP or an inpatient rehabilitation program, for the prescribing of methadone in a patient with a diagnosis of opioid addiction. Although methadone is commonly used and can legally be prescribed for the treatment of chronic pain, methadone maintenance for the treatment of addiction cannot legally be managed by a regular outpatient medical practice. This patient has a history of heroin addiction and has been on methadone maintenance through an OTP, so this prescription should not be assumed under the guise of treatment for chronic pain. Although implementing multidisciplinary care is likely an excellent strategy, it should not be combined with methadone treatment in this situation. Prescribing an opioid for pain in a patient with a history of addiction is at the provider's discretion and may depend on the clinical circumstances, but a prescription of an extended-release opioid for pain would not likely have improved safety in this patient compared with the closely monitored setting of an OTP. Furthermore, conversion of methadone to other opioids is problematic due to significant interpatient variability in methadone pharmacodynamics.

FURTHER READING

Herron A, Brennan T (Eds.). *The ASAM Essentials of Addiction Medicine.* 2nd ed. Chevy Chase, MD: American Society of Addiction Medicine; 2015:Chap. 50.
Ries R, Fiellin D, Miller S, et al. (Eds.). *The ASAM Principles of Addiction Medicine.* 5th ed. Chevy Chase, MD: American Society of Addiction Medicine; 2014:Chap. 50.

29. ANSWER: A

The Harrison Act was passed in 1914 and was primarily focused on regulating commerce surrounding opioid prescribing and dispensing in the United States. A clause applying to doctors allowed distribution "in the course of his professional practice only." This was interpreted to mean that a doctor could not prescribe opioids for the treatment of addiction because addiction at that time was not considered a disease. In 1919, this was upheld by the Supreme Court, reinforcing that physicians could not legally prescribe opioids for the maintenance of addiction. The Narcotic Addict Treatment Act of 1974 was the first law to address legitimate medical maintenance treatment for addiction, and it required that physicians obtain a separate registration to prescribe methadone to an opioid-addicted patient and also that they adhere to a set of treatment standards. The Anti-Drug Abuse Act of 1986 was focused on reducing illicit drug use and increasing prison sentencing for those found in possession of illicit drugs, especially cocaine. DATA 2000 allows for physicians in a regular medical office to dispense or prescribe Schedule III, IV, and V opioid medications that have been approved by the FDA for the treatment of addiction (i.e., buprenorphine/naloxone), although with some restrictions.

FURTHER READING

Center for Substance Abuse Treatment (CSAT). *Clinical Guidelines for the Use of Buprenorphine in the Treatment of Opioid Addiction.* Treatment Improvement Protocol (TIP) Series 40. Rockville, MD: CSAT; 2004.
Center for Substance Abuse Treatment (CSAT). *Medication-Assisted Treatment for Opioid Addiction in Opioid Treatment Programs.* Treatment Improvement Protocol (TIP) Series 43. Rockville, MD: CSAT; 2005:Chap. 2.
White W. *Slaying the Dragon: The History of Addiction Treatment and Recovery in America.* Bloomington, IL: Chestnut Health Systems/Lighthouse Institute; 1998.

30. ANSWER: C

Although it may seem important to notify the patient's employer of risky behavior related to drug use, in the medical profession in the United States, confidentiality is sacrosanct, and reporting this finding to the patient's employer or law enforcement would violate medical confidentiality laws. This patient has not specifically expressed intent to inflict harm on a third party, so a "duty to warn" obligation would likely not apply.

According to the National Conference of State Legislatures (http://www.ncsl.org/research/health/lb-duty-to-warn.aspx),

Doctors and mental health professionals are responsible for maintaining confidentiality of patient information based on the ethical standards of their profession. This concept in health care can be traced to the Roman Hippocratic Oath taken by doctors. These ethical standards have been codified into state and federal law over time, making professionals legally liable for breaching confidentiality. In an effort to protect potential victims from a patient's violent behavior, however, *Tarasoff v. The Regents of the University of California* in 1976 imposed a legal duty on psychotherapists to warn third parties of potential threats to their safety.

In the clinical situation presented in this question, actively helping the patient to find appropriate treatment for opioid addiction would likely be considered an appropriate step by a medical provider to "protect" both the patient and society from potential harm related to illicit drug use. Physicians are encouraged to check state laws regarding specific exceptions to confidentiality rules and can consult with their institution's ethics committee for further guidance when needed.

Immediate discharge from the practice will likely not be helpful in guiding this patient to the appropriate treatment. A nonconfrontational interview with the patient may be useful for collecting more information about illicit drug use and encouraging the patient to seek treatment. It is not advisable to prescribe an opioid to a patient with a known diagnosis of opioid addiction, except as part of a methadone treatment program or buprenorphine office-based program.

FURTHER READING

Herron A, Brennan T (Eds.). *The ASAM Essentials of Addiction Medicine.* 2nd ed. Chevy Chase, MD: American Society of Addiction Medicine; 2015:Chaps. 109–110.
Ries R, Fiellin D, Miller S, et al. (Eds.). *The ASAM Principles of Addiction Medicine.* 5th ed. Chevy Chase, MD: American Society of Addiction Medicine; 2014:Chaps. 109–110.

31. ANSWER: D

Patients with active addiction will tend to have a preference for short-acting formulations with routes of the most rapid onset, such as IV administration. A rapid rise in blood levels of a substance will boost the psychoactive, euphoric effect of the drug. Significant fluctuations in blood levels of an opioid will also lead to emotional lability and swings in anxiety and pain. Extended-release oral formulations, when used properly, will not result in such fluctuations and will have limited euphoric effects compared to short-acting formulations, but they will still have utility in the treatment of pain if titrated safely and appropriately. Sublingual buprenorphine is used for medical maintenance of opioid addiction. Due to a long half-life and only partial opioid agonism, it is less likely to produce significant euphoria compared to short-acting opioid agonists. Buprenorphine has been shown to have significant pain-relieving properties. Short-acting oral formulations will not provide as rapid a rise in blood levels as IV formulations; therefore, they may be less desired by patients who are inclined to abuse substances. When possible, transitioning patients with acute and subacute pain to extended-release oral formulations may optimize pain control while not enabling the disease of addiction.

FURTHER READING

Ries R, Fiellin D, Miller S, et al. (Eds.). *The ASAM Principles of Addiction Medicine*. 5th ed. Chevy Chase, MD: American Society of Addiction Medicine; 2014:Chap. 93.

8.

PHARMACOLOGY

Ryan Nobles

INTRODUCTION

This chapter focuses on principles of pharmacokinetics; pharmacodynamics; adverse effects; drug interactions; and common indications in regard to opioids, nonsteroidal anti-inflammatory agents, acetaminophen, anticonvulsants, and antidepressants. The questions are formulated to focus on the most relevant topics that may be tested on the listed medications, but this chapter is not a comprehensive review. The information provided should be supplemented with additional study of the cited literature in the Further Reading section for each question.

QUESTIONS

1. Which of the following manifestations in nervous system activity following nerve injury would not contribute to propagation of a chronic pain state?

    A. Increased spinal glutamate that leads to tactile allodynia from NMDA activation

    B. Increased spinal dynorphin leading to increased release of spinal γ-aminobutyric acid (GABA)

    C. Upregulation of spinal sodium channels and downregulation of potassium channels

    D. Increased activation of spinal microglia and astrocytes in segments that receive input from injured nerves

2. Which of the following explains the role of GABA and glycine in propagation of the chronic pain state following nerve injury?

    A. Agonist activity at the $GABA_A$ or glycine receptor produces a potent tactile allodynia.

    B. There is increased GABA and glycine activity with inhibitory control over Aβ primary afferent terminals following nerve injury.

    C. $GABA_A$ and glycine receptor activation becomes paradoxically excitatory following nerve injury.

    D. Nerve injury results in increased chloride transporter activity and decreases intracellular chloride.

3. Opioids have been shown to exert both spinal and supraspinal actions in modulating pain perception. Which of the following is incorrect in describing opioid's actions on neural systems?

    A. Opioid agonists inhibit injury-provoked discharge of dorsal horn neurons propagated by C fibers.

    B. Opioids postsynaptically inhibit voltage-sensitive calcium channels and reduce the binding of primary afferent peptide transmitters.

    C. Opioids activate postsynaptic potassium channels and block excitation of dorsal horn neurons by glutamate.

    D. Opioids promote outflow from the periaqueductal gray, activating ascending serotonin and noradrenergic pathways to modulate emotional response to pain.

4. Of the functions of opioid receptors listed here, which is incorrectly matched with its activity?

    A. κ receptor—thermal nociception and chemical visceral pain

    B. μ receptor—respiratory depression

    C. δ receptor—constipation

    D. μ receptor—analgesia and physical dependence

5. A 74-year-old patient who is on a 50-μg/hr fentanyl patch for lumbar post-laminectomy syndrome has noted decreased effectiveness in his pain control after starting a new medication. Which medication is most likely responsible for this change?

    A. Phenytoin

    B. Azithromycin

C. Baclofen
D. Fluconazole

6. A 68-year-old female patient with a history of type 1 diabetes has been increasingly somnolent during the past month. She is on chronic narcotic therapy for complex regional pain syndrome, type I of the right lower extremity. A recent visit to her primary care physician revealed a creatinine of 1.8 mg/dl. Which of the following medications is most likely not responsible for her sedation?

A. Morphine
B. Baclofen
C. Fentanyl
D. Hydromorphone

7. A 57-year-old male patient with chronic pancreatitis and a history of sleep apnea is being considered for long-term narcotic therapy for abdominal pain. To which of the following adverse effects of opioids does tolerance not develop?

A. Pruritis
B. Nausea and vomiting
C. Sedation
D. Constipation
E. Respiratory depression

8. A 35-year-old patient with HIV secondary to contaminated blood transfusion presents to your clinic for evaluation. He has severe neuropathic pain in his bilateral feet, is on warfarin for recurrent deep vein thrombosis, and is taking gabapentin 1200 mg three times daily with minimal relief. You are considering methadone for pain control. Which of the following immunologic effects of opioid receptor binding is incorrect?

A. μ—decreases natural killer (NK) cell activity
B. μ—promotes T cell proliferation
C. δ—increases NK cell activity
D. κ—pronounced suppression of humoral immunity

9. A 42-year-old male with daily pain from lumbar post-laminectomy syndrome has been taking methadone for the past year with adequate analgesic response. However, he has begun reporting significant side effects that are concerning. Which of the following side effects is most likely not attributable to chronic methadone therapy?

A. Decreased libido
B. Erectile dysfunction
C. Gynecomastia
D. Nocturnal emissions

10. A 48-year-old male continues to experience significant pain following a right total knee replacement despite escalating doses of hydrocodone. Which of the following of his other medications is most likely not responsible for this lack of effect of hydrocodone?

A. Quinidine
B. Fluoxetine
C. Azithromycin
D. Buproprion

11. Which of the following is a feature of morphine 6-glucuronide (M6G) and not morphine 3-glucuronide (M3G)?

A. Analgesia
B. Allodynia
C. Myoclonus
D. Seizures

12. Which feature of oxycodone results in an increased potency compared with morphine?

A. Increased lipophilicity
B. Induction of CYP2D6 enzyme
C. Higher bioavailability
D. Increased presence of active metabolites

13. A 69-year-old patient with a history of renal cell carcinoma with metastases to her lumbar spine was admitted for seizures after starting a new outpatient chronic opioid regimen. Her creatinine on admission was found to be 2.3 mg/dl. Which of the following metabolites is most likely not the cause of her seizures?

A. Morphine 3-glucuronide
B. Normeperidine
C. Hydromorphone 3-glucuronide
D. Oxymorphone

14. Which of the following is not a feature of methadone?

A. μ and δ receptor agonism
B. NMDA antagonism
C. Serotonin reuptake inhibition
D. Active metabolites

15. A 52-year-old male with left upper extremity brachial plexopathy from a motor vehicle trauma has lost his methadone prescription. He has been off the medication for 3 days but is denying any symptoms of withdrawal. What feature of methadone is responsible for this presentation?

A. Long alpha elimination phase
B. Long beta elimination phase

C. Slow renal excretion
D. Metabolism separate from the 2D6 and 3A4 CYP enzymes

16. The patient from Question 15 has a complex medical history, including coronary artery disease with multiple drug-eluting stents, schizoaffective disorder currently managed with amitriptyline, and renal failure secondary to a history of cocaine abuse. Which feature of methadone is most likely at highest risk for the patient?

A. QT prolongation
B. Active metabolite accumulation secondary to renal failure
C. Direct cardiac toxicity due to action on fast Na^+ channels
D. Acidic urinary pH levels leading to increased circulating levels

17. A new patient presents to your clinic and is taking oxymorphone 10 mg by mouth every 12 hours for chronic breast pain following mastectomy for intraductal carcinoma. Which of the following is not true in regard to oxymorphone?

A. It is 1.5 times as potent as morphine in oral formulations.
B. It is the end product of 3-O-demethylation by CYP2D6 of oxycodone.
C. It is a potent μ agonist with two to five times higher affinity than morphine.
D. It accounts for approximately 10% of oxycodone metabolites.

18. A 47-year-old patient with chronic intercostal neuralgia calls your clinic because he ran out of his current prescription for narcotics and would like a new prescription ordered by phone to his pharmacy. Which of the following medications was reclassified from Schedule III to Schedule II in 2014 due to concerns voiced by governmental regulatory commissions?

A. Tramadol
B. Oxycodone
C. Hydrocodone
D. Hydromorphone

19. Which of the following is not a shared common feature of tramadol and methadone?

A. Serotonin reuptake inhibition
B. NMDA antagonism
C. μ receptor agonist
D. Available in extended-release formulations

20. A 45-year-old male with diabetic neuropathic pain in the feet was recently started on a new medication regimen for pain, including tramadol 100 mg by mouth every 8 hours. The patient reports symptoms of racing heartbeat, shortness of breath, and tremor after being on the regimen for 1 week. Which of the following medications is most likely a part of the patient's home regimen resulting in the reported side effects?

A. Baclofen
B. Gabapentin
C. Venlafaxine
D. Carbamazepine

21. Which of the following is true regarding tramadol's pharmacologic actions?

A. Maximum serum concentration or oral dose reached in 6 hours
B. Bioavailability of 90–100% following multiple doses
C. Cannot cross the placenta
D. Metabolism primarily by spontaneous degradation and renal excretion

22. A 57-year-old female with hepatitis C and cervical post-laminectomy syndrome admits to consuming more than 20 oxycodone/acetaminophen 10/325 mg tablets per day for the past week. Through what mechanism of acetaminophen metabolism do toxic metabolites accumulate?

A. Glucuronidation and conjugation by CYP3A4 and CYP2D6 to acetophenitidin
B. Oxidative metabolism via CYP2E1 and CYP1A2 to N-acetyl-benzoquinone imine
C. Excess glutathione production and depletion of procoagulant liver enzymes
D. Renal transformation of acetaminophen to toxic metabolites phenacetin and nor-acetaminophen

23. Which of the following is not an adverse side effect attributed to acetaminophen?

A. Elevated serum alanine transaminase (ALT) with acute use of recommended doses
B. Depletion of glutathione reserves with chronic use greater than 4 g/day
C. Normal liver function transaminase with chronic use
D. Increased levels of serum opioids due to hepatic dysfunction with doses less than 4 g/day

24. According to the most recent clinical studies, which of the following patients would most likely benefit from acetaminophen over nonsteroidal anti-inflammatory agents?

A. 70-year-old type I diabetic with history of four-vessel coronary bypass at age 50 years now on daily aspirin therapy with creatinine of 0.8 mg/dl complaining of right knee pain
B. 48-year-old type II diabetic with gastroesophageal reflux disease complaining of severe left hip pain with recent X-ray demonstrating osteoarthritis in the joint
C. 67-year-old HIV patient with end-stage renal disease and hepatocellular carcinoma with right shoulder pain
D. 32-year-old patient with severe thoracic spine pain secondary to ankylosing spondylitis

25. A 63-year-old female presents with burning pain in her chest wall secondary to postherpetic neuralgia. You have decided to add a tricyclic antidepressant (TCA) for adjunctive pain control. Which of the following is not a proposed mode of TCAs analgesic action?

A. Interaction with α_2 receptors
B. Interference with serotonin reuptake
C. Propagation of sodium channels
D. Alteration of NMDA binding characteristics

26. Duloxetine has been approved by the US Food and Drug Administration (FDA) to treat all of the following pain conditions except:

A. Osteoarthritis
B. Fibromyalgia
C. Median nerve mononeuropathy
D. Painful diabetic neuropathy

27. A 45-year-old male with diabetic neuropathic pain in the feet, peptic ulcer disease, and obesity is being considered for adjunct therapy with an antidepressant. Which of the following is an incorrect side effect of TCAs and selective serotonin reuptake inhibitors (SSRIs)?

A. TCA use may be complicated by cholinergic side effects (dry mouth and urinary retention).
B. TCAs cause weight gain more frequently than SSRIs.
C. TCAs have a higher number of deaths per million prescriptions.
D. TCAs are associated with a higher incidence of peptic ulcer disease compared to SSRIs.

28. The binding of the calcium channel modulators (gabapentin and pregabalin) to what subunit of L-type voltage calcium channels results in the decreased release of glutamate, norepinephrine, and substance P?

A. $\alpha_3\delta$
B. $\alpha_2\delta$
C. $\alpha_2\gamma$
D. $\alpha_3\gamma$

29. A 52-year-old male with diabetic neuropathy is being evaluated for non-opioid medication management. To date, the patient has only taken nonsteroidal anti-inflammatory drugs (NSAIDs) and the occasional hydrocodone/acetaminophen for his pain. You are considering therapy with gabapentin. Which of the following is correct in regard to gabapentin?

A. Rapid dose titration over 1 week to 3600 mg/day in naive patients due to lack of significant side effects
B. Increased dosage required in patients with renal insufficiency
C. FDA approved for treatment of postherpetic neuralgia up to 1800 mg/day
D. Has not been studied as treatment for opioid-induced hyperalgesia

30. In considering the previously discussed patient with painful diabetic neuropathy, you realize he may be a candidate for pregabalin instead of gabapentin. Which of the following is not an advantage of pregabalin in comparison to gabapentin?

A. More rapid onset of pain relief
B. No need for dosing adjustments in renal insufficiency
C. Linear pharmacokinetics and minimal interpatient variability
D. Less dose-related adverse effects

31. A 25-year-old female with cervical spinal cord syrinx reports to your clinic for evaluation of bilateral lower extremity burning-type neuropathic pain. She has failed treatment with methadone and oxycodone. A spinal cord stimulator trial provided no relief. After doing some research on the Internet, she is interested in ziconotide as an intrathecal therapy. Which of the following side effects is not associated with ziconotide?

A. Dizziness and confusion
B. Hallucinations
C. Respiratory depression
D. Elevations in creatine kinase (CK)

32. A 61-year-old patient with a history of leukemia presents to your clinic with a new diagnosis of trigeminal neuralgia. Her sharp stabbing pain has been

unresponsive to trials of gabapentin and pregabalin. You are considering a sodium channel-modulating anticonvulsant for her next line of therapy. Which side effect is most often associated with oxcarbazepine (Trileptal) versus carbamazepine (Tegretol)?

A. Hyponatremia (<125 mmol/l)
B. Pancytopenia
C. Stevens–Johnson syndrome
D. Toxic epidermal necrolysis

33. A 37-year-old female patient with a history of migraines that started in her 20s and have become an everyday occurrence presents to your clinic seeking treatment. She has tried triptans, over-the-counter remedies, and botulinum toxin injections without benefit. You are considering topiramate (Topamax) for migraine prophylaxis. Which of the following is not a mechanism of action for topiramate?

A. Binds GABA$_A$ receptors and increases opening frequency of chloride ion channels
B. Decreases activity of L-type calcium channels
C. Carbonic anhydrase inhibitor
D. Direct antagonist of NMDA receptors

34. Which of the following clinical scenarios is not true in regard to the pharmacokinetics of NSAIDs?

A. Hypoalbuminemia will not affect pharmacokinetics because most of the plasma concentration is in unbound form proteins.
B. Because NSAIDs are rapidly absorbed following oral and rectal administration, patients with impaired gastrointestinal (GI) absorption may report poor effectiveness.
C. Renal failure mainly influences clearance of NSAIDs that form acyl glucuronides as a major elimination pathway.
D. Biotransformation in the liver is the major elimination pathway for most NSAIDs through cytochrome P450 metabolism.

35. All of the following NSAIDs are reversible cyclo-oxygenase inhibitors except:

A. Ibuprofen
B. Meloxicam
C. Aspirin
D. Clopidogrel

36. Which of the following statements is true in regard to ketorolac (Toradol)?

A. Minor binding to plasma proteins resulting in increased potency compared to other NSAIDs
B. Extensive metabolism via spontaneous plasma degradation with the production of toxic renal metabolites
C. Analgesic effect within 30 minutes, with peak effect in 1 or 2 hours in the parenteral form
D. Lack of GI adverse effects due to intravenous (IV) administration

37. A 57-year-old male is being evaluated in your clinic for new-onset lumbar radiculopathy from a far lateral right disc protrusion at L5–S1. He has started physical therapy and presents to you for initial medication management. He has a significant medical history of gastroesophageal reflux disease, coronary artery disease with drug-eluting stent placement, and diabetes mellitus type II. He is currently taking aspirin, atorvastatin, metformin, and famotidine. You elect to start him on ibuprofen and gabapentin. Which of the following is true regarding his new medication regimen?

A. Increased risk of stroke due to intravascular depletion secondary to gabapentin-related renal effects
B. Increased risk of myocardial infarction secondary to ibuprofen administration
C. Decreased risk of stroke due to cardioprotective effects of gabapentin
D. Decreased risk of renal insufficiency due to renal blood flow protective effects of ibuprofen

38. A 72-year-old patient with rheumatoid arthritis presents to your clinic for evaluation for bilateral knee pain. He is having difficulty keeping track of his medications during the day. He is currently taking ibuprofen 600 mg every 8 hours for his pain with moderate relief. You are considering switching him to meloxicam as an alternative NSAID. Which of the following is not true regarding meloxicam's profile?

A. COX-1 preferential with less GI toxicity than nonselective NSAIDs
B. 20-hour half-life making it available in once-daily dosing
C. Linear pharmacokinetics over 7.5- to 30-mg dosages
D. Near complete absorption with metabolization to four inactive metabolites

39. Which of the following is true regarding celecoxib?

A. Preferential COX-1 nonselective NSAID
B. Interferes with platelet function and contraindicated in the perioperative period

C. Half-life of 11 hours with peak plasma levels in 3 hours
D. Metabolized mainly by renal glomerular filtration and excretion

40. Which of the following statements correctly characterizes the hematologic pathways and subsequent effects by NSAIDs?

A. Endoperoxides are converted in platelets to PGI_2, which causes vasoconstriction and further platelet activation.
B. Endoperoxides are converted in endothelium to TXA_2, which causes vasodilation and inhibition of platelets.
C. All NSAIDs result in irreversible COX enzyme inhibition for the life of the platelet.
D. Platelets cannot regenerate COX enzyme.

41. A 55-year-old male with a history of coronary artery disease with three drug-eluting stents presents to your clinic complaining of acute lumbar radicular pain. His lumbar magnetic resonance image shows a paracentral disc protrusion at right L3–L4 with mild to moderate neuroforaminal narrowing. In addition to gabapentin and physical therapy, you decide to place him on a short-term NSAID regimen before proceeding with injection therapy. Which of the following NSAIDs has the least associated risk of adverse cardiac events according to recent studies?

A. Ibuprofen
B. Naproxen
C. Celecoxib
D. Meloxicam

42. A 68-year-old male with severe bilateral knee osteoarthritis presents to your clinic for evaluation. He has a history of opioid dependence and refuses to take oral narcotics. He has tried acetaminophen, gabapentin, and tizanidine for his pain without success. Knee steroid injections provide only approximately 1 week of relief. Bilateral genicular nerve blocks were unsuccessful. He has a negative cardiac history but does have a history of gastroesophageal reflux. You are considering an NSAID for his treatment. Which of the following is incorrect regarding gastrointestinal side effects of NSAIDs?

A. Ulceration is caused by epithelial lining irritation and inhibition of prostaglandin synthesis.
B. COX-2 inhibitors are preferred in patients with a history of coronary artery disease and peptic ulcer disease.
C. Alterations in platelet function secondary to NSAIDs may contribute to gastric bleeding in patients with ulcers.
D. Risk factors for adverse effects include concomitant anticoagulant use, tobacco abuse, and advanced age.

43. Which of the following is true regarding the renal effects of NSAIDs?

A. Congestive heart failure and lupus are not risk factors for renal toxicity associated with NSAIDs.
B. Alterations in prostaglandin-related blood flow are most likely responsible for adverse renal effects from NSAIDs.
C. COX-2 inhibitors are not associated with hypertension and edema.
D. Aspirin potentiates the effects of diuretics.

ANSWERS

1. ANSWER: B

Spinal glutamate may increase dramatically following neuronal insult secondary to increased spontaneous activity of the primary afferent and a loss of intrinsic inhibition that would normally modify resting glutamate levels. Evidence shows that intrathecal glutamate promotes tactile allodynia and thermal hyperalgesia through NMDA and non-NMDA mechanisms.

Spinal dynorphin appears to initiate concurrent release of glutamate and result in enhanced tactile allodynia.

Neural insult results in upregulation in multiple sodium channels and downregulation of potassium channels. One example is an increase in the expression of the $\alpha_2\delta$ subunit. Highly selective binding with gabapentin blocks the allodynic effects produced by the upregulation of the subunit.

By observation of an increasing amount of markers denoting their presence following neuronal injury, astrocytes and microglia contribute to the propagation of the chronic pain state. Astrocytes and microglia release neural-modulating substances (chemokines, proteases, nitric oxide, and cytokines) that increase spinal expression of cyclooxygenase, nitric oxide synthetase, and glutamate transporters.

FURTHER READING

Benzon H, Rathmell JP, Wu CL, et al. (Eds.). *Practical Management of Pain*. 5th ed. Philadelphia, PA: Mosby; 2014.

2. ANSWER: C

Interneurons in the dorsal horn form presynaptic terminal complexes that modulate large Aβ primary afferents through GABA and glycine. Studies have shown that antagonists to the GABA$_A$ or glycine receptor produce a potent tactile allodynia. Following neuronal injury, GABA$_A$ and glycine receptor activation becomes paradoxically excitatory. The responsible receptors are chloride ionophores, which maintain a transmembrane gradient by the export of chloride. Nerve injury results in decreased chloride transporter activity and increases in intracellular chloride. Now, when afferent input activates GABA and glycine activity, an exaggerated response to the Aβ primary afferents is observed.

FURTHER READING

Benzon H, Rathmell JP, Wu CL, et al. (Eds.). *Practical Management of Pain*. 5th ed. Philadelphia, PA: Mosby; 2014.

3. ANSWER: B

Opioid agonists are responsible for inhibition of injury-provoked discharge of dorsal horn neurons propagated by C fibers. Dorsal horn neurons also receive afferent Aβ input that does not appear to be blocked by opioids. Opioids block the activation of voltage-sensitive calcium channels and thereby reduce the presynaptic release of primary afferent peptide transmitters (substance P). Opioids activate postsynaptic potassium channels and counteract the excitatory actions of glutamate in dorsal horn neurons.

Opioids also have multiple supraspinal mechanisms that modify pain behaviors. Opioids act on presynaptic GABA terminals, blocking their inhibitory effect on outflow from periaqueductal gray neurons. Uninhibited periaqueductal gray outflow activates serotonin and noradrenergic pathways projecting into the limbic forebrain, which influences the emotional response to pain.

SUGGESTED READING

Benzon H, Rathmell JP, Wu CL, et al. (Eds.). *Practical Management of Pain*. 5th ed. Philadelphia, PA: Mosby; 2014.

4. ANSWER: C

The three best characterized opioid receptors (μ, δ, and κ) belong to a family of guanine protein-coupled receptors located pre- and postsynaptically at sites in the central nervous system (CNS) and peripheral tissues. The κ receptor is similar to the μ receptor in that it influences thermal nociception but, in addition, it also modulates chemical visceral pain. The δ receptor influences mechanical and inflammatory pain. A study with μ knockout mice found that they have no response to morphine regarding analgesia, respiratory depression, constipation, or physical dependence.

FURTHER READING

Benzon H, Rathmell JP, Wu CL, et al. (Eds.). *Practical Management of Pain*. 5th ed. Philadelphia, PA: Mosby; 2014.
Keiffer BL. Opioids: First lessons from knockout mice. *Trends Pharmacol Sci*. 1999;20:19–26.
Martin M, Matifas A, Maldonado R, et al. Acute antinociceptive responses in single and combinatorial opioid receptor knockout mice: Distinct mu, delta and kappa tones. *Eur J Neurosci*. 2003;24:198–205.

5. ANSWER: A

The cytochrome P450 system is responsible for the metabolism of certain opioids. Two isoforms of CYP have been studied in regard to opioid biotransformation: 2D6 and 3A4. 2D6 is responsible for biotransformation of codeine, oxycodone, and hydrocodone. 3A4 is responsible for rendering fentanyl and methadone to their inactive forms. Certain drugs can affect the ability of 3A4's action on opioids. Macrolide antibiotics (erythromycin, clarithromycin, azithromycin, etc.) appear to decrease the clearance of methadone and fentanyl. Anticonvulsants (phenytoin) induce activation of the enzyme and increase clearance.

FURTHER READING

Benzon H, Rathmell JP, Wu CL, et al. (Eds.). *Practical Management of Pain*. 5th ed. Philadelphia, PA: Mosby; 2014.
Labroo RB, Paine MF, Thummel KE, et al. Fentanyl metabolism by human hepatic and intestinal cytochrome P4503A4: Implications for interindividual variability in disposition, efficacy, and drug interactions. *Drug Metab Dispos*. 1997;25:1072–1080.
Tempelhoff R, Modica PA, Spitznagel EL. Anticonvulsant therapy increases fentanyl requirements during anaesthesia for craniotomy. *Can J Anaesth*. 1990;37:327–332.

6. ANSWER: C

Many medications used for chronic pain management may undergo transformation to active metabolites that can accumulate in the setting of renal insufficiency. Opioids with hydroxyl groups (morphine and hydromorphone) undergo hepatic metabolism via uridine disphosphate glucuronosyltransferase enzymes, which converts the opioids to glucuronide metabolites. These metabolites then undergo renal excretion. In patients with renal insufficiency, metabolites may accumulate, leading to an increased incidence of adverse events.

Fentanyl mainly undergoes hepatic biotransformation through the CYP3A4 enzyme to norfentanyl.

Baclofen is primarily a GABA$_B$ agonist and should be used with caution in patients with renal insufficiency.

FURTHER READING

Benzon H, Rathmell JP, Wu CL, et al. (Eds.). *Practical Management of Pain*. 5th ed. Philadelphia, PA: Mosby; 2014.
Mervyn D. Opioids in renal failure and dialysis patients. *J Pain Symptom Manage*. 2004;28:497–504.

7. ANSWER: D

All of the listed side effects of opioids are commonly encountered. Pruritis occurs more frequently with intravenous and neuraxial opioids and appears to be secondary to histamine release activating C-fiber itch receptors. It can be treated with antihistamines or low dosages of nalbuphine (κ receptor agonist). Nausea and vomiting typically may last 2 or 3 days. Causative factors include activation in the medullary chemoreceptor trigger zone, stimulation in the vestibular apparatus, and constipation. Sedation usually occurs in opioid-naive patients or those undergoing dose escalations, and it abates at approximately 7 days. Sedation that persists may be secondary to other medications (benzodiazepines, tricyclics, and muscle relaxants) or hepatic/renal insufficiency. Respiratory depression is secondary to μ receptor-induced depression of brainstem centers that control respiratory drive. Naloxone should be administered in patients who cannot be aroused with careful titration to avoid withdrawal symptoms, seizures, and severe pain.

Constipation is the most common side effect of opioids, and tolerance does not usually develop. The mechanism is secondary to opioid binding to receptors in the antrum of the stomach and proximal small bowel. Current data on transdermal opioids have not proven a decreased incidence of constipation.

FURTHER READING

Benzon H, Rathmell JP, Wu CL, et al. (Eds.). *Practical Management of Pain*. 5th ed. Philadelphia, PA: Mosby; 2014.
Charuluxananan S, Kyokong O, Somboonviboon W, et al. Nalbuphine versus ondansetron for prevention of intrathecal morphine-induced pruritus after cesarean delivery. *Anesth Analg*. 2003;96:1789–1793.
Choi YS, Billings JA. Opioid antagonists: A review of their role in palliative care, focusing on use in opioid-related constipation. *J Pain Symptom Manage*. 2002;24:71–79.
Holtzman M, Fishman SM. Opioid receptors. In: Benzon HT, Raja SN, Molloy RE, et al. (Eds.), *Essentials of Pain and Regional Anesthesia*. Philadelphia, PA: Churchill Livingstone; 2005:87–93.
Simoneau II, Hamza MS, Mata HP, et al.: The cannabinoid agonist WIN55,212–2 suppresses opioid-induced emesis in ferrets. *Anesthesiology*. 2001;94:882–887.
Zacny JP. A review of the effects of opiates on psychomotor and cognitive functioning in humans. *Exp Clin Psychopharmacol*. 1995;3:432–466.

8. ANSWER: B

Opioids have complex and varying effects on the immune response. Despite the observation that exogenous opioids may result in immunosuppression, endorphins appear to be immune system stimulators. Short- and long-term opioid use negatively effects antibody responses, natural killer cell activity, cytokine expression, and phagocytic activity. Opioids appear to induce a central influence on the immune system through the hypothalamic–pituitary–adrenal axis and autonomic nervous system. The actions of different opioid receptors on the immune system are outlined in Table 8.1.

Table 8.1 OPIOID RECEPTORS ACTIONS ON THE IMMUNE SYSTEM

RECEPTOR	ACTIVITY
μ	Decreases NK cell activity (central) Macrophage phagocytosis (central) Inhibits T cell proliferation (central) Nitric oxide release (peripheral)
δ	Increases NK cell activity (central) Potentiates humoral immune response Decreases plaque-forming cell response
δ antagonist	At low dose, inhibits delayed hypersensitivity reaction
κ	Pronounced suppression of humoral immunity
κ antagonist	Increases plaque-forming cell response Suppression of humoral immune response

FURTHER READING

Benyamin R, Trescot A, Datta S, et al. Opioid complications and side effects. *Pain* Physician. 2008;11:S105–S120.

Chuang TK, Killam KF Jr, Chuang LF, et al. Mu opioid receptor gene expression in immune cells. *Biochem Biophys Res Commun.* 1995;216:922–930.

Dimitrijevic M, Stanojevic S, Kovacevic-Jovanovic V, et al. Modulation of humoral immune responses in the rat by centrally applied met-enk and opioid receptor antagonists: Functional interactions of brain OP1, OP2 and OP3 receptors. *Immunopharmacology.* 2000;49:255–262.

Peterson PK, Molitor TW, Chao CC. The opioid–cytokine connection. *J Neuroimmunol.* 1998;83:63–69.

Radulovic J, Jankovic BD. Opposing activities of brain opioid receptors in the regulation of humoral and cell-mediated immune responses in the rat. *Brain Res.* 1994;661:189–195.

Stephanou A, Fitzharris P, Knight RA, et al. Characteristics and kinetics of proopiomelanocortin mRNA expression by human leucocytes. *Brain Behav Immun.* 1991;5:319–327.

9. ANSWER: D

The troublesome sexual side effects of chronic opioid therapy have been related to hypogonadism. Testosterone levels are lowered 1–4 hours after initial administration of opioids, with resumption normally 24 hours after opioid cessation. The testosterone effects have been more strongly associated with methadone and may not completely manifest themselves with other opioids. However, androgen-related side effects have been observed with other opioids.

Women are not exempt from hormonal side effects of opioids. Due to a reduction in estrogen levels in women on methadone therapy, side effects of depression, dysmenorrhea, sexual dysfunction, and reduced bone mineral density have been described.

FURTHER READING

Benyamin R, Trescot A, Datta S, et al. Opioid complications and side effects. *Pain Physician*. 2008;11:S105–S120.

Daniell HW. Opioid endocrinopathy in women consuming prescribed sustained-action opioids for control of nonmalignant pain. *J Pain.* 2008;9:28–36.

Woody G, McLellan AT, O'Brien C, et al. Hormone secretion in methadone-dependent and abstinent patients. *NIDA Res Monogr.* 1988;81:216–223.

10. ANSWER: C

Codeine is an alkaloid derived from morphine and often administered in combination with acetaminophen. It is a weak μ opioid agonist with a 2.5- to 3-hour half-life. Evidence suggests that the analgesic effect is dependent on the conversion of codeine to morphine by the CYP2D6 enzyme through O-demethylation. A genetic polymorphism is responsible for an altered response to the medication. Also, some medications may result in a lack of efficacy of codeine secondary to inhibition of the CYP2D6 enzyme, including quinidine, paroxetine, fluoxetine, and buproprion.

FURTHER READING

Benzon H, Rathmell JP, Wu CL, et al. (Eds.). *Practical Management of Pain.* 5th ed. Philadelphia, PA: Mosby; 2014.

Eckhardt K, Li S, Ammon S, et al. Same incidence of adverse drug events after codeine administration irrespective of the genetically determined differences in morphine formation. *Pain.* 1998;76:27–33.

11. ANSWER: A

Metabolism of morphine to its metabolites occurs mainly in the liver. M6G is a μ and δ agonist and accounts for 5–15% of morphine's metabolites. M6G results in analgesia and other typical side effects of opioids. M3G comprises approximately 50% of morphine's metabolites and produces effects that oppose morphine's analgesic actions, including allodynia, hyperalgesia, myoclonus, and seizures. Oral morphine appears to produce more M3G and M6G compared to IV, intramuscular, or rectal routes due to bypass of hepatic metabolism. Chronic oral administration may result in higher circulating levels of M3G and M6G than parent compound, and the metabolites may undergo deconjugation back to the parent compound by colonic flora and be reabsorbed as morphine. Also, the metabolites are excreted by the kidneys and may accumulate in the setting of renal insufficiency.

FURTHER READING

Benzon H, Rathmell JP, Wu CL, et al. (Eds.). *Practical Management of Pain.* 5th ed. Philadelphia, PA: Mosby; 2014.

Janicki PK, Parris WC. Clinical pharmacology of opioids. In: Smith HS (Ed.), *Drugs for Pain*. Philadelphia, PA: Hanley & Belfus; 2003:97–118.

12. ANSWER: C

Oxycodone is a semisynthetic opioid that has a higher bio-availability compared to morphine (60% vs. 33% in oral formulations). It may be administered in conjunction with acetaminophen (Percocet, Roxicet, and Endocet) or aspirin (Percodan). Oxycontin utilizes sustained-release technology to increase duration of action. After undergoing hepatic metabolism by CYP2D6, it is converted to its active metabolite oxymorphone and inactive metabolite noroxycodone.

FURTHER READING

Benzon H, Rathmell JP, Wu CL, et al. (Eds.). *Practical Management of Pain*. 5th ed. Philadelphia, PA: Mosby; 2014.

13. ANSWER: D

Multiple opioids are reduced to active metabolites with deleterious side effects. Of these compounds, several have been implicated in causing CNS hyperactivity and seizures. Meperidine is hepatically demethylated to the neurotoxic metabolite normeperidine, which has a 12- to 16-hour half-life. Likewise, hydromorphone is metabolized in the liver to hydromorphone 3-glucuronide, which potentiates allodynia, myoclonus, and seizures in patients with renal insufficiency. Morphine is metabolized into morphine 3- and 6-glucuronide. M3G shares similar side effects with H3G. Oxymorphone is a μ opioid agonist and is the active metabolite of oxycodone.

FURTHER READING

Benzon H, Rathmell JP, Wu CL, et al. (Eds.). *Practical Management of Pain*. 5th ed. Philadelphia, PA: Mosby; 2014.
Inturrisi CE. Clinical pharmacology of opioids for pain. *Clin J Pain*. 2002;18:S3–S13.

14. ANSWER: D

Methadone is unique among the opioids secondary to its many interesting properties. It is both a μ and a δ receptor agonist and displays NMDA antagonism and serotonin reuptake blockade. It possesses no known neurotoxic or active metabolites.

FURTHER READING

Benzon H, Rathmell JP, Wu CL, et al. (Eds.). *Practical Management of Pain*. 5th ed. Philadelphia, PA: Mosby; 2014.

15. ANSWER: B

Methadone's variable elimination half-life may reach up to 27 hours secondary to its lipophilicity and tissue distribution. In addition, it also undergoes biphasic elimination. The alpha elimination period ranges from 8 to 12 hours and mirrors the analgesic half-life of 6–8 hours. However, the beta elimination phase ranges from 30 to 60 hours and can prevent withdrawal symptoms upon cessation.

Methadone is susceptible to multiple drug interactions secondary to the CYP system, including the 2D6 and 3A4 subtypes.

Decreased gastric pH will result in increased methadone absorption. However, renal failure does not alter excretion of methadone, but it is affected by urinary pH increases (which decrease methadone clearance in urine). Urine pH higher than 6 can nearly eliminate clearance and result in increased levels.

FURTHER READING

Benzon H, Rathmell JP, Wu CL, et al. (Eds.). *Practical Management of Pain*. 5th ed. Philadelphia, PA: Mosby; 2014.
Fishman SM, Wilsey B, Mahajan G, et al. Methadone reincarnated: Novel clinical applications with related concerns. *Pain Med*. 2002;3:339–348.
Mahajan G, Fishman SM. Major opioids in pain management. In: Benzon HT, Raja SN, Molloy RE, et al. (Eds.), *Essentials of Pain and Regional Anesthesia*. Philadelphia, PA: Churchill Livingstone; 2005:94–105.

16. ANSWER: A

A possible source of methadone-related mortality includes torsades de pointes arrhythmias secondary to QT prolongation induced by methadone. There is a potential additive effect of QT prolongation when other agents that affect this conduction variable are present (e.g., tricyclic antidepressants).

FURTHER READING

Benzon H, Rathmell JP, Wu CL, et al. (Eds.). *Practical Management of Pain*. 5th ed. Philadelphia, PA: Mosby; 2014.
Gil M, Sala M, Anguera I, et al. QT prolongation and torsades de pointes in patients infected with human immunodeficiency virus and treated with methadone. *Am J Cardiol*. 2003;92:995–997.

Krantz MJ, Lewkowiez L, Hayes H, et al. Torsades de pointes associated with very high dose methadone. *Ann Intern Med.* 2002;137:501–504.

17. ANSWER: A

Oxycodone undergoes oxidative metabolism by N-demethylation through CYP3A4 to noroxycodone (weak μ affinity) and by O-demethylation to oxymorphone (strong μ affinity—two to five times higher affinity than morphine). Oxymorphone is available in immediate and extended-release formulations and is approximately six times as potent as oral morphine in an equianalgesic dose. Oxymorphone comprises approximately 10% of oxycodone metabolites.

FURTHER READING

Benzon H, Rathmell JP, Wu CL, et al. (Eds.). *Practical Management of Pain.* 5th ed. Philadelphia, PA: Mosby; 2014.
Heiskanen T, Olkkola KT, Kalso E. Effects of blocking CYP2D6 on the pharmacokinetics and pharmacodynamics of oxycodone. *Clin Pharmacol Ther.* 1998;64:603–611.

18. ANSWER: C

As of October 2014, hydrocodone was the most prescribed opioid in the United States with 137 million prescriptions in 2013. An FDA advisory committee recommended the Drug Enforcement Administration change the schedule of hydrocodone from III to II in 2013 following a review of prescribing practices and patient misuse. Key changes included no more phone-in refills and a restriction to a 30-day supply per prescription. Combination drugs that paired hydrocodone with acetaminophen were altered to limit the acetaminophen content per pill to 325 mg.

Hydrocodone is six to eight times more potent than codeine and undergoes CYP2D6 metabolism to hydromorphone and CYP3A4 metabolism to noroxycodone. It is approximately half as potent as morphine with regard to receptor affinity. An extended-release formulation of hydrocodone alone is now commercially available.

FURTHER READING

Benzon H, Rathmell JP, Wu CL, et al. (Eds.). *Practical Management of Pain.* 5th ed. Philadelphia, PA: Mosby; 2014.
Throckmorton DC. Re-scheduling prescription hydrocodone combination drug products: An important step toward controlling misuse and abuse. Available at http://blogs.fda.gov/fdavoice/index.php/2014/10/re-scheduling-prescription-hydrocodone-combination-drug-products-an-important-step-toward-controlling-misuse-and-abuse.

19. ANSWER: D

Tramadol has an interesting variety of clinical mechanisms for its unique analgesic effects. It is a weak agonist of the μ receptor but is only partially blocked by naloxone. It has an inhibitory effect on central norepinephrine and serotonin reuptake. Some data also suggest it has a concentration-dependent antagonism of NMDA receptors. It is available in immediate, sustained-release (12-hour), and extended-release (24-hour) formulations.

Methadone shows affinity for the μ and δ opioid receptors. It also has features of serotonin reuptake blockade and NMDA antagonism. Its prevention of withdrawal symptoms after cessation is related to its biphasic elimination, with the beta elimination phase lasting 30–60 hours. It is not available in extended-release formulations.

FURTHER READING

Benzon H, Rathmell JP, Wu CL, et al. (Eds.). *Practical Management of Pain.* 5th ed. Philadelphia, PA: Mosby; 2014.
Hara K, Minami K, Sata T. The effects of tramadol and its metabolite on glycine, gamma-aminobutyric acid A, and *N*-methyl-D-aspartate receptors expressed in *Xenopus* oocytes. *Anesth Analg.* 200;100(5):1400–1405.
Hennies HH, Friderichs E, Schneider J. Receptor binding, analgesic and antitussive potency of tramadol and other selected opioids. *Arzneimittelforschung.* 1988;38:877–880.
Mahajan G, Fishman SM. Major opioids in pain management. In: Benzon HT, Raja SN, Molloy RE, et al. (Eds.), *Essentials of Pain and Regional Anesthesia.* Philadelphia, PA: Churchill Livingstone; 2005;94–105.

20. ANSWER: C

Serotonin toxicity is characterized by a triad consisting of neuromuscular hyperactivity (tremor, clonus, and hyperreflexia), autonomic hyperactivity (diaphoresis, fever, tachycardia, and tachypnea), and altered mental status (agitation, excitement, and confusion). Pathophysiology is not completely defined but appears to involve overstimulation of central serotonin receptors. Serotonin syndrome may be secondary to concomitant use of multiple drugs affecting the serotonergic system (Table 8.2). Although overdose of amitriptyline alone does not appear to precipitate serotonin toxicity, venlafaxine is more often the cause of serotonin toxicity compared to SSRIs, possibly related to mechanisms separate from serotonin reuptake.

FURTHER READING

Bamigbade TA, Davidson C, Langord RM, et al. Actions of tramadol, its enantiomers and principal metabolite, *O*-desmethyltramadol, on serotonin (5-HT) efflux and uptake in the rat dorsal raphe nucleus. *Br J Anaesth.* 1997;79:352–356.

Table 8.2 **SPECTRUM OF SEROTONIN SYNDROME**

MILD STATE OF SEROTONIN-RELATED SYMPTOMS	SEROTONIN SYNDROME (FULL-BLOWN FORM)		TOXIC STATES
Single symptom may predominate	At least four major or three major and two minor of the following:		Coma

Most common are
    Tremor
    Myoclonus
    Diaphoresis and shivering
	Major
	
	Mental symptoms
	    Impaired consciousness
	    Elevated mood
	Neurologic symptoms
	    Myoclonus
	    Tremor
	    Shivering
	    Rigidity
	    Hyperreflexia
	Vegetative symptoms
	    Fever
	    Sweating
		Minor
		
		Restlessness
		Insomnia
		Incoordination
		Dilated pupils
		Akathisia
		Tachycardia
		Tachypnea, dyspnea
		Diarrhea
		Hypertension, hypotension
			Generalized tonic–clonic seizures
			Fever (may exceed 40°C)
			Disseminated intravascular coagulation and renal failure

SOURCE: From Gnanadesigan N, Espinoza RT, Smith R, et al. Interaction of serotonergic antidepressants and opioid analgesics: Is serotonin syndrome going undetected? *J Am Med Dir Assoc.* 2005;6(4):265–269.

Benzon H, Rathmell JP, Wu CL, et al. (Eds.). *Practical Management of Pain.* 5th ed. Philadelphia, PA: Mosby; 2014.

Dawson AH. Cyclic antidepressant drugs. In Dart RC (Ed.), *Medical Toxicology.* 3rd ed. Baltimore, MD: Lippincott Williams & Wilkins; 2004:834–843,

Gillman PK, Whyte IM. Serotonin syndrome. In: Haddad P, Dursun S, Deakin B (Eds.), *Adverse Syndromes and Psychiatric Drugs.* Oxford, UK: Oxford University Press; 2004:37–49.

21. ANSWER: B

Maximum serum concentration of tramadol is reached in approximately 2 hours. Following multiple doses, bioavailability increases from 68% to 90–100%. It can cross the placenta and is bound to plasma proteins by 20%. Primary metabolism is via CYP enzymes to multiple metabolites, with the primary being *O*-desmethyltramadol (also known as M1). Poor metabolizers with a polymorphism of CYP2D6 may require higher loading doses and more frequent rescue analgesia.

FURTHER READING

Benzon H, Rathmell JP, Wu CL, et al. (Eds.). *Practical Management of Pain.* 5th ed. Philadelphia, PA: Mosby; 2014.

Lee CR, McTavish D, Sorkin EM. Tramadol: A preliminary review of its pharmacodynamic and pharmacokinetic properties, and therapeutic potential in acute and chronic pain states. *Drugs.* 1993;46:313–340.

Liao S, Hill JF, Nayak RK. Pharmacokinetics of tramadol following single and multiple oral doses in man [abstract]. *Pharm Res.* 1992;9(Suppl.):308.

Lintz W, Barth H, Osterloh G, et al. Bioavailability of enteral tramadol formulations: 1st communication: Capsules. *Arzneimittelforschung.* 1986;36:1278–1283.

Stamer UM, Lehnen K, Hothker F, et al. Impact of CYP2D6 genotype on postoperative tramadol analgesia. *Pain.* 2003;105:231–238.

Wu WN, McKown LA, Liao S. Metabolism of the analgesic drug Ultram (tramadol hydrochloride) in humans: API-MS and MS/MS characterization of metabolites. *Xenobiotica.* 2002;32:411–425.

22. ANSWER: B

Acetaminophen has analgesic and antipyretic actions in vivo without a clear mechanism of pharmacologic activity. Its half-life ranges from 1.25 to 3 hours, with 25% of the dose undergoing first-pass metabolism in the liver. Approximately 90% is metabolized in the hepatic system to nontoxic metabolites. Approximately 10% transforms through oxidative metabolism via CYP2E1 and CYP1A2 to the hepato/nephrotoxic metabolite *N*-acetyl-*p*-benzoquinone imine (NAPQI). Once the gluronoidation and sulfonation enzyme system for 90% of the drug is saturated, the total fraction of NAPQI increases. Glutathione detoxifies accumulated NAPQI. Patients with depleted glutathione levels (HIV, cirrhosis, and hepatitis C) may be at increased risk for adverse events.

There appears to be association in the literature with elevated international normalized ratio (INR) secondary to concomitant acetaminophen and oral anticoagulant interactions; however, no randomized controlled studies have provided evidence of statistically significant differences in INR.

FURTHER READING

Benzon H, Rathmell JP, Wu CL, et al. (Eds.). *Practical Management of Pain.* 5th ed. Philadelphia, PA: Mosby; 2014.

Gadisseur AP, Van Der Meer FJ, Rosendaal FR. Sustained intake of paracetamol (acetaminophen) during oral anticoagulant therapy with coumarins does not cause clinically important INR changes: A randomized double-blind clinical trial. *J Thromb Haemost.* 2003;1:714–717.

Toes MJ, Jones AL, Prescott L: Drug interactions with paracetamol. *Am J Ther.* 2005;12:56–66.

23. ANSWER: D

A study of healthy adults given 4 g of acetaminophen per day for 14 days found that 31–44% had elevated ALT up to three times the upper limit of normal. Glutathione reserves are depleted with chronic use of acetaminophen and may lead to hepatic and renal toxicity. Liver function transaminases are not routinely elevated possibly due to cellular adaptation, resulting in increased glutathione production. Opioids were not found to have additional effect on ALT levels and do not appear to be altered by concomitant use of acetaminophen.

FURTHER READING

Benzon H, Rathmell JP, Wu CL, et al. (Eds.). *Practical Management of Pain.* 5th ed. Philadelphia, PA: Mosby; 2014.

Shayiq RM, Roberts DW, Rothstein K, et al. Repeat exposure to incremental doses of acetaminophen provides protection against acetaminophen-induced lethality in mice: An explanation for high acetaminophen dosage in humans without hepatic injury. *Hepatology.* 1999;29:451–463.

Watkins PB, Seeff LB. Drug-induced liver injury. *Hepatology.* 2006;43:618–631.

24. ANSWER: A

Superiority of acetaminophen to NSAIDs for managing osteoarthritis-type pain is controversial. Examining a patient's total clinical picture is key to developing an appropriate regimen. With a history of heart disease but normal hepatic and renal function, acetaminophen would probably be the preferred agent to treat right knee pain. Symptoms of gastric reflux can be managed with a selective COX-2 inhibitor or the addition of a proton pump inhibitor to a patient's regimen. Acetaminophen and NSAIDs should most likely be avoided in end-stage renal and hepatic disease. Ankylosing spondylitis is responsive to the anti-inflammatory effects of NSAIDs, which are considered first-line treatment.

FURTHER READING

Benzon H, Rathmell JP, Wu CL, et al. (Eds.). *Practical Management of Pain.* 5th ed. Philadelphia, PA: Mosby; 2014.

Fored CM, Ejerblad E, Lindblad P, et al. Acetaminophen, aspirin, and chronic renal failure. *N Engl J Med.* 2001;345:1801–1808.

Pincus T, Koch G, Lei H, et al. Patient preference for Placebo, Acetaminophen (Paracetamol) or Celecoxib Efficacy Studies (PACES): Two randomised, double blind, placebo controlled, cross-over clinical trials in patients with knee or hip osteoarthritis. *Ann Rheum Dis.* 2004;63:931–939.

Rohekar S, Chan J, Tse SM, et al. 2014 Update of the Canadian Rheumatology Association/Spondyloarthritis Research Consortium of Canada treatment recommendations for the management of spondyloarthritis: Part II. Specific management recommendations. *J Rheumatol.* 2015;42(4):665–681.

Towheed TE, Judd MJ, Hochberg MC, et al. Acetaminophen for osteoarthritis. *Cochrane Database Syst Rev.* 2003;2.

25. ANSWER: A

In animal models, antinociceptive effects of TCAs are inhibited in the presence of 5-HT antagonists and central 5-HT depletion. Similarly, antinociception with TCAs is inhibited with coadministration with the α_1 and α_2 receptor antagonist phentolamine, but analgesia is observed in the presence of TCA and selective α blockers. Sodium channel blockade appears to be a component of the analgesic actions of TCAs. Amitriptyline has the most potent sodium channel blocking ability and has been demonstrated to show antinociceptive effects in murine models of pain. Studies of rat models demonstrated prevention of calcium influx into neurons produced by NMDA with TCAs, resulting in alteration of NMDA binding characteristics.

Strong evidence has been presented for pain relief with TCAs in patients with postherpetic neuralgia and diabetic neuropathy. Less conclusive evidence has been found for their use in spinal cord injury pain and fibromyalgia. There does not appear to be significant relief when TCAs are used for cancer-related neuropathic pain or HIV neuropathy.

FURTHER READING

Ansuategui M, Naharro L, Feria M. Noradrenergic and opioidergic influences on the antinociceptive effect of clomipramine in the formalin test in rats. *Psychopharmacology.* 1989;98:93–96.

Ardid D, Guilbaud G. Antinociceptive effects of acute and "chronic" injections of tricyclic antidepressant drugs in a new model of mononeuropathy in rats. *Pain.* 1992;49:279–287.

Benzon H, Rathmell JP, Wu CL, et al. (Eds.). *Practical Management of Pain.* 5th ed. Philadelphia, PA: Mosby; 2014.

Dick IE, Brochu RM, Purohit Y, et al. Sodium channel blockade may contribute to the analgesic efficacy of antidepressants. *J Pain.* 2007;8:315–324.

Paudel KR, Das BP, Rauniar GP, et al. Antinociceptive effect of amitriptyline in mice of acute pain models. *Indian J Exp Biol.* 2007;45:529–531.

Reynolds IJ, Miller RJ. Tricyclic antidepressants block N-methyl-D-aspartate receptors: Similarities to the action of zinc. *Br J Pharmacol.* 1988;95:95–102.

Sierralta F, Pinardi G, Miranda HF. Effect of p-chlorophenylalanine and alpha-methyltyrosine on the antinociceptive effect of antidepressant drugs. *Pharmacol Toxicol.* 1995;77:276–280.

26. ANSWER: C

Duloxetine is a serotonin–norepinephrine reuptake inhibitor with a 10-fold selectivity for 5-HT. It has been extensively studied in patients with painful diabetic neuropathy, fibromyalgia, musculoskeletal back pain, and osteoarthritis, with FDA approval for the preceding indications. It appears to be most effective at doses of 60–120 mg/day, with nausea being one of the most common side effects in this dose range. For fibromyalgia, duloxetine reduces pain, quantity of palpable tender points, and stiffness scores.

FURTHER READING

Arnold LM, Lu Y, Crofford LJ, et al. A double-blind, multicenter trial comparing duloxetine with placebo in the treatment of fibromyalgia patients with or without major depressive disorder. *Arthritis Rheum.* 2004;50:2974–2984.

Benzon H, Rathmell JP, Wu CL, et al. (Eds.). *Practical Management of Pain.* 5th ed. Philadelphia, PA: Mosby; 2014.

Rashkin J, Pritchett YL, Wang F, et al. A double-blind, randomized multicenter trial comparing duloxetine with placebo in the management of diabetic peripheral neuropathic pain. *Pain Med.* 2005;6:346–356.

Smith TR: Duloxetine in diabetic neuropathy. *Expert Opin Pharmacother.* 2006;7:215–223.

27. ANSWER: D

TCAs often result in cholinergic side effects and have increased risk of these side effects in studies comparing them to SSRIs. Weight gain is more likely to occur in association with TCA therapy than SSRIs. A study from the United Kingdom illuminated a much higher death rate per million prescriptions for TCAs than SSRIs, and a US study found TCAs to be the most commonly used antidepressant for suicide attempts. In a study of incidence of peptic ulcer disease, SSRIs with or without NSAIDs were correlated with a much higher incidence in ulcers compared to TCAs.

SUGGESTED READING

Benzon H, Rathmell JP, Wu CL, et al. (Eds.). *Practical Management of Pain.* 5th ed. Philadelphia, PA: Mosby; 2014.

Buckley NA, McManus PR. Fatal toxicity of serotonergic and other antidepressant drugs: Analysis of United Kingdom mortality data. *Br Med J.* 2002;325:1332–1333.

De Jong JC, Van den Berg PB, Tobi H, et al. Combined use of SSRIs and NSAIDs increases the risk of gastrointestinal adverse effects. *Br J Clin Pharmacol.* 2003;55:591–595.

Fava M: Weight gain and antidepressants. *J Clin Psychiatry.* 2006; 11:S37–S41.

Vieweg WV, Linker JA, Anum ES, et al. Child and adolescent suicides in Virginia: 1987–2003. *J Child Adolesc Psychopharmacol.* 2005;15:6556–6563.

28. ANSWER: B

The calcium channel modulators gabapentin and pregabalin are structurally derived from GABA, but neither display activity at the GABA receptor, with no influence on uptake or metabolism of GABA. Both modulators bind to the $\alpha_2\delta$ subunit of L-type voltage-gated calcium channels to exert their effects. The L-type calcium channel is a type of high-voltage-activated channel. This type of channel requires a large membrane depolarization and is the primary proponent of calcium entry and subsequent release of presynaptic neurotransmitters. L-type channels are concentrated in skeletal, neuronal, and smooth muscle.

FURTHER READING

Benzon H, Rathmell JP, Wu CL, et al. (Eds.). *Practical Management of Pain.* 5th ed. Philadelphia, PA: Mosby; 2014.

Fink K, Dooley D, Meder W, et al. Inhibition of neuronal Ca^{2+} influx by gabapentin and pregabalin in the human neocortex. *Neuropharmacology.* 2002;42:229–236.

Taylor C. The biology and pharmacology of calcium channel alpha2-delta proteins. *CNS Drug Rev.* 2004;10:183–188.

Yamakage M, Namiki A. Calcium channels—Basic aspects of their structure, function and gene encoding; Anesthetic action on the channels—A review. *Can J Anaesth.* 2002;49:151–164.

29. ANSWER: C

Gabapentin is usually started in a naive patient at 100–300 mg per day and titrated in 300-mg increments every 2–5 days to avoid adverse effects. The most common adverse effects are fatigue, somnolence, and dizziness. A reduced dosing regimen is recommended for patients with renal insufficiency. Gabapentin is FDA approved for treatment of postherpetic neuralgia up to 1800 mg/day, but it has been extensively studied for other pain conditions, including complex regional pain syndrome, painful diabetic neuropathy, various causes of neuropathic pain, and opioid-induced hyperalgesia. In a study of gabapentin in patients with lumbar spinal stenosis, the following outcomes were noted: a decrease in pain scores, higher walking distances, and diminished sensory and motor deficits.

FURTHER READING

Backonja M, Beydoun A, Edwards K, et al. Gabapentin monotherapy for the treatment of painful neuropathy: A multicenter, double-blind, placebo-controlled trial in patients with diabetes mellitus. *JAMA.* 1998;280:1831–1836.

Benzon H, Rathmell JP, Wu CL, et al. (Eds.). *Practical Management of Pain.* 5th ed. Philadelphia, PA: Mosby; 2014.

Compton P, Kehoe P, Sinha K, et al. Gabapentin improves cold-pressor pain responses in methadone-maintained patients. *Drug Alcohol Depend*. 2010;109:213–219.

Rowbotham M, Harden N, Stacey B, et al. Gabapentin for the treatment of postherpetic neuralgia: A randomized controlled trial. *JAMA*. 1998;280:1837–1842.

Yaksi A, Ozgonenel L, Ozgonenel B. The efficacy of gabapentin therapy in patients with lumbar spinal stenosis. *Spine*. 2007;32:939–942.

FURTHER READING

Benzon H, Rathmell JP, Wu CL, et al. (Eds.). *Practical Management of Pain*. 5th ed. Philadelphia, PA: Mosby; 2014.

Klotz U. Ziconotide—A novel neuron-specific calcium channel blocker for the intrathecal treatment of severe chronic pain: A short review. *Int J Clin Pharmacol Ther*. 2006;44:478–483.

Rauck R, Wallace M, Leong M, et al. A randomized, double-blind, placebo-controlled study of intrathecal ziconotide in adults with severe chronic pain. *J Pain Symptom Manage*. 2006;5:393–406.

30. ANSWER: B

Pregabalin shares the same mechanism of action as gabapentin by binding at the $\alpha_2\delta$ subunit of L-type calcium channels. Initial dosing is 150 mg/day in two or three divided doses, and it can be titrated up to 600 mg/day. Dose must be adjusted in patients with renal insufficiency. In some trials, patients have responded to the analgesic effect within the first week of treatment. Pregabalin also seems to lack the variability between effective dose and dose at which side effects occur that seems to plague gabapentin therapy. The most common adverse dose-related effects with pregabalin are somnolence and dizziness. Pregabalin is approved by the FDA for treatment of postherpetic neuralgia, painful diabetic neuropathy, and spinal cord injury neuropathic pain.

FURTHER READING

Benzon H, Rathmell JP, Wu CL, et al. (Eds.). *Practical Management of Pain*. 5th ed. Philadelphia, PA: Mosby; 2014.

Gilron I, Wajsbrot D, Therrien F, et al. Pregabalin for peripheral neuropathic pain: A multicenter, enriched enrollment randomized withdrawal placebo-controlled trial. *Clin J Pain*. 2011;27:185–193.

Sills G. The mechanism of action of gabapentin and pregabalin. *Curr Opin Pharmacol*. 2006;6:108–113.

Van Seventer R, Feister H, Young J, et al. Efficacy and tolerability of twice-daily pregabalin for treating pain and related sleep interference in postherpetic neuralgia: A 13-week, randomized trial. *Curr Med Res Opin*. 2006;22:1202–1208.

31. ANSWER: C

Ziconotide is a peptide isolated from the venom of *Conus magus* marine snail, and it blocks N-type calcium channels in the spinal cord's dorsal horn. It is administered intrathecally. It does not cause tolerance or dependence, and it can be stopped immediately in the event of adverse effects without risk of withdrawal symptoms. It does not cause respiratory depression. Common side effects include dizziness, confusion, and ataxia, which can result from overly rapid dose titration. Rare, but reported, side effects include hallucinations and elevated CK. The mechanism of CK elevation is unknown. It has been studied in randomized, placebo-controlled trials for severe chronic pain refractory to other modes of treatment.

32. ANSWER: A

Both carbamazepine and oxcarbazepine have been studied for the treatment of trigeminal neuralgia. However, both medications are limited by their respective side effect profiles. Carbamazepine's common side effects include sedation, dizziness, and nausea/vomiting. Serious adverse effects that have been reported with carbamazepine include pancytopenia, Stevens–Johnson syndrome, and toxic epidermal necrolysis. Blood monitoring should be performed every 2–4 months because the number needed to harm for adverse effects is 24.

Oxcarbazepine is a keto-analogue of carbamazepine and lacks the hematologic side effects. It has also been found to be effective for patients with trigeminal neuralgia who had no benefit from carbamazepine. A serious adverse effect that may develop with oxcarbazepine is hyponatremia, usually during the initial 3 months. Blood sodium monitoring is required when initiating therapy. It shares the common adverse effects of sedation and nausea/vomiting with carbamazepine.

FURTHER READING

Benzon H, Rathmell JP, Wu CL, et al. (Eds.). *Practical Management of Pain*. 5th ed. Philadelphia, PA: Mosby; 2014.

Gomez-Arguelles JM, Dorado R, Sepulveda JM, et al. Oxcarbazepine monotherapy in carbamazepine-unresponsive trigeminal neuralgia. *J Clin Neurosci*. 2008;15:516–519.

Gronseth G, Cruccu G, Alksne J, et al. Practice parameter—The diagnostic evaluation and treatment of trigeminal neuralgia (an evidence-based review): Report of Quality Standards Subcommittee of the American Academy of Neurology and the European Federation of Neurological Societies. *Neurology*. 2008;71:1183–1190.

33. ANSWER: D

Topiramate was FDA approved for migraine prophylaxis after compelling evidence accrued in some large clinical trials. It has multiple mechanisms of action. It increases GABA activity by binding receptors and increasing opening frequency of embedded chloride ion channels, which is independent from benzodiazepine and barbiturate-related

GABA mechanisms. It also inhibits voltage-sensitive sodium channels and prevents sustained repetitive firing. It is an inhibitory modulator of glutamate at its receptor. It decreases activity of L-type calcium channels and is a carbonic anhydrase inhibitor.

Topiramate possesses linear pharmacokinetics with a half-life of 19–25 hours. Oral bioavailability is approximately 85%.

FURTHER READING

Benzon H, Rathmell JP, Wu CL, et al. (Eds.). *Practical Management of Pain*. 5th ed. Philadelphia, PA: Mosby; 2014.
Brandes JL, Saper JR, Diamond M, et al. Topiramate for migraine prevention: A randomized controlled trial. *JAMA*. 2004;291:965–973.

34. ANSWER: A

Peak plasma concentrations of most NSAIDs are reached within 2 or 3 hours secondary to rapid GI absorption. The extent of drug absorption from the GI system is more important than the rate. Rectal and oral routes are similar with regard to NSAID systemic absorption.

Regarding distribution, most NSAIDs are highly bound to plasma proteins, with less than 1% unbound. Albumin is the major binder of NSAIDs, and disease states involving hypoalbuminemia result in increased unbound form, affecting distribution and elimination.

Renal failure has variable effects on NSAID kinetics. Absorption is not affected, but plasma protein binding is compromised, which results in an increased unbound portion of the drugs. Clearance of NSAIDs that rely on the formation of acyl glucuronides as an elimination pathway is impaired in patients with renal failure (naproxen, indoprofen, and ketoprofen). Effects on other NSAIDs are minimal (ibuprofen) if they are metabolized through oxidative routes.

Most NSAIDs undergo hepatic biotransformation through oxidation, glucuronide conjugation, or both in the cytochrome P450 system. Renal excretion of nonmetabolized drug is a lesser elimination pathway.

FURTHER READING

Benzon H, Rathmell JP, Wu CL, et al. (Eds.). *Practical Management of Pain*. 5th ed. Philadelphia, PA: Mosby; 2014.
Cooke AR, Hunt JN. Relationship between pH and absorption of acetylsalicylic acid from the stomach. *Gut*. 1969;10:77–78.
Davies NM, Skjodt NM. Choosing the right nonsteroidal anti-inflammatory drug for the right patient: A pharmacokinetic approach. *Clin Pharmacokinet*. 2000;38:377–392.
Evans AM, Hussein Z, Rowland M. Influence of albumin on the distribution and elimination kinetics of diclofenac in the isolated perfused rat liver: Analysis by the impulse-response technique and the dispersion model. *J Pharm Sci*. 1993;82:421–428.

Gibaldi M. Drug distribution in renal failure. *Am J Med*. 1977;62:471–474.

35. ANSWER: C

Aspirin is an irreversible cyclooxygenase inhibitor. It has a variable dose-dependent elimination half-life of 2.5–19 hours. It attains peak plasma levels 1 hour after rapid absorption from the stomach and small intestine. Platelets cannot synthesize new COX, and the inhibition exerted on their function is present for the 10- to 14-day life cycle of the platelet.

FURTHER READING

Benzon H, Rathmell JP, Wu CL, et al. (Eds.). *Practical Management of Pain*. 5th ed. Philadelphia, PA: Mosby; 2014.

36. ANSWER: C

Ketorolac (Toradol) is nearly completely bound to plasma proteins with major metabolization by hepatic conjugation with renal excretion. Duration of analgesia is 4–6 hours, and it onsets within 30 minutes and peaks in 1 or 2 hours. Current recommendations advise limiting therapy to less than 5 days due to adverse effects of GI bleeding. Deaths have also been reported secondary to operative site bleeding following administration.

SUGGESTED READING:

Benzon H, Rathmell JP, Wu CL, et al. (Eds.). *Practical Management of Pain*. 5th ed. Philadelphia, PA: Mosby; 2014.
Gills JC, Brogden RN. Ketorolac: A reappraisal of its pharmacodynamics and pharmacokinetic properties and therapeutic use in pain management. *Drugs*. 1997;53:139–188.
Strom BL, Berlin JA, Kinman JL, et al. Parenteral ketorolac and risk of gastrointestinal and operating site bleeding: A postmarketing surveillance study. *JAMA*. 1996;275:376–382.

37. ANSWER: B

Ibuprofen is a propionic acid derivative and commonly used NSAID for multiple complaints. Peak plasma levels occur 1 or 2 hours after an oral dose with a 3.5-hour half-life. Most metabolization occurs in the liver. With a regimen of 800 mg every 8 hours, gastrointestinal side effects are prominent and may include nausea and GI upset. Renal adverse effects have not been reported at over-the-counter dosage recommendations and only seem problematic in elderly patients with decreased cardiac output at doses greater than 1600 mg/day. However, a concerning adverse effect of ibuprofen is the antagonism of irreversible aspirin-induced platelet inhibition. Cardioprotective effects of aspirin are compromised with concurrent usage of ibuprofen.

FURTHER READING

Benzon H, Rathmell JP, Wu CL, et al. (Eds.). *Practical Management of Pain*. 5th ed. Philadelphia, PA: Mosby; 2014.

Catella-Lawson F, Reilly MP, Kapoor SC, et al. Cyclooxygenase inhibitors and the antiplatelet effect of aspirin. *N Engl J Med*. 2001;345:1809–1817.

Mann JF, Goerig M, Brune K, et al. Ibuprofen as an over-the-counter drug: Is there a risk for renal injury? *Clin Nephrol*. 1993;39:1–6.

38. ANSWER: A

Meloxicam is a COX-2 preferential NSAID that also inhibits prostanoid synthesis in inflammatory cells. Recent trials have shown it to be as effective as piroxicam, diclofenac, and naproxen for osteoarthritis with less adverse GI events, including bleeding and perforation. It is available in 7.5- and 15-mg tablets with a half-life of 20 hours, rendering it useful for once-daily dosing. It displays linear pharmacokinetics and reaches steady-state plasma concentration in 3–5 days. It is metabolized to four inactive metabolites and then excreted in urine and feces.

FURTHER READING

Benzon H, Rathmell JP, Wu CL, et al. (Eds.). *Practical Management of Pain*. 5th ed. Philadelphia, PA: Mosby; 2014.

Gates BJ, Nguyen TT, Setter SM, et al. Meloxicam: A reappraisal of pharmacokinetics, efficacy and safety. *Expert Opin Pharmacother*. 2005;6:2117–2140.

Vidal L, Kneer W, Baturone M, et al. Meloxicam in acute episodes of soft tissue rheumatism of the shoulder. *Inflamm Res*. 2001;50:S24–S29.

39. ANSWER: C

Celecoxib is a selective COX-2 inhibitor that does display some inhibition of COX-1 at high doses. It does not affect platelet function and can be administered in the perioperative period. Celecoxib reaches peak plasma levels approximately 3 hours after an oral dose and is 97% protein bound. Half-life is approximately 11 hours, and it is contraindicated in the presence of sulfonamide allergies. Adverse effects of the drug in clinical trials were headache, edema, diarrhea, nausea, and sinusitis. It is metabolized mainly by the liver via the cytochrome P450 system and eliminated via the biliary system.

FURTHER READING

Benzon H, Rathmell JP, Wu CL, et al. (Eds.). *Practical Management of Pain*. 5th ed. Philadelphia, PA: Mosby; 2014.

Dembo G, Park SB, Kharasch ED. Central nervous system concentration of cyclooxygenase-2 inhibitors in humans. *Anesthesiology*. 2005;102:409–415.

Kessenich C. Cyclooxygenase 2 inhibitors: An important new drug classification. *Pain Manage Nurs*. 2001;2:13–18.

Leese PT, Hubbard RC, Karim A, et al. Effects of celecoxib, a novel cyclooxygenase-2 inhibitor, on platelet function in healthy adults: A randomized, controlled trial. *J Clin Pharmacol*. 2000;40:124–132.

40. ANSWER: D

Platelet activity is mediated by the balance of the conversion of prostaglandin endoperoxides (derived from arachidonic acid) into PGI_2 in endothelium and TXA_2 in platelets. PGI_2 is a vasodilator and platelet inhibitor, and it is balanced by the vasoconstricting, platelet-activating properties of TXA_2. The irreversible COX inhibitor aspirin results in platelet aggregation inhibition for the life of the platelet (7–10 days) because platelets cannot regenerate COX enzyme. NSAID COX inhibition is transient and reverses following drug elimination. Studies are mixed regarding increased bleeding risk in the perioperative period.

FURTHER READING

Benzon H, Rathmell JP, Wu CL, et al. (Eds.). *Practical Management of Pain*. 5th ed. Philadelphia, PA: Mosby; 2014.

Schafer A. Effects of nonsteroidal anti-inflammatory drugs on platelet function and systemic hemostasis. *J Clin Pharmacol*. 1995;35:209–219.

41. ANSWER: B

NSAID administration may result in an altered balance of PGI_2 and TXA_2, leading to an increase in cardiovascular thrombosis. Long-term administration of COX-2 inhibitors may result in increased blood pressure, promotion of atherosclerosis, and aberrations in vascular responses. Rofecoxib and celecoxib studies were halted prematurely due to an increase in cardiovascular events. In 2005, an FDA review led to recommendations and warnings regarding new development of hypertension, exacerbation of preexisting disease, and elevated incidence of cardiovascular events. A review of 51 observational studies that included more than 3 million patients stratified NSAIDs based on incidence of usage and cardiovascular events. Adverse cardiovascular effects were least in association with naproxen.

FURTHER READING

Benzon H, Rathmell JP, Wu CL, et al. (Eds.). *Practical Management of Pain*. 5th ed. Philadelphia, PA: Mosby; 2014.

Egan KM, Wang M, Fries S, et al. Cyclooxygenases, thromboxane, and atherosclerosis: Plaque destabilization by cyclooxygenase-2 inhibition combined with thromboxane receptor antagonism. *Circulation*. 2005;111:334–342.

Levesque LE, Brophy JM, Zhang B. The risk of myocardial infarction with cyclooxygenase-2 inhibitors: A population study of elderly adults. *Ann Intern Med*. 2005;142:481–489.

McGettigan P, Henry D. Cardiovascular risk with non-steroidal anti-inflammatory drugs: Systematic review of population-based controlled observational studies. *PLoS Med*. 2011;8:e1001098.

Solomon SD, McMurray JV, Pfeffer MA, et al.; for the Adenoma Prevention with Celecoxib (APC) Study Investigators. Cardiovascular risk associated with celecoxib in a clinical trial for colorectal adenoma prevention. *N Engl J Med*. 2005;352:1071–1080.

US Food and Drug Administration. Memorandum: Analysis and recommendations for agency action regarding non-steroidal anti-inflammatory drugs and cardiovascular risk. 2005.

42. ANSWER: B

Risk factors for gastric ulceration secondary to NSAID use include advanced age, ulceration history, increased dose of NSAIDs, multiple NSAID use, concurrent anticoagulant use, tobacco abuse, alcohol use, and coexisting *Helicobacter pylori* infection. NSAIDs are responsible for direct epithelial lining irritation and result in an inability of the gastric mucosa to regulate bicarbonate, vascular flow, and epithelial regeneration. Alterations in platelet function can contribute to preexisting ulcer bleeding. Due to the increased incidence of cardiovascular events associated with their use, COX-2 inhibitors should be avoided in patients with a history of cardiovascular disease. In patients with cardiovascular risk and GI risk factors, a nonselective NSAID coupled with a proton pump inhibitor is recommended.

FURTHER READING

Amer M, Bead V, Bathon J. Use of NSAIDs in patients with cardiovascular disease. *Cardiol Rev*. 2010;18:204–212.

Benzon H, Rathmell JP, Wu CL, et al. (Eds.). *Practical Management of Pain*. 5th ed. Philadelphia, PA: Mosby; 2014.

Hawkey CJ, Hawthrone AB, Hudson N, et al. Separation of the impairment of hemostasis by aspirin from mucosal injury in the human stomach. *Clin Sci*. 1991;81:565–573.

Wallace JL, McCafferty DM, Carter L, et al. Tissue-selective inhibition of prostaglandin synthesis in rat by tepoxalin: Anti-inflammatory without gastropathy. *Gastroenterology*. 1993;105:1630–1636.

43. ANSWER: B

The proposed mechanism for NSAID-related renal toxicity is disruption of autoregulation of renal blood flow secondary to blockade of renal production of prostaglandins. Also, COX-2 inhibition results in sodium retention, and COX-1 and -2 inhibition causes changes in glomerular filtration rate. NSAIDs of all mechanisms of action are associated with edema and hypertension. Risk factors for NSAID-mediated renal adverse effects are chronic and multiple NSAID use, dehydration, intravascular depletion, congestive heart failure, peripheral vascular disease, shock, sepsis, systemic lupus erythematosus, liver disease, and advanced age.

FURTHER READING

Barkin RL, Buvanendran A. Focus on the COX-1 and COX-2 agents: Renal events of nonsteroidal and anti-inflammatory drugs—NSAIDs. *Am J Ther*. 2004;11:124–129.

Benzon H, Rathmell JP, Wu CL, et al. (Eds.). *Practical Management of Pain*. 5th ed. Philadelphia, PA: Mosby; 2014.

Taber SS, Mueller BA. Drug-associated renal dysfunction. *Crit Care Clin*. 2006;22:357–374.

9.

MISCELLANEOUS PHARMACOLOGY

Ramana K. Naidu

INTRODUCTION

This chapter discusses the unique and miscellaneous drugs that play a role in chronic pain management. The therapies can be used for analgesia, to address comorbidities associated with chronic pain, and to manage side effects associated with commonly used analgesics. Essentially, this is a diverse group of pharmacological questions that are important for the armamentarium of the pain physician. Topics range from neuroleptics to antispasticity drugs and sympatholytic drugs. Knowledge of these sometimes rarely used drugs can be highly useful in challenging situations.

QUESTIONS

1. Which of the following steroids commonly used for interventional pain management has the smallest particulates when used for epidural injection?

 A. Methylprednisolone (Solu-Medrol)
 B. Triamcinolone (Kenalog)
 C. Commercial betamethasone (Celestone)
 D. Compounded betamethasone
 E. Dexamethasone (Decadron)

2. Which of the following drugs has the highest affinity to the mu opioid receptor?

 A. Naloxone
 B. Tramadol
 C. Buprenorphine
 D. Hydromorphone
 E. Nalbuphine

3. Which of the following is the reason why one should consider switching from gabapentin to pregabalin?

 A. Reduced creatinine clearance
 B. Impaired intestinal transport limiting bioavailability

 C. Hepatic dysfunction
 D. Hypoalbuminemia
 E. Cost

4. The muscle relaxant carisoprodol produces a metabolite that has the potential for addiction. What is the name of this metabolite?

 A. Methylamine
 B. Mexilitene
 C. Meprobamate
 D. Metaxolone
 E. Meperidine

5. Chlorzoxazone is a centrally acting muscle relaxant that has all of the following properties Except:

 A. It is not a tricyclic antidepressant.
 B. It can rarely cause hepatotoxicity.
 C. It is an α_2 agonist.
 D. It is less sedating than carisoprodol.
 E. It is not a benzodiazepine.

6. Which of the following drugs is closest in action to lidocaine?

 A. Levetiracetam
 B. Lamotrigine
 C. Procainamide
 D. Thiothixene
 E. Mexiletine

7. Respiratory depression due to buprenorphine is rare, but when it occurs, it can be difficult to reverse. Which of the following is a respiratory stimulant that can be used to maintain minute ventilation due to buprenorphine-related respiratory depression?

 A. Doxapram
 B. Naltrexone

C. Naloxone
D. Donepezil
E. Acetazolamide

8. Methadone is not metabolized through which of the following cytochrome P450 systems?

A. CYP2B6
B. CYP2C9
C. CYP2C19
D. CYP2A6
E. CYP2C8

9. A 39-year-old woman with a history of bipolar depression with psychotic features overdoses on risperidone. Features of neuroleptic malignant syndrome include all of the following except:

A. Tachycardia
B. Raised plasma creatine phosphokinase
C. Severe muscle rigidity
D. Leukopenia
E. Pyrexia

10. Mexiletine is an antiarrhythmic that works as a:

A. Nav1.7-specific sodium channel blocker
B. N-type calcium channel blocker
C. Potassium channel blocker
D. Nonselective sodium channel blocker
E. Ligand-gated sodium channel blocker

11. Which of the following drugs does not have *N*-methyl-D-aspartate (NMDA) antagonist properties?

A. D-Alanine
B. Levorphanol
C. Xenon
D. D-Methadone
E. Memantine

12. A 37-year-old woman undergoes a total hip arthroplasty for avascular necrosis. Her history is significant for asthma as a child and severe migraine headaches. On postoperative day 1, she is found seizing in her room. Withdrawal from which of the following medications is most likely the cause of her condition?

A. Sumatriptan
B. Naproxen
C. Fioricet (acetaminophen/butalbital/caffeine)
D. Calcitonin
E. Gabapentin

13. It is estimated that the risk of developing rash when starting lamotrigine is approximately 10%. When discussing the risk of Stevens–Johnson syndrome associated with the initiation of lamotrigine, what is the approximate reported incidence to explain to patients?

A. 18% (1/5.5)
B. 8% (1/12.5)
C. 0.8% (1/125)
D. 0.08% (1/1250)
E. 0.008% (1/12,500)

14. Ziconitide is derived from the venom of *Conus magus* and blocks calcium influx into which of the following types of calcium channels?

A. L-type
B. N-type
C. P-type
D. R-type
E. T-type

15. As a membrane stabilizer, oxcarbazepine has some advantages compared to carbamazepine; however, there are still potentially harmful side effects. Which of the following lab values should be monitored after initiation of oxcarbazepine?

A. Complete blood count
B. Aspartate transaminase/alanine transaminase
C. International normalized ratio
D. Sodium
E. Creatinine

16. Intrathecal baclofen is used as an antispasticity agent by acting as an agonist at which of the following receptors?

A. $GABA_A$
B. $GABA_B$
C. $GABA_C$
D. α_2
E. Muscarinic

17. Cyclobenzaprine is structurally related to which of the following drugs?

A. Amitriptyline
B. Tizanidine
C. Diazepam
D. Baclofen
E. Methocarbamol

18. The following side effects should be discussed with patients receiving frequent epidural steroid injections except:

A. Bone demineralization
B. Hyperglycemia
C. Menstrual irregularities
D. Diuresis
E. Allergic reaction

19. Intravenous regional anesthesia using guanethidine has been administered in sympathetically mediated pain syndromes. Guanethidine works by depleting which of the following neurotransmitters?

A. Epinephrine
B. Dopamine
C. Serotonin
D. Norepinephrine
E. Substance P

20. Orphenadrine is a muscle relaxant that has all of the following pharmacological properties Except:

A. H1 receptor antagonist
B. NMDA receptor antagonist
C. mACh receptor antagonist
D. Norepinephrine reuptake inhibitor
E. H2 receptor antagonist

21. Which of the following pair of steroids has the highest relative glucocorticoid potency?

A. Methylprednisolone and dexamethasone
B. Prednisone and betamethasone
C. Triamcinolone and hydrocortisone
D. Betamethasone and dexamethasone
E. Dexamethasone and hydrocortisone

22. Metabolism through which of the following cytochrome P450 pathways can alter the plasma concentration of tricylic antidepressants due to genetic or other drug influences?

A. 3A4
B. 2C9
C. 2D6
D. 2B6
E. 1A2

23. Which two local anesthetics are implicated in the development of methemoglobinemia?

A. Procaine and benzocaine
B. Prilocaine and benzocaine
C. Lidocaine and mepivacaine
D. Tetracaine and prilocaine
E. Procaine and lidocaine

24. Caffeine is often added to commonly used analgesics such as acetaminophen/paracetamol, ibuprofen, and diclofenac. A Cochrane Review of the use of caffeine as an analgesic concluded which of the following?

A. The addition of caffeine (≥100 mg) to a standard dose of commonly used analgesics provides a small but important increase in the proportion of participants who experience a good level of pain relief.
B. The addition of caffeine (≥100 mg) to a standard dose of commonly used analgesics provides a large and important increase in the proportion of participants who experience a good level of pain relief.
C. The addition of caffeine (≥100 mg) is helpful only when combined with acetaminophen and not with COX inhibitory drugs.
D. The addition of caffeine (≥100 mg) to a standard dose of commonly used analgesics has no impact on pain and is used only for its central nervous system (CNS) stimulant properties.
E. The addition of caffeine (≥100 mg) to a standard dose of commonly used analgesics does not have any role in pain or as a CNS stimulant.

25. A patient visits the pain clinic complaining of fevers, stiff muscles, and a racing heart rate. She was started on olanzapine for refractory migraine. All of the following are potential treatments for this condition except:

A. Dantrolene
B. Bromocriptine
C. Amantadine
D. Benzodiazepines
E. Morphine

26. Which of the following drugs used for opioid-induced pruritus is on the American Geriatric Society's Beers criteria, a list of medications that are relatively and absolutely contraindicated in patients older than age 65 years?

A. Nalbuphine
B. Naloxone
C. Ondansteron
D. Propofol
E. Hydroxyzine

27. What is the proposed mechanism of action of magnesium in pain management?

A. AMPA antagonist
B. Neurokinin-1 agonist
C. NMDA antagonist

D. Substance P antagonist

E. Cholecystokinin analogue

28. An adjuvant is added to a regional blockade involving bupivacaine. A week later, the patient reports that she noticed the block lasts longer by a few hours than previous blocks with local anesthetic only. In addition, she reports having a dry mouth, decreased heart rate, and dizziness when going from sitting to standing suddenly. What is the adjuvant?

A. Clonidine

B. Magnesium

C. Dexamethasone

D. Ketorolac

E. Buprenorphine

29. Which of the following NMDA receptor subunits has promise as a target of the modulation of pain?

A. NR2A

B. NR2B

C. NR2C

D. NR2D

E. NR3A

ANSWERS

1. ANSWER: C

In Benzon et al.'s study, the particle sizes of commonly used steroids for interventional pain management are photographed and categorized by particle size. Dexamethasone does not have any particulate; therefore, of the particulate steroids, commercially prepared betamethasone has the smallest particulate size. Interestingly, betamethasone sodium phosphate by itself is also a nonparticulate. Compounded betamethasone has a higher percentage of particles that are larger than 50 μm. Knowing the particulate size of injectates is important because this indicates how they are made and whether they impose increased risk to patients. The importance of this was highlighted in the New England Compounding Center fungal outbreak of October 2012 related to lots of methylprednisolone.

FURTHER READING

Benzon H, Chew TL, McCarthy RJ, et al. Comparison of the particle sizes of different steroids and the effect of dilution: A review of the relative neurotoxicities of the steroids. *Anesthesiology*. 2007;106:331–338.

2. ANSWER: C

Of the opioids listed, buprenorphine has the highest affinity to the mu opioid receptor. It is one of the properties of buprenorphine that makes it beneficial in that patients who try to abuse other opioids will not obtain any pleasure or reward from these drugs. On the other hand, it can also be detrimental, such as in acute pain management of a patient already on a relatively high dose of buprenorphine—for example, a patient entering the emergency department who is on sublingual buprenorphine (Suboxone, Subutex, Zubsolv, or Bunavail) therapy. The commonly used opioids for analgesia—fentanyl, hydromorphone, morphine, hydrocodone, and oxycodone—may require significantly higher doses to achieve effect.

FURTHER READING

Freye E. *Opioids in Medicine*. New York, NY: Springer; 2008:118.

3. ANSWER: B

The gabapentinoids, gabapentin and pregabalin, are similar in their mechanism of action as $\alpha_2\delta$ ligand calcium channel modulators. The bioavailability of pregabalin (90%) is much higher than that of gabapentin (30–60%). The reason for this discrepancy is the intestinal system L transporter, which is saturable. Gabapentin relies solely on this transport mechanism, whereas pregabalin uses this as well as nonsaturable absorption. Therefore, patients who reach a ceiling effect with escalating doses of gabapentin may be candidates for a pregabalin trial.

Choices A, C, and D impact both gabapentinoids. Choice D is a reason to switch from pregabalin to gabapentin because pregabalin is more expensive due to the later development and its patent. Over time, the economics of these drugs may invert in their pricing, but currently pregabalin (Lyrica) is more expensive than gabapentin; therefore, gabapentin is generally preferred when costs/insurance coverage are an issue.

FURTHER READING

Toth C. Pregabalin: Latest safety evidence and clinical implications for the management of neuropathic pain. *Ther Adv Drug Saf.* 2014;5(1):38–56.

4. ANSWER: C

Methylamine is a colorless gas that is a derivative of ammonia. It gained notoriety in pop culture through the show *Breaking Bad*. Mexilitene is a class Ib antiarrhythmic and is not a metabolite of carisoprodol. Meprobamate is the metabolite of carisoprodol that is responsible for its addictive qualities. Meprobamate itself is a Schedule IV drug and has been associated with withdrawal syndromes when patients discontinue carisoprodol abruptly. Metaxolone is another drug in the muscle relaxant class. Meperidine is a mu opioid that has local anesthetic properties and atropine-like effects.

FURTHER READING

Bramness J, Skurtveit S, Fauske L, et al. Association between blood carisoprodol:meprobamate concentration ratios and CYP2C19 genotype in carisoprodol-drugged drivers: Decreased metabolic capacity in heterozygous CYP2C19*1/CYP2C19*2 subjects? *Pharmacogenetics*. 2003;13(7):383–388.

5. ANSWER: C

Chlorzoxazone is a central-acting drug in the class of antispasmodics/muscle relaxant. Although its exact mechanism is unclear, it appears to have a role in changing the conductance of calcium-activated potassium channels, which may impact muscle relaxation. It is not an α_2 agonist. The drug in this category that does have α_2 agonist properties is tizanidine (Zanaflex). Furthermore, it is not a tricyclic antidepressant.

FURTHER READING

Liu YC, Lo YK, Wu SN. Stimulatory effects of chlorzoxazone, a centrally acting muscle relaxant, on large conductance calcium-activated potassium channels in pituitary GH3 cells. *Brain Res*. 2003;959:86–97.
National Institutes of Health, US National Library of Medicine. Drug label information. Available at http://dailymed.nlm.nih.gov/dailymed/drugInfo.cfm?id=15262.

6. ANSWER: E

Lidocaine was the first amide local anesthetic to be developed, which occurred in the 1940s in Sweden. Its mechanism of action is in blocking fast voltage-gated sodium channels in the cell membranes of neurons and of the myocardium; it is also a class Ib antiarrhythmic and has been used for ventricular arrhythmias. Mexiletine is also a class Ib antiarrhythmic and can be used for sodium channelopathies such as erythromelalgia. Levetiracetam is a membrane stabilizer used in the treatment of epilepsy and for neuropathic pain management. Lamotrigine is a sodium channel membrane stabilizer that is used for neuropathic pain management. Procainamide is also a class Ib antiarrhythmic but is not used as an analgesic. Thiothixene is a typical antipsychotic that can be used for the treatment of schizophrenia. It is in the thixanthene class of drugs and was developed in 1967. Mexiletine is a class Ib antiarrhythmic voltage-gated sodium channel antagonist with analgesic properties, like lidocaine.

7. ANSWER: A

Due to the higher affinity of buprenorphine to the mu receptor compared to the commonly used antagonist naloxone, other agents may be required to help with respiratory stimulation. The analeptic doxapram can be administered intravenously at a dose of 1–1.5 mg/hr to provide respiratory stimulation. If naloxone is used, much higher doses may need to be used, such as 4–8 mg/hr continuous infusion. Both naloxone and naltrexone are not respiratory stimulants. In one study, donepezil was examined as a buprenorphine-induced respiratory depression therapy in a rabbit model. Acetazolamide has not been reported to be of any benefit in this situation.

FURTHER READING

Foster B, Twycross R, Mihalyo M, et al. Therapeutic reviews: Buprenorphine. *J Pain Symptom Manage*. 2013;45(5):939–949.
Sakuraba S, Tsujita M, Arisaka H, et al. Donepezil reverses buprenorphine-induced central respiratory depression in anesthetized rabbits. *Biol Res Santiago*. 2009;42(4):469–475.

8. ANSWER: D

Methadone has variable bioavailability due in part to its multiple pathways of metabolism. Of the listed pathways, CYP2A6 is not one of the pathways that methadone utilizes for metabolism. It does get metabolized by all of the others, with rank order described by Chang et al.:

$$CYP2B6 > 3A4 > 2C19 > 2D6 > 2C18, 3A7 > 2C8, 2C9, 3A5$$

Kharasch et al. found that 2B6 is the most important determinant of metabolism of methadone in humans.

FURTHER READING

Chang Y, Fang W, Lin SN, et al. Stereo-selective metabolism of methadone by human liver microsomes and cDNA-expressed cytochrome P450s: A reconciliation. *Basic Clin Pharmacol Toxicol*. 2011;108:55–62.
Kharasch ED, Regina KJ, Blood J, et al. Methadone pharmacogenetics: CYP2B6 polymorphisms determine plasma concentrations, clearance, and metabolism. *Anesthesiology*. 2015;123(5):1142–1153.
Lugo R, Satterfield KL, Kern SE. Pharmocokinetics of methadone. *J Pain Palliat Care Pharmacother*. 2005;19(4):13–24.

9. ANSWER: D

Neuroleptic malignant syndrome is a potentially life-threatening condition and requires understanding of the signs and symptoms to diagnose and treat it. Because your patients may be on antipsychotics for psychiatric comorbidities or neuropathic pain, it is important to understand these signs and symptoms. The features of neuroleptic malignant syndrome include the following:

1. Fever
2. Tachycardia
3. Severe muscle rigidity
4. Altered mental status
5. Raised plasma creatine phosphokinase
6. Leukocytosis
7. Impaired liver function tests
8. Renal impairment
9. Electrocardiogram abnormalities

FURTHER READING

Howard P, et al. Therapeutic reviews: Antipsychotics. *J Pain Palliat Care Pharmacother*. 2011;41(5):956–964.

Trollor JN, Chen X, Sachdev PS. Neuroleptic malignant syndrome associated with atypical antipsychotic drugs. *CNS Drugs*. 2009;23(6):477–492.

10. ANSWER: A

Mexiletine is a class Ib antiarrythmic that is a voltage-gated sodium channel blocker; it is not a nonselective or ligand-gated channel agonist/antagonist. It has been used for neuropathic pain syndromes including erythromelalgia, which is related to SCN9A loss-of-function mutations resulting in aberrant signaling from Nav1.7 channels.

The N-type or neural-type calcium channels consist of α_1, $\alpha_2\delta$, β_1, β_3, and β_4 subunits. The $\alpha_2\delta$ subunit is modulated by gabapentinoids. The entire receptor is antagonized by ziconotide. The class III antiarrhythmics are potassium channel blockers.

FURTHER READING

Cregg R, Cox JJ, Bennett DL, et al. Mexiletine as a treatment for primary erythromelalgia: Normalization of biophysical properties of mutant L858F NaV 1.7 sodium channels. *Br J Pharmacol*. 2014;171(19):4455–4463.

11. ANSWER: A

Several NMDA antagonists have roles in medicine. The NMDA receptor, which is agonized by glutamate, is important in playing a role in wind-up, tolerance, and opioid-induced hyperalgesia. Some of the NMDA antagonists that have been trialed in pain management include ketamine, magnesium, dextromethorphan, nitrous oxide, xenon, amantadine, memantine, ketobemidone, levorphanol, D-methadone, and, to a lesser extent, L-methadone. D-Alanine is an NMDA agonist.

FURTHER READING

Traynelis SF, Wollmuth LP, McBain CJ, et al. Glutamate receptor ion channels: Structure, regulation, and function. *Pharmacol Rev*. 2010;62(3):405–496.

12. ANSWER: C

Fioricet is a combination of butalbital, a barbiturate, acetaminophen, and caffeine. The sudden withdrawal of Fioricet has resulted in seizure activity, and this is a major reason why headache specialists are prescribing it less often or are restricting its use. Cessation of the migraine abortive agents sumatriptan and naproxen can lead to rebound headaches. Gabapentin, although an antiepileptic, potentially can lead to a withdrawal syndrome resulting in seizures; the propensity to do so is less than that of butalbital. Calcitonin has been trialed for migraine therapy, but abstinence of calcitonin has not been related to seizure activity.

FURTHER READING

Micieli G, Cavallini A, Martignoni E, et al. Effectiveness of salmon calcitonin nasal spray preparation in migraine treatment. *Headache*. 1988;28(3):196–200.

Romero CE, Baron JD, Knox AP, et al. Barbiturate withdrawal following Internet purchase of Fioricet. *Arch Neurol*. 2004;61(7):1111–1112.

13. ANSWER: D

Lamotrigine may be a useful neuropathic pain agent; however, the rare risk of toxic epidermal necrolysis is very serious and needs to be disclosed and discussed with patients embarking on this therapy. It is estimated to occur in 0.08% or 1 out of 1250 patients.

FURTHER READING

Benzon H, Raja SN, Liu SS, et al. *Essentials of Pain Medicine*. 3rd ed. Philadelphia, PA: Saunders; 2011:120.

14. ANSWER: B

Ziconotide (Prialt) is the ω-toxin peptide derived from the snail *Conus magus*. It is one of several types of conotoxins. It exerts its effect at the N-type calcium channel. It has a unique role in intrathecal drug delivery for neuropathic pain with a narrow therapeutic index. It is one of three currently US Food and Drug Administration (FDA) approved intrathecal drug therapies, with the other two being morphine and baclofen.

FURTHER READING

Benzon H, Raja SN, Liu SS, et al. *Essentials of Pain Medicine*. 3rd ed. Philadelphia, PA: Saunders; 2011:129.

15. ANSWER: D

Oxcarbazepine has potential advantages compared to carbamazepine regarding major side effects such as aplastic anemia and agranulocytosis. However, the prospect of developing hyponatremia exists, and it usually manifest in the first months after initiation of this drug. It is recommended that patients be aware of the signs and symptoms of hyponatremia, including lethargy, seizure, and coma, and be tested for plasma sodium levels in the first several weeks after initiation. Generally, patients reach their nadir in the first several months after initiation, and then their plasma sodium level is stabilized on their regimen over time.

FURTHER READING

Benzon H, Raja SN, Liu SS, et al. *Essentials of Pain Medicine*. 3rd ed. Philadelphia, PA: Saunders; 2011:125.

16. ANSWER: B

Baclofen is derived from γ-aminobutyric acid (GABA) and agonizes the $GABA_B$ receptor. It is used for spasticity associated with cerebral palsy, multiple sclerosis, and spinal cord injury. Abrupt withdrawal of continuous intrathecal baclofen therapy can be dangerous, even life threatening. Benzodiazepines agonize the $GABA_A$ receptor. $GABA_C$ receptors are now labeled as $GABA_A$ rho receptors, which have high expression in the retina of vertebrates and are not responsive to benzodiazepines, barbiturates, or baclofen. $α_2$ agonists include clonidine, dexmedetomidine, and tizanidine. Muscarinic antagonists used in pain management include scopolamine and atropine.

17. ANSWER: A

Cyclobenzaprine is structurally related to tricyclic antidepressants. Among the answer choices, amitriptyline is the only tricyclic antidepressant listed. Tizanidine is a muscle relaxant with $α_2$ agonist properties. Diazepam is a benzodiazepine. Baclofen, as in Question 16, is a $GABA_B$ agonist. Methocarbamol is another muscle relaxant that is derived from guaifenesin.

FURTHER READING

Benzon H, Raja SN, Liu SS, et al. *Essentials of Pain Medicine*. 3rd ed. Philadelphia, PA: Saunders; 2011:143.

18. ANSWER: D

Steroid therapy has been utilized in pain management for decades. Knowledge of the myriad potential consequences of steroid therapy is paramount. Rather than frank diuresis, steroids can lead to fluid retention. In addition, steroids can lead to the following:

- Bone demineralization
- Hyperglycemia
- Menstrual irregularities
- Allergic reaction
- Elevated blood pressure
- Generalized erythema/flushing
- Gastritis/peptic ulcer disease
- Hypothalamic–pituitary–adrenal axis suppression
- Cushing's syndrome
- Steroid myopathy

It is important to discuss and disclose all of these risks when providing repetitive therapies on a cyclical basis. Although the risks may be minimal with the initial steroid injection, subsequent injections increase risks over time; therefore, it is important to use the lowest reasonable dose, possibly even none, as frequently as possible and to routinely assess and ensure improvements in functional benchmarks.

FURTHER READING

Benzon H, Raja SN, Liu SS, et al. *Essentials of Pain Medicine*. 3rd ed. Philadelphia, PA: Saunders; 2011:152.

19. ANSWER: D

Guanethedine is a sympatholytic that has been trialed as a means to reduce pain associated with complex regional pain syndrome via intravenous regional anesthesia. It reduces the release of norepinephrine (NE) and takes the place of NE in transmitted vesicles. The drug has been used as an antihypertensive resistant to other therapies; however, it is not widely used for this purpose.

20. ANSWER: E

Orphenadrine is an antihistamine, related to diphenhydramine, that has been used as a muscle relaxant. It does not have H2 receptor antagonism, although like diphenhydramine, it has several pharmacologic actions, including the following:

1. H1 receptor antagonism without H2 receptor antagonism
2. NMDA receptor antagonism
3. mACh receptor antagonism

4. Norepinephrine reuptake inhibitor
5. Nav1.7, Nav1.8, and Nav1.9 sodium channel blocker
6. HERG potassium channel blocker

FURTHER READING

Benzon H, Raja SN, Liu SS, et al. *Essentials of Pain Medicine*. 5th ed. Philadelphia, PA: Mosby; 2014.

Desaphy JF, Dipalma A, De Bellis M, et al. Involvement of voltage-gated sodium channels blockade in the analgesic effects of orphenadrine. *Pain*. 2009;142(3):225–235.

Kapur S, Seeman P. NMDA receptor antagonists ketamine and PCP have direct effects on the dopamine D(2) and serotonin 5-HT(2) receptors—Implications for models of schizophrenia. *Mol Psychiatry*. 2002;7(8):837–844.

Kornhuber J, Parsons CG, Hartmann S, et al. Orphenadrine is an uncompetitive *N*-methyl-D-aspartate (NMDA) receptor antagonist: Binding and patch clamp studies. *J Neural Transm Gen Sect*. 1995;102(3):237–246.

Pubill D, Canudas AM, Pallàs M, et al. Assessment of the adrenergic effects of orphenadrine in rat vas deferens. *J Pharm Pharmacol*. 1999;51(3):307–312.

Rumore MM, Schlichting DA. Analgesic effects of antihistaminics. *Life Sci*. 1985;36(5):403–416.

Scholz EP, Konrad FM, Weiss DL, et al. Anticholinergic antiparkinson drug orphenadrine inhibits HERG channels: Block attenuation by mutations of the pore residues Y652 or F656. *Naunyn-Schmiedeberg's Arch Pharmacol*. 2007. 376 (4): 275–284.

Syvälahti EK, Kunelius R, Laurén L. Effects of antiparkinsonian drugs on muscarinic receptor binding in rat brain, heart and lung. *Pharmacol Toxicol*. 1988;62(2):90–94.

21. ANSWER: D

According to Benzon et al., both betamethasone and dexamethasone have the highest glucocorticoid potency, with betamethasone edging out dexamethasone 33 to 27 (Table 9.1). In *Stoelting's Pharmacology and Physiology in Anesthetic Practice*, the two have equal glucocorticoid activity. Among commonly used steroids for interventional pain management, these are the two with the highest relative glucocorticoid potency.

Table 9.1 **COMPARISON OF THE DIFFERENT STEROIDS IN TERMS OF GLUCORTICOID POTENCIES**

STEROID	RELATIVE GLUCOCORTICOID POTENCY
Prednisone	(4)
Methylprednisolone	5
Triamcinolone	5
Betamethasone	33
Dexamethasone	27

SOURCE: Adapted from Benzon H, Chew TL, McCarthy RJ, et al. Comparison of the particle sizes of different steroids and the effect of dilution: A review of the relative neurotoxicities of the steroids. *Anesthesiology*. 2007;106:331–338.

FURTHER READING

Benzon H, Chew TL, McCarthy RJ, et al. Comparison of the particle sizes of different steroids and the effect of dilution: A review of the relative neurotoxicities of the steroids. *Anesthesiology*. 2007;106:331–338.

Flood P, Rathmel JP, Shafer S. (Eds.). *Stoelting's Pharmacology and Physiology in Anesthetic Practice*. 5th ed. Philadelphia, PA: Wolters Kluwer; 2015.

22. ANSWER: C

Several CYP450 enzymes are important for the metabolism of drugs involved in pain management. Understanding these differences and the impact of genetics and other agents is important to the pain physician. CYP450 2D6 is important in the metabolism of tricyclic antidepressants, as it is for codeine, hydrocodone, and oxycodone. There is a range of patients who are poor metabolizers, extensive metabolizers, rapid metabolizers, and ultrarapid metabolizers, affecting the plasma concentrations of the desired therapeutic. 2C9 is important for the metabolism of commonly used cyclooxygenase inhibitors (nonsteroidal anti-inflammatory drugs), such as celecoxib and naproxen. 2B6 is a major determinant of methadone metabolism. In addition to knowing which CYP450 systems are involved in a drug's metabolism (substrates), it is also important to know whether substances inhibit or induce metabolism through these pathways. A commonly cited example is grapefruit juice being an inhibitor of the 3A4 system, which may have an impact on warfarin metabolism and, therefore, efficacy versus adverse effects.

FURTHER READING

Brunton LL, Chabner B, Knollman B. *Goodman and Gilman's The Pharmacological Basis of Therapeutics*. 12th ed. New York, NY: McGraw-Hill; 2012:412.

23. ANSWER: B

Among local anesthetics, prilocaine and benzocaine can both result in methemoglobinemia. Lidocaine has also been implicated, but mepivacaine and procaine have not. Methemoglobinemia is formed from ferric (Fe^{3+}) rather than ferrous (Fe^{2+}) iron, which makes the functioning ferrous units have higher affinity to oxygen, thus shifting the oxygen–hemoglobin dissociation curve to the left. This can cause tissue hypoxia, resulting in altered mental status, cyanosis, shortness of breath, and fatigue. It is generally clinically benign, although there have been several case reports of clinical sequelae from the use of topical benzocaine

(HurriCaine spray) resulting in cyanosis. The life-saving therapy, when there is fulminant tissue hypoxia, is the intravenous administration of methylene blue.

FURTHER READING

Hegedus F, Herb K. Benzocaine-induced methemoglobinemia. *Anesth Prog.* 2005;52(4):136–139.

24. ANSWER: A

Caffeine, a methylxanthine, has been added to several analgesics for the treatment of headache and other acute pains. This Cochrane Review examined several studies comparing analgesics with (vs. without) caffeine and concluded that the addition of caffeine (≥100 mg) to a standard dose of commonly used analgesics provides a small but important increase in the proportion of participants who experience a good level of pain relief. Caffeine may play a direct role as an analgesic in addition to being a CNS stimulant and vasoconstrictor.

FURTHER READING

Derry CJ, Derry S, Moore RA. Caffeine as an analgesic adjuvant for acute pain in adults. Cochrane Database Syst Rev. 2012;14(3):CD009281.

25. ANSWER: E

Antipsychotics may be used in specific challenging pain management situations, especially in the setting of psychotic symptoms or comorbid psychotic diseases. The atypical antipsychotics may have a reduced side effect profile but still can cause neuroleptic malignant syndrome. Several therapies may be employed, including dantrolene, the dopamine agonist bromocriptine, amantadine, and benzodiazepines. Morphine does not have a role as an antidote in this syndrome.

FURTHER READING

Trollor JN, Chen X, Sachdev PS. Neuroleptic malignant syndrome associated with atypical antipsychotic drugs. *CNS Drugs.* 2009;23(6):477–492.

26. ANSWER: E

The Beers criteria from the American Geriatric Society are a list of medications that are potentially harmful for patients older than age 65 years. With a growing "baby boomer" population, it is important to limit the adverse reactions associated with these drugs. The antihistamines have the risk for development of delirium and should be avoided in the elderly.

Furthermore, antihistamines typically address peripheral opioid-induced pruritus caused by histaminergic release and may be ineffective for opioid-induced pruritus. If there are no histaminergic signs or symptoms, such as urticarial, flushing, and erythema, it is unwise to employ an antihistamine for this condition. The other answer choices have merit but may be limited by routes of administration, cost, and monitoring, although these choices are relatively safe in the geriatric population when administered at the correct doses.

FURTHER READING

Campanelli CM. American Geriatrics Society updated Beers criteria for potentially inappropriate medication use in older adults: The American Geriatrics Society 2012 Beers Criteria Update Expert Panel. *J Am Geriatr Soc.* 2012;60(4):616–631.

27. ANSWER: C

Magnesium is a NMDA antagonist that has had a checkered past regarding its efficacy in acute postoperative pain management. A meta-analysis by De Oliveira et al. gave credence to its use in the perioperative period, especially given its low side effect profile in the face of opioid escalation. It is important to note that there are several NMDA subunits, which explains why only certain NMDA antagonists have a role in the modulation of nociception and pain and others do not.

FURTHER READING

De Oliveira Jr GS, Castro-Alves LJ, Khan JH, et al. Perioperative systemic magnesium to minimize postoperative pain: A meta-analysis of randomized controlled trials. *Anesthesiology.* 2013;119:178–190.
Naidu R, Flood P. Magnesium: Is there a signal in the noise? *Anesthesiology.* 2013;119:13–15.
Petrenko AB, Yamakura T, Baba H, et al. The role of N-methyl-D-aspartate (NMDA) receptors in pain: A review. *Anesth Analg.* 2003;97:1108–1116.

28. ANSWER: A

Several adjuvants have been used to prolong the duration of neural blockade by local anesthetics. Although the evidence regarding their use is mixed, it is important to know the potential side effects of each adjuvant. Clonidine, an α_2 agonist, can cause bradycardia, dry mouth, and orthostatic hypotension when used as an adjuvant. It is not FDA approved for this indication; it is FDA approved for hypertension and for pediatric attention deficit hyperactivity disorder (2010). It has also been used for anxiety disorders and for withdrawal symptoms associated with opioids, alcohol, benzodiazepines, and nicotine. Per Popping et al., the average extension of duration of regional blockade was 2 hours when added to intermediate-acting local anesthetics.

FURTHER READING

Popping DM, Elia N, Marret E, et al. Clonidine as an adjuvant to local anesthetics for peripheral nerve and plexus blocks: A meta-analysis of randomized trials. *Anesthesiology.* 2009;111:406–415.

29. ANSWER: B

One of the primary reasons why the group of medications known as NMDA antagonists have disparate effects is that all these drugs may affect different subunits and therefore may have a unique therapeutic benefit or adverse effect profile. The NR2B appears to play a role as an anti-hyperalgesic and may continue to be a target of therapeutics development for chronic pain.

FURTHER READING

Petrenko AB, Yamakura T, Baba H, et al. The role of *N*-methyl-D-aspartate (NMDA) receptors in pain: A review. *Anesth Analg.* 2003;97:1108–1116.

NEUROMODULATION

Bryan Covert and Marc A. Huntoon

INTRODUCTION

Although one could argue that all facets of pain medicine are, in essence, a form of neuromodulation, this chapter seeks to address the indications for, and complications related to, surgical, pharmacologic, and adjunctive neuromodulation therapy. Many forms of neuromodulation therapy find their inspiration from the landmark work by Melzack and Wall in 1965 that described the gate theory of pain. More than 50 years later, technological and pharmaceutical progress leads the charge in this exciting field within pain medicine. As our understanding of the generation, transmission, and interpretation of pain signaling expands, the options for interventional and medical therapy will surely follow suit. These advancements are a welcome addition as the aging population meets a medical community seeking to curb chronic opioid therapy. The questions in this chapter serve as a guide to the salient neuromodulation techniques, but an emphasis should be placed on the suggested readings for this chapter to develop a more thorough understanding on the topic and variety of techniques and pharmacotherapy not covered here.

FURTHER READING

Melzack R, Wall PD. Pain mechanisms: A new theory. *Science.* 1965;150(3699):971–979.

QUESTIONS

1. Transcutaneous electrical nerve stimulation (TENS) is postulated to work peripherally by stimulation of which of the following?

A. M_2 muscarinic receptors at the motor end plate
B. Aβ sensory afferent fibers
C. Myelinated Aδ fibers
D. Peripheral C fibers

2. After 30 minutes of low-frequency (2 Hz) transcutaneous electrical nerve stimulation, reversal of the induced analgesic effects would be expected with the administration of:

A. Flumazenil
B. Intrathecal cholecystokinin (CCK) antagonist
C. Naloxone
D. High-dose fluoxetine

3. Burst programming for spinal cord stimulation is characterized by the use of a stimulus frequency of:

A. 10,000 Hz
B. 10–20 Hz
C. 250–500 Hz
D. 1000–2000 Hz

4. The mechanism of analgesia with spinal cord stimulation is mediated by which of the following neurotransmitters?

A. Glutamate
B. Calcitonin gene-related peptide
C. Norepinephrine
D. γ-Aminobutyric acid (GABA)

5. In patients carrying the following diagnoses, which would be the least likely to achieve significant reduction in pain with spinal cord stimulation therapy?

A. Failed back surgery syndrome without a radicular component with pain of 17 years' duration
B. Complex regional pain syndrome type 1 in the right upper extremity
C. Painful diabetic neuropathy
D. Postherpetic neuralgia

6. High-frequency stimulation offers the advantage over conventional spinal cord stimulation of:

A. Longer implantable pulse generator (IPG) battery life
B. Improved results when applied to post-thoracotomy pain syndrome
C. Paresthesia-free pain relief
D. Lower complication rates

7. A 73-year-old male presents to the pain clinic for follow up 6 days after a spinal cord stimulator trial for post-laminectomy syndrome with radicular pain. He has a significant past medical history of type 2 diabetes, hypertension, and coronary artery disease. He reports excellent coverage of his pain and plans to proceed to permanent spinal cord stimulator implantation. The leads are removed without complication. Four hours later, he calls and reports that he has noticed increased pain at the site of lead removal and progressive leg weakness since leaving the clinic. What is the next best step in management?

A. Instruct him to return to the clinic for evaluation immediately.
B. Arrange for stat magnetic resonance imaging (MRI) and neurosurgeon consultation, and meet the patient at the hospital.
C. Reassure the patient that this is common, but ask him to monitor for further changes over the next few hours.
D. Instruct him to go to the nearest emergency room for evaluation.

8. What is the least likely complication associated with spinal cord stimulator implantation?

A. Unwanted stimulation
B. Infection
C. Hardware malfunction
D. Lead fracture

9. Risk factors for accidental dural puncture during spinal cord stimulator implantation include all of the following except:

A. Midline interlaminar approach
B. Low body mass index
C. Scoliosis
D. Retrograde approach

10. Generally accepted indications for peripheral nerve stimulation include all of the following except:

A. Complex regional pain syndrome (CRPS) type II in a patient with an indwelling spinal cord stimulator

B. Tibial neuralgia after tarsal tunnel surgery
C. Diabetic polyneuropathy
D. Transformed migraine

11. Identify the perineurium in Figure 10.1, which represents a short-axis cross-sectional view of a peripheral nerve.

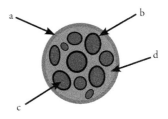

Figure 10.1 A short-axis cross-sectional view of a peripheral nerve.

12. Ziconotide inhibits pain primarily through modulation of what receptor type?

A. G protein-coupled receptor
B. Voltage-gated calcium channel
C. Glutamatergic receptor
D. GABA$_B$ receptor

13. A 73-year-old male is being treated for cancer pain with intrathecal (IT) morphine via a drug delivery system. He presents to your clinic for a refill. During the past year, his IT dose has increased 1 mg/day, and he has noticed a marked increase in pain during the past month with concomitant abdominal pain and diarrhea during the past week. He denies any loss of bowel or bladder function but does note some subjective lower extremity weakness. On exam, you appreciate loss of sensory function as tested to light touch in an L5 dermatomal distribution. What would be the next best step in management?

A. Send for MRI of the abdomen to assess for progression of malignant disease
B. Perform computed tomography myelogram of the spine
C. Refill his catheter with a higher concentration of morphine
D. Add ziconotide to the intrathecal infusion

14. For which of the following patients would the use of targeted intrathecal opioid delivery be most indicated?

A. A 27-year-old male with metastatic rhabdomyosarcoma on oral opioid therapy experiencing constipation and sedation but effective pain control
B. A 75-year-old female with chronic low back pain with post-laminectomy syndrome on escalating

doses of chronic opioid therapy without side effects or effective pain relief

C. A 53-year-old homeless male with pancreatic adenocarcinoma with life expectancy less than 3 months

D. A 43-year-old female with fibromyalgia and multiple somatic complaints on pregabalin, milnacipran, and a combination of sustained-release and immediate-release opioids totaling a morphine equivalent dose of 250 mg daily

15. Which of the following opioids is the least lipophilic?

A. Morphine
B. Fentanyl
C. Sufentanil
D. Hydromorphone

16. Which of the following drugs binds to the α subunit of voltage-gated sodium channels and may augment analgesia in patients with IT morphine therapy?

A. Gabapentin
B. Baclofen
C. Bupivacaine
D. Adenosine

17. Which of the following is a commonly described side effect related to IT opioid drug delivery?

A. Acalculous cholecystitis
B. Hypogonadotropic hypogonadism

C. Diabetes insipidus
D. Anhydrosis

18. Which of the following, when infused intrathecally, complements spinal cord stimulation therapy by acting on G protein-coupled receptors in the dorsal horn?

A. Midazolam
B. Baclofen
C. Gabapentin
D. Droperidol

19. For which of the following patients would dorsal root entry zone lesioning be most effective?

A. A 17-year-old male with T10 spinal cord transection with paroxysmal, lancinating pain in a dermatomal pattern immediately above the area affected by his injury

B. A 65-year-old female with facial pain in a V2 distribution secondary to trauma

C. A 53-year-old male with phantom limb pain following a traumatic amputation

D. A 45-year-old female with occipital neuralgia following a motor vehicle collision

20. With what diagnosis would microvascular decompression be expected to be most efficacious?

A. Trigeminal neuralgia
B. Postherpetic neuralgia
C. Occipital neuralgia
D. Neurogenic thoracic outlet syndrome

ANSWERS

1. ANSWER: B

The mechanism of action of TENS is complex and likely through multiple pathways, but one of the most widely accepted mechanisms is based on the gate control theory, originally described by Melzack and Wall in 1965. Following this theory, stimulation of Aβ (large-diameter, myelinated sensory afferent) fibers propagates antidromic activation of ascending pathways and antagonizes Aδ and C fibers via orthodromic stimulation of descending inhibitory interneurons. Ultimately, this theoretical mechanism of TENS therapy for pain relief occurs at the spinal cord level in the substantia gelatinosa. This modality and applied theory have led to the development of sophisticated dorsal column spinal cord stimulator technologies for more complex pain syndromes.

FURTHER READING

Claydon LS, Chestert L, Johnson MI, et al. Transcutaneous electrical nerve stimulation (TENS) for neuropathic pain in adults. *Cochrane Database Syst Rev Protoc.* 2010;10.

Melzack R, Wall PD. Pain mechanisms: A new theory. *Science.* 1965;150(3699):971–979.

2. ANSWER: C

Numerous studies have examined the role of endogenous opioid-mediated analgesia in TENS. Specifically, animal studies have shown increased concentrations of opioid peptides immediately following short sessions of both low-frequency (2 Hz) and high-frequency (100 Hz) TENS. Proenkephalin-derived peptides have been shown to be increased in rat cerebrospinal fluid (CSF) following low-frequency TENS. Supporting the involvement of these peptides in the induced analgesic effect is the reversibility of this analgesia with the μ receptor antagonist naloxone. Interestingly, this naloxone-mediated reversal is not observed reliably following high-frequency (100 Hz) TENS therapy, which suggests a separate physiologic mechanism for TENS-induced analgesia. Naltrindole, a δ opioid receptor antagonist, has been shown to reverse high-frequency TENS analgesia in animal models. Electroacupuncture and TENS may induce the release of CCK into the CSF, causing a tolerance-like effect that can be reversed in part by injection of CCK-A and CCK-B antagonists. Although some studies have shown paradoxical pain induced by high-dose serotonin–norepinephrine reuptake inhibitors therapy, this has not been correlated in the setting of TENS-mediated analgesia.

FURTHER READING

DeSantana JM, da Silva LFS, Sluka KA. Cholecystokinin receptors mediate tolerance to the analgesic effect of TENS in arthritic rats. *Pain.* 2010;148(1):84–93.

Han JS, Chen XH, Sun SL, et al. Effect of low- and high-frequency TENS on Met-enkephalin-Arg-Phe and dynorphin A immunore-activity in human lumbar CSF. *Pain.* 1991;47(3):295–298.

Kalra A, Urban MO, Sluka KA. Blockade of opioid receptors in rostral ventral medulla prevents antihyperalgesia produced by transcutaneous electrical nerve stimulation (TENS). *J Pharmacol Exp Ther.* 2001;298(1):257–263.

3. ANSWER: C

Neurons controlling pain perception fire in both a tonic, continuous manner and in groups of action potentials with periods of quiescence. Burst programming was developed with the understanding that activating both of these groups can provide more effective pain relief. In addition, burst stimulation has been reported to more effectively activate the cerebral cortex, which can cause pain relief at amplitudes below the threshold of paresthesia. The basic controls of spinal cord stimulation programming involve pulse width (ms), which defines the length of the pulse; amplitude (mA), representing the magnitude of the pulse; and frequency (Hz), which defines the number of pulses delivered per second. Specifically excluded from the answer choices is 40–50 Hz because this would create confusion. Burst is designed to deliver bursts of pulses at a low frequency of 40–50 Hz. The bursts contain impulses within that are delivered at a high frequency (500 Hz) within each pulse. See Figure 10.2 for further understanding.

FURTHER READING

De Ridder D, Vanneste S, Plazier M, et al. Burst spinal cord stimulation: Toward paresthesia-free pain suppression. *Neurosurgery.* 2010;66(5):986–990.

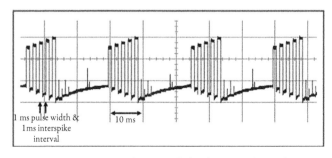

Figure 10.2 Constant current burst mode (mA): 1-ms spikes with a 1-ms spike interval (500-Hz spike mode) and 5-ms charge balance firing at 40 Hz (40-Hz burst mode).

SOURCE: Reprinted with permission from De Ridder D, Vanneste S, Plazier M, van der Loo E, Menovsky T. Burst spinal cord stimulation: toward paresthesia-free pain suppression. *Neurosurgery.* 2010;66(5):986–990. doi:10.1227/01.NEU.0000368153.44883.B3.

4. ANSWER: D

Animal models of neuropathic pain have shown that coadministration of low doses of GABA and adenosine A1 receptor agonists potentiate the effects of spinal cord stimulation-mediated reduction in allodynia. Extracellular GABA has also been measured in animal models for neuropathic pain states in the dorsal horn before and during spinal cord stimulation therapy. GABA levels were found to be significantly lower in those with induced neuropathic pain compared to controls and significantly higher following spinal cord stimulation therapy. This further supports the theory that inhibitory interneurons play a key role in the analgesic effect of spinal cord stimulation.

FURTHER READING

Cui JG, Meyerson BA, Sollevi A, et al. Effect of spinal cord stimulation on tactile hypersensitivity in mononeuropathic rats is potentiated by simultaneous GABA(B) and adenosine receptor activation. *Neurosci Lett*. 1998;247(2–3):183–186.
Stiller CO, Cui JG, O'Connor WT, et al. Release of gamma-aminobutyric acid in the dorsal horn and suppression of tactile allodynia by spinal cord stimulation in mononeuropathic rats. *Neurosurgery*. 1996;39(2):365–367.

5. ANSWER: A

Although post-laminectomy syndrome has been shown to be responsive to spinal cord stimulator therapy, a number of patient-related factors play in a role in the likelihood of long-term success of spinal cord stimulation therapy. Extensive evidence showing a favorable response to spinal cord stimulation therapy in cases of failed back surgery syndrome (FBSS), CRPS, postherpetic neuralgia, and painful diabetic neuropathy, and even angina and peripheral vascular disease. Factors that have suggested a lower probability of significant pain relief with spinal cord stimulator therapy include older age, somatization, catastrophizing thoughts, and pain duration longer than 15 years. In 2004, Cameron described the success rate of spinal cord stimulation in various diagnoses. Specifically, the reported success rate of FBSS/low back and leg pain was 62%, whereas the rate of success for CRPS I and II together was 84%, and that for postherpetic neuralgia was 82%. Patient selection is crucial in risk:benefit and cost:benefit optimization in spinal cord stimulator therapy, so an understanding of the most up-to-date criteria for patient selection should consistently be sought.

FURTHER READING

Borjesson M, Andrell P, Lundberg D, et al. Spinal cord stimulation in severe angina pectoris—A systematic review based on the Swedish Council on Technology assessment in health care report on long-standing pain. *Pain*. 2008;140(3):501–508.
Cameron T. Safety and efficacy of spinal cord stimulation for the treatment of chronic pain: A 20-year literature review. *J Neurosurg*. 2004;100(3 Suppl Spine):254–267.
Claeys LG, Berg W, Jonas S. Spinal cord stimulation in the treatment of chronic critical limb ischemia. *Acta Neurochir Suppl*. 2007;97 (Pt 1):259–265.
Jeon YH. Spinal cord stimulation in pain management: A review. *Korean J Pain*. 2012;25(3):143.
Kumar K, Hunter G, Demeria D. Spinal cord stimulation in treatment of chronic benign pain: Challenges in treatment planning and present status, a 22-year experience. *Neurosurgery*. 2006;58(3):481–496.
Kumar K, Toth C, Nath RK, et al. Epidural spinal cord stimulation for treatment of chronic pain—Some predictors of success: A 15-year experience. *Surg Neurol*. 1998;50(2):110–111.
Van Buyten JP, Van Zundert J, Vueghs P, et al. Efficacy of spinal cord stimulation: 10 years of experience in a pain centre in Belgium. *Eur J Pain*. 2001;5(3):299–307.

6. ANSWER: C

Emerging therapies using high-frequency spinal cord stimulation show promise in the treatment of chronic pain. High-frequency stimulation using frequencies of 10,000 Hz conveys the benefit of paresthesia-free stimulation while adding the additional benefit of better efficacy for axial low back pain. It is postulated that high-frequency stimulation more selectively activates Aβ fibers, allowing it to provide better relief of pain at amplitudes that are below the threshold for induced paresthesia. It may not be surprising, given these findings, that patients who failed conventional stimulation therapy were able to achieve significant pain reduction with high-frequency stimulation modes. Use of high-frequency stimulation offers the additional benefit of time saved during implantation because lead placement is made anatomically without additional sensory paresthesia testing. This therapy has shown promise in FBSS, radicular pain, and axial back pain but has not yet shown that it is better for post-thoracotomy pain. In addition, the complication rates are similar to those of conventional stimulation.

FURTHER READING

Al-Kaisy A, Van Buyten J-P, Smet I, et al. Sustained effectiveness of 10 kHz high-frequency spinal cord stimulation for patients with chronic, low back pain: 24-month results of a prospective multicenter study. *Pain Med*. 2014;15(3):347–354.
Kapural L, Yu C, Doust MW, et al. Novel 10-kHz high-frequency therapy (HF10 therapy) is superior to traditional low-frequency spinal cord stimulation for the treatment of chronic back and leg pain: The SENZA-RCT randomized controlled trial. *Anesthesiology*. 2015;123(4):851–860.

7. ANSWER: B

The symptoms described as well as the patient history suggesting potential antiplatelet drug use are concerning for a developing epidural hematoma. Spinal cord stimulator trial and permanent implantation represent high-risk procedures for bleeding in the setting of concomitant anticoagulant use. In this clinical scenario, the potential hematoma seems to have developed at the time of lead removal, which represents a lower risk; however, a rigid spinal cord stimulator lead can disrupt vessels in the epidural venous plexus upon implantation or removal. Time is of the essence in this clinical scenario because patients who develop epidural hematoma require surgical evacuation, and when this is done outside of 8 hours from presentation, the probability for poor neurologic outcome is significantly higher. The diagnosis and management of a suspected epidural hematoma require collaboration between the implanting physician, radiologist, and spine surgeon. Although this disastrous complication is rare in regional neuraxial anesthesia (1:150,000–1:200,000), the size and rigidity of the lead and level of manipulation required during implantation may increase this incidence during spinal cord stimulator implantation. Asking the patient to monitor for ongoing neurologic changes may delay diagnosis. Although evaluating the patient personally is important, obtaining stat imaging and arranging for surgical help are most critical.

FURTHER READING

Deer TR, Stewart CD. Complications of spinal cord stimulation: Identification, treatment, and prevention. *Pain Med.* 2008;9 (Suppl 1): S93–S101.
Narouze S, Benzon HT, Provenzano DA, et al. Interventional spine and pain procedures in patients on antiplatelet and anticoagulant medications: Guidelines from the American Society of Regional Anesthesia and Pain Medicine, the European Society of Regional Anaesthesia and Pain Therapy, the American Academy of Pain Medicine, the International Neuromodulation Society, the North American Neuromodulation Society, and the World Institute of Pain. *Reg Anesth Pain Med.* 2015;40(3):182–212.
Vandermeulen EP, Van Aken H, Vermylen J. Anticoagulants and spinal-epidural anesthesia. *Anesth Analg.* 1994;79(6):1165–1177.

8. ANSWER: A

There are a number of complications related to spinal cord stimulator implantation. The most likely complication overall and the most frequently associated complication with reoperation is lead migration. Since the advent of multipolar stimulation technology, this complication has required reoperation less often because reprogramming can typically salvage the system and provide the desired pain coverage. Another complication frequently requiring reprogramming is epidural fibrosis. As fibrosis develops, reprogramming is often required. Stimulus amplitude may need to be increased if analgesia is diminished in some cases. In addition, surgical revision may be required in cases in which current transfer is made preferentially to the lateral nerve roots and spinal structures as fibrotic tissue increases resistance to flow. Lead fracture is a complication that can be associated with surgical trauma to the lead or the anatomical location of lead implantation. It is more likely with cervical or retrograde implantation approaches. Despite careful surgical technique and prophylactic measures, infection is a well-described but rare complication related to the IPG pocket site or the implanted leads. Of all the complications listed, unwanted stimulation is the least likely. In 2004, Cameron reviewed approximately 30,000 cases described in the literature to evaluate the major rate of complications related to spinal cord stimulation therapy. The most common complication listed in this study was lead migration at 13.2%, whereas lead fracture was the second most common complication. Infection rates have been described in the literature to range from 2% to 6%, although it appears that these percentages are decreasing, approaching similar rates of infection as those of other surgical interventions.

FURTHER READING

Cameron T. Safety and efficacy of spinal cord stimulation for the treatment of chronic pain: A 20-year literature review. *J Neurosurg.* 2004;100(3 Suppl Spine):254–267.
Deer TR, Stewart CD. Complications of spinal cord stimulation: Identification, treatment, and prevention. *Pain Med.* 2008; 9(Suppl 1):S93–S101.

9. ANSWER: B

Although protective of resultant postdural puncture headache (PDPH), obesity is described as a risk factor for accidental dural puncture, not low body mass index. Accidental dural puncture is the most common neurological insult from spinal cord stimulator implantation. Given the type and gauge of the needle used, the likelihood of postdural puncture headache following identified accidental dural puncture is high (likely >50%). Typically, conservative management of PDPH, such as caffeine, hydration, oral analgesics, abdominal binders, and/or encouraging supine positioning, will suffice. However, epidural blood patch has been described as a therapy for patients with indwelling spinal cord stimulator leads. Caution should be exercised because the blood may serve as a medium for bacterial growth. Other complications related to dural puncture have been described during spinal cord stimulation, including unexpected paresthesias that may be explained by conductance of simulation pulses through the CSF directly.

Deer TR, Stewart CD. Complications of spinal cord stimulation: Identification, treatment, and prevention. *Pain Med.* 2008;9(Suppl 1):S93–S101.

Eldrige JS, Weingarten TN, Rho RH. Management of cerebral spinal fluid leak complicating spinal cord stimulator implantation. *Pain Pract.* 2006;6(4):285–288.

10. ANSWER: C

Although the indications for peripheral nerve stimulation are less well vetted from an efficacy or cost perspective than spinal cord stimulation, a number of clinical indications are commonly accepted for this therapy. A review of available publications regarding the use of peripheral nerve stimulation found that 60–70% of patients with occipital neuralgia, transformed migraine, and neuropathic pain confined to a single nerve distribution may respond (CRPS II or CRPS I with symptoms of a single nerve distribution). Peripheral nerve stimulation can be combined with spinal cord stimulation therapy for additive analgesia. In patients with CRPS with symptoms in more than one peripheral nerve, a poor response to peripheral nerve stimulation was noted. Diabetic peripheral neuropathy is a polyneuropathy by definition and would not be expected to respond as well as the clinical syndromes listed in this question.

Bittar RG, Teddy PJ. Peripheral neuromodulation for pain. *J Clin Neurosci Off J Neurosurg Soc Australas.* 2009;16(10):1259–1261.

Hassenbusch SJ, Stanton-Hicks M, Schoppa D, et al. Long-term results of peripheral nerve stimulation for reflex sympathetic dystrophy. *J Neurosurg.* 1996;84(3):415–423.

11. ANSWER: B

Understanding peripheral neural anatomy is critical to the understanding of the concept of peripheral nerve stimulation-induced analgesia and implementing it in practice. Answer choice A shows the epineurium surrounding the perineural space. Answer B shows the perineurium, which encapsulates bundles of fascicles. Answer choice C shows these bundles of fascicles, and answer choice D is the perineural space. Peripheral nerve stimulation works by direct inhibition of primary nociceptive afferents, which causes suppression of induced central sensitization by disrupting peripheral input. Complex studies regarding the influence of peripheral nerve organization on the sensitivity to electrical stimulation have shown that size and number of fascicles within a nerve directly correlate with the ease of stimulation of each fascicle within that nerve. This may help explain why stimulation of a peripheral nerve below a threshold for paresthesia is still able to produce reliable analgesia. Ultrasound may be used for a trial of peripheral nerve stimulation or as a mapping procedure prior to implantation. Unfortunately, peripheral nerve stimulation is currently an off-label indication because no complete generator and lead combination system is available.

Grinberg Y, Schiefer MA, Tyler DJ, et al. Fascicular perineurium thickness, size, and position affect model predictions of neural excitation. *IEEE Trans Neural Syst Rehabil Eng.* 2008;16(6):572–581.

Huntoon MA, Huntoon EA, Obray JB, et al. Feasibility of ultrasound-guided percutaneous placement of peripheral nerve stimulation electrodes in a cadaver model: Part one, lower extremity. *Reg Anesth Pain Med.* 2008;33(6):551–557.

12. ANSWER: B

Ziconotide inhibits presynaptic N-type calcium channel and is US Food and Drug Administration approved for intrathecal use. High-density N-type and P/Q-type calcium channels are primarily located at presynaptic terminals. The blockade of N-type calcium channels in the dorsal horn inhibits the release of excitatory neurotransmitters such as substance P and glutamate from primary afferent neurons. Ziconotide was isolated from marine cone snail venom and has a unique structure preventing oral use and resisting metabolism in the CSF. Ziconotide is an amino peptide that would be readily broken down in the gastrointestinal tract if administered orally, but it is relatively resistant to CSF peptidases; therefore, its clearance from spinal cord is mediated by CSF flow, not metabolism. Ziconotide has shown promise in the treatment of chronic cancer, AIDS, and neuropathic pain. However, widespread implementation has been limited by serious side effects and a narrow therapeutic window. Common side effects described are abnormal gait, amblyopia, dizziness, nausea, nystagmus, mood or psychiatric disturbances, hallucinations, urinary retention, and vomiting. These side effects have been described as dose-dependent and entirely reversible with discontinuation or dose reduction. Ziconotide has been used primarily as a single agent for pain control, but recent studies have suggested a synergistic effect in reduction in pain scores and total daily opioid dose. However, the amino-peptide structure of ziconotide makes it relatively unstable in combination with other medications, which may necessitate earlier pump refill. Despite dose-dependent serious side effects, ziconotide shows promise as a complimentary agent in the treatment of chronic malignant and nonmalignant pain unresponsive to conventional therapy.

FURTHER READING

Lawson EF, Wallace MS. Current developments in intraspinal agents for cancer and noncancer pain. *Curr Pain Headache Rep.* 2010;14(1):8–16.

Rauck RL, Wallace MS, Leong MS, et al. A randomized, double-blind, placebo-controlled study of intrathecal ziconotide in adults with severe chronic pain. *J Pain Symptom Manage.* 2006;31(5):393–406.

Smith HS, Deer TR. Safety and efficacy of intrathecal ziconotide in the management of severe chronic pain. *Ther Clin Risk Manage.* 2009;5(3):521–534.

Staats PS, Yearwood T, Charapata SG, et al. Intrathecal ziconotide in the treatment of refractory pain in patients with cancer or AIDS: A randomized controlled trial. *JAMA.* 2004;291(1):63–70.

Wallace MS, Rauck R, Fisher R, et al. Intrathecal ziconotide for severe chronic pain: Safety and tolerability results of an open-label, long-term trial. *Anesth Analg.* 2008;106(2):628–637.

Webster LR, Fakata KL, Charapata S, et al. Open-label, multicenter study of combined intrathecal morphine and ziconotide: Addition of morphine in patients receiving ziconotide for severe chronic pain. *Pain Med.* 2008;9(3):282–290.

but include progressively increasing doses of morphine dose, decreased therapeutic response to medication, onset of pain with new characteristics or location, neurologic deficit or dysfunction, and generalized weakness/muscle weakness. When a catheter-tip granuloma is suspected, especially when there are signs of neurologic compromise, consensus guidelines offer a clinical algorithm for further management. This algorithm is depicted in Figure 10.3.

FURTHER READING

Deer TR, Prager J, Levy R, et al. Polyanalgesic Consensus Conference—2012: Consensus on diagnosis, detection, and treatment of catheter-tip granulomas (inflammatory masses). *Neuromodulation.* 2012;15(5):483–496.

Duarte RV, Raphael JH, Southall JL, et al. Intrathecal inflammatory masses: Is the yearly opioid dose increase an early indicator? *Neuromodulation.* 2010;13(2):109–113.

13. ANSWER: B

Catheter-tip granuloma formation is a serious complication related to long-term intrathecal drug delivery. These inflammatory masses are described as spherical collections of macrophages, plasma cells, eosinophils, or lymphocytes. Granuloma formation is an infrequent complication related to intrathecal drug delivery, but reports of this potentially devastating complication have increased in recent years. Granuloma formation is described as being related to the migration of mast cells from the meningeal vasculature and appears to be drug related. IT opioid therapy is the only agreed upon etiology of true granuloma formation. Although there exist case reports of granuloma formation following IT baclofen monotherapy, the accuracy of the diagnosis of granuloma has been questioned. Risk factors for granuloma formation are high drug concentration (>25 mg/ml for morphine), high total dose of infused opioid, low CSF flow rates, and low drug flow rate. Strategies used to reduce the incidence of granuloma formation include minimizing the dose and concentration of intrathecal opioids, using intermittent bolus dosing strategies, and use of adjuvant intrathecal medications to limit dose and concentration of the total opioid analgesic dose. In a retrospective analysis of patients receiving long-term IT drug therapy, there was a significant correlation between opioid dose increase per year and the development of granuloma. The mean morphine dose increase over a year period in patients who developed a granuloma was 0.88 mg/day compared to 0.22 mg/day increase in those who did not develop a granuloma. Morphine is the most likely drug implicated in granuloma formation either as monotherapy or combination therapy, followed by hydromorphone. No cases of IT granuloma formation have been described with either fentanyl or sufentanil. Signs/symptoms of granuloma formation are varied

14. ANSWER: A

Although patient selection for IT opioid therapy is a topic of ongoing investigation, general selection criteria are well circulated. The selection of a patient for IT opioid therapy is multifaceted and must acknowledge both the source of the pain and patient-specific factors that may influence the rate of successful implantation. The aim of IT opioid therapy is to minimize the side effects associated with high-dose oral opioids, such as excessive sedation, respiratory depression, and constipation, while providing improved pain relief and improved overall function. In a large randomized controlled study evaluating the efficacy of IT therapy compared to comprehensive medical management, Smith et al. found that IT therapy showed significantly improved pain, decreased drug-related side effects, and a trend toward increased survival at 6 months. Deer et al. reported similar findings of increased survival, which may be related to decreased side effects from oral opioid therapy. In response to these reports, the 2012 Polyanalgesic Consensus Conference report suggests that the belief that a patient must have a greater than 3-month life expectancy may need reconsideration. Although more robust evidence exists for the utilization of IT opioid therapy in cancer pain, there is emerging evidence for the use of IT opioid therapy in other situations. In addition, many authors acknowledge that cancer pain is predominantly nociceptive or mixed nociceptive–neuropathic in etiology. This may shed light on the nonmalignant conditions amenable to IT opioid therapy. The ideal candidate for IT opioid therapy would have proven analgesic benefit (albeit suboptimal) with oral opioid therapy, poor response to other conservative therapy (including relatively noninvasive interventional techniques), experienced dose-dependent opioid-related side effects, and nearly round-the-clock oral opioid

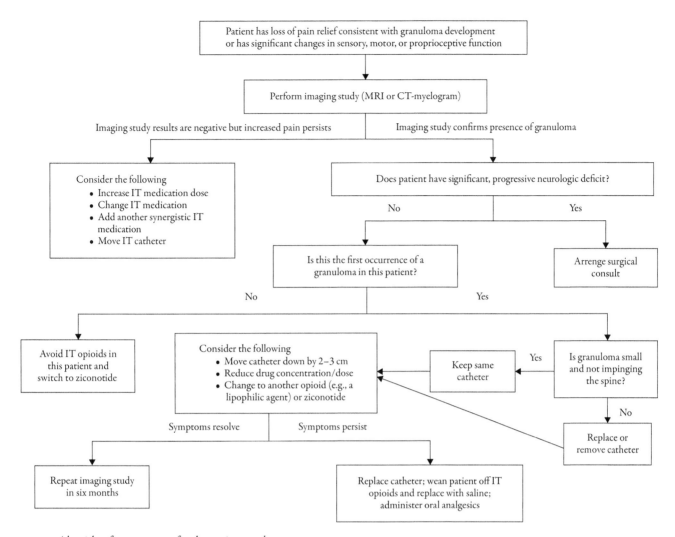

Figure 10.3 Algorithm for treatment of catheter-tip granuloma.

SOURCE: Reprinted with permission from Deer TR, Prager J, Levy R, et al. Polyanalgesic Consensus Conference—2012: Consensus on diagnosis, detection, and treatment of catheter-tip granulomas (inflammatory masses). *Neuromodulation*. 2012;15(5):483–496. doi:10.1111/j.1525–1403.2012.00449.x.

therapy. Patients without proven analgesic benefit, stable social situations, good personal hygiene, or a pain syndrome that is not secondary to a clear organic pain generator represent poor candidates for IT opioid therapy.

FURTHER READING

Cohen SP, Dragovich A. Intrathecal analgesia. *Anesthesiol Clin.* 2007;25(4):863–882, viii.

Deer TR, Prager J, Levy R, et al. Polyanalgesic Consensus Conference 2012: Recommendations for the management of pain by intrathecal (intraspinal) drug delivery—Report of an interdisciplinary expert panel. *Neuromodulation.* 2012;15(5):436.

Deer TR, Smith HS, Burton AW, et al. Comprehensive consensus based guidelines on intrathecal drug delivery systems in the treatment of pain caused by cancer pain. *Pain Physician.* 2011;14(3):E283–E312.

Smith TJ, Staats PS, Deer T, et al. Randomized clinical trial of an implantable drug delivery system compared with comprehensive medical management for refractory cancer pain: Impact on pain, drug-related toxicity, and survival. *J Clin Oncol.* 2002;20(19):4040–4049.

15. ANSWER: A

When utilizing IT opioid therapy, it is crucial to have an understanding of the relevant pharmacologic properties of the drugs being employed. Opioid medications exert their analgesic effects in the substantia gelatinosa in the spinal cord, binding to opioid receptors there. These receptors are divided into three major subtypes: μ, δ, and κ. These G protein-coupled receptors are located pre- and postsynaptically. Presynaptic opioid receptor agonism results in inhibition of substance P and calcitonin gene-related peptide release through inhibition of voltage-gated calcium channels. Postsynaptic opioid receptors exert their analgesia through inhibition of adenyl cyclase, and this results in potassium influx and neuronal hyperpolarization.

The overall analgesic effect of the IT opioid is determined by the specific drug's receptor affinity as well as its ability to reach the target receptors at the appropriate level in the spinal cord. Depending on the position of an

IT catheter and the target fibers, rostral spread within the CSF may be desired. There is a direct correlation between the water solubility at physiologic pH and a drug's ability to spread within the CSF. Studies have demonstrated that the degree of rostral spread of epidural and IT concentrations of opioids is based on the relative hydrophobicity of the opioids. Morphine is the most water-soluble opioid used in IT therapy. It acts primarily via the μ opioid receptor. Hydromorphone is less hydrophilic; acts on the μ, κ, and δ opioid receptors; and is 4 or 5 times more potent than morphine. Fentanyl and sufentanil are 100 and 1000 times more potent than morphine and are relatively lipophilic opioids. The more lipophilic opioids highlight the importance for deliberate catheter tip placement to treat specific pain complaints. Although there is a significant difference in the rostral spread of opioid medications based on their relative hydrophillicity, animal models continue to show that catheter tip location is critical even for morphine. Pig models have shown a 5- to 10-fold difference in concentration of IT opioids within 5–10 cm of the catheter tip.

An understanding of the pharmacodynamics and pharmacokinetics with non-opioid analgesics being used for IT therapy is equally important. The principal pharmacologic factors related to ziconotide are detailed in Question 12.

FURTHER READING

Bernards CM, Shen DD, Sterling ES, et al. Epidural, cerebrospinal fluid, and plasma pharmacokinetics of epidural opioids: Part 1. Differences among opioids. *Anesthesiology*. 2003;99(2):455–465.

Cohen SP, Dragovich A. Intrathecal analgesia. *Anesthesiol Clin*. 2007;25(4):863–882, viii.

Flack SH, Anderson CM, Bernards C. Morphine distribution in the spinal cord after chronic infusion in pigs. *Anesth Analg*. 2011;112(2):460–464.

16. ANSWER: C

All local anesthetics work by binding to the α subunit of intracellular voltage-gated sodium channels in neurons. By binding to the sodium channel, local anesthetics prevent sodium influx and eventual action potentials. These drugs block with variable selectivity nociceptive, sympathetic, and motor fibers within nerves. Bupivacaine is an amide local anesthetic that is commonly used for IT therapy in acute surgical analgesia and chronic pain management. Select studies have shown bupivacaine to be helpful as an adjunct to IT opioid therapy. In a retrospective analysis of 109 patients with failed back surgery syndrome or cancer-related pain, patients with both IT bupivacaine and opioid therapy had better pain control, 23% lower total morphine dose, and higher satisfaction than those with IT opioids alone, suggesting a synergistic effect related to this combination therapy. Other studies have shown a less robust improvement in pain but significant differences in quality-of-life scores. The 2012 polyanalgesic consensus panel lists IT bupivacaine as a first- and second-line drug as an adjunct to IT opioid therapy in neuropathic as well as nociceptive pain states, respectively. The recommended starting dose for IT bupivacaine is 1–4 mg/day.

FURTHER READING

Deer TR, Caraway DL, Kim CK, et al. Clinical experience with intrathecal bupivacaine in combination with opioid for the treatment of chronic pain related to failed back surgery syndrome and metastatic cancer pain of the spine. *Spine J*. 2002;2(4):274–278.

Deer TR, Prager J, Levy R, et al. Polyanalgesic Consensus Conference 2012: Recommendations for the management of pain by intrathecal (intraspinal) drug delivery—Report of an interdisciplinary expert panel. *Neuromodulation*. 2012;15(5):436.

Mironer YE, Haasis JC, Chapple I, et al. Efficacy and safety of intrathecal opioid/bupivacaine mixture in chronic nonmalignant pain: A double blind, randomized, crossover, multicenter study by the National Forum of Independent Pain Clinicians (NFIPC). *Neuromodulation*. 2002;5(4):208–213.

17. ANSWER: B

In a study of 73 patients that was published in 2000, Abs et al. showed that most men and all women developed hypogonadotropic hypogonadism that was proven by serum androgen levels in men and serum luteinizing hormone, progesterone, and estradiol levels in women. It is suggested that this goes largely unrecognized in clinical practice. A publication developed by the 2012 Polyanalgesic Consensus Conference makes specific recommendations to limit morbidity related to implantation and maintenance of IT drug delivery systems. For example, to reduce the adverse event of respiratory depression, the authors suggest optimizing coexisting pulmonary disease using expert consultation, advising smoking cessation, expert optimization for those with risk factors for or known history of obstructive sleep apnea, and discontinuing benzodiazepines prior to implantation. The other listed answer choices are not described complications associated with IT opioid therapy. Although morphine has been described as causing sphincter of Oddi contraction, the clinical translation of this temporary effect has not been substantiated. Sweating is listed as a common side effect with IT opioid therapy, not anhydrosis. Diabetes insipidus is not described as a common side effect associated with IT opioid therapy. On the contrary, animal studies and human studies have shown peripheral edema to be a common side effect, especially in those with preexisting venous stasis disease during the early phases of therapy. There is some suggestion that modulation of antidiuretic hormone plays a role in this side effect.

Abs R, Verhelst J, Maeyaert J, et al. Endocrine consequences of long-term intrathecal administration of opioids. *J Clin Endocrinol Metab.* 2000;85(6):2215–2222.

Cohen SP, Dragovich A. Intrathecal analgesia. *Anesthesiol Clin.* 2007;25(4):863–882, viii.

Deer TR, Levy R, Prager J, et al. Polyanalgesic Consensus Conference 2012: Recommendations to reduce morbidity and mortality in intrathecal drug delivery in the treatment of chronic pain. *Neuromodulation.* 2012;15(5):467–482.

human subjects have not been completely demonstrated. Midazolam acts as a $GABA_A$ agonist. $GABA_A$ is a ligand-gated chloride channel. Use of midazolam in acute pain management has been described, but safety concerns with chronic IT midazolam therapy, particularly in the setting of concurrent IT opioid therapy, have hampered its widespread adoption as an adjunct to continuous IT therapy. Gabapentin acts as an L-type voltage-gated calcium channel blocker at the alpha $\alpha_2\delta$ subunit, not on GABA receptors. Droperidol acts predominantly as a dopaminergic antagonist at D2 receptors.

18. ANSWER: B

Baclofen acts as a $GABA_B$ receptor agonist, serving as an inhibitory neurotransmitter in the spinal cord. $GABA_B$ receptors are G protein-coupled receptors that act by modulating the activity of presynaptic potassium and calcium channels, as well as postsynaptic inhibition of adenylate cyclase activity. In animal models using immunohistological staining techniques, the position of $GABA_B$ receptors appears to be well situated to produce analgesic effects in the dorsal horn and the dorsal root ganglion. In addition, $GABA_B$ receptors are found on interneurons in the spinal cord. The presumed effect of pain relief from intrathecally administered baclofen therapy based on their concentration in these key anatomic locations has been well demonstrated in animal models in both acute and chronic pain states. These findings have not been demonstrated as effectively in human studies. Interestingly, in a pilot study with a small cohort of patients, Lind et al. found that the addition of IT baclofen to spinal cord stimulation (SCS) therapy provided additional pain relief compared to either SCS or IT baclofen therapy alone. This supports not only the model of $GABA_B$ receptor-mediated analgesia but also the $GABA_B$0mediated effect of SCS therapy in interneurons. Whereas investigation of the use of baclofen for chronic nociceptive and neuropathic pain is emerging, the role for baclofen for spasticity-related pain is well established. The crossover between chronic pain and spasticity requires that a pain specialist be familiar with the appropriate use and potential complications associated with IT baclofen therapy. The most serious of these complications is acute baclofen withdrawal syndrome. Presentations of this potentially fatal syndrome range from anxiety, increased spasticity, and disorientation to hyperthermia, myoclonus, seizures, rhabdomyolysis, disseminated intravascular coagulation, multisystem organ failure, and coma. When acute baclofen withdrawal syndrome is suspected, patients should be supplemented with oral baclofen therapy and may require intensive care and high-dose benzodiazepines. The other answer choices for this question describe therapies that may have some benefit when administered intrathecally, but the magnitude of their effect and safety in

Engle MP, Gassman M, Sykes KT, et al. Spinal nerve ligation does not alter the expression or function of GABA(B) receptors in spinal cord and dorsal root ganglia of the rat. *Neuroscience.* 2006;138(4):1277–1287.

Hammond DL, Drower EJ. Effects of intrathecally administered THIP, baclofen and muscimol on nociceptive threshold. *Eur J Pharmacol.* 1984;103(1–2):121–125.

Hwang JH, Yaksh TL. The effect of spinal GABA receptor agonists on tactile allodynia in a surgically-induced neuropathic pain model in the rat. *Pain.* 1997;70(1):15–22.

Lind G, Meyerson BA, Winter J, et al. Intrathecal baclofen as adjuvant therapy to enhance the effect of spinal cord stimulation in neuropathic pain: A pilot study. *Eur J Pain.* 2004;8(4):377–383.

Mohammed I, Hussain A. Intrathecal baclofen withdrawal syndrome— A life-threatening complication of baclofen pump: A case report. *BMC Clin Pharmacol.* 2004;4:6.

19. ANSWER: A

Although neuroablative surgical techniques have largely been replaced by therapies such as SCS and IT neuromodulation, it is important to identify patients who may benefit from these neurosurgical techniques. Dorsal root entry zone lesioning procedures still have a place in certain pain syndromes. Although they have been used in a wide range of pain states, the best evidence for their use is in "boundary" zone pain related to spinal cord injury. Dorsal root entry zone (DREZ) lesioning relieves pain by disrupting signals into and out of the superficial layers of the spinal cord dorsal horn. Afferent nociceptive fibers terminate and ascending nociceptive fibers originate in this location. DREZ lesioning is most effective for relief of paroxysmal neuropathic pain as opposed to continuous neuropathic pain.

Deer TR, Leong MS, Buvanendran A, et al. *Comprehensive Treatment of Chronic Pain by Medical, Interventional, and Integrative Approaches: The American Academy of Pain Medicine Textbook on Patient Management.* New York, NY: Springer; 2013.

Sindou M. Microsurgical DREZotomy (MDT) for pain, spasticity, and hyperactive bladder: A 20-year experience. *Acta Neurochir (Wien)*. 1995;137(1–2):1–5.

20. ANSWER: A

Microvascular decompression is a surgical technique that is most commonly used to relieve trigeminal neuralgia (TN) or glossopharyngeal neuralgia (GN). The rationale behind the procedure is to relieve neural compression from adjacent blood vessels as they enter the brainstem. Although trigeminal neuralgia and glossopharyngeal neuralgia may alternatively be treated using rhizotomy and percutaneous ablative techniques, microvascular decompression can provide relief without any induced sensory deficit. Pain relief is achieved at a high rate (>90%), and this technique is generally believed to provide the longest-lasting pain relief of all of the interventional approaches to treat TN and GN.

FURTHER READING

Deer TR, Leong MS, Buvanendran A, et al. *Comprehensive Treatment of Chronic Pain by Medical, Interventional, and Integrative Approaches: The American Academy of Pain Medicine Textbook on Patient Management*. New York, NY: Springer; 2013.

Kalkanis SN, Eskandar EN, Carter BS, et al. Microvascular decompression surgery in the United States, 1996 to 2000: Mortality rates, morbidity rates, and the effects of hospital and surgeon volumes. *Neurosurgery*. 2003;52(6):1251–1252.

11.

PAIN MANAGEMENT TECHNIQUES

Maureen F. McClenahan and William Beckman

INTRODUCTION

This chapter provides a broad review of various interventional pain management procedures with a focus on indications, anatomy, and complications. Specific techniques reviewed include transforaminal epidural steroid injection, lumbar sympathetic block, stellate ganglion block, cervical and lumbar radiofrequency ablation, gasserian ganglion block, sacroiliac joint injection, celiac plexus block, lateral femoral cutaneous nerve block, ilioinguinal block, lumbar medial branch block, obturator nerve block, ankle block, occipital nerve block, superior hypogastric plexus block, spinal cord stimulation, and intrathecal drug delivery systems. The chapter reviews contrast agents, neurolytic agents, botulinum toxin use, corticosteroids, and ziconotide pharmacology and side effects in addition to diagnosis and management of local anesthetic toxicity syndrome. It also discusses indications for neurosurgical techniques, including dorsal root entry zone lesioning. In addition, information on radiation safety and the use of anticoagulants with neuraxial blocks is covered.

QUESTIONS

1. A 37-year-old female with low back pain and radicular symptoms in the L5 distribution is scheduled to receive an L5–S1 transforaminal steroid injection. Traditionally, placement of the needle in which location within the triangle of Kambin ("safe triangle") will minimize the possibility of spinal nerve root or radicular artery injury?

A. Superior aspect of the intervertebral foramen, inferior to the pedicle, and inferolateral to the pars interarticularis
B. Inferior aspect of the intervertebral foramen, inferior to the pedicle, and inferolateral to the pars interarticularis

C. Superior aspect of the intervertebral foramen, inferior to the pedicle, and inferomedial to the pars interarticularis
D. In the midportion of the foramen, inferomedial to the pars interarticularis

2. A 53-year-old male with complex regional pain syndrome of the left lower extremity underwent a lumbar sympathetic block with phenol after receiving excellent but short-duration pain relief with bupivacaine. One week post-procedure, he is complaining of sharp pain radiating to the anterior thigh and groin. What is the most likely etiology of these new-onset symptoms?

A. Myofascial pain secondary to injection of neurolytic into the psoas muscle
B. Lumbar plexopathy
C. Genitofemoral neuralgia
D. Retrograde ejaculation

3. All of the following are reported complications related to cervical transforaminal steroid injections except:

A. Death
B. Cortical blindness
C. Chronic gait disturbance
D. Cerebellar infarct

4. A 45-year-old female sustained a traumatic brachial plexus root avulsion injury and now has intractable right upper extremity pain. She is scheduled to undergo cervical dorsal root entry zone (DREZ) lesioning. All of the following are true regarding this procedure except:

A. The DREZ lesion targets Lissauer's tract, which is composed of the small lightly or unmyelinated fibers that enter the dorsal entry zone from the lateral aspect of the DREZ.

B. The DREZ lesion attempts to preserve those fibers that reside on the medial aspect of the dorsal root entry zone. These fibers are involved in proprioception and touch and are destined for the dorsal column pathways.

C. The trigeminal nucleus caudalis, the cranial continuation of the dorsal horn, receives a large proportion of nociceptive signaling from the trigeminal system and is therefore the target structure in the treatment of facial pain.

D. Motor complications range from 0% to 69% due to the presence of the corticospinal tract that resides just medial to the dorsal horn.

5. A 54-year-old male who underwent an L2–L3 fusion is now experiencing lower back pain radiating to the posterior and lateral aspects of the thigh. He underwent bilateral L3–L5 median branch blocks with greater that 50% relief of pain and has returned to the clinic for radiofrequency ablation. The following are all true statements except:

A. Provocative maneuvers to aid in the diagnosis of facet syndrome include pain with flexion, contralateral bending, and ipsilateral bending.

B. Tenderness to palpation in the cervical and lumbar paraspinous region was found to be a positive predictor of outcome in two large, retrospective studies.

C. False-positive rates for medial branch blocks range from 25% to 40% in the lumbar spine and 25% to 30% in the cervical spine.

D. Multiple retrospective studies have found a difference in successful pain relief following radiofrequency ablation when using 80% rather than 50% relief after medial branch block.

6. A 44-year-old female underwent C4–C7 radiofrequency ablation for chronic cervicalgia. She presents to the clinic 1 week after the procedure with complaints of a sunburned feeling over her neck in the region treated. Her motor and sensory exam of the upper and lower extremities is otherwise normal. She is afebrile without any nausea, vomiting, or constitutional signs or symptoms. Which of the following is the most likely etiology for her symptoms?

A. The patient is experiencing thermal neuritis of the ventral nerve root.

B. The patient has an epidural abscess and needs emergent magnetic resonance imaging (MRI).

C. The patient is experiencing post-denervation neuritis.

D. You suspect the radiofrequency probe may have injured the cervical spinal cord and your patient is in need of emergent MRI.

7. You are consenting a patient for an L5–S1 interlaminar epidural steroid injection. Which of the following is a false statement regarding use of contrast agents?

A. Osmotoxic reactions include pain on injection, hemolysis, endothelial damage with capillary leak and edema, flushing, warmth, hypotension, cardiovascular collapse, and hypervolemia.

B. Ionic iodinated contrast agents are the agents of choice for interventional pain procedures due to their higher osmolality.

C. No studies have demonstrated a decreased incidence of reaction in patients with a previous reaction to a non-ionized contrast agent despite treatment with steroid and antihistamines.

D. Gadolinium can be considered as an alternative agent for high-risk patients.

8. A 65-year-old male with diabetes and hypertension presents to your clinic after receiving three epidural steroid injections during the past 12 months and would like to discuss whether further treatment with steroid is available to him now. All of the following are true statements regarding the use of corticosteroids except:

A. Potential adverse systemic reactions include elevated blood pressure, fluid retention, and hyperglycemia.

B. Sterile meningitis and arachnoiditis have been reported following intrathecal injection of methylprednisolone.

C. The mechanism of action for corticosteroid therapy includes local and systemic reduction of inflammatory mediator production, reduction in ectopic discharge rates seen following nerve injury, and reversible inhibition of nociceptive C fiber transmission.

D. The use of particulate corticosteroid has not been implicated in spinal cord infarction after placement of epidural steroid.

9. You have just performed a gasserian ganglion block with local anesthetic for a 64-year-old female with intractable tic douloureux who has failed pharmacologic management. You are called to the recovery after your nurse states, "It looks like her eye is protruding!" All of the following are true statements regarding complications associated with gasserian ganglion blocks except:

A. Radiofrequency lesioning, glycerol rhizotomy, and balloon compression have complication rates of 29.2%, 24.8%, and 16.1%, respectively.

B. Retrobulbar hematoma with secondary exophthalmos is a possible complication if the needle passes into the retrobulbar space.

C. Anesthesia dolorosa manifests with mild to moderate post-procedure pain and is thought to be secondary to complete destruction of the ganglion.
D. Loss of corneal reflex, keratitis, and ulceration are observed in 3–15% of patients following neurolysis.

10. A 34-year-old female presents to your clinic with persistent right-sided lumbosacral pain that extends into the right buttock and leg. She has a known leg length discrepancy as a result of a past femoral shaft fracture sustained in a motor vehicle accident. You suspect that she has sacroiliac (SI) joint dysfunction. Which of the following is a true statement?

A. The etiology of sacroiliac joint pain can be from either intra-articular or extra-articular sources.
B. Sacroiliac-mediated pain may be reliably diagnosed through history and physical exam.
C. Sacroiliac-mediated pain has pathognomonic pain referral patterns as well as highly sensitive and specific radiological imaging findings.
D. Radiofrequency ablation techniques are more effective for the treatment of intra-articular sources of SI joint pain.

11. You have just completed a right-sided lumbar sympathetic block with 20 ml of bupivacaine for a 33-year-old female with complex regional pain syndrome of the right foot. Your patient begins to complain of dizziness and perioral numbness. She loses consciousness and begins to experience generalized tonic–clonic activity. Based on your suspected diagnosis, which of the following statements is true?

A. Bupivacaine, secondary to its potent lipophilicity, exhibits less cardiotoxicity compared to ropivacaine.
B. Local anesthetic systemic toxicity syndrome (LAST) usually presents first with cardiovascular signs and symptoms followed by central nervous system effects.
C. Cardiovascular effects of LAST syndrome include hypertension, vasoconstriction, and a hyperdynamic cardiac state.
D. The use of 20% intralipid has been shown to be effective for resuscitation from bupivacaine-induced cardiac toxicity.

12. A 35-year-old male presents to your clinic for his first right-sided stellate ganglion block. The following are all important considerations when performing this procedure except:

A. Ultrasound guidance, compared to fluoroscopy, provides the additional advantage of direct visualization of the thyroid gland, vertebral artery, esophagus, and pleura.

B. In approximately 10% of cases, the vertebral artery may enter the vertebral transverse foramen at C5 or higher.
C. The appearance of Horner's syndrome signifies a successful sympathetic blockade of the ipsilateral upper extremity.
D. Most of the indications for stellate ganglion block are based on case reports and case series with the exception of Raynaud's and complex regional pain syndromes, which do have outcome studies.

13. A 76-year-old female with end-stage colon cancer has an implanted intrathecal drug delivery system infusing a combination of morphine and clonidine for intractable abdominal pain. She presents to your clinic with worsening back pain that extends into her lower extremities. She states that her legs have become progressively weak, and she has lost urinary continence several times in the past 12 hours. What is the most appropriate first step in management?

A. Obtain an emergent MRI of the lumbar spine.
B. Decrease the dose of intrathecal morphine/clonidine.
C. Increase the dose of intrathecal morphine/clonidine.
D. Obtain a routine MRI.

14. You are managing a 46-year-old female with multiple sclerosis with an implanted intrathecal drug delivery system that was placed for refractory neuropathic pain symptoms involving the lower extremities. She has been experiencing increasing pain symptoms resulting in frequent dose escalations of morphine. As a result, you are considering rotation to intrathecal ziconotide. Which of the following is true regarding intrathecal use of ziconotide?

A. Animal studies show that ziconotide reduces tactile and mechanical allodynia in a dose-independent manner.
B. Ziconotide has a large therapeutic window attributable to its low side effect profile.
C. Ziconotide can be abruptly terminated without withdrawal effects.
D. Ziconotide is considered a first-line agent for the treatment of neuropathic pain in patients with complicated past psychiatric history.

15. A 75-year-old female with pancreatic cancer suffers from chronic intractable abdominal pain that has been refractory to pharmacologic management. She underwent celiac plexus neurolysis this morning and has now presented to the emergency department with increasing back pain and orthostasis. Which of the following

statements is false regarding potential complications related to this procedure?

A. Orthostatic hypotension can occur in 10–15% of patients and can last up to 2 weeks.
B. Retroperitoneal hemorrhage must be considered in any patient presenting with backache with or without orthostasis.
C. Paraplegia and transient motor paralysis have been reported after celiac plexus block, which is thought to be due in part to spasm of the lumbar segmental arteries.
D. Near fatal dehydration secondary to diarrhea after a celiac plexus block has been reported.

16. A 68-year-old male patient with a herniated lumbar disk and lower extremity radicular pain is referred to you for a lumbar epidural steroid injection. While taking the history and performing the physical, you learn that the patient is taking the antiplatelet medication clopidogrel, which he has been taking for several months. He is not on any other antiplatelet or anticoagulant medications. Which of the following is incorrect regarding antiplatelet therapy and the performance of neuraxial procedures?

A. Neuraxial procedures can be safely performed if a patient is taking ibuprofen, but 24-hour stoppage may be warranted for higher risk procedures.
B. It is recommended that clopidogrel be stopped at least 7 days prior to a neuraxial procedure.
C. It is safe to go ahead with the procedure without stopping clopidogrel as long as meticulous attention is paid to the technique.
D. Clopidogrel acts by inhibiting adenosine diphosphate (ADP) receptor-mediated platelet activation.

17. Which of the following is correct concerning radiation safety while performing interventional pain medicine procedures using fluoroscopy?

A. Changing the position of the X-ray source by moving the C-arm does not alter the radiation exposure of the practitioner or the patient.
B. Wearing thyroid shields can help prevent thyroid cancer.
C. Wearing a lead apron is necessary only if the procedure is expected to take a long time.
D. Wearing leaded gloves allows the practitioner to have the hands in the exposure field without concern for radiation exposure.

18. A patient is referred to you for evaluation for a spinal cord stimulator (SCS) placement. Which of the following is correct?

A. If the history and physical exam point to a pain condition that is amenable to SCS therapy, it is not necessary to perform a trial period initially.
B. Psychological evaluation of potential SCS candidates is not recommended.
C. SCS therapy is recommended as an initial treatment, so more conservative treatments are not necessary prior to considering SCS.
D. Although the gate theory has been proposed as the mechanism of action by which SCS provides relief, the exact mechanism is not completely clear.

19. Which of the following is incorrect regarding performing a neurolytic superior hypogastric plexus block?

A. The superior hypogastric plexus is located bilaterally between the lower third of L5 and the upper third of S1 in the retroperitoneal space just anterior to the vertebral bodies.
B. Correct needle tip placement for the block is anterolateral to the L5–S1 disc space verified in two views.
C. Transdiscal and transvenous approaches have been described but are less desirable for neurolytic block.
D. Flow of contrast posteriorly toward the L5 nerve roots is acceptable when verifying needle tip placement prior to injecting the neurolytic agent.

20. Which of the following statements is incorrect regarding botulinum toxin?

A. Botulinum toxin blocks presynaptic acetylcholine release.
B. The denervation induced by botulinum toxin is temporary.
C. Botulinum toxin decreases the amount of substance P.
D. The functional denervation caused by botulinum toxin usually lasts 3–4 months.

21. You are seeing a patient diagnosed with occipital neuralgia who reports having received significant relief with occipital nerve blocks in the past. Which of the following statements is correct?

A. Occipital nerve blocks are not useful in the treatment of occipital neuralgia.
B. The greater occipital nerve is usually medial to the occipital artery.
C. The greater occipital nerve derives from the medial branch of the dorsal ramus of C2 between the C2 and C3 vertebra.
D. Entrance into the foramen magnum is not a concern when performing a greater occipital nerve block.

22. Which of the following statements concerning agents used for neurolytic blocks is correct?

    A. Glycerol and phenol are the two agents commonly used for epidural or intrathecal neurolytic blocks.

    B. The use of ethyl alcohol is characteristically associated with a painless, warm feeling on injection.

    C. Phenol is also commonly used as a neurolytic agent for the treatment of trigeminal neuralgia.

    D. It takes 3–5 days for the full effect of ethyl alcohol to manifest.

23. A 68-year-old female presents with a complaint of chronic left foot pain due to diabetic neuropathy. She has received relief previously with intermittent ankle blocks. Which of the following statements concerning ankle blocks is correct?

    A. The sciatic nerve is the source of all of the terminal nerves of the foot.

    B. The saphenous nerve is located posterior to the medial malleolus.

    C. The sural nerve is located anterior to the lateral malleolus.

    D. The posterior tibial nerve is located posterior to the medial malleolus.

24. Which of the following is incorrect regarding lumbar sympathetic blocks?

    A. The lumbar sympathetic chains are located anterolaterally to the vertebral bodies.

    B. The best location for the needle tip is the lower portion of L1.

    C. A rise in the skin temperature indicates successful sympathetic blockade.

    D. If the needle is advanced too far anteriorly, vascular puncture may occur.

25. Which of the following statements is correct regarding an obturator nerve block?

    A. The obturator nerve arises from L1–L4.

    B. The obturator nerve innervates the lateral thigh.

    C. The obturator nerve provides innervation to the hip joint.

    D. Potential for vascular injury is not a concern when performing this block.

26. Which of the following is not a technique to decrease the false-positive rate when performing a lumbar medial branch block?

    A. Avoiding sedation

    B. Minimize the amount of local anesthetic for the skin

    C. Limit the injected volume to no more than 0.5 ml

    D. Target a point high on the transverse process

27. You are seeing a 42-year-old otherwise healthy male who has had persistent right groin pain for 5 months since his right inguinal hernia repair. After a thorough history and physical exam, you are planning to perform a diagnostic block. Which of the following statements is incorrect?

    A. Needle entry point is classically 2 in. medial and 2 in. inferior to the anterior superior iliac spine.

    B. The ilioinguinal nerve arises from L3.

    C. One potential complication is blockade of the femoral nerve.

    D. If the diagnostic block is ineffective, one should consider a radiculopathy of L1 in the differential diagnosis.

28. Which of the following is not a contraindication to the placement of an intrathecal drug delivery system?

    A. Systemic infection

    B. Uncorrected coagulopathy

    C. Lack of response during a trial to the medication to be infused

    D. Maximal medical therapy that has not provided adequate relief

29. Which of the following statements regarding minimizing radiation exposure risk while using fluoroscopic X-rays is incorrect?

    A. Larger patients result in higher dose rates.

    B. Maximize the distance between the patient and the X-ray tube.

    C. Maximize the distance between the patient and the image intensifier.

    D. Minimize the beam-on time.

30. A 42-year-old obese male presents with complaints of bilateral thigh numbness for several months. He also notes that clothes overlying the area produce an unpleasant sensation. On physical exam, you note that there is decreased sensation to light touch over the lateral aspect of the thigh bilaterally. Conservative treatment to date has not produced any relief. Which of the following statements is correct regarding the nerve block that can be performed for this condition?

    A. Needle entry point is usually 2 cm medial and caudal to the anterior superior iliac spine.

    B. Due to the vascular structures in the vicinity of this nerve, there is a high risk of vascular injury.

C. Needle entry point is usually 2 cm medial and 2 cm inferior to the pubic tubercle.

D. Needle entry point is usually 2 cm superior and 2 cm lateral to the anterior superior iliac spine.

31. You are seeing a patient referred to you for intractable pain due to a unilateral lower extremity malignancy. Conservative therapy has not been successful in alleviating the patient's pain. After a complete history and physical exam, you are discussing treatment options with the patient, including the possibility of a cordotomy procedure. Which of the following statements about the cordotomy procedure is correct?

A. Pain relief for a successful cordotomy occurs at the same dermatomal level at which the cordotomy is performed.

B. The success rate for cordotomy is the same whether the etiology of the pain is cancer-related or not.

C. Recurrence of the pain is a significant potential limiting factor.

D. Bilateral upper cervical cordotomy is an appropriate treatment option for patients with severe respiratory impairment.

32. A 67-year-old male with diabetes, chronic obstructive pulmonary disease, hypertension, and a history of a myocardial infarction (MI) is scheduled to undergo cingulotomy for intractable malignant pain. All of the following are true statements regarding the preoperative evaluation except:

A. Functional capacity is vital information because exercise capacity is a reliable predictor of perioperative cardiac events.

B. The stability and timing of a recent myocardial infarction do not impact the incidence of perioperative morbidity and mortality.

C. A recent MI, defined as having occurred within 6 months of noncardiac surgery, is an independent risk factor for perioperative stroke, which is associated with an eightfold increase in the perioperative mortality rate.

D. More postoperative complications, increased length of hospitalization, and inability to return home after hospitalization were more pronounced among "frail" (e.g., those with impaired cognition and with dependence on others in instrumental activities of daily living), older adults (>70 years of age).

ANSWERS

1. ANSWER: A

The exiting spinal nerve root typically exits in the inferior portion of the intervertebral foramen. Needle placement in the safe triangle has traditionally been advocated in order to avoid injury to the exiting spinal nerve. In an anteroposterior view, its upper border is a transverse line underneath the pedicle extending from mid-pedicle to the lateral pedicular line. The lateral border is a line extending craniocaudad from the lateral aspect of the pedicle to the exiting spinal nerve root. The hypotenuse lies parallel to the spinal nerve root and connects the former two lines. Figure 11.1 illustrates proper positioning of the needle in the safe triangle while performing a lumbar transforaminal steroid injection.

The "magnus ramus radicularis anterior," or artery of Adamkiewicz (AKA), is the major branch of the anterior spinal artery providing arterial blood supply to the thoracolumbar spinal cord. Eighty percent of the time, it is located between T9 and T12. Work by Murthy and colleagues suggests that the AKA is often in the upper and midportion of the foramina and often within the safe triangle.

FURTHER READING

Landers M, Jones R, Rosenthal R, et al. Lumbar spinal neuraxial procedures. In: Raj P (Ed.), *Interventional Pain Management: Image Guided Procedures*. 2nd ed. Philadelphia, PA: Saunders; 2008:323–324.

Murthy NS, Maus TP, Behrns CL. Intraforaminal location of the great anterior radiculomedullary artery (artery of Adamkiewicz): A retrospective review. *Pain Med*. 2010;11:1756–1764.

2. ANSWER: C

Genitofemoral neuralgia presents with groin and/or anterior thigh pain, sensory loss, or weakness. The genitofemoral nerve is most susceptible at the L4–L5 level, where it has emerged from the psoas muscle and is now anterior to the fascia. Mild neuralgias are most commonly transient and can be treated with non-opioid analgesics. Severe neuralgias can be treated with transcutaneous electrical nerve stimulation, tricyclic antidepressants, antiepileptic agents, and intravenous lidocaine (1–2 ml/kg). Genitofemoral involvement usually occurs with too far lateral or posterior placement of the needle, which results in deposition of the injectate into the psoas muscle. Proper needle placement when performing a lumbar sympathetic block is illustrated in Figure 11.2.

Deposition of injectate into the psoas muscle can also involve the lumbar plexus, which can present with more widespread lower extremity involvement of pain, sensory loss, or motor weakness. Retrograde ejaculation is a rare complication and most often occurs with bilateral sympathectomies.

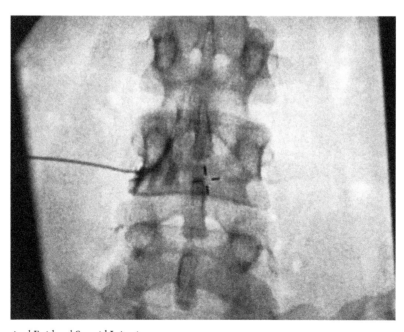

Figure 11.1 Lumbar Transforaminal Epidural Steroid Injection

SOURCE: Reprinted with permission from Sekhadia M, Benzon H. Peripheral selective nerve root blocks and transforaminal epidural steroid injections. In: Benzon H, Raja S, Fishman S (Eds.), *Essentials of Pain Management*. 3rd ed. Philadelphia, PA: Saunders; 2011;316,Figure 45–2.

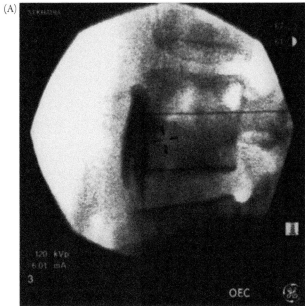

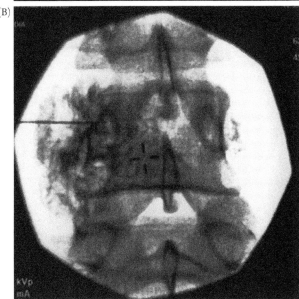

Figure 11.2 (A) Lateral image of correct placement and contrast pattern for lumbar sympathetic block. (B) Correct anteroposterior position of needle for lumbar sympathetic block.
SOURCE: Reprinted with permission from Sekhadia M, Nader A. Peripheral sympathetic blocks. In: Benzon H, Raja S, Fishman S (Eds.), *Essentials of Pain Management*. 3rd ed. Philadelphia, PA: Saunders; 2011:625, Figures 79–3 and 79–4.

FURTHER READING

Niv D, Gofeld M. Lumbar sympathetic blocks. In: Raj P (Ed.), *Interventional Pain Management: Image Guided Procedures*. 2nd ed. Philadelphia, PA: Saunders; 2008:318.

3. ANSWER: C

The estimated incidence of permanent cord or other neurologic complications for cervical transforaminal epidural steroid injection is 1 in 10,000. Paraplegia, quadriplegia,

spinal cord infarction, cortical blindness, and cerebellar infarction have all been reported. These outcomes are secondary to inadvertent intravascular injections or embolization of particulate matter found in corticosteroid through the radicular or vertebral arteries. The use of blunt tip needles may reduce the incidence of vascular penetration and subsequent intravascular injection.

Relevant anatomic relationships to consider include the location of the vertebral artery, which lies medial to the lateral border of the mid-cervical spine from C3 to C6 and anterior to the nerve roots. It is prudent to avoid anterior or more medial placement of the needle in the intervertebral foramen in order to minimize the possibility of injection into the vertebral artery. The use of contrast and fluoroscopy may reduce the chance of complications related to intravascular injection. Figure 11.3 shows proper needle placement while performing cervical transforaminal steroid injections.

The use of methylprednisolone is not recommended when performing cervical transforaminal epidural steroid injections. Methylprednisolone has the largest particle size of all the steroids and easily precipitates. If injected into a vascular structure, it can result in segmental spinal cord or brain infarction. In animal studies, in addition to particles, the carrier solution for methylprednisolone has also been implicated in injury. Betamethasone has the smallest particle size of the particulates, but dexamethasone is a nonparticulate steroid and should be used to decrease risk.

FURTHER READING

Dawley JD, Moeller-Bertram T, Wallace MS, et al. Intra-arterial injection in the rat brain: Evaluation of steroids used for transforaminal epidurals. *Spine*. 2009;34:1638–1644.
Hammer M, Noe C, Racz G, et al. Spinal neuraxial procedures of the head and neck. In: Raj P (Ed.), *Interventional Pain Management: Image Guided Procedures*. 2nd ed. Philadelphia, PA: Saunders; 2008:144–151.
Murthy NS, Maus TP, Behrns CL. Intraforaminal location of the great anterior radiculomedullary artery (artery of Adamkiewicz): A retrospective review. *Pain Med*. 2010;11:1756–1764.
Sekhadia M. Selective nerve root blocks and transforaminal epidural steroid injections. In: Benzon H, Raja S, Fishman S, et al. (Eds.), *Essentials of Pain Management*. 3rd ed. Philadelphia, PA: Saunders; 2011:318.

4. ANSWER: D

DREZ lesioning was first performed by Sindou in 1972 using coagulation as his neurodestructive technique, followed by Nashold and Ostdahl in 1974 using radiofrequency ablation. Lesioning of the small, lightly myelinated or unmyelinated nerve fibers is performed along the inferolateral aspect of the DREZ. Fibers that lie on the medial

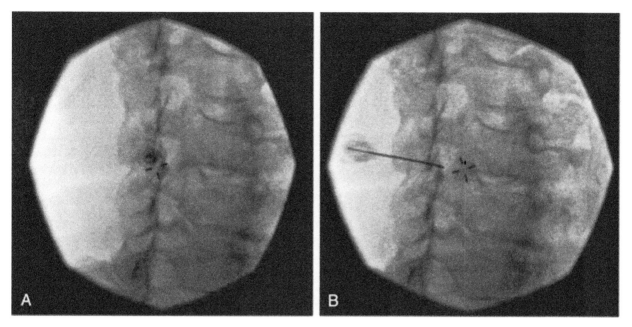

Figure 11.3 (A) Initial needle placement posterior over the superior articular process. (B) Needle walked anteriorly off of the superior articular process.

SOURCE: Reprinted with permission from Sekhadia M, Benzon H. Peripheral selective nerve root blocks and transforaminal epidural steroid injections. In: Benzon H, Raja S, Fishman S (Eds.), *Essentials of Pain Management*. 3rd ed. Philadelphia, PA: Saunders; 2011:316, Figure 45–5.

aspect of the DREZ are avoided in order to preserve dorsal column functions, including proprioception and touch.

Motor complications range from 0% to 69% due to the close proximity of the corticospinal tract that lies just lateral to the dorsal horn. Additional variables that contribute to the motor complication rate are vasculature supply disruption with resultant spinal cord ischemia and the variable size and angulation of the dorsal horn and entry zone found at each spinal level.

The nucleus caudalis extends from the upper cervical spinal cord to the brainstem. The target lesion for facial pain is at the upper rootlets of C2. Due to the proximity of the spinocerebellar tract, lesioning of the caudalis was complicated by a high rate of ataxia (up to 90%). With the development of angulated, insulated radiofrequency needles, the chance of damaging this tract had been reduced, and rates of ataxia have been reduced to approximately 39%.

FURTHER READING

Rosenow J. Neurosurgical procedures for treatment of intractable pain. In: Benzon H, Raja S, Fishman S, et al. (Eds.), *Essentials of Pain Management*. 3rd ed. Philadelphia, PA: Saunders; 2011:162–164.

5. ANSWER: D

When performing diagnostic medial branch blocks, retrospective studies have shown no difference in using 50% or 80% symptom improvement as a cutoff value for patient selection for radiofrequency ablation.

Clinical symptoms and pain referral patterns for facet syndrome lack specificity. "Facet loading" and "facet syndrome" were named based on small retrospective studies; however, subsequent larger and well-designed studies did not validate these findings. The L4–L5 and L5–S1 levels experience the greatest amount of strain with forward flexion. The L3–S1 levels also experience strain with contralateral bending, whereas the L1–L2 and L2–L3 levels are strained with ipsilateral bending.

Typical pain referral patterns have emerged that can be helpful in the evaluation despite substantial overlap between different spinal levels. The upper lumbar facets can refer pain to the hip and upper anterolateral thigh. The lower lumbar facets can refer pain to the posterolateral thigh and calf. The upper cervical facets can refer pain to the upper neck and occiput, the middle cervical facets to the lower neck and supraclavicular area, and the lower cervical facets to the lower aspect of the neck and periscapular region.

Potential causes of false-positive results include excess sedation, large amounts of local anesthetic used for skin localization that can result in spread to other structures implicated in the pain syndrome, or placebo. Dreyfuss et al. found that aiming for a target lower on the transverse process rather than the typical target at the superomedial aspect of the transverse process reduced epidural spread of the local anesthetic. In the cervical spine, Cohen et al. found that a greater than 50% decrease in spread to

adjacent structures was achieved by using 0.25 ml compared with 0.5 ml. Ackerman et al. found a fivefold increase
in false-positive rates with injection of lidocaine down to
the facet joint compared to superficial saline. Box 11.1 summarizes modalities to reduce the false-positive rate for lumbar medial branch blocks.

FURTHER READING

Ackerman WE, Munir MA, Zhang JM, et al.: Are diagnostic lumbar
facet injections influenced by pain of muscular origin?. Pain Pract.
2004;4:286–291.
Brummett C, Cohen S, Facet syndrome: Facet joint injections, medial
branch blocks, and radiofrequency denervation. In: Benzon H, Raja
S, Fishman S, et al. (Eds.), Essentials of Pain Management. 3rd ed.
Philadelphia, PA: Saunders; 2011:322–327.
Cohen SP, Strassels SA, Kurihara C, et al.: Randomized study assessing
the accuracy of cervical facet joint nerve (medial branch) blocks using
different injectate volumes. Anesthesiology. 2010;112:144–152.
Dreyfuss P, Schwarzer AC, Lau P, et al. Specificity of lumbar medial
branch and L5 dorsal ramus blocks. A computed tomography study.
Spine. 1997;22:895–902.

6. ANSWER: C

Radiofrequency of the medial branches is associated with
few complications; however, the most common complication following conventional radiofrequency ablation is post-
denervation neuritis that can last days to a week or more.
Patients will present with dysesthesias often described as a
sunburn and allodynia that involves the skin overlying the
levels treated. This is thought to be due to thermal injury to
the lateral branch of the corresponding level that provides
sensation to the overlying skin and soft tissue. Significant
post-procedure pain occurs in less than 10% of patients.

Thermal injury to the exiting spinal nerve root occurs
uncommonly due to the motor testing that is done at 2
Hz at no less than three times the sensory threshold or 3
V. Injury to a spinal nerve should be suspected with new

onset of radicular pain with or without radiculopathy (dermatomal or myotomal sensory or motor deficit) at the level
treated.

Epidural abscess is a rare complication that is typically
reported in the context of perioperative epidural catheter
infusions. It is rarely reported as a complication after an epidural steroid injection and is predominately associated with
Staphylococcus species in immunocompromised patients
(mostly patients with diabetes or cancer). Patients will usually present within 2 weeks with back pain. The presence of
a high clinical index of suspicion accompanied by elevated
erythrocyte sedimentation rate or C-reactive protein may
be more useful than white blood cell count in screening.

FURTHER READING

Brummett C, Cohen S. Facet syndrome: Facet joint injections, medial
branch blocks, and radiofrequency denervation. In: Benzon H, Raja
S, Fishman S, et al. (Eds.), Essentials of Pain Management. 3rd ed.
Philadelphia, PA: Saunders; 2011:329.
Obray J, Huntoon M. Interlaminar and transforaminal epidural steroid
injections. In: Benzon H, Rathmell JP, Wu CL, et al. (Eds.), Raj's
Practical Management of Pain. 4th ed. Philadelphia, PA: Mosby;
2008:999.
Rathmell J. Facet injection: Intra-articular injection, medial branch
block, and radiofrequency treatment. In: Rathmell J (Ed.), Atlas
of Image-Guided Intervention in Regional Anesthesia and Pain
Medicine. 2nd ed. Philadelphia, PA: Wolters Kluwer; 2012:80–117.

7. ANSWER: B

Non-ionic contrast agents are considered the agent of choice
for interventional pain procedures secondary to their low
osmolality, which reduces the potential for osmotoxic reactions. Non-ionic agents are hydrophilic; therefore, after
intravascular injection, these agents are rapidly redistrib-
uted to the extracellular space and undergo renal elimination without resorption and minimal metabolism. The
elimination half-life is 2 hours in patients with normal
renal function; however, excretion can last weeks in patients
with renal dysfunction.

Potential osmotoxic reactions that can occur when
using ionic iodinated contrast agents, include pain on injection, hemolysis, endothelial damage with capillary leak and
edema, flushing, warmth, hypotension, cardiovascular collapse, and hypervolemia.

Compared to non-ionic contrast agents, ionic agents
have four times the incidence of idiosyncratic and potentially severe anaphylactic reactions. Minor reactions occur
in 3–12% of patients and severe reaction in 0.06–0.2%.
Severe reactions include anaphylactic or anaphylactoid reactions that can present with laryngeal or pulmonary edema,
hypotension, bronchospasm, convulsions, cardiac dys-
rhythmias, or cardiac arrest. Severe reactions are typically

dose independent, with symptom onset usually within 1 hour of dose administration. Risk factors include patients with a prior reaction to an ionic contrast agent, asthma, atopy, or advanced heart disease. Delayed hypersensitivity reactions can also occur and are twice as frequent with non-ionic dimers compared to non-ionic monomers. Treatment prophylaxis protocols include antihistamines, adrenergic agents, and corticosteroids. There is established efficacy in prophylaxis when using ionic contrast agents but not when using non-ionic agents.

Some recommend the use of gadolinium-containing contrast for patients who are high risk for a severe reaction. Dose reduction is warranted in patients with moderate to severe renal impairment because it has been implicated in the development of nephrogenic systemic fibrosis.

FURTHER READING

Botelho R, Sitzman B. Pharmacology for the interventional pain physician. In: Benzon H, Raja S, Fishman S, et al. (Eds.), *Essentials of Pain Management*. 3rd ed. Philadelphia, PA: Saunders; 2011:147–149.

8. ANSWER: D

Several cases of central nervous system injury have been reported after transforaminal epidural steroid injections resulting in paraplegia or embolic cerebrovascular accidents. The injuries occurred after injection of steroid, local anesthetic, and dye. The suspected mechanisms of injury include proximal intraneural spread of injectate, embolization of particulate steroid to the vascular supply to the spinal cord or brain, or spasm or injury to these vessels. Supporting these hypotheses, cadaver studies suggest that the entry of the ascending cervical and deep cervical arteries in the posterior portion of the cervical intervertebral foramen lies within a few millimeters of the needle path utilized in the transforaminal approach to epidural steroid injections. These findings were confirmed by Hoeft and colleagues.

Short courses of steroids (<2 or 3 weeks) are usually very safe, and side effects are rare. These effects may include fluid retention, hyperglycemia, elevated blood pressure, mood changes, menstrual irregularities, gastritis, Cushing's syndrome, increased appetite, weight gain, increased infections, and delayed wound healing. More serious side effects may occur with long-term and high-dose regimens.

Sterile meningitis and arachnoiditis have been reported following intrathecal injection of methylprednisolone; however, this was thought to be due to the polyethylene preservative.

Therapeutic effects of glucocorticoids include gene regulation and anti-inflammatory effects that occur via multiple mechanisms involving cytokines, inflammatory mediators, inflammatory cells, nitric oxide synthase, and adhesion molecules. It has been demonstrated that these agents have membrane-stabilizing effects that can suppress spontaneous ectopic neural discharge from neuromas and prevent the subsequent development of ectopic impulse discharge in a newly injured nerve. Topical application has been shown to block C fibers but not Aβ fibers.

FURTHER READING

Hoeft MA, Rathmell JP, Monsey RD, et al. Cervical transforaminal injection and the radicular artery: Variation in anatomical location within the cervical intervertebral foramina. Reg Anesth Pain Med 2006;31:270–274.
Variakojis R, Benzon H. Pharmacology for the interventional pain physician. In: Benzon H, Rathmell JP, Wu CL, et al. (Eds.), *Raj's Practical Management of Pain*. 4th ed. Philadelphia, PA: Mosby; 2008:722–723, 726.

9. ANSWER: C

Dysesthesias including anesthesia dolorosa may occur in up to 6% of patients who undergo neurodestructive procedures of the gasserian ganglion and are thought to be due to the incomplete destruction of the ganglion. Mild dysesthesias are characterized by a pulling or burning sensation, whereas anesthesia dolorosa manifests with severe post-procedure pain.

Facial hematoma and subscleral hematoma of the eye are common sequelae to the gasserian ganglion block due to the highly vascular pterygopalatine space and the closely approximated middle meningeal artery.

Corneal anesthesia can result from anesthetic involvement of the ophthalmic division of the trigeminal nerve. If left untreated, this can result in keratitis or ulceration. Corneal sensation should be tested with a cotton swab after performing a gasserian ganglion block, and if present, sterile ophthalmic ointment should be used and the affected eye patched to avoid damage. This should be continued until corneal anesthesia has resolved. Consultation with ophthalmology is recommended.

Radiofrequency lesioning, glycerol rhizotomy, and balloon compression have complication rates of 29.2%, 24.8%, and 16.1%, respectively.

FURTHER READING

Day M, Justiz R. Head and neck blocks. In: Benzon H, Raja S, Fishman S, et al. (Eds.), *Essentials of Pain Management*. 3rd ed. Philadelphia, PA: Saunders; 2011:541–542.
Waldman S. Gasserian ganglion block. In: Waldman S (Ed.), *Atlas of Interventional Pain Management*. 4th ed. Philadelphia, PA: Saunders; 2015:34.

10. ANSWER: A

Pain syndromes involving the sacroiliac joint can be categorized into intra- and extra-articular sources. Intra-articular sources include infection and arthritis, whereas extra-articular sources include enthesopathy, fractures, ligamentous injury, and myofascial pain. Differentiating between intra- and extra-articular sources can have implications when deciding on treatment strategy. Dreyfuss et al. found that multisite lateral branch blocks were more effective at blocking pain from ligamentous probing than for discomfort elicited during capsular distention. Extra-articular mediated pain is more likely to be unilateral, present in younger patients, have more tenderness, and be related to an inciting event.

Multiple studies have shown that no single historical or physical examination sign can reliably diagnose a painful sacroiliac joint. The results of reviews have been mixed regarding the ability of provocative physical exam maneuvers to diagnose or differentiate sacroiliac-mediated pain from other sources. History and physical exam are used to aid in the selection for diagnostic sacroiliac joint injections. Additional useful findings in patients being considered for SI joint injection include pain located below L5, increased pain when rising from a sitting position, and tenderness that overlies the joint.

There are no pathognomonic pain referral patterns for SI joint pain. In a retrospective review of 50 patients with injection-confirmed SI joint pain, Slipman et al. found the most common referral patterns to be to the buttock (94%), lower lumbar region (72%), ipsilateral lower extremity (50%), groin (14%), pain below the knee (28%), and foot pain (12%). Cohen et al. also noted variable pain referral patterns, including the lower leg (23%) and groin (20%). Radiologic imaging techniques are plagued by poor sensitivities and/or specificities. Slipman et al. and Maigne et al. reported sensitivities of 13% and 46%, respectively, for the use of radionuclide bone scanning for the diagnosis of SI joint pain. In a retrospective review, Elgafy et al. reported that computed tomography (CT) imaging carried a sensitivity of 69% and specificity of 57.5%.

Anatomic studies have shown that the lateral branches of the SI joint vary in number and location, from side to side, and from level to level. Due to the small single lesion diameter of 3 or 4 mm, this variability creates a challenge when performing conventional radiofrequency ablation techniques targeting the lateral branches. Controlled and uncontrolled studies support the use of cooled radiofrequency, which increases lesion diameter by 200–300%. Radiofrequency techniques target the posterior nerve supply, which will not affect pain originating from the ventral aspect of the joint. Cohen et al. identified demographic and clinical factors in patients undergoing denervation techniques who experienced greater than 50% relief at 6 months post-procedure. Age older than 65 years, higher pre-procedure pain score, opioid usage, and pain extending below the knee were all associated with treatment failure. A weak association was found between positive outcome and cooled radiofrequency.

FURTHER READING

Cohen S. Pain originating from the buttock: Sacroiliac joint syndrome and piriformis syndrome. In: Benzon H, Raja S, Fishman S, et al. (Eds.), *Essentials of Pain Management*. 3rd ed. Philadelphia, PA: Saunders; 2011:330–333.

Cohen SP, Strassels S, Kurihara C, et al. Outcome predictors for sacroiliac (lateral branch) radiofrequency denervation. Reg Anesth Pain Med. 2009;34:206–206.

Dreyfuss P, Snyder BD, Park K, et al. The ability of single site, single depth sacral lateral branch blocks to anesthetize the sacroiliac joint complex. Pain Med. 2008;9:844–850.

Elgafy H, Semaan HB, Ebraheim NA, et al. Computed tomography findings in patients with sacroiliac pain. Clin Orthop. 2001;382:112–118.

Maigne JY, Boulahdour H, Chatellier G. Value of quantitative radionuclide bone scanning in the diagnosis of sacroiliac joint syndrome in 32 patients with low back pain. Eur Spine J. 1998;7:328–331.

Slipman CW, Jackson HB, Lipetz JS, et al. Sacroiliac joint pain referral zones. Arch Phys Med Rehabil. 2000;81:334–338.

11. ANSWER: D

The incidence of systemic local anesthetic toxicity is 7–20/10,000 for peripheral nerve blocks and 4/10,000 for epidural blocks. Toxic levels are usually associated with excessive dose, intravascular injection, medical comorbidities that lower the seizure threshold, or aberrations with metabolism or elimination. Manifestation of local anesthetic toxicity most often begins with central nervous system side effects followed by cardiovascular effects. Central nervous system symptoms include metallic taste, perioral numbness, dizziness, muscle twitching, and seizures. Cardiovascular effects include arrhythmias, cardiac depression, hypotension, vasodilation, cardiac arrest, and collapse. Potent lipophilic local anesthetics, including bupivacaine, are more cardiotoxic than the less lipophilic agents, such as ropivacaine. These agents also can be refractory to the usual resuscitative measures. The use of 20% intralipid has been shown to be effective for resuscitation from bupivacaine-mediated cardiac toxicity through its proposed extraction of the lipophilic agent. A proposed intralipid regimen begins with a bolus of 1.2–2.0 ml/kg followed by an infusion of 0.25–0.5 ml/kg.

FURTHER READING

Botelho R, Sitzman B. Pharmacology for the interventional pain physician. In: Benzon H, Raja S, Fishman S, et al. (Eds.), *Essentials of Pain Management*. 3rd ed. Philadelphia, PA: Saunders; 2011:150.

12. ANSWER: C

Compared to the head and neck structures, the appearance of Horner's syndrome does not indicate complete sympathetic blockade of the upper extremity when performing a stellate ganglion block. This is due to the fact that all preganglionic fibers that affect the head and neck structures synapse or pass through the stellate ganglion. In comparison, sympathetic input to the upper extremity also may include branches from the brachial plexus and the first to third intercostal nerves via postganglionic fibers from the gray rami. These fibers are termed Kuntz's nerves and can result in incomplete sympathectomy of the upper extremity despite the presence of a Horner's sign.

The stellate ganglion, or cervicothoracic ganglion, is a fusion of the inferior cervical and first thoracic ganglions of the sympathetic trunk. Based on extensive anatomic studies using dissection, MRI, and CT, it is most often located at C7, along the lateral border of the longus colli, anterior to the neck of the first rib, and posterior to the vertebral vessels. Recent studies have described the subfascial position below the prevertebral fascia. Ultrasound guidance provides the added benefit of visualization of major vasculature and soft tissue structures, including the prevertebral fascia, longus colli muscle, thyroid, and esophagus, and it allows for the accurate placement of local anesthetic in a subfascial plane, with avoidance of intramuscular placement into the longus colli. It enables the identification of a needle trajectory that can avoid inadvertent esophageal puncture or vasculature disruption, including the inferior thyroid artery, which can result in mediastinitis or hematoma/ hemorrhage, respectively. In 90% of patients, the vertebral artery lies anterior to the stellate ganglion at C7 and enters the transverse vertebral foramen, posterior to the anterior tubercle of C6. In 10% of cases, the artery may enter at C5 or higher, which leaves the artery susceptible to injury, especially with blind or fluoroscopically guided procedures. Figure 11.4 illustrates the visualization of soft tissue and vascular structures that can be avoided when performing a stellate ganglion block with ultrasound guidance. The following list includes some of the indications based on case reports or case series with the exception of complex regional pain syndrome and Raynaud's disease, which are supported by outcome studies:

- Complex regional pain syndrome
- Vascular insufficiency—Raynaud's syndrome, vasospasm, vascular disease
- Accidental intra-arterial injection of drug
- Postherpetic neuralgia and acute herpes zoster
- Phantom pain
- Frostbite
- Complex regional pain syndrome, breast and postmastectomy pain
- Quinine poisoning
- Hyperhidrosis of upper extremity
- Cardiac arrhythmias
- Angina
- Vascular headaches
- Neuropathic pain syndromes including central pain
- Cancer pain
- Facial pain—atypical and trigeminal neuralgia

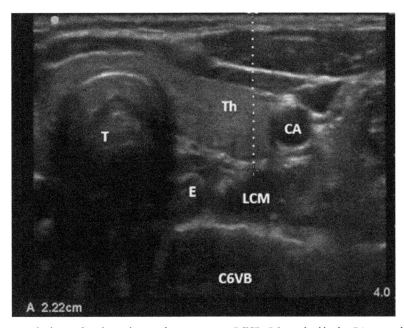

Figure 11.4 Sonogram of anterior neck obtained with gentle transducer pressure. C6VB, C6 vertebral body; CA, carotid artery; E, esophagus; LCM, longus colli muscle; T, trachea; Th, thyroid; white dotted line, skin-to-target distance (2.2 cm).

SOURCE: Reprinted with permission from Gofeld M, Shankar H. Ultrasound-guided sympathetic blocks: Stellate ganglion and celiac plexus block. In: Benzon H, Raja S, Fishman S (Eds.), *Essentials of Pain Management*. 3rd ed. Philadelphia, PA: Saunders; 2011:496, Figure 67–3.

• Hot flashes

This list of potential indications for stellate ganglion blockade is reprinted with permission from Sekhadia M. Peripheral sympathetic blocks. In: Benzon H, Raja S, Fishman S, et al. (Eds.), *Essentials of Pain Management*. 3rd ed. Philadelphia, PA: Saunders; 2011:622, Table 79–1.

FURTHER READING

Gofeld M, Shankar H. Ultrasound-guided sympathetic blocks: Stellate ganglion and celiac plexus block. In: Benzon H, Raja S, Fishman S, et al. (Eds.), *Essentials of Pain Management*. 3rd ed. Philadelphia, PA: Saunders; 2011:496.

Sekhadia M, Nader A, Benzon H. Peripheral sympathetic blocks. In: Benzon H, Raja S, Fishman S, et al. (Eds.), *Essentials of Pain Management*. 3rd ed. Philadelphia, PA: Saunders; 2011:621–623, 628.

13. ANSWER: A

Once thought to be rare, it is now believed that as many as 1 in 20 patients treated with intrathecal opioids will develop an intrathecal granuloma at the catheter tip. Large granulomas can result in spinal cord or nerve root compression that may manifest as worsening pain, new radicular symptoms, weakness, sensory deficits, loss of bladder or bowel function, or paralysis. With rapid- or acute-onset neurologic deterioration, emergent surgical decompression is warranted in order to prevent permanent neurologic compromise. In patients who have already developed neurologic deficits and then undergo surgical decompression, one-third make a complete recovery, one-third are able to remain ambulatory, and one-third remain either nonambulatory or paralyzed.

In this case, an emergent MRI is warranted due to the patient's rapidly deteriorating neurologic exam. Conversely, asymptomatic granulomas can be managed by discontinuation of the infusion, which frequently results in either stabilization or regression of the granuloma. Hypertonic saline administration after opioid cessation has been shown to be effective. Most commonly, the catheter tip is pulled back one or two spinal levels, usually resulting in granuloma resolution.

An increase in pain in the setting of an abnormal neurologic exam does not warrant an increase in intrathecal opioid or clonidine. Imaging is indicated in order to rule out compressive pathology. Increasing opioid doses due to new painful sensations in a dermatomal distribution near the level of the catheter tip should raise suspicion for the development of a granuloma. Although decreasing the dose of morphine may lessen the propensity of granuloma formation in the future, the current symptoms mandate an urgent MRI to evaluate for granuloma or other causes. The neurologic exam should be followed closely with vigilance for subtle changes resulting from the slow-growing nature of catheter tip granulomas. Changes in the neurologic exam warrant follow-up imaging (MRI or CT myelogram) to assess for granuloma formation.

FURTHER READING

Nanney A. Implanted drug delivery systems for the control of chronic pain. In: Benzon H, Raja S, Fishman S, et al. (Eds.), *Essentials of Pain Management*. 3rd ed. Philadelphia, PA: Saunders; 2011:459–460.

14. ANSWER: C

Ziconotide is a 25-amino acid peptide derived from marine snail venom. It is a highly selective N-type voltage-sensitive calcium channel antagonist found on the presynaptic terminals in the dorsal horn. Animal studies show that ziconotide reduces tactile and mechanical allodynia in a dose-dependent manner. In addition, randomized, placebo-controlled, double-blind trials have established its efficacy in patients with severe neuropathic pain and chronic malignant and nonmalignant pain.

Ziconotide has a narrow therapeutic window between doses, resulting in side effects compared to the dose required for analgesia. This results in a high-risk profile for side effects, which have been shown to occur in 15–99% of patients. Side effects include dizziness, confusion, ataxia, nystagmus, memory impairment, dysmetria, sedation, agitation, hallucinations, nausea, vomiting, urinary retention, somnolence, and coma. These effects most frequently occur with higher initial dosing scales or with rapid dose escalation.

Ziconotide should be avoided in patients with a history of psychosis or a complex past psychiatric history. It has the potential to cause serious psychiatric and neurologic impairment, especially with high initial dosing or rapid dose escalation. Consequently, it is recommended that ziconotide be initiated at a low dose with slow upward titration to minimize risk of developing these adverse side effects.

FURTHER READING

Nanney A. Implanted drug delivery systems for the control of chronic pain. In: Benzon H, Raja S, Fishman S, et al. (Eds.), *Essentials of Pain Management*. 3rd ed. Philadelphia, PA: Saunders; 2011:459–460.

15. ANSWER: A

Orthostatic hypotension can occur in 1–3% of patients undergoing a celiac plexus block and can last for up to 2 weeks. Treatment consists of bed rest and fluid replacement.

For patients who need to ambulate during the first week, compression bandages applied to the lower extremities have been used with some success.

Retroperitoneal hemorrhage is a rare complication; however, it must be considered in any patient presenting with backache with or without orthostasis. These patients should have serial hematocrit measurements. If a low or decreasing value is noted, imaging is warranted to evaluate for the source of blood loss, which could include injury to the kidneys, aorta, or other vascular structures.

Paraplegia and transient motor paralysis, thought to be secondary to spasm of the lumbar segmental arteries, have been reported after celiac plexus block. Animal studies revealed that the degree of spasm was directly related to the concentration of phenol and inversely related to the concentration of alcohol. Additional factors likely play a role and may include direct injury to a vascular or neurologic structure as well as spread of neurolytic to the spinal cord.

Near fatal dehydration secondary to diarrhea after a celiac plexus block has been reported. Diarrhea is a result of the sympathectomy involving the intestinal tract. Treatment consists of hydration and antidiarrheals such as loperamide.

FURTHER READING

Erdek M, deLeon-Casasola O. Neurolytic visceral sympathetic blocks. In: Benzon H, Raja S, Fishman S, et al. (Eds.), *Essentials of Pain Management*. 3rd ed. Philadelphia, PA: Saunders; 2011:526–527.

16. ANSWER: C

Although aspirin (acetylsalicylic acid (ASA)) and nonsteroidal anti-inflammatory drugs (NSAIDs) affect platelet function, their risks are less clear than those for drugs such as clopidogrel. New guidelines recommend cessation of ASA for 6 days when used for primary prophylaxis in higher risk procedures such as spinal stimulation. Shared decision-making between the pain physician and other physicians involved in anticoagulant use is always important. NSAIDs may require stoppage but have more variable effects due to different half-lives.

Clopidogrel is a thienopyridine medication that works by interfering with ADP receptor-mediated platelet activation. Ticlopidine is another thienopyridine medication, and it should be stopped at least 14 days prior to a neuraxial procedure.

FURTHER READING

Benzon H. Anticoagulants and neuraxial and peripheral nerve blocks. In: Benzon H, Raja S, Fishman S, et al. (Eds.), *Essentials of Pain Medicine*. 3rd ed. Philadelphia, PA: Saunders; 2011:629–636.

Narouze S, Benzon H, Provenzano D, et al. Interventional spine and pain procedures in patients on antiplatelet and anticoagulant medications: Guidelines from the American Society of Regional Anesthesia and Pain Medicine, the European Society of Regional Anaesthesia and Pain Therapy, the American Academy of Pain Medicine, the International Neuromodulation Society, the North American Neuromodulation Society, and the World Institute of Pain. *Reg Anesth Pain Med*. 2015;40:182–212.

17. ANSWER: B

When performing interventional pain procedures utilizing fluoroscopy, it is imperative to understand the potential radiation risks posed to the patient, the practitioner, as well as others in the room. The optimal position is for the X-ray tube on the fluoroscopy unit to be underneath the table on which the patient is positioned and to be as far away from the patient as possible. This means the image intensifier is above the patient and as close to the patient as possible without interfering in the performance of the procedure. The practitioner and others in the room should wear lead aprons and thyroid shields at all times. Leaded eyeglasses provide additional protection for the practitioner's eyes.

The dose of radiation decreases with the square of the distance from the X-ray source, so doubling the distance from the X-ray source results in a decrease in radiation dose by a factor of four. Conversely, rotating the C-arm such that the X-ray source moves out from under the table increases the radiation dose to the patient as well as the practitioner (if the X-ray source is moved toward the practitioner). The practitioner should step away from the source in these situations when the beam is on to minimize his or her exposure.

Although wearing leaded gloves would seem to decrease the radiation exposure, it can actually increase the radiation output from the machine if the hands are in the exposure field while the beam is on. This occurs in units that have automatic brightness control because they will automatically increase the radiation output in response the leaded gloves being in the field due to the higher density of the gloves. This increase in radiation output can eliminate the protective effects of the leaded gloves.

FURTHER READING

Rathmell J. Radiation safety and use of radiographic contrast agents in pain medicine. In: Benzon H, Rathmell J, Wu C, et al. (Eds.), *Practical Management of Pain*. 5th ed. Philadelphia, PA: Mosby; 2014:981–986.

18. ANSWER: D

Although SCS can be a tremendous benefit to patients, patient selection is a critical element in determining which patients are appropriate candidates. Evaluation includes determining if a patient's pain condition is appropriate for SCS, having the patient undergo a psychological evaluation, examination of radiographic studies to check for any potential anatomic impediments to safe lead placement, and the performance of a trial period. Although the gate theory was initially proposed to explain the mechanism by which SCS provides pain relief, the specific mechanism is not entirely understood.

FURTHER READING

Hurley R, Burton A. Spinal cord and peripheral nerve stimulation. In: Benzon H, Rathmell J, Wu C, et al. (Eds.), *Practical Management of Pain*. 5th ed. Philadelphia, PA: Mosby; 2014:939–951.

19. ANSWER: D

The superior hypogastric plexus is a retroperitoneal structure that is situated bilaterally between the lower third of the fifth lumbar vertebral body and upper third of the first sacral vertebral body. When performing a superior hypogastric plexus block, the needle tip should be anterolateral to the L5–S1 intervertebral disc space and be verified in both the anteroposterior and lateral planes with fluoroscopy. Both transvenous and transdiscal approaches are described, but during neurolysis, meticulous care should be taken to not inject into those structures. Flow of the contrast agent back to the nerve roots is not desired because injection of the neurolytic agent in such circumstances would lead to deficits in the distribution of the nerve root.

FURTHER READING

LoDico M, de Leon-Casasola O. Neurolysis of the sympathetic axis for cancer pain management. In: Benzon H, Rathmell J, Wu C, et al. (Eds.), *Practical Management of Pain*. 5th ed. Philadelphia, PA: Mosby; 2014:798–801.

20. ANSWER: B

Botulinum toxin blocks the presynaptic release of acetylcholine by irreversibly binding to presynaptic cholinergic neurons. Because this binding is irreversible, it results in permanent denervation. Although this is permanent, new axons and synapses will form, allowing for a functional recovery and thus making the overall effect transient. The clinical effect usually lasts 3 to 4 months. In addition, botulinum toxin-A has been shown to inhibit the release of glutamate, which decreases the amount of substance P. Doses

Table 11.1 ONABOTULINUM TOXIN A DOSING FOR CHRONIC MIGRAINE BY MUSCLE USING THE PREEMPT INJECTION PARADIGM

HEAD/NECK AREA	RECOMMENDED DOSE: TOTAL DOSAGE (NO. OF SITES[*])
Frontalis[†]	20 units (in four sites)
Corrugators[†]	10 units (in two sites)
Procerus	5 units (in one site)
Occipitalis[†]	30 units (in six sites), rebreak up to 40 units in 8 sites
Temporalis[†]	40 units (in eight sites), rebreak up to 50 units in 10 sites
Trapezius[†]	30 units (in six sites), rebreak up to 50 units in 10 sites
Cervical paraspinal muscle[†]	20 units (in five sites)

TOTAL dose range: 155–195 units.

[*]EACH intramuscular injection site = 0.1 ml = 5 U onabotulinum toxin A.

[†]DOSE distributed bilaterally for the minimum 155 U dose.

SOURCE: Reprinted from Anitescu A, Benzon HT, Variakojis R. Pharmacology for the interventional pain physician. In: Benzon H, Rathmell J, Wu C, et al. (Eds.), *Practical Management of Pain*, 596–614 (2014) with permission from Elsevier.

for some common injection sites used in the treatment of migraine headaches are listed in Table 11.1.

FURTHER READING

Anitescu M, Benzon H, Variakojis R. Pharmacology for the interventional pain physician. In: Benzon H, Rathmell J, Wu C, et al. (Eds.), *Practical Management of Pain*. 5th ed. Philadelphia, PA: Mosby; 2014:606–610.

21. ANSWER: B

Occipital nerve blocks can be an effective treatment for occipital neuralgia. There is some support for its use in cervicogenic headaches as well as cluster headaches. Anatomically, the greater occipital nerve is generally medial to the occipital artery (Figure 11.5). It is the medial branch of the dorsal primary ramus of C2, arising between C1 and C2, and on ultrasound imaging may be seen emerging under the obliquus capitus inferior muscle. One can palpate the occipital artery at the superior nuchal ridge and then direct the needle medial to that point. One must be careful not to inject too far inferiorly when performing this block due to the risk of the needle entering the foramen magnum.

FURTHER READING

Candido K, Day M. Nerve blocks of the head and neck. In: Benzon H, Rathmell J, Wu C, et al. (Eds.), *Practical Management of Pain*. 5th ed. Philadelphia, PA: Mosby; 2014:706–707.

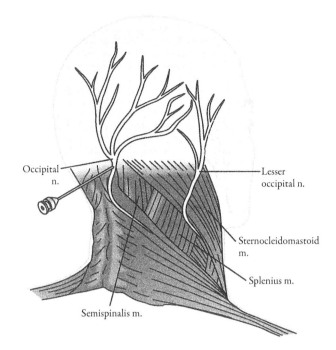

Occipital n.

Lesser occipital n.

Sternocleidomastoid m.

Splenius m.

Semispinalis m.

Figure 11.5 The anatomy and site of nerve blocking for the great occipital nerve.
SOURCE: Reprinted with permission from Candido K, Day M. Nerve blocks of the head and neck. In: Benzon H, Rathmell J, Wu C, et al. (Eds.), *Practical Management of Pain*. 5th ed. Philadelphia, PA: Mosby; 2014:706.

22. ANSWER: D

Whereas glycerol is used in the treatment of trigeminal neuralgia, ethyl alcohol and phenol are the two agents commonly employed for epidural or intrathecal neurolytic blocks. As noted in Table 11.2, which lists the characteristics of these agents, ethyl alcohol is generally associated with a burning sensation on injection. The full effect of ethyl alcohol generally occurs in 3–5 days.

FURTHER READING

Adams M, Benzon H, Hurley R. Chemical neurolytic blocks. In: Benzon H, Rathmell J, Wu C, et al. (Eds.), *Practical Management of Pain*. 5th ed. Philadelphia, PA: Mosby; 2014:782–793.

23. ANSWER: D

Five terminal nerve branches innervate the foot: the posterior tibial nerve, the superficial peroneal nerve, the deep peroneal nerve, the sural nerve, and the saphenous nerve. The first four arise from the sciatic nerve, whereas the saphenous nerve arises from the femoral nerve. Anatomically, the posterior tibial nerve is located just posterior to the medial malleolus, and the saphenous nerve is located anterior to the medial malleolus. The sural nerve is located posterior to the lateral malleolus, and the superficial peroneal nerve is located anterior to the lateral malleolus. The deep peroneal

Table 11.2 **CHARACTERISTICS OF CHEMICAL NEUROLYTIC AGENTS**

	ALCOHOL	PHENOL
Physical properties	Low water solubility	Absorbs water on air exposure
Stability at room temperature	Unstable	Stable
Concentration	100%	4–8%
Diluent	None	Glycerin
Relative to CSF	Hypobaric	Hyperbaric
Injection sensation	Burning pain	Painless, warm feeling
Onset of neurolysis	Immediate	Delayed (15 min)
CSF uptake ends	30 minutes	15 minutes
Full effect of neurolysis	3–5 days	1 day

CSF, cerebrospinal fluid.

SOURCE: Reprinted from Adams MCB, Benzon HT, Hurley RW. Chemical neurolytic blocks. In: Benzon H, Rathmell J, Wu C, et al. (Eds.), *Practical Management of Pain*, 784–793 (2014) with permission from Elsevier.

nerve is located anteriorly between the extensor digitorum longus tendon and the extensor hallucis longus tendon. The innervation of the cutaneous areas is shown in Figure 11.6.

FURTHER READING

Brown D. *Atlas of Regional Anesthesia*. 4th ed. Philadelphia, PA: Saunders; 2010:136–138.
Shastri U, Kwofie K, Salviz E, et al. Lower extremity nerve blocks. In: Benzon H, Rathmell J, Wu C, et al. (Eds.), *Practical Management of Pain*. 5th ed. Philadelphia, PA: Mosby; 2014:742–744.
Tureanu L, Ganapathy S, Nader A. Sciatic nerve block and ankle block. In: Benzon H, Raja S, Fishman S, et al. (Eds.), *Essentials of Pain Medicine*. 3rd ed. Philadelphia, PA: Saunders; 2011:616–620.

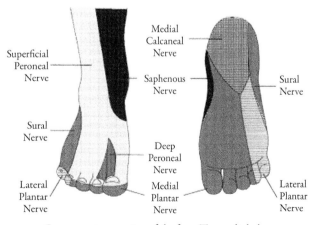

Superficial Peroneal Nerve

Sural Nerve

Lateral Plantar Nerve

Medial Calcaneal Nerve

Saphenous Nerve

Deep Peroneal Nerve

Medial Plantar Nerve

Sural Nerve

Lateral Plantar Nerve

Figure 11.6 Cutaneous innervation of the foot. The medial plantar nerve, lateral plantar nerve, and medial calcaneal nerve are branches of the posterior tibial nerve.
SOURCE: Reprinted with permission from Tureanu L, Ganapathy S, Nader A. Sciatic nerve block and ankle block. In: Benzon H, Raja S, Fishman S, et al. (Eds.), *Essentials of Pain Medicine*. 3rd ed. Philadelphia, PA: Saunders; 2011:617.

24. ANSWER: B

The lumbar sympathetic chains run bilaterally along the anterolateral vertebral bodies, generally from the lower third of the second lumbar vertebral body to the upper third of the third lumbar vertebral body. The needle tip should be positioned near the lower portion of L2 or the upper portion of L3. Just anterior to the vertebral bodies are the aorta and the inferior vena cava, so advancing the needle too far anteriorly could result in the puncture of one of these vessels. Skin temperature is commonly used as an indicator of a successful sympathetic block.

FURTHER READING

Brown D. *Atlas of Regional Anesthesia*. 4th ed. Philadelphia, PA: Saunders; 2010:336–338.
Sekhadia M, Nader A, Benzon H. Peripheral sympathetic blocks. In: Benzon H, Raja S, Fishman S, et al. (Eds.), *Essentials of Pain Medicine*. 3rd ed. Philadelphia, PA: Saunders; 2011:624–626.

25. ANSWER: C

The obturator nerve arises from L2–L4 (although largely from L3–L4). It provides innervation to the medial thigh as well as the hip joint and adductor muscles. There are vascular structures in the vicinity of the obturator nerve, so vascular injury, hematoma, or intravascular injection are potential risks and complications.

FURTHER READING

Brown D. *Atlas of Regional Anesthesia*. 4th ed. Philadelphia, PA: Saunders; 2010:126–128.
Perlas A, Factor D, Candido K, et al. Blocks of the lumbar plexus and its branches. In: Benzon H, Raja S, Fishman S, et al. (Eds.), *Essentials of Pain Medicine*. 3rd ed. Philadelphia, PA: Saunders; 2011:602–604.

26. ANSWER: D

When performing lumbar medial branch blocks, false-positive rates can be as high as 40%. Steps to reduce the incidence of false-positive results include not using sedation or analgesic medication during the procedure. In addition, limiting the injected volume to no more than 0.5 ml as well as minimizing the amount of local anesthetic used for the skin can help. The target area should be lower on the transverse process, not higher, if one desires to reduce false-positive rates.

FURTHER READING

Brummett C, Cohen S. Facet syndrome: Facet joint injections, medial branch blocks, and radiofrequency denervation. In: Benzon H,

Raja S, Fishman S, et al. (Eds.), *Essentials of Pain Medicine*. 3rd ed. Philadelphia, PA: Saunders; 2011:322–329.

27. ANSWER: B

The ilioinguinal nerve arises from L1. When performing an ilioinguinal block, the needle entry point is 2 in. medial and 2 in. inferior to the anterior superior iliac spine. Potential complications include entering the peritoneal cavity and perforating the intestine as well as inadvertent blockade of the femoral nerve.

FURTHER READING

Rahangdale R, Tureanu L, Molloy R. Truncal blocks: Intercostal, paravertebral, interpleural, suprascapular, ilioinguinal, and iliohypogastric nerve blocks. In: Benzon H, Raja S, Fishman S, et al. (Eds.), *Essentials of Pain Medicine*. 3rd ed. Philadelphia, PA: Saunders; 2011:592–593.
Waldman S. *Atlas of Interventional Pain Management*. 5th ed. Philadelphia, PA: Elsevier; 2015:431–435.

28. ANSWER: D

Answers A–C are all contraindications to the placement of an intrathecal drug delivery system. Any systemic infection must first be treated and resolved prior to implantation or the device may become seeded, necessitating removal. Any coagulopathy must be corrected to avoid potential hemorrhagic complications or possible hematoma formation, which could lead to devastating neurologic events. Permanent placement of an intrathecal drug delivery system should be preceded by a trial with the agent to be administered. Failure of a favorable response during the trial is a contraindication to implantation. Failure of maximal medical therapy should be demonstrated prior to consideration of implanting the system, and it would be an indication for implanting an intrathecal drug delivery system.

FURTHER READING

Nanney A, Muro K, Levy R. Implanted drug delivery systems for the control of chronic pain. In: Benzon H, Raja S, Fishman S, et al. (Eds.), *Essentials of Pain Medicine*. 3rd ed. Philadelphia, PA: Saunders; 2011:451–461.

29. ANSWER: C

When performing procedures and using an X-ray source such as fluoroscopy, it is important to take steps that minimize the radiation exposure of the patient, the provider, and anyone in the procedure room as much as possible. Some steps to help reduce radiation exposure include collimating down to the area of interest, minimizing beam-on time, and maximizing the distance between the X-ray source and the patient. Larger patients do result in higher dose rates.

FURTHER READING

Chung B, Benzon H. Fluoroscopy and radiation safety. In: Benzon H, Raja S, Fishman S, et al. (Eds.), *Essentials of Pain Medicine*. 3rd ed. Philadelphia, PA: Saunders; 2011:502–510.

30. ANSWER: A

The patient appears to be suffering from meralgia paresthetica. The correct approach using surface landmarks for blocking the lateral femoral cutaneous nerve is to go 2 cm medial and 2 cm inferior to the anterior superior iliac spine. The landmarks in choice C describe the approach for an obturator nerve block. Although unintended blockade of the femoral and obturator nerves can occur with this block, there are not any significant vascular structures in the immediate vicinity of the lateral femoral cutaneous nerve, so there is not a high risk of vascular injury with this block.

FURTHER READING

Minieka M, Nishida T, Benzon H. Entrapment neuropathies. In: Benzon H, Raja S, Fishman S, et al. (Eds.), *Essentials of Pain Medicine*. 3rd ed. Philadelphia, PA: Saunders; 2011:400–401.
Perlas A, Factor D, Candido K, et al. Blocks of the lumbar plexus and its branches. In: Benzon H, Raja S, Fishman S, et al. (Eds.), *Essentials of Pain Medicine*. 3rd ed. Philadelphia, PA: Saunders; 2011:601–602.
Shastri U, Kwofie K, Salviz E, et al. Lower extremity nerve blocks. In: Benzon H, Rathmell J, Wu C, et al. (Eds.), *Practical Management of Pain*. 5th ed. Philadelphia, PA: Mosby; 2014:735–736.

31. ANSWER: C

The cordotomy procedure disrupts the pain projection pathways in the anterolateral spinal cord. The specific targets are the spinothalamic and spinoreticular tracts. Due to the manner in which the spinothalamic axons cross over from the contralateral cord, pain relief typically occurs two to three spinal segments below where the cordotomy lesion is introduced. In addition, in the upper cervical spinal cord, the spinothalamic tract is just lateral to the reticulospinal tract, which carries respiratory fibers. Thus, it is generally not advisable to perform bilateral upper cervical cordotomy, and in patients with severe respiratory impairment, even unilateral upper cervical cordotomy is not recommended.

Cordotomy can be an extremely effective technique to address pain emanating from the lower trunk or lower extremities. Although success rates vary, there is a higher immediate success rate for cancer-related pain compared to pain that is not cancer-related. Over time, the percentage of patients with continued pain relief decreases regardless of the etiology of the pain, so recurrence of the pain is a significant potential drawback. Other complications include ataxia and paresis (which are the most common and usually resolve over time), urinary and fecal incontinence, as well as impotence. There is increased occurrence of these complications when a bilateral procedure is performed. Respiratory failure occurs less frequently but is a potentially life-threatening complication.

FURTHER READING

Dubuisson D, Bajwa Z. Neurosurgical treatment of pain. In: Warfield C, Bajwa Z (Eds.), *Principles and Practice of Pain Medicine*. 2nd ed. New York, NY: McGraw-Hill; 2004. Available at http://accessanesthesiology.mhmedical.com/content.aspx?bookid=411&Sectionid=40429871. Accessed December 15, 2015.
Rosenow J. Neurosurgical procedures for treatment of intractable pain. In: Benzon H, Raja S, Fishman S, et al. (Eds.), *Essentials of Pain Medicine*. 3rd ed. Philadelphia, PA: Saunders; 2011:166–167.

32. ANSWER: B

Major adverse cardiac event (MACE) after non-cardiac surgery is often associated with prior coronary artery disease events. The stability and timing of a recent MI impact the incidence of perioperative morbidity and mortality. A retrospective review demonstrated that postoperative MI rates decreased as the time from MI to surgical date increased, and the 30-day mortality rate also decreased. This risk was affected by the presence and type of coronary revascularization that occurred at the time of the MI.

The Revised Cardiac Risk Index is a simple, validated, and accepted tool to assess perioperative risk of major cardiac complications (MI, pulmonary edema, ventricular fibrillation or primary cardiac arrest, and complete heart block). It has six predictors of risk for major cardiac complications, only one of which is based on the procedure.

FURTHER READING

Fleisher LA, Fleischmann KE, Auerbach AD, et al. 2014 ACC/AHA guideline on perioperative cardiovascular evaluation and management of patients undergoing noncardiac surgery: A report of the American College of Cardiology/American Heart Association Task Force on Practice Guidelines. *J Am Coll Cardiol*. 2014;64(22):e77–e137.

12.

MUSCULOSKELETAL PAIN

M. Gabriel Hillegass, Anthony A. Tucker, and Antonio Quidgley-Nevares

INTRODUCTION

This chapter on musculoskeletal pain is composed of a question-and-answer bank that encompasses the breadth of the fund of knowledge required for the evaluation and management of various chronic musculoskeletal pain syndromes. Not only do probing questions with concise and informative answer explanations challenge the reader's knowledge base but also references for further reading and mastery of the subject are provided. Topics covered include epidemiology, disability, rehabilitation, anatomy and physiology (including neurophysiology and mediators of inflammation), and the musculoskeletal exam. The pathophysiology, diagnosis, and management of musculoskeletal pain conditions such as common orthopedic and occupational injuries, osteoarthritis, chronic tissue pain states, and various autoimmune diseases (e.g., rheumatoid arthritis) are also expertly reviewed. These high-yield questions correspond to the musculoskeletal pain section of the American Board of Medical Specialties' Pain Medicine Content Outline.

QUESTIONS

1. Which of the following muscles is most commonly involved in rotator cuff tendinitis?

A. Supraspinatus
B. Infraspinatus
C. Teres minor
D. Teres major
E. Subscapularis

2. Clinical features of myofascial pain syndrome may include all of the following except:

A. Myofascial trigger points
B. Palpable taut bands of skeletal muscle

C. Sensory abnormalities
D. Trophic changes of the skin
E. Referred autonomic phenomena

3. Treatment for chronic myofascial pain syndrome in a patient with significant pain and disability should include:

A. Implementation of an active exercise program
B. Therapeutic physical modalities such as heat as well as muscle and nerve stimulation
C. Physical therapy techniques such as targeted stretching, strengthening, and correction of aggravating postural and biomechanical factors
D. Cognitive–behavioral therapy addressing fear avoidance, poor coping skills, and other maladaptive behaviors and thought patterns
E. All of the above

4. According to the US Department of Labor, Bureau of Labor Statistics, repetitive strain injuries have the highest incidence in which of the following industries?

A. Service
B. Health care
C. Manufacturing
D. A and C
E. B and C

5. All of the following are criteria used by the Office of Disability in the Social Security Administration for determining disability based on the diagnosis of chronic pain syndrome except:

A. Limited daily activities due to pain
B. Inability to maintain employment in the preceding 12 months
C. Excessive use of medication and medical services
D. Behavioral changes including depression and anxiety
E. Six months of intractable pain

6. A patient presents with pain, stiffness, and swelling involving the metocarpophalangeal and proximal interphalangeal joints bilaterally, with plain radiographs revealing diffuse periarticular osteopenia. Which of the following is a possible treatment option over the anticipated course of this disease?

A. Nonsteroidal anti-inflammatory drugs (NSAIDs)
B. Low-dose systemic corticosteroids
C. Low-dose weekly methotrexate
D. Tumor necrosis factor (TNF) antagonists
E. All of the above

7. All of the following statements regarding the treatment of knee osteoarthritis are true except:

A. Muscle strengthening and aerobic exercise reduce symptoms and improve functional capacity.
B. Transcutaneous electrical nerve stimulation (TENS) reduces pain during active use.
C. COX-2 inhibitors have superior efficacy with respect to analgesia compared to nonselective COX inhibitors.
D. Intra-articular viscosupplementation with hyaluronic acid has not demonstrated significant clinical efficacy.
E. Adaptive equipment (e.g., cane or walker) use with proper training can reduce pain and prevent falls.

8. Which of the following neurophysiologic processes contributes to the development of chronic neuropathic pain states?

A. Activation of "on" cells in the rostral ventral medulla and subsequent increased facilitatory effects of descending modulation
B. Upregulation of spinal dynorphin and subsequent increased release of excitatory neurotransmitters from primary afferent neurons
C. Suppression of "off" cells in the rostral ventral medulla and subsequent decreased inhibitory effects of descending modulation
D. A and C
E. A, B, and C

9. Which of the following sequences correctly identifies the order and character of somatosensory events during patient contact with a brief, intense heat stimulus such as a flame?

A. Aδ fiber pricking pain; Aβ fiber pressure sensation; C fiber burning pain
B. Aβ fiber pressure sensation; Aδ fiber pricking pain; C fiber burning pain
C. Aδ fiber pricking pain; C fiber burning pain; Aβ fiber pressure sensation

D. Aβ fiber pressure sensation; C fiber burning pain; Aδ fiber pricking pain
E. C fiber burning pain; Aδ fiber pricking pain; Aβ fiber pressure sensation

10. All of the following are inflammatory mediators and play a role in peripheral nociceptor activation except:

A. Bradykinin
B. Adenosine
C. Serotonin
D. Glycine
E. Histamine

11. The Apley "Scratch" test is performed to evaluate a patient's shoulder. Which of the following is a correct component of the Apley "Scratch test?

A. Reach behind his head and touch the superior medial angle of the ipsilateral scapula to evaluate the shoulder's abduction and internal rotation.
B. Reach in front of his head and touch the opposite acromion to evaluate the shoulder's internal rotation and abduction.
C. Reach behind his head and touch the superior medial angle of the opposite scapula to evaluate the shoulder's adduction and internal rotation.
D. Reach behind his back to touch the inferior angle of the opposite scapula to evaluate the shoulder's internal rotation and adduction.
E. Reach in front of his head and touch the opposite acromion to evaluate the shoulder's external rotation and adduction.

12. A patient complains of anterior dull knee pain. The pain is worse when walking down stairs and when standing after sitting for a prolonged period of time. Which physical exam finding may confirm the diagnosis?

A. Positive O'Brien test
B. Positive Lachman test
C. Femoral anteversion
D. Positive J sign
E. Positive McMurray sign

13. A 58-year-old male presents with a complaint of right anterior groin pain of an insidious onset. There is loss of internal and external rotation of the hip. Plain radiographs of the right hip show an irregular, mottled appearance of the right femoral head. The best treatment option at this time would be:

A. Physical therapy
B. Intra-articular steroid injection
C. Traction of the hip

D. Total hip arthroplasty
E. Osteotomy of the femoral head

14. The process of joint destruction in rheumatoid arthritis includes all the following except:

A. Initial injury to the synovial microvasculature
B. Synoviocyte activation via class III HLA antigens leading to synovial cell proliferation
C. T lymphocyte infiltration
D. Atrophy of the synovium
E. Joint ankylosis with advanced disease

15. The American College of Rheumatology's diagnostic criteria for rheumatoid arthritis include all of the following except:

A. Morning stiffness in the joints that must last at least 1 hour before maximal improvement
B. Arthritis in three or more joints simultaneously with soft tissue swelling or fluid
C. Consistently asymmetric arthritis and subcutaneous nodules in extensor surfaces
D. Radiologic changes showing erosions, bony decalcification, and joint space narrowing on hand and wrist
E. Positive serum rheumatoid factor

16. Disability due to knee osteoarthritis is most likely to be secondary to which of the following?

A. Increasing age
B. Sports-related joint injury
C. Being a marathon runner
D. Morbid obesity
E. Sedentary work

17. An amateur golfer presents to you with pain in the lateral aspect of the elbow. The pain is worse with hand gripping. Which of the following is the best answer?

A. The pathology is due to repetitive valgus stress of the elbow.
B. The pathology is due to microtears of the tendon of the extensor carpi radialis brevis.
C. Plain radiographs of the elbow will confirm the diagnosis.
D. This condition may lead to osteochondritis dissecans of the capitellum.
E. Ulnar neuropathy may occur if not addressed.

18. A patient presents with pain and tenderness over the radial aspect of the wrist. On examination, the symptoms are reproduced with passive ulnar deviation of the wrist with the thumb flexed into the palm while making a fist. Treatment may include all of the following interventions except:

A. NSAIDs
B. Thumb spica splint to immobilize the thumb
C. Neutral wrist splint
D. Corticosteroid injection
E. Surgical intervention

19. A 22-year-old male presents with low back pain and morning stiffness in the low back for more than 1 year. It had an insidious onset. On examination, there is tenderness over the bilateral sacroiliac joints. There is also a decrease in range of motion of the lumbar spine. Lab work was positive for HLA-B27. Other findings consistent with this condition include all of the following except:

A. Iritis
B. Radiologic finding of bilateral sacroiliac joint narrowing
C. Radiologic finding of calcification of the anterior spinal ligament and ankylosis of the apophyseal joints
D. Increased chest expansion
E. Schober test changes indicating disease progression

20. Musculoskeletal complications of sickle cell disease include all of the following except:

A. Pain predominately in the small joints
B. Osteonecrosis
C. Dactylitis
D. Osteomyelitis
E. Pain in the abdomen, chest, and back

21. In epidemiologic studies, low back pain is associated with all of the following factors except:

A. Poor job satisfaction
B. Smoking
C. Occupational setting
D. Psychological distress
E. Poor overall health

22. Which statement is false regarding COX-1 and COX-2 enzymes?

A. COX-2 inhibits prostaglandin synthesis.
B. COX-1 has a primary role in modulating physiologic processes.
C. The substrate for COX-1 and COX-2 is arachidonic acid.
D. COX-1 and COX-2 are expressed in the dorsal root ganglion (DRG) neurons and in the spinal cord.
E. COX-2 can be induced in the peripheral and central nervous system.

23. Which of the following statements are true regarding the immune system and pain?

A. Interleukin (IL)-1 receptor antagonism increases hyperalgesia.
B. Peripheral nerve damage leads to peripheral and central immune responses.
C. Microglial activation increases central sensitization and allodynia.
D. A and B
E. B and C

24. A 24-year-old long-distance runner complains of chronic right lateral hip and knee pain that worsens during runs and is associated with a "snapping sound." Which of the following statements best relates to the patient's medical condition?

A. This syndrome is often associated with abnormal reflexes.
B. The patient usually has significant symptoms at rest and with performing activities of daily living.
C. This syndrome is the most common cause of lateral knee pain in runners.
D. Another name for this condition is internal snapping hip syndrome.
E. The snapping sound results from the iliopsoas tendon rubbing over the iliopectineal eminence or the femoral head.

25. When considering supraspinal processing of nociceptive input from muscle, all of the following statements are true except:

A. Chronic deep somatic pain can lead to cortical sensitization.
B. The lateral spinothalamic tract and spinomesencephalic tract transmit nociceptive input.
C. Over time, patients with chronic muscular pain have been shown to lose both white and gray matter.
D. The periaqueductal gray receives nociceptive input.
E. The parabrachial nucleus receives nociceptive input from the spinoparabrachial tract.

26. Which neural structures are thought to be involved in receiving nociceptive input from muscle tissue?

A. The thalamus
B. The periaqueductal gray
C. The parabrachial nucleus
D. Insular cortex
E. All of the above

27. For fibromyalgia syndrome (FMS), all of the following are true except:

A. The 2010 diagnostic criteria are based on symptom severity index and widespread pain index scores.

B. The 2010 diagnostic criteria require a tender point exam.
C. Fibromyalgia patients have increased substance P in their cerebrospinal fluid (CSF).
D. Temporomandibular joint syndrome is a common comorbidity.
E. Dysfunction of the descending inhibitory pain pathways is a likely etiology for pain in FMS.

28. You are evaluating a new patient with chronic low back pain, and the patient would like to know the cause of the pain. Which statement best describes a response that fits into the biopsychosocial model for pain?

A. Chronic pain is a result of organic dysfunction or injury.
B. Spinal imaging identifies the cause of chronic low back pain in most cases.
C. Chronic pain is a subjective result of the dynamic interaction between sensory input and the body's modulation of the input based on genetics, learned behaviors, expectations, health state, mood, culture, and social environment.
D. If the history, physical examination, and diagnostic evaluations fail to identify a source of pain, then the etiology is most likely due to a psychological condition.
E. Pain treatment focuses on the use of medications or procedural interventions to block the dysfunctional pain pathways.

29. Primary sacroiliac joint pain/dysfunction is commonly characterized by all of the following clinical and objective findings except:

A. Positive antalgic gait
B. Elevated alkaline phosphatase
C. Positive Fortin finger sign
D. Positive diagnostic sacroiliac joint injection
E. Positive FABER test

30. Important features of polymyalgia rheumatica include all of the following except:

A. Elevated erythrocyte sedimentation rate (ESR)
B. Chronic myalgias with significant muscle weakness
C. Bilateral stiffness
D. Symptoms affect primarily shoulder and pelvic girdles
E. Generalized fatigue

31. Rehabilitation for chronic discogenic lumbar pain should include all of the following except:

A. General conditioning
B. Ergonomic workplace modifications
C. Assessment of functional goals
D. Passive treatment modalities
E. Lumbar stabilization plan

ANSWERS

1. ANSWER: A

The supraspinatus muscle is most commonly involved due to impingement and subsequent inflammation caused by the acromion, coracoacromial ligament, acromioclavicular joint, and/or coracoid process. Impingement syndrome is defined as anterior shoulder pain with forward arm flexion as a result of acromial compression on the supraspinatus tendon. A subacromial local anesthetic injection may help differentiate a rotator cuff tear from tendinitis because the patient's pain and performance with muscle strength testing will likely improve with the latter condition. The teres major muscle is not part of the rotator cuff.

FURTHER READING

Bowen J, Malanga G. Rotator cuff tendinitis. In: Frontera W, Silver J, Rizzo T (Eds.), *Essentials of Physical Medicine and Rehabilitation*. 2nd ed. Philadelphia, PA: Saunders; 2008:71–76.

2. ANSWER: D

Myofascial pain syndrome may be a primary disorder causing local, regional, or general musculoskeletal pain and dysfunction, or it may be a secondary disorder resulting from another condition, such as lumbar facet syndrome. Typically, both motor (trigger points and taut bands) and sensory (decreased pain threshold and referred pain) abnormalities exist. Associated autonomic phenomenon may include piloerection, sweating, and skin blood flow changes resulting in regional skin temperature changes. Trophic changes of the skin and nails are not associated with this syndrome.

FURTHER READING

Childers M, Feldman J, Guo H. Myofascial pain syndrome. In: Frontera W, Silver J, Rizzo T (Eds.), *Essentials of Physical Medicine and Rehabilitation*. 2nd ed. Philadelphia, PA: Saunders; 2008:529–538.

3. ANSWER: E

A functional restoration approach to rehabilitation that focuses on cognitive–behavioral therapies combined with physical therapy modalities and techniques as well as patient adoption of a low-impact active exercise program is the treatment of choice for those with significant pain and disability due to myofascial pain syndrome. This involves efforts of an interdisciplinary team consisting of a physician, psychologist, and/or psychiatrist and physical therapist. This is an example of the biopsychosocial approach to treatment as opposed to the biomedical approach.

FURTHER READING

Childers M, Feldman J, Guo H. Myofascial pain syndrome. In: Frontera W, Silver J, Rizzo T (Eds.), *Essentials of Physical Medicine and Rehabilitation*. 2nd ed. Philadelphia, PA: Saunders; 2008:529–538.

4. ANSWER: D

Repetitive strain injuries account for approximately 65% of reported cases of occupational illness annually. These injuries are defined as nonspecific upper extremity pain that commonly results from repetitive motion of the arm or wrist, movements that require extremes of hand or arm position, prolonged static postures, and vibration. These injuries are often multifactorial. Other contributing factors include a poor ergonomic work environment, task invariability, lack of autonomy, and high psychological stress at work. The service and manufacturing industries have a high demand for upper extremity-intensive tasks and often involve computer processing and keyboard use, thus making them at greatest risk. The health care industry has a higher incidence of back-related injuries.

FURTHER READING

McInnis K. Repetitive strain injuries. In: Frontera W, Silver J, Rizzo T (Eds.), *Essentials of Physical Medicine and Rehabilitation*. 2nd ed. Philadelphia, PA: Saunders; 2008:539–544.

5. ANSWER: B

The Social Security Administration's Office of Disability does not consider employment history when determining disability status. Applicants for disability must meet all six of the following criteria: 6 months of intractable pain; limited activities of daily living secondary to pain; excessive use of medication and medical services; behavioral changes including depression and anxiety; lack of clear relationship of pain to an organic disorder; and history of multiple diagnostic tests, unsuccessful treatments, and surgeries.

FURTHER READING

Mostoufi S. Chronic pain syndrome. In: Frontera W, Silver J, Rizzo T (Eds.), *Essentials of Physical Medicine and Rehabilitation*. 2nd ed. Philadelphia, PA: Saunders; 2008:505–510.

6. ANSWER: E

Early rheumatoid arthritis (RA) is characterized by the clinical presentation presented in this question. Advanced RA is characterized by joint laxity and a multitude of deformities caused by chronic synovitis and subsequent destruction of capsuloligamentous and tendinous structures. NSAIDs may be helpful in reducing inflammation and pain, but they do not impede synovial proliferation and eventual bone and joint destruction. Low-dose corticosteroids and methotrexate, as well as targeted biologics such as TNF antagonists (e.g., etanercept, infliximab, and adalimumab), all reduce synovial proliferation and can slow disease progression. Other biologics used to treat RA include an inhibitor of T cell costimulation (abtacept) and a monoclonal anti-B cell antibody (rituximab).

FURTHER READING

Ring D, Kay J. Hand rheumatoid arthritis. In: Frontera W, Silver J, Rizzo T (Eds.), *Essentials of Physical Medicine and Rehabilitation*. 2nd ed. Philadelphia, PA: Saunders; 2008:161–166.

7. ANSWER: C

There is no evidence that COX-2 inhibitors are more effective than nonselective COX inhibitors in providing analgesia for knee osteoarthritis, although the side effect profile may be more tolerable in the former. Patient selection and education is key because chronic NSAID use may lead to serious cardiovascular, gastrointestinal, hematologic, and renal complications. Maintaining activity with static and dynamic quadriceps strengthening combined with aerobic exercise reduces pain and improves proprioception and functional outcomes in knee osteoarthritis. Water aerobics, exercise bicycles, and other low-impact activities should be utilized.

FURTHER READING

Wilkins A, Phillips E. Knee osteoarthritis. In: Frontera W, Silver J, Rizzo T (Eds.), *Essentials of Physical Medicine and Rehabilitation*. 2nd ed. Philadelphia, PA: Saunders; 2008:345–354.

8. ANSWER: E

All of the physiologic changes in nociceptive processing listed in answers A, B, and C can contribute to chronic neuropathic pain states such as allodynia, hyperalgesia, and even opioid-induced hyperalgesia. With chronic pain, the affective pain pathway can be altered such that cortical and limbic structures (prefrontal cortex, anterior cingulate cortex, and amygdala) that project to the periaqueductal gray and subsequently to the rostral ventral medulla undergo plastic changes resulting in the overall facilitation of pain processing via the mechanisms mentioned in the answer choices. Chronic opioid exposure can similarly alter the "on" and "off" cell balance, thus facilitating nociception. It is believed that "on" cell activation plays a more predominant role in the establishment of chronic pain states.

FURTHER READING

Raja S, Dougherty P. Anatomy and physiology of somatosensory and pain processing. In: Benzon H, Raja S, Fishman S, et al. (Eds.), *Essentials of Pain Medicine*. 3rd ed. Philadelphia, PA: Saunders; 2011:1–7.

9. ANSWER: B

The conduction velocity of peripheral nerve fibers depends primarily on their degree of myelination. Aβ fibers are heavily myelinated and the largest fibers; thus, they are the fastest (up to 120 m/s conduction velocity). These fibers do not transmit nociceptive inputs but, rather, relay light touch, pressure, proprioception, and hair movement. Aδ fibers are smaller and have less myelination and thus have slower conduction velocities (5–20 m/s). Accordingly, they transmit the "first pain" sensations such as a sharp, pricking painful stimulus in this case. C fibers have no myelin and are the smallest in size. They conduct most slowly (<2 m/s) and convey the burning "second pain" sensation.

FURTHER READING

Raja S, Dougherty P. Anatomy and physiology of somatosensory and pain processing. In: Benzon H, Raja S, Fishman S, et al. (Eds.), *Essentials of Pain Medicine*. 3rd ed. Philadelphia, PA: Saunders; 2011:1–7.

10. ANSWER: D

Glycine is present within the central nervous system and is the main inhibitory amino acid at the spinal level. It acts at two different receptors: a chloride-linked strychnine-sensitive receptor and a strychnine-insensitive site on the NMDA glutamate receptor. All of the following "inflammatory soup" mediators play a role peripherally in nociception: bradykinin, hydrogen ions (low pH), serotonin, histamine, eicosanoids (prostaglandins, thromboxanes, and leukotrienes), nitric oxide, adenosine, ATP, cytokines (IL-1β, IL-6, and TNF-α), nerve growth factor, matrix metalloproteinases, and other proteinases (thrombin, trypsin, and tryptase).

FURTHER READING

Dougherty P, Raja S, Boyette-Davis J. Neurochemistry of somatosensory and pain processing. In: Benzon H, Raja S, Fishman S, et al. (Eds.), *Essentials of Pain Medicine*. 3rd ed. Philadelphia, PA: Saunders; 2011:8–15.

11. ANSWER: D

The Apley "Scratch" test is the quickest active way to evaluate a patient's range of motion. First, to test abduction and external rotation, ask the patient to reach behind his head and touch the superior medial angle of the opposite scapula. Next, to determine the range of internal rotation and adduction, instruct the patient to reach in front of his head and touch the opposite acromion. Third, to further test internal rotation and adduction, have the patient reach behind his back to touch the inferior angle of the opposite scapula. Observe the patient's movement during all phases of testing for any limitation of motion or for any break of normal rhythm or symmetry.

FURTHER READING

Hoppenfeld S. Physical Examination of the Spine and Extremities. 1st ed. Norwalk, CT: Appleton-Century-Crofts: 1976:21.

12. ANSWER: D

The patient reports symptoms suggestive of patellofemoral pain syndrome. The J sign is the lateral tracking of the patella as the knee moves from flexion to terminal extension, which will confirm the diagnosis. The O'Brien test is used for labral lesions of the shoulder. The Lachman test is used to test for injury to the anterior cruciate ligament. Femoral anteversion is seen in children when the femur has a distal internal rotation. The McMurray test helps identify meniscal injuries.

FURTHER READING

Braddom R (Ed.). *Physical Medicine and Rehabilitation*. 4th ed. Philadelphia, PA: Saunders; 2010:817, 855–858.

13. ANSWER: A

The patient most likely is suffering from avascular necrosis of the hip. In the adult population, the most common risk factors are steroid use and alcohol consumption. The goal of treatment is to keep the femoral head within the acetabulum. The first step will be a course of physical therapy. Traction is not indicated. Intra-articular steroid injections increase the risk of worsening of the avascular necrosis. Osteotomy may help improve pain and function of symptomatic patients. Total hip arthroplasty is typically not a first-line treatment option.

FURTHER READING

Cuccurullo S (Ed.). *Physical Medicine and Rehabilitation Board Review*. 2nd ed. New York, NY: Demos; 2010:222–223.

14. ANSWER: D

All are correct with the exception of synovial atrophy. The steps described in the answer choices lead to synovial hypertrophy and cartilage destruction, which subsequently lead to pannus formation. Pannus is a membrane of granulation tissue that covers the articular cartilage. Joint integrity is gradually destroyed as the pannus invades the periarticular bone and cartilage at the joint margins. Joint ankylosis may occur at the end stage of joint destruction.

FURTHER READING

Braddom R (Ed.). *Physical Medicine and Rehabilitation*. 4th ed. Philadelphia, PA: Saunders; 2010:771–773.
Cuccurullo S (Ed.). *Physical Medicine and Rehabilitation Board Review*. 2nd ed. New York, NY: Demos; 2010:95–97.

15. ANSWER: C

Rheumatoid arthritis is almost always symmetric. Other criteria include the following: morning stiffness in the joints that must last at least 1 hour before maximal improvement (hand stiffness usually improves in 1 or 2 hours for rheumatoid arthritis and in less than 30 minutes for osteoarthritis), arthritis in three or more joints simultaneously with soft tissue swelling or fluid, consistently symmetric arthritis and subcutaneous nodules in extensor surfaces, radiologic changes showing erosions, bony decalcification and joint space narrowing in the hand and wrist, and a positive rheumatoid factor.

FURTHER READING

Braddom R (Ed.). *Physical Medicine and Rehabilitation*. 4th ed. Philadelphia, PA: Saunders; 2010:775.

16. ANSWER: D

Morbid obesity has the highest correlation with disability due to knee osteoarthritis. The correlation is less with increased age and sports-related injury. There is no correlation with running or sedentary work.

FURTHER READING

Cuccurullo S (Ed.). *Physical Medicine and Rehabilitation Board Review*. 2nd ed. New York, NY: Demos; 2010:108.

17. ANSWER: B

The patient most likely has a diagnosis of lateral epicondylitis. The mechanism of injury is an overload of the extensor and supinator tendons due to overuse and poor mechanics. This leads to microtears of the extensor carpi radialis brevis. Plain radiographs are not indicated unless there is suspicion of arthritis or a loose body. Repetitive valgus stress of the elbow may lead to medial epicondylitis, which in turn may lead to osteochondritis dissecans of the capitellum. Ulnar neuropathy may occur with medial epicondylitis due to valgus stretch of the nerve.

FURTHER READING

Braddom R (Ed.). *Physical Medicine and Rehabilitation*. 4th ed. Philadelphia, PA: Saunders; 2010:151, 323, 826–827.

18. ANSWER: C

This patient has symptoms suggestive of De Quervain tenosynovitis or radial styloid tenosynovitis. The described physical exam test is the Finkelstein test. Treatment is conservative and includes NSAIDs and immobilization with a thumb spica splint. A neutral wrist splint will not provide sufficient immobilization. If there is no improvement with more conservative measures, a corticosteroid injection may be considered. Surgical intervention may be considered in extreme cases that failed conservative management.

FURTHER READING

Braddom R (Ed.). *Physical Medicine and Rehabilitation*. 4th ed. Philadelphia, PA: Saunders; 2010:195–196, 832.
Cuccurullo S (Ed.). *Physical Medicine and Rehabilitation Board Review*. 2nd ed. New York, NY: Demos; 2010:100, 195–196.

19. ANSWER: D

The patient is likely suffering from ankylosing spondylitis. As this disease progresses, there is a decrease in chest expansion leading to restrictive pulmonary disease. Iritis is the most common extraskeletal manifestation of ankylosing spondylitis. The radiological findings listed in the answer choices are consistent with this condition. The Schober test is useful for detecting limitations in lumbar flexion and extension range of motion.

FURTHER READING

Braddom R (Ed.). *Physical Medicine and Rehabilitation*. 4th ed. Philadelphia, PA: Saunders; 2010:900–901.
Cuccurullo S (Ed.). *Physical Medicine and Rehabilitation Board Review*. 2nd ed. New York, NY: Demos; 2010:117–119.

20. ANSWER: A

Sickle cell crisis results in pain in the large joints from juxta-articular joint infarcts with synovial ischemia. Osteonecrosis is due to local hypoxia with occlusion of the vascular system. The most common joints affected are the femoral head and the humeral head. Dactylitis is a painful, nonpitting swelling of the hands and feet that is often the first symptom of sickle cell disease in children. Osteomyelitis is a complication of sickle cell disease. Pain in the abdomen, chest, and back is also common.

FURTHER READING

Cuccurullo S (Ed.). *Physical Medicine and Rehabilitation Board Review*. 2nd ed. New York, NY: Demos; 2010:134.

21. ANSWER: C

A 2010 analysis of 24 workplace studies strongly concluded that occupational setting is not associated with low back pain. However, research has shown that dissatisfied workers are twice as likely to develop low back pain. Predictors for chronic low back pain include psychological distress, poor general health, low levels of physical activity, smoking, dissatisfaction with employment, and clinical factors.

FURTHER READING

Mcfarlane G, McBeth J, Jones G. Epidemiology of pain. In: McMahon S, Koltzenburg M, Tracey I, et al. (Eds.), *Wall and Melzack's Textbook of Pain*. 6th ed. Philadelphia, PA: Saunders; 2013:232–247.

22. ANSWER: A

COX-1 and COX-2 enzymes are both responsible for catalyzing the initial steps in prostaglandin synthesis. Both COX-1 and COX-2 are expressed constitutively in DRG neurons and in the spinal cord. In general, COX-1 is considered to have a housekeeping (constitutive) role in most parts of the body. COX-1 induces prostanoids that modulate physiologic processes in the stomach, lung, kidneys, and platelet aggregation. COX-2 expression is usually minimal unless there is inflammation. COX-2 is induced by inflammatory cytokines, growth factors, and neurotransmitters in both the peripheral nervous system and the central nervous system.

FURTHER READING

Birmingham B, Buvanendran A. Nonsteroidal anti-inflammatory drugs, acetaminophen and COX-2 inhibitors. In: Benzon H, Rathmell J, Wu C, et al. (Eds.), *Practical Management of Pain*. 5th ed. Philadelphia, PA: Mosby; 2014:553–568.

23. ANSWER: E

Antagonism of IL-1 receptor decreases hyperalgesia. Peripheral nerve damage triggers lymphocytes, macrophages, and granulocytes in the peripheral immune system. Peripheral nerve injury also triggers the central immune response via microglial activation. Allodynia and central sensitization are the result of microglial activation. Microglia activation results in the release of brain-derived neurotrophic factor, increasing allodynia and central sensitization.

FURTHER READING

Apkarian A. Pain and brain changes. In: Benzon H, Rathmell J, Wu C, et al. (Eds.), *Practical Management of Pain*. 5th ed. Philadelphia, PA: Mosby; 2014:113–131.

24. ANSWER: C

Iliotibial band syndrome (ITBS) usually affects athletes from sports that involve much running. It does not typically affect activities of daily living. ITBS is the most common cause of lateral knee pain in runners. The iliotibial band is a strong fascial band that runs along the lateral aspect of the thigh from the level of the greater trochanter to the proximal anterolateral tibia. Neurologic examination is typically normal. An audible snap can sometimes be heard due to the ITB rubbing over the greater trochanter. ITBS is sometimes referred to as lateral snapping hip syndrome. By contrast, internal snapping hip syndrome occurs when the iliopsoas tendon rubs over the iliopectineal eminence or the femoral head, causing the snapping sound.

FURTHER READING

Hansen P, Willick S. Musculoskeletal disorders of the lower extremity. In: Braddom R (Ed.), *Physical Medicine and Rehabilitation*. 4th ed. Philadelphia, PA: Saunders; 2010:843–870.

25. ANSWER: C

In patients with chronic deep somatic pain, such as low back pain and fibromyalgia, the cortical representation of the painful body part can expand. This represents cortical sensitization. In addition to the lateral spinothalamic tract, the spinomesencephalic tract transmits nociceptive information to the periaqueducal gray in the mesencephalon. The spinoparabrachial tract transmits nociceptive signals to the parabrachial nucleus in the pons. The parabrachial nucleus is an important center for nociception from deep somatic tissue, including muscle. At least one study has shown that patients with chronic pain can lose 5–11% of gray cortical matter. There is no evidence that chronic pain causes white matter degeneration.

FURTHER READING

Mense S. Basic mechanisms of muscle. In: McMahon S, Koltzenburg M, Tracey I, et al. (Eds.), *Wall and Melzack's Textbook of Pain*. 6th ed. Philadelphia, PA: Saunders; 2013:620–628.

26. ANSWER: E

There is evidence that the thalamus receives nociceptive input from muscle in the ventral posterior lateral nucleus and the ventral posterior medial nucleus. The periaqueducal gray receives nociceptive input from muscle via the spinothalamic tract. The parabrachial nucleus is an important center for nociception from deep somatic tissue, including muscle, and receives input via the spinobrachial tract. The insular cortex receives thalamic pain projections and projects to limbic structures, such as the amygdala. It is involved in the emotional–affective component of pain and in the autonomic response to nociception.

FURTHER READING

Mense S. Basic mechanisms of muscle. In: McMahon S, Koltzenburg M, Tracey I, et al. (Eds.), *Wall and Melzack's Textbook of Pain*, 6th ed. Philadelphia, PA: Saunders; 2013:620–628.

27. ANSWER: B

According to the 2010 American College of Rheumatology diagnostic criteria for FMS, a patient must have either a widespread pain index of at least 7 and a symptom severity score of at least 5 or a widespread pain index of at least 3 and a symptom severity score of at least 9. The new criteria do not include a tender point exam as described in the 1990 criteria. Common symptoms reported by FMS patients include fatigue, stiffness, anxiety, depression, and temporomandibular joint pain. FMS patients have been found to have higher levels of substance P in their CSF. In addition, altered serotonin (5-HT) levels likely have a pathologic role. These neurochemical derangements lead to dysfunction of the descending antinociceptive pathways, which is the most likely mechanism for the pain of FMS.

FURTHER READING

Childers M, Feldman J, Guo H. Myofascial pain syndrome. In: Frontera W, Silver J, Rizzo T, et al. (Eds.), *Essentials of Physical Medicine and Rehabilitation*. 3rd ed. Philadelphia, PA: Saunders; 2015:520–526.

Hong C. Muscle pain syndromes. In: Braddom R (Ed.), *Physical Medicine and Rehabilitation*. 4th ed. Philadelphia, PA: Saunders; 2010:971–1001.

28. ANSWER: C

The traditional biomedical model of pain is based on the assumption that pain results from a specific disease state represented by dysfunctional anatomy and physiology. Objective tests are sought to confirm the pathology and physical impairment. Medical interventions are subsequently performed to target the organic dysfunction or source of pathology. In up to 86% of cases of chronic low back pain, the etiology is undetermined despite extensive imaging of the spine. Moreover, up to 35% of asymptomatic patients have significant radiologic spinal pathologic findings. A substantial number of patients with chronic pain do not exhibit significant psychopathology. In contrast to the biomedical approach, the integrative biopsychosocial perspective views pain as a subjective perception that results from the transduction, transmission, and modulation of sensory input filtered through a person's genetic composition and previous learning history that is modulated further by the person's current physiologic state, idiosyncratic appraisals, expectations, present mood state, and sociocultural environment.

FURTHER READING

Turk D. Psychosocial aspects of chronic pain. In: Benzon H, Rathmell J, Wu C, et al. (Eds.), *Practical Management of Pain*. 5th ed. Philadelphia, PA: Mosby; 2014:139–148.

29. ANSWER: B

Patients with sacroiliac joint pain often present with an antalgic gait. With the advent of fluoroscopy, diagnostic infiltration of the sacroiliac joint with local anesthetic may be a more reliable indicator of the pain generator than traditional physical exam tests such as the Patrick/FABER test and Fortin finger sign. In the Fortin finger sign, the patient points to the area of pain with one finger. The result is positive if the site is within 1 cm of the posterior superior iliac spine, generally inferomedial to it. In the Patrick/FABER test, the patient lies supine. The ipsilateral heel is placed on the contralateral thigh proximal to the knee, and the ipsilateral knee is then guided toward the examining table while counterpressure is applied to the contralateral anterior superior iliac spine. The result is positive if pain is elicited along the ipsilateral sacroiliac joint.

FURTHER READING

Simon S. Sacroiliac joint pain and related disorders. In: Waldman S (Ed.), *Pain Management*. 2nd ed. Philadelphia, PA: Saunders; 2011:757–762.

30. ANSWER: B

Polymyalgia rheumatica is characterized by four main features: (1) bilateral, symmetric musculoskeletal symptoms affecting the shoulder and pelvic girdles; (2) stiffness that is particularly worse after rest; (3) unaffected muscle strength; and (4) systemic symptoms such as fatigue, weight loss, elevated ESR, and low-grade fever.

FURTHER READING

Hazelman B. Polymyalgia rheumatica. In: Waldman S (Ed.), *Pain Management*. 2nd ed. Philadelphia, PA: Saunders; 2011:413–415.

31. ANSWER: D

Rehabilitation programs for chronic low back pain from disc degeneration should include a detailed assessment of functional limitations and specific treatment goals. A general conditioning program, workplace modifications, footwear modifications, and a lumbar stabilization plan focused on postural stability are important. Active modalities are preferred over passive modalities such as ultrasound, except in acute pain cases.

FURTHER READING

Schaufele M, Tate J. Lumbar degenerative disease. In: Frontera W, Silver J, Rizzo T (Eds.), *Essentials of Physical Medicine and Rehabilitation*. 3rd ed. Philadelphia, PA: Saunders; 2015:225–232.

13.

PHYSICAL MEDICINE AND REHABILITATION AND ELECTRODIAGNOSIS

Aaron Jay Yang

INTRODUCTION

This chapter focuses on the principles of physical modalities, exercise therapy, mobilization, massage, traction, spinal orthoses, and electrodiagnosis. The questions focus on the most relevant and timely topics that may be tested within this section, and most answers are highlighted by important key facts that are associated with the tested questions. This chapter is by no means a comprehensive review of the field of physical medicine and rehabilitation. Rather, it is a guide to some of the main principles that may fall under this field in regard to the examination. For a more comprehensive overview on a certain topic, the reader should consult the Further Reading sections that follow each answer.

QUESTIONS

1. A 78-year-old male is currently experiencing chronic low back pain and has been using therapeutic heat in the form of heating pads. What type of heat transfer is this considered?

A. Radiation
B. Convection
C. Conduction
D. Conversion
E. Evaporation

2. Which of the following is not a contraindication for use of therapeutic ultrasound in physical therapy?

A. Prior laminectomy site
B. Prosthetic cement around the hip
C. Open epiphysis in adolescent
D. Contracture
E. Pacemaker

3. Which modality utilizes an electrical field to move charged particles across a biologic membrane?

A. Iontophoresis
B. Shortwave diathermy
C. Phonophoresis
D. Fluidotherapy
E. Low-energy laser

4. Transcutaneous electrical nerve stimulation (TENS) is based on the theory of stimulating which nerve fibers in order to close the "gate" on pain transmission?

A. Myelinated Aμ fibers
B. Myelinated Aβ fibers
C. Myelinated Aδ fibers
D. Unmyelinated C fibers

5. Which of the following is not a contraindication to TENS therapy?

A. Pregnancy
B. Cancer
C. Rheumatoid arthritis
D. Pacemaker
E. Vascular disease

6. A 46-year-old female presents for evaluation and management of a right C6 cervical radiculopathy. In considering cervical traction, which of the following may be the most optimal angle for traction?

A. 5–10° of flexion
B. 10–15° of extension
C. 20–30° of flexion
D. 0–5° of extension
E. 40–50° of flexion

7. In regard to counseling a patient who is considering cervical or lumbar traction, which of the following is not a contraindication to traction?

A. Osteoporosis
B. Pregnancy
C. Active peptic ulcer disease
D. Lumbar fusion
E. Lumbar radiculopathy

8. When considering potential massage therapy for a patient, which of the following does not describe a massage technique?

A. Articulatory treatment
B. Effleurage
C. Pétrissage
D. Tapotement
E. Friction massage

9. Which of the following is not a contraindication for high-velocity manipulation?

A. Paget's disease
B. Myofascial pain syndrome
C. Acute cervical radiculopathy
D. Osteomyelitis
E. Benign bone tumor

10. Which massage technique utilizes rhythmic, alternating contact of varying pressure between the hands of the therapist and the soft tissue of the patient?

A. Friction massage
B. Pétrissage
C. Tapotement
D. Rolfing structural integration
E. Feldenkrais pattern

11. An 85-year-old male is involved in a car accident and is admitted due to an unstable cervical fracture. Considering a cervical orthosis, which of the following is most restrictive in terms of range of motion?

A. Philadelphia collar
B. Sternal–occipital mandibular immobilizer (SOMI) brace
C. Halo device
D. Four-poster brace
E. Soft collar

12. A 70-year-old female with a history of osteoporosis presents with an acute lower thoracic compression fracture. Which of the following braces would you recommend?

A. Jewett brace
B. Thoracolumbosacral orthosis (TLSO)
C. Milwaukee brace
D. Taylor brace
E. Miami J

13. A 32-year-old male develops numbness after improper use of crutches following a right knee injury. Which nerve is most likely to be affected?

A. Radial nerve
B. Posterior interosseous nerve
C. Axillary nerve
D. Musculocutaneous nerve
E. Suprascapular nerve

14. A 82-year-old male patient who recently started to use a single-point cane asks you how he would know if his cane is at the correct height. Which of the following would be a correct response?

A. The elbow should be extended in standing position.
B. The elbow should be flexed at 45° with the cane at the level of the iliac crest.
C. The elbow should be flexed to 30° with the cane at the level of the umbilicus.
D. The elbow should be flexed to 20° with the cane at the level of the greater trochanter.
E. The elbow should be extended with the cane at the level of the iliac crest.

15. A 60-year-old male presents with osteoarthritis involving the medial compartment of the knee. Which type of shoe modification would be the most appropriate recommendation?

A. Lateral wedge
B. Rocker bottom sole
C. Medial wedge
D. Solid ankle cushioned heel
E. Metatarsal pads

16. A 38-year-old female presents to your clinic with lateral epicondylosis (tennis elbow). Which type of exercises would be most appropriate for this patient?

A. Closed kinetic chain exercises
B. Open kinetic chain exercises
C. Eccentric-based exercises
D. Concentric-based exercises
E. Flexibility based exercises

17. An 82-year-old female with rheumatoid arthritis was admitted as an inpatient for pneumonia and subsequently is being evaluated by therapy for

deconditioning. Which type of therapy would be most recommended for this patient at this time?

A. Isometric-based exercises
B. Isotonic-based exercises
C. Isokinetic-based exercises
D. Open kinetic chain exercises

18. A 30-year-old female presents to your clinic with radicular leg pain on the left that is worse with lumbar flexion-based activities. Which type of therapy may be the most recommended at this time?

A. Mechanical diagnosis and treatment therapy
B. Proprioceptive neuromuscular facilitation
C. Myofascial release therapy
D. Iontophoresis therapy
E. Feldenkrais therapy

19. A 60-year-old male suffered a traumatic brain injury due to a motor vehicle accident. He subsequently could not return to work as a construction manager due to his cognitive status. His loss of job is an example of which of the following?

A. Disease
B. Disability
C. Impairment
D. Handicap

20. You are observing a 45-year-old female during her gait and notice a pelvic drop and a lateral trunk lean over the contralateral side. Therapy should focus on strengthening which of the following muscles?

A. Quadratus lumborum
B. Gluteus maximus
C. Rectus abdominis
D. Gluteus medius
E. Quadriceps

21. Which of the following tests has been found to be most sensitive in diagnosing lower lumbar radicular nerve pain due to a disc herniation?

A. Seated slump test
B. Straight leg raise
C. Patrick's test
D. Femoral stretch test
E. Thompson test

22. A 25-year-old male was involved in a motor vehicle accident and sustained a crush injury to the right wrist. Subsequent electrodiagnostic studies demonstrated axonal injury to the median nerve. What is the growth of axons at the wrist following this crush injury?

A. 1 mm/day
B. 10 mm/day
C. 2 cm/day
D. 1 cm/day
E. 1 in./day

23. Electrodiagnostic testing evaluates which of the following nerve fibers?

A. Unmyelinated C fibers
B. Myelinated Aδ fibers
C. Myelinated Aβ fibers
D. Myelinated Aα fibers

24. When performing a electrodiagnostic evaluation on a patient with cool limbs, it is important to acknowledge that decreasing temperature can have what effect on nerve conduction waveform characteristics?

A. Decrease in amplitude
B. Decrease in duration
C. Prolong the latency
D. Increase the conduction velocity

25. A 47-year-old male presents to your clinic with acute low back pain and what clinically presents like a right L4 radiculopathy with foot drop. Approximately how long will it take to observe reinnervation potentials on electromyography?

A. 5–7 days
B. 2 weeks
C. 6 months
D. 5 weeks
E. 3 months

26. An 85-year-old female presents to your clinic with a left L5 radiculopathy. Which of the following proximal muscles would be an appropriate L5 innervated muscle to test with needle electromyography?

A. Gluteus medius
B. Iliopsosas
C. Gluteus maximus
D. Adductor longus

27. A 27-year-old volleyball player presents with right-sided shoulder pain with weakness with shoulder external rotation only. Which of the following would most likely explain her symptoms?

A. Axillary neuropathy at the humeral head
B. Suprascapular neuropathy at the spinoglenoid notch

C. Suprascapular neuropathy at the suprascapular notch
D. Radial neuropathy along the spiral groove

28. An unmyelinated C fiber has a membrane action potential conduction velocity of approximately how many meters/second?

A. 100 m/s
B. 50 m/s
C. 25 m/s
D. 10 m/s
E. 1 m/s

29. A 72-year-old male underwent a left total hip replacement. Which of the following is the most commonly injured nerve following surgery?

A. Femoral nerve
B. Sciatic nerve
C. Tibial nerve
D. Superior gluteal nerve
E. Obturator nerve

30. Median mononeuropathy at the wrist (carpal tunnel syndrome) would not affect which of the following muscles?

A. Abductor pollicis brevis
B. Flexor pollicis brevis
C. First and second lumbricals
D. Flexor digitorum superficialis
E. Opponens pollicis

31. What nerve roots supply innervation to the lateral femoral cutaneous nerve?

A. L1–L2
B. L3–L4
C. L4–L5
D. L2–L3

32. A 34-year-old male was involved in a motor vehicle accident and subsequently presents to your clinic a few weeks later with shoulder abduction weakness and forearm extended and pronated with wrist in flexed position. Which of the following nerve root or

peripheral nerve damage would most likely explain his presentation?

A. Radial neuropathy
B. C8–T1 plexopathy
C. Axillary neuropathy
D. C5–C6 plexopathy
E. Median neuropathy

33. Which of the following statements about laser-evoked potentials is false?

A. Aδ and C fibers are primarily activated.
B. CO_2 laser is used to generate potentials.
C. This study can be used to evaluate visceral pain.
D. Superficial burns are one of the risks involved with this test.
E. Laser evoked potentials can be used to assess syringomyelia.

34. Which of the following is not considered an advantage of quantitative sensory testing (QST) over conventional nerve conduction studies?

A. Ability to assess small fiber nerve function
B. Allows the ability to gather objective data
C. Can assess central pathway function
D. Can detect both negative and positive sensory symptoms

35. Which of the following muscles has the highest innervation ratio (muscle fiber:axon)?

A. Gastrocnemius
B. Abductor pollicis brevis
C. Brachioradialis
D. Triceps
E. Extensor hallucis longus

36. Which of the following regarding the sympathetic skin response is false?

A. Response can be obtained by an audible noise.
B. Response can be easily obtained over the forearm or axilla.
C. Response can be highly variable.
D. Response is affected by temperature.
E. Response is a low-frequency potential.

ANSWERS

1. ANSWER: C

Heat application can be divided into superficial and deep heat and is dependent on the depth of heat and form of transfer of heat. Heat transfer can occur through conversion, convection, conduction, and radiation. *Conduction* is the most commonly encountered type of heat transfer and involves the transfer of thermal energy between two bodies in direct contact. Examples include heating pads, hot packs, and paraffin baths. *Convection* uses movement of a medium to transfer thermal energy, and examples of this are contrast baths and hydrotherapy. *Conversion* refers to the transformation of energy to heat, such as ultrasound and microwave diathermy. *Radiation* involves thermal radiation emitted from any surface or body with a temperature above absolute zero.

KEY FACTS: PRECAUTIONS FOR USE OF THERAPEUTIC HEAT

- Acute inflammation
- Bleeding disorder or hemorrhage
- Malignancy
- Impaired sensation
- Vascular disease
- Scars or atrophic skin
- Inability to respond to pain

FURTHER READING

Stanos SP, Rivers E, Prather H, et al. Physical medicine and rehabilitation approaches to pain management. In: Benzon H, Raja H, Fishman S, et al. (Eds.), *Essentials of Pain Medicine*. 3rd ed. Philadelphia, PA: Saunders; 2011.

Webber DC, Hoppe KM. Physical agent modalities. In: Braddom R, et al. (Eds.), *Physical Medicine & Rehabilitation*. 3rd ed. Philadelphia, PA: Saunders; 2007.

2. ANSWER: D

Therapeutic ultrasound is a type of deep heat that transforms energy to heat. Heating is greatest at the bone–tissue interface and uses a higher frequency than diagnostic ultrasound to produce a deeper tissue response. Common indications for therapeutic ultrasound include tendonitis, arthritis, contractures, and subacute trauma. General precautions are listed under Key Facts. Of note, ultrasound therapy is safe near metal implants, but caution must be used near arthroplasties that use prosthetic cements that do not readily dissipate heat.

KEY FACTS: CONTRAINDICATIONS FOR USE OF THERAPEUTIC ULTRASOUND

- Malignancy
- Open epiphysis
- Pacemaker
- Near heart, eyes, reproductive organs, and carotid sinus
- Laminectomy site
- Total hip prosthesis

FURTHER READING

Stanos SP, Rivers E, Prather H, et al. Physical medicine and rehabilitation approaches to pain management. In: Benzon H, Raja H, Fishman S, et al. (Eds.), *Essentials of Pain Medicine*. 3rd ed. Philadelphia, PA: Saunders; 2011.

Webber DC, Hoppe KM. Physical agent modalities. In: Braddom R, et al. (Eds.), *Physical Medicine & Rehabilitation*. 3rd ed. Philadelphia, PA: Saunders; 2007.

3. ANSWER: A

Iontophoresis uses an electric field to move various medications such as corticosteroids or lidocaine across a biologic membrane to directly deliver medications to soft tissues. For example, dexamethasone is commonly placed on the electrode of the same polarity with opposite electrodes placed on the skin. A current is applied to drive the medication away from the electrode into the tissue, thus minimizing systemic side effects. Shortwave diathermy is a rarely used modality that produces deep heating via conversion. Phonophoresis involves the use of ultrasound to transfer topically applied medications into the skin. Fluidotherapy is a dry heating modality that transfers superficial heat by convection. Last, low-energy laser therapy utilizes a lower power to cause nonthermal physiologic effects within tissues.

KEY FACTS: CLINICAL INDICATIONS FOR IONTOPHORESIS

- Plantar fasciitis
- Lateral epicondylitis
- Achilles tendonitis
- Patellar tendonitis
- Subacromial bursitis
- Greater trochanteric bursitis

FURTHER READING

Stanos SP, Rivers E, Prather H, et al. Physical medicine and rehabilitation approaches to pain management. In: Benzon H, Raja H,

Fishman S, et al. (Eds.), *Essentials of Pain Medicine*. 3rd ed. Philadelphia, PA: Saunders; 2011.

Webber DC, Hoppe KM. Physical agent modalities. In: Braddom R, et al. (Eds.), *Physical Medicine & Rehabilitation*. 3rd ed. Philadelphia, PA: Saunders; 2007.

4. ANSWER: B

The TENS unit is a programmable device that uses electrical fields to stimulate nerve fibers in order to affect pain transmission. Based on the gate control theory proposed by Melzack and Wall in 1965, TENS stimulates the large, myelinated Aβ afferent nerve fibers, which in turn inhibit the smaller Aδ and C fibers from transmitting pain to the thalamus. Different types of TENS delivery exist, including conventional, acupuncture-like, burst modes, and hyperstimulation. Conventional is the most commonly used type, which provides a high-frequency, low-intensity stimulation that is better tolerated and provides quicker analgesia.

FURTHER READING

Stanos SP, Rivers E, Prather H, et al. Physical medicine and rehabilitation approaches to pain management. In: Benzon H, Raja H, Fishman S, et al. (Eds.), *Essentials of Pain Medicine*. 3rd ed. Philadelphia, PA: Saunders; 2011.

Webber DC, Hoppe KM. Physical agent modalities. In: Braddom R, et al. (Eds.), *Physical Medicine & Rehabilitation*. 3rd ed. Philadelphia, PA: Saunders; 2007.

5. ANSWER: C

TENS units have been used in a variety of medical conditions. Some indications for the use of TENS therapy include general neuropathic pain, trigeminal neuralgia, rheumatoid arthritis, diabetic neuropathy, and other musculoskeletal pain conditions. Of note, treatment time for TENS therapy ranges from 30 minutes to a maximum of 2 hours per session. Intensity of the TENS therapy should be monitored because patients may develop skin irritation or general discomfort.

KEY FACTS: CLINICAL CONTRAINDICATIONS FOR TENS THERAPY

- Pacemaker
- Pregnancy
- Malignancy
- Active hemorrhage
- Circulatory impairment
- Decreased skin sensation
- Seizure disorder

FURTHER READING

Stanos SP, Rivers E, Prather H, et al. Physical medicine and rehabilitation approaches to pain management. In: Benzon H, Raja H, Fishman S, et al. (Eds.), *Essentials of Pain Medicine*. 3rd ed. Philadelphia, PA: Saunders; 2011.

Webber DC, Hoppe KM. Physical agent modalities. In: Braddom R, et al. (Eds.), *Physical Medicine & Rehabilitation*. 3rd ed. Philadelphia, PA: Saunders; 2007.

6. ANSWER: C

Cervical traction can be provided manually or with a device, and it is often used for treatment of nerve root compression, muscle spasm, and musculoskeletal pain. Elongation of the cervical spine and vertebral joint distraction can occur with traction force of at least 25 pounds. For treatment of cervical radiculopathy, the neck is in a flexion position of approximately 20–30°, which optimally opens up the intervertebral foramen. Of note, traction can be continuous or intermittent, with intermittent traction commonly being used for neural compression where greater pull may be of benefit. This is opposed to continuous traction, which is more beneficial for prolonged muscle stretch and may be beneficial for myofascial pain.

KEY FACTS: PRESCRIPTION PARAMETERS FOR CERVICAL TRACTION

- Positioning: Neck in flexion with the patient supine or seated with optimal angle of pull between 20° and 30°.
- Amount of traction: At least 25 pounds for optimal distraction. Weights greater than 50 pounds have not been shown to confer any additional benefit.
- Intermittent versus continuous: Continuous traction provides prolonged muscle stretch, whereas intermittent traction may provide a greater pull and help with neural foraminal opening.

FURTHER READING

Strax TE, Grabois M, Gonzalez P, et al. Physical modalities. In: Cucurillo S (Ed.), *Physical Medicine and Rehabilitation Board Review*. 2nd ed. New York, NY: Demos; 2010.

Wolf CJ, Brault JS. Manipulation, traction, and massage. In: Braddom R, et al. (Eds.), *Physical Medicine & Rehabilitation*. 3rd ed. Philadelphia, PA: Saunders; 2007.

7. ANSWER: E

Cervical and lumbar traction may be indicated for a variety of medical conditions. Traction may benefit those with cervical or lumbar radicular pain or radiculopathy by reducing nerve root compression and subsequent nerve irritation. In addition, it may also loosen adhesions in the dural sleeves. Traction may also assist in soft tissue and joint mobilization, which would be helpful for myofascial pain conditions in the cervical or lumbar spine. Contraindications for spinal traction are listed under Key Facts.

KEY FACTS: CONTRAINDICATIONS TO CERVICAL AND LUMBAR SPINE TRACTION

- Atlantoaxial subluxation
- Active peptic ulcer disease
- Vertebrobasilar insufficiency
- Aortic aneurysm
- Pregnancy
- Restrictive lung disease
- Cauda equina syndrome
- Osteomyelitis or diskitis
- Osteoporosis
- Malignancy with spine involvement
- Ligamentous instability: Marfan syndrome, rheumatoid arthritis, Ehlers–Danlos syndrome

FURTHER READING

Strax TE, Grabois M, Gonzalez P, et al. Physical modalities. In: Cucurillo S (Ed.), *Physical Medicine and Rehabilitation Board Review*. 2nd ed. New York, NY: Demos; 2010.
Wolf CJ, Brault JS. Manipulation, traction, and massage. In: Braddom R, et al. (Eds.), *Physical Medicine & Rehabilitation*. 3rd ed. Philadelphia, PA: Saunders; 2007.

8. ANSWER: A

Massage can be described as a group of procedures that manipulate the soft tissues of the body that can have multiple therapeutic benefits. Performed most commonly with the hands, massage can have reflexive effects that may include improved circulation due to vasodilation of blood vessels, mechanical effects through increased venous blood return from the periphery, decreasing muscle tightness and increasing lymphatic drainage, and loosening muscle adhesions. In addition, simply laying of the hands can have psychologic benefits as well. Some of the common techniques utilized through therapeutic massage are included under Key Facts. Of note, articulatory treatment is not a massage technique but, rather, more utilized as part of osteopathic manipulative treatment with the goal of increasing joint range of motion by using low-velocity and high-amplitude forces across a joint.

KEY FACTS: COMMON THERAPEUTIC MASSAGE TECHNIQUES

- Effleurage: Utilizes gliding movements over the skin with varying degrees of pressure without deep muscle involvement, which is helpful for muscle relaxation
- Pétrissage: Kneading movements performed with varying depths of pressure, which can determine the mechanical effects
- Tapotement: Percussion type of massage that alternates varying pressure between the hands and soft tissue of the patient; often used in conjunction with chest therapy for postural drainage
- Friction massage: Prevents or breaks muscle adhesions and applies massage force in transverse or perpendicular plane to the target muscle, tendon, or ligament
- Myofascial release: Light pressure applied in specific direction of the fascia for prolonged periods in order to stretch or release fascial tightness

FURTHER READING

Strax TE, Grabois M, Gonzalez P, et al. Physical modalities. In: Cucurillo S (Ed.), *Physical Medicine and Rehabilitation Board Review*. 2nd ed. New York, NY: Demos; 2010
Wolf CJ, Brault JS. Manipulation, traction, and massage. In: Braddom R, et al. (Eds.), *Physical Medicine & Rehabilitation*. 3rd ed. Philadelphia, PA: Saunders; 2007.

9. ANSWER: B

Manual medicine techniques can be classified in multiple different ways, and the terms *indirect* and *direct* are used to classify the techniques. Direct technique involves the operator moving the body part in the direction of restriction, whereas indirect technique means the operator moves the body part away from the restrictive barrier. Direct techniques involve thrust, articulation, muscle energy, and direct myofascial release, whereas indirect techniques include craniosacral therapy, strain–counterstrain, and indirect myofascial release. Spinal manipulation, typically inferring high-velocity manipulation, can have complications, with the most serious involving cervical manipulation and stroke. Common side effects include local discomfort, tiredness, headache, and radiating discomfort.

KEY FACTS: CONTRAINDICATIONS FOR SPINAL MANIPULATION

- Acute fracture or dislocation
- Osteomyelitis
- Active inflammatory arthropathy
- Ligamentous laxity

- Spinal tumor
- Osteoporosis
- Cauda equina syndrome
- Myelopathy
- Acute compression fracture
- Bleeding disorder

FURTHER READING

Drake DF, Schulman RA, Daimaru D. Integrative medicine in reha-
bilitation. In: Braddom R, et al. (Eds.), *Physical Medicine &
Rehabilitation*. 3rd ed. Philadelphia, PA: Saunders; 2007.
Wolf CJ, Brault JS. Manipulation, traction, and massage. In: Braddom
R, et al. (Eds.), *Physical Medicine & Rehabilitation*. 3rd ed.
Philadelphia, PA: Saunders; 2007.

10. ANSWER: C

Tapotement is a massage technique that utilizes rhythmic
alternating contact of varying pressure between the soft
tissue and the hands of the therapist. Various techniques
are utilized with this type of massage, including clapping,
beating, pounding, and hacking. This type of massage technique is often utilized in chest therapy to assist in postural
drainage of patients with disease processes such as cystic
fibrosis. Friction massage involves various methods of
applying pressure to the soft tissue with the goal of breaking down adhesions or loosening trigger points. Pétrissage
is a compression type of massage that utilizes kneading
movements to have a mechanical effect on the soft tissues.
Rolfing uses superficial and then deeper friction massage
to stretch fascia and help muscles to lengthen and relax.
Last, the Feldenkrais method uses multiple repetitions of
functional movements in order to increase proprioceptive
awareness with the goal to increase functional movements
with reduction in pain.

FURTHER READING

Strax TE, Grabois M, Gonzalez P, et al. Physical modalities.
In: Cucurillo S (Ed.), *Physical Medicine and Rehabilitation Board
Review*. 2nd ed. New York, NY: Demos; 2010.
Wolf CJ, Brault JS. Manipulation, traction, and massage. In: Braddom
R, et al. (Eds.), *Physical Medicine & Rehabilitation*. 3rd ed.
Philadelphia, PA: Saunders; 2007.

11. ANSWER: C

Cervical orthoses can be indicated for vertebral fracture,
spinal column instability, or ligamentous injury involving
the spine. The halo device is mostly used for unstable cervical fractures or postoperative management, and it is the
most restrictive in terms of range of motion of the cervical spine (Table 13.1). The halo device includes a ring that
attaches to the skull through pins, vest, and superstructure.
This device is used for approximately 3 months. One of the
most commonly used cervical orthoses is the Philadelphia
collar, which is used for stable bony or ligamentous injuries
and limits mostly flexion and extension. It is also used during emergency transport or after cervical fusion.

Table 13.1 **EFFECTS OF ORTHOSES ON RANGE
OF MOTION**

CERVICAL ORTHOSIS	MEAN OF NORMAL MOTION (%)		
	FLEXION/ EXTENSION	LATERAL BENDING	ROTATION
Normal	100	100	100
Soft collar	74.2	92.3	82.6
Philadelphia collar	28.9	66.4	43.7
SOMI brace	27.7	65.6	33.6
Halo device	4.0	4.0	1.0

FURTHER READING

Norbury JW, Tilley E, Moore DP. Spinal orthoses in rehabilitation.
In: Braddom R, et al. (Eds.), *Physical Medicine & Rehabilitation*. 3rd
ed. Philadelphia, PA: Saunders; 2007.
Uustal H, Baerga E. Prosthetics and orthotics. In: Cucurillo S (Ed.),
Physical Medicine and Rehabilitation Board Review. 2nd ed.
New York, NY: Demos; 2010.

12. ANSWER: A

The Jewett brace is used to treat lower thoracic or upper
lumbar compression fractures. This brace prevents flexion
of the thoracolumbar region with a three-point pressure
system. This brace is not indicated for burst fractures or any
unstable fractures. The TLSO extends from the sacrum to
the inferior angle of the scapula and decreases load on the
spine by increasing intra-abdominal pressure. This brace is
commonly used for postoperative stabilization following
spine surgery. The Taylor brace is similar to the TLSO in
limiting flexion and extension, and it is primarily used to
treat kyphosis from osteoporotic compression fractures.
Due to better control of the spine, most clinicians prefer the
TLSO over the Taylor brace. The Milwaukee brace spans
the entire spine segment and includes a cervical ring that is
usually indicated for scoliosis that is 25–40° with the apex
of the curve superior to the T8 vertebral body. Last, the
Miami J collar is a cervical collar that mainly limits cervical
flexion and extension and is used for cervical strain or stable
cervical fractures.

FURTHER READING

Norbury JW, Tilley E, Moore DP. Spinal orthoses in rehabilitation. In: Braddom R, et al. (Eds.), *Physical Medicine & Rehabilitation*. 3rd ed. Philadelphia, PA: Saunders; 2007.

Uustal H, Baerga E. Prosthetics and orthotics. In: Cucurillo S (Ed.), *Physical Medicine and Rehabilitation Board Review*. 2nd ed. New York, NY: Demos; 2010.

13. ANSWER: C

Use of axillary crutches requires good strength and range of motion of the upper extremities. A proper-fitting crutch length is determined by measuring the distance from the axillary fold to 6 inches lateral to the fifth toe with the patient in the standing position. The hand piece should allow the elbow to be flexed to 30° and wrist in extension and fingers in fist formation around the hand piece. The patient should be able to raise his or her body several inches by extending the elbow. Improper use may place the patient at risk of causing axillary nerve compression. Contrary to popular belief, crutches are not designed to support the patient's body weight, and extra padding of the axillary area should not be added because this may further risk nerve injury. The axillary nerve innervates the deltoid and teres minor muscles and provides sensation to the lateral shoulder. The patient may complain of weakness with shoulder abduction and external rotation.

KEY FACTS: PROPER CRUTCH PRESCRIPTION

- Proper length is measured from the axillary fold to 6 inches lateral to the fifth toe with the patient standing.
- Elbow should be flexed to 30° with the wrist in extension and hand formed in a fist around the hand piece.
- Patient should be able to lift his or her body several inches with elbow extension.
- Patient should not add any axillary padding to avoid resting his or her body weight on the crutches and thus avoid any potential axillary nerve injury.

FURTHER READING

Hennessey WJ, Uustal H. Lower limb orthoses. In: Braddom R, et al. (Eds.), *Physical Medicine & Rehabilitation*. 3rd ed. Philadelphia, PA: Saunders; 2007.

Uustal H, Baerga E. Prosthetics and orthotics. In: Cucurillo S (Ed.), *Physical Medicine and Rehabilitation Board Review*. 2nd ed. New York, NY: Demos; 2010.

14. ANSWER: D

Canes are typically prescribed to reduce weight-bearing forces across injured joints or structures, improve balance, provide stability for weakened muscles, and decrease pain. The cane should function by increasing the base of support, provide sensory feedback, and reduce weight bearing of the lower extremities. A proper-fitting cane should be assessed by first measuring the tip of the cane to the level of the greater trochanter with the patient standing upright. The elbow should be flexed approximately 20°. In general, the cane should be held in the hand opposite of the affected lower limb and is advanced with the affected limb. When climbing up and down stairs, patients should be counseled to ascend stairs with the strong and unaffected limb and descend with the affected limb.

KEY FACTS: PROPER CANE PRESCRIPTION

- Proper cane length is determined by measuring the tip of the cane to the greater trochanter with the patient standing and elbow flexed to 20°.
- The cane should be held in the hand opposite of the affected limb and advanced with the affected limb.
- Patient should be advised to always have the unaffected lower limb assume the first full weight-bearing load. The patient should start with the unaffected limb when ascending stairs; when descending stairs, the patient should start with the affected limb.

FURTHER READING

Hennessey WJ, Uustal H. Lower limb orthoses. In: Braddom R, et al. (Eds.), *Physical Medicine & Rehabilitation*. 3rd ed. Philadelphia, PA: Saunders; 2007.

Uustal H, Baerga E. Prosthetics and orthotics. In: Cucurillo S (Ed.), *Physical Medicine and Rehabilitation Board Review*. 2nd ed. New York, NY: Demos; 2010.

15. ANSWER: A

Lateral shoe wedges can alter the ground reaction forces, thus affecting loading more proximally across the knee. Patients with a genu varum deformity may develop osteoarthritis involving the medial compartment of the knee. A lateral wedge could be considered to prevent further genu varum of the knee and could be considered for conservative treatment. The wedge is typically ¼-inch thick along the lateral border of the shoe and may widen the patient's gait. A medial wedge would increase genu varum of the knee, thus worsening medial compartment loading. Metatarsal pads reduce weight across the metatarsal heads and are used for forefoot pain, whereas rocker bottom soles assist in relieving metatarsal pain and quicken the gait cycle.

Table 13.2 TYPES OF STRENGTHENING EXERCISES

ISOMETRIC	ISOKINETIC	ISOTONIC
• No visible joint movement	• Visible joint movement	• Visible joint movement
• External force cannot be overcome	• Constant speed	• Variable speed
• Done in static position	• Variable external resistance	• Constant external resistance or weight
• Example: Pushing against a wall	• Example: Nautilus machine	• Example: Bicep curls

FURTHER READING

Hennessey WJ. Lower limb orthoses. In: Braddom R, et al. (Eds.), *Physical Medicine & Rehabilitation*. 3rd ed. Philadelphia, PA: Saunders; 2007.

Uustal H, Baerga E. Prosthetics and orthotics. In: Cucurillo S (Ed.), *Physical Medicine and Rehabilitation Board Review*. 2nd ed. New York, NY: Demos; 2010.

16. ANSWER: C

Rehabilitation exercises can be classified into multiple different categories. Closed kinetic chain (CKC) exercises involve a distal extremity in which it is in constant contact with an immobile surface such as a machine surface or ground, thus reducing the amount of shear forces across a joint as opposed to open kinetic chain exercises, in which the distal extremity is free to move in space. CKC exercises are often considered more functional and exercise more than one muscle group at a time. Examples of CKC exercise are push-ups, squats, and dead lifts. Concentric-based exercises involve muscle shortening against resistance and the subject is able to overcome the resistance. An example of this type of exercise is bicep curls. Eccentric-based exercises involve lengthening of the muscle under tension, often against a force that cannot be overcome, which causes increased tissue destruction. Muscle soreness is often seen following these types of exercises. Lateral epicondylosis is a degenerative tendinosis for which eccentric-based exercises are commonly used as first-line treatment based on the belief that these types of exercises reorganize tendon structure through formation of new fibrous tissue.

FURTHER READING

Cullinane FL, Boocock MG, Trevelyan FC. Is eccentric exercise an effective treatment for lateral epicondylitis? A systematic review. *Clin Rehabil*. 2014;28(1):3–19.

Finnoff JT. Musculoskeletal disorders of the upper limb. In: Braddom R, et al. (Eds.), *Physical Medicine & Rehabilitation*. 3rd ed. Philadelphia, PA: Saunders; 2007.

Strax TE, Grabois M, Gonzalez P, et al. Physical modalities. In: Cucurillo S (Ed.), *Physical Medicine and Rehabilitation Board Review*. 2nd ed. New York, NY: Demos; 2010.

17. ANSWER: A

Isotonic exercises involve visible joint movement with variable speed and constant external resistance or weight (Table 13.2). An example of this is bicep curls with barbells during which the elbow joint is flexing and extending with variable speed but the weight of the barbell does not change with the repetition. Isokinetic exercises also involve visible joint movement at a constant speed that may have variable external resistance. Although not as commonly seen or utilized, this type of exercise is seen with the use of a Nautilus machine. Last, isometric exercises do not involve any visible joint movement due to an external force that cannot be overcome. This type of exercise can also be performed by holding a joint in static position—for example, pushing against a wall. This type of exercise may be preferred when joint mobilization may be contraindicated due to an inflammatory condition such as rheumatoid arthritis. This type of exercise does not alter synovial fluid composition, which would be ideal in patients with inflammatory arthritis.

FURTHER READING

Hicks JE, Joe GO, Gerber LH. Rehabilitation of the patient with inflammatory arthritis and connective-tissue disease. In: DeLisa JA, Gans BM, Walsh NE (Eds.), *Physical Medicine and Rehabilitation: Principles and Practice*. 4th ed. Philadelphia: Lippincott Williams & Wilkins; 2005.

Strax TE, Grabois M, Gonzalez P, et al. Physical modalities. In: Cucurillo S (Ed.), *Physical Medicine and Rehabilitation Board Review*. 2nd ed. New York, NY: Demos; 2010.

Wilder RP, Jenkins JG, Seto CK, et al. Therapeutic exercise. In: Braddom R, et al. (Eds.), *Physical Medicine & Rehabilitation*. 3rd ed. Philadelphia, PA: Saunders; 2007.

18. ANSWER: A

Mechanical diagnosis and treatment (MDT), also known as the McKenzie method, is based on the idea that patients may present with a "directional preference" in which movement in a specific direction may eliminate pain and restore function. Focusing on spine treatment, the assessment explores different positions and movements that may exacerbate the patient's pain and may develop a treatment plan based on repetitive movements in the patient's directional preference. The majority of spine patients have a preference for extension-based movements; the patient in this case may benefit from this type of therapy. Proprioceptive neuromuscular facilitation is a type of rehabilitation training that focuses on stretching and range of motion to improve motor performance, most often following a stroke. Myofascial release therapy and Feldenkrais therapy could be considered but may not be the first option in this particular patient. Last, iontophoresis uses an electric field to move various medications such as corticosteroids or lidocaine across a biologic membrane to directly deliver them to soft tissues and would not be recommended for this patient.

KEY FACTS: MDT OR MCKENZIE THERAPY

- MDT was developed by Robin McKenzie in the 1980s.
- It is focuses on a "directional preference" in which repetitive movements in a preferable direction may help alleviate or eliminate the patient's pain.
- The majority of spine patients have a preference for extension-based exercises.
- Centralization of the patient's pain can be seen in which the radiating pain in the extremity retreats to the midline; this has been shown to be an accurate predictor of successful outcome with this type of therapy.

FURTHER READING

Stanos SP, Rivers E, Prather H, et al. Physical medicine and rehabilitation approaches to pain management. In: Benzon H, Raja H, Fishman S, et al. (Eds.), *Essentials of Pain Medicine*. 3rd ed. Philadelphia, PA: Saunders; 2011.
Wilder RP, Jenkins JG, Seto CK, et al. Therapeutic exercise. In: Braddom R, et al. (Eds.), *Physical Medicine & Rehabilitation*. 3rd ed. Philadelphia, PA: Saunders; 2007.

19. ANSWER: D

The definitions of disability, impairment, and handicap are important to differentiate as they apply to patients and society (Table 13.3). According to American Medical Association (AMA) guidelines, *disability* is defined by an alteration of an individual's capacity to meet personal, social, or occupational demands due to impairment. Disability relates to function relative to activities of daily living or work. An example of a disability is the inability to ambulate due to paraplegia. *Impairment* is defined by the AMA as a loss, loss of use, or derangement of any body part, organ system, or organ function. Examples are paraplegia due to a stroke or inability to write due to carpal tunnel syndrome. Last, *handicap* is the inability to fulfill a societal role as a result of the impairment and disability. An example is loss of a job as construction worker due to paraplegia.

FURTHER READING

Serrousi RE, Robinson JP. Impairment rating and disability determination. In: Braddom R, et al. (Eds.), *Physical Medicine & Rehabilitation*. 3rd ed. Philadelphia, PA: Saunders; 2007.
Strax TE, Grabois M, Gonzalez P, et al. Physical modalities. In: Cucurillo S (Ed.), *Physical Medicine and Rehabilitation Board Review*. 2nd ed. New York, NY: Demos; 2010.

20. ANSWER: D

Trendelenburg gait occurs with weakness of the hip abductors, which primarily include the gluteus medius and minimus muscles. With weakness, there is contralateral pelvic drop due to poor activation of the stabilizing hip abductors, and the patient may compensate by leaning laterally over the weakened hip abductors. For example, if a patient is standing on his or her right leg and the left pelvis drops, this indicates weakness of the right hip abductors due to inability to stabilize the pelvis to prevent the pelvic drop. In order to compensate for this, the patient may lean his or her body toward the right in order to keep the center of gravity over the unaffected side.

KEY FACTS: CAUSES OF TRENDELENBURG GAIT

- Lumbar radiculopathy (L5 or S1)
- Congenital hip dislocation
- Hip dysplasia
- Hip osteoarthritis
- Fractures of the greater trochanter
- Poliomyelitis
- Slipped capital femoral epiphysis
- Superior gluteal neuropathy

Table 13.3 DEFINING IMPAIRMENT, DISABILITY, AND HANDICAP

IMPAIRMENT	DISABILITY	HANDICAP
• Physical or psychological abnormality as a result of injury or disease • Example: Paraplegia due to a stroke	• Alteration of individual's capacity to meet personal, social, or occupational demands due to impairment • Example: Inability to ambulate due to stroke	• Inability to fulfill a societal role due to impairment and disability • Example: Loss of job as construction worker

Table 13.4 NEURAL TENSION TESTS FOR THE LUMBAR SPINE

SEATED SLUMP TEST	STRAIGHT LEG RAISE	FEMORAL STRETCH TEST
• Provocative test for lower lumbar disc herniation • May help differentiate hamstring tightness from lumbosacral radicular pain • Found to be more sensitive than the straight leg raise	• Provocative test for lower lumbar disc herniation • Positive test is considered if pain is reproduced between 30° and 70° of flexion • Found to be more specific than the seated slump test	• Provocative test for upper lumbar disc herniation • May have false positives from other etiologies, such as a femoral neuropathy, quadriceps tightness, or hip pathology

FURTHER READING

Brown DP, Freeman ED, Cucurillo S. Musculoskeletal medicine. In: Cucurillo S (Ed.), *Physical Medicine and Rehabilitation Board Review*. 2nd ed. New York, NY: Demos; 2010.

Esquenazi A, Talaty M. Gait analysis: Technology and clinical applications. In: Braddom R, et al. (Eds.), *Physical Medicine & Rehabilitation*. 3rd ed. Philadelphia, PA: Saunders; 2007.

21. ANSWER: A

In the setting of lumbar radicular leg pain, provocative tests that provide neural tension may play an important part of the physical examination in order to provide appropriate treatment including image-guided injections (Table 13.4). The seated slump test has been shown to have greater sensitivity than the straight leg raise in patients with symptoms from a lumbar disc herniation. This test is performed with the patient seated with arms behind her back and legs together and knees against the examining table. The patient slumps forward as much as possible and then is asked to flex her head while the examiner applies further light pressure to flex the neck. While maintaining full spine and neck flexion, the affected knee is extended, and the patient is asked whether her pain is concordant to her symptoms. Sensitivity can be increased by adding foot dorsiflexion. The patient is then asked to extend her neck, and relief of her symptoms with neck extension correlates with a positive test. As with the straight leg raise test, this test is more useful when the lower lumbosacral nerve roots are involved. Of note, the straight leg raise test has been shown to be slightly more specific than the seated slump test. The femoral stretch test is more useful for upper lumbar nerve root irritation from the L2, L3, or L4 levels, whereas Patrick's test is used to diagnose sacroiliac joint-related pain, and the Thompson test is used to test the integrity of the Achilles tendon.

FURTHER READING

Barr KP, Harrast MA. Low back pain. In: Braddom R, et al. (Eds.), *Physical Medicine & Rehabilitation*. 3rd ed. Philadelphia, PA: Saunders; 2007.

Majlesi J, Togay H, Ünalan H, et al. The sensitivity and specificity of the Slump and the Straight Leg Raising tests in patients with lumbar disc herniation. *J Clin Rheumatol*. 2008;14(2):87–91.

Malanga GA, Nadler S. Physical examination of the lumbar spine. In: *Musculoskeletal Physical Examination: An Evidence-Based Approach*. Philadelphia, PA: Mosby; 2006.

22. ANSWER: A

Peripheral nerve injuries can be classified by Seddon's classification, which has three stages of injury: neurapraxia, axonotmesis, and neurotmesis (Table 13.5). Neuropraxia is characterized by local myelin injury due to nerve compression with intact axons causing a focal conduction block. Muscle atrophy is not typically seen, and recovery may occur in weeks to months. Axonotmesis is characterized by disruption of the axons due to nerve crush injury with subsequent Wallerian degeneration. The endoneurium remains intact, which allows the axon to regenerate along its previous course. The rate of axonal regeneration is generally estimated to be 1 mm/day. It is important to emphasize that axonal regeneration is not synonymous with return of function. Last, neurotmesis is complete disruption of the axons and surrounding connective tissue due to nerve transection. This is a poor prognosis often requiring surgical reapproximation of the nerve.

Table 13.5 CLASSIFICATION OF NERVE INJURIES

SEDDON'S CLASSIFICATION	SUNDERLAND'S CLASSIFICATION	NERVE TISSUES INJURED
Neurapraxia	Grade 1	Myelin
Axonotmesis	Grade 2	Axon and myelin
Neurotmesis	Grade 3	Axon, myelin, endoneurium
	Grade 4	Axon, myelin, endoneurium, perineurium
	Grade 5	Axon, myelin, endoneurium, perineurium, epineurium

FURTHER READING

Dumitru D, Andary M. Electrodiagnostic medicine I: Fundamental principles. In: Braddom R, et al. (Eds.), *Physical Medicine & Rehabilitation*. 3rd ed. Philadelphia, PA: Saunders; 2007.

Dumitru D, Zwarts MJ, Amato A. Peripheral nervous system's reaction to injury. In: *Electrodiagnostic Medicine*. 2nd ed. Philadelphia, PA: Hanley & Belfus; 2002.

Freeman TL, Johnson EW, Freeman ED, et al. Electrodiagnostic medicine and clinical neuromuscular physiology. In: Cucurillo S (Ed.), *Physical Medicine and Rehabilitation Board Review*. 2nd ed. New York, NY: Demos; 2010.

Preston D, Shapiro B. Approach to nerve conduction studies and electromyography. In: *Electromyography and Neuromuscular Disorders*. 3rd ed. Philadelphia, PA: Saunders; 2013.

23. ANSWER: D

Peripheral nerves can be classified as myelinated or unmyelinated, autonomic or somatic, sensory or motor, and based on the size of their diameter. There is a direct relationship between the diameter of the nerve fiber and conduction velocity, in which the nerves with the fastest conduction velocity also have the largest diameter. During clinical nerve conduction studies, the large myelinated nerve fibers are studied, whereas the smaller myelinated fibers (Aβ and Aδ) and unmyelinated C fibers are not recorded. As a result, small fiber neuropathies may not be detected with routine electrodiagnostic testing.

FURTHER READING

Preston D, Shapiro B. Anatomy and neurophysiology. In: *Electromyography and Neuromuscular Disorders*. 3rd ed. Philadelphia, PA: Saunders; 2013.

24. ANSWER: C

Skin temperature is one of the most important physiologic factors when performing nerve conduction studies. In general, the temperature of the upper extremities should be greater than 33°C, and that of the lower extremities should be greater than 31°C. As the temperature drops below ideal conditions, this can affect waveform characteristics of the action potential due to delayed opening and closing of sodium channels (Table 13.6). The distal latency becomes prolonged, the amplitude of the sensory or motor action potential increases, the duration of the action potential increases, and the conduction velocity is decreased. Slowing of the conduction velocity or latency prolongation can lead to the wrong diagnosis of a peripheral neuropathy or mononeuropathy and may lead to unnecessary intervention. As a result, extremities should be warmed to appropriate temperatures using warm water, blankets, or heating pads.

Table 13.6 DECREASE IN TEMPERATURE AND WAVEFORM PARAMETERS

WAVEFORM	CHANGE IN PARAMETERS
Distal latency	Prolonged
Duration	Increased
Conduction velocity	Decreased
Amplitude (motor or sensory)	Increased

FURTHER READING

Dumitru D, Zwarts MJ, Amato A. Nerve conduction studies. In: *Electrodiagnostic Medicine*. 2nd ed. Philadelphia, PA: Hanley & Belfus; 2002.

Freeman TL, Johnson EW, Freeman ED, et al. Electrodiagnostic medicine and clinical neuromuscular physiology. In: Cucurillo S (Ed.), *Physical Medicine and Rehabilitation Board Review*. 2nd ed. New York, NY: Demos; 2010.

Preston D, Shapiro B. Basic nerve conduction studies. In: *Electromyography and Neuromuscular Disorders*. 3rd ed. Philadelphia, PA: Saunders; 2013.

25. ANSWER: D

In neuropathic lesions such as a lumbosacral radiculopathy, the time required to see denervation and reinnervation in the affected muscle is dependent on the distance between the lesion and the muscle (Table 13.7). From the onset of an acute injury, it may take 10–14 days to see denervation in the muscles beginning in the proximal lumbar paraspinal muscles closest to the lesion site. Approximately 2 or 3 weeks later, the proximal muscles become affected, and 3 or 4 weeks after the injury, the distal innervated muscles will show denervation potentials. Reinnervation potentials are not typically seen until 5 or 6 weeks after the injury and begin in the proximal innervated muscles.

Table 13.7 TIMETABLE OF ELECTROMYOGRAPHY FINDINGS WITH RADICULOPATHY

TIME	ELECTROMYOGRAPHY FINDINGS
Day of injury	Decreased recruitment of motor units
1 week	Denervation seen in the paraspinal muscles
2 weeks	Denervation seen in the proximal innervated muscles
3–4 weeks	
5–6 weeks	Denervation seen in the distal innervated muscles
	Reinnervation potentials seen starting proximally

FURTHER READING

Freeman TL, Johnson EW, Freeman ED, et al. Electrodiagnostic medicine and clinical neuromuscular physiology. In: Cucurillo S (Ed.), *Physical Medicine and Rehabilitation Board Review*. 2nd ed. New York, NY: Demos; 2010.

Preston D, Shapiro B. Radiculopathy. In: *Electromyography and Neuromuscular Disorders*. 3rd ed. Philadelphia, PA: Saunders; 2013.

Tubbs S, Rizk E, Shoja MM, et al. Nerve injuries in sports. In: *Nerves and Nerve Injuries*. Oxford, UK: Elsevier; 2015.

26. ANSWER: A

The gluteus medius muscle is an L5 and S1 innervated muscle with innervation from the superior gluteal nerve. Due to the proximal location of this muscle, it is often included in radiculopathy screening during electromyography testing because denervation and reinnervation potentials are seen earlier than the distal L5 innervated muscles. The gluteus maximus muscle is an S1 and S2 innervated muscle with peripheral innervation from the inferior gluteal nerve. The iliopsoas muscle is an L2 and L3 innervated muscle with peripheral innervation by the Femoral nerve. Last, the adductor longus muscle is an L2, L3, and L4 innervated muscle with peripheral innervation by the obturator nerve.

FURTHER READING

Perotto A, et al. Thigh and pelvis and hip joint. In: *Anatomical Guide for the Electromyographer*. 5th ed. Springfield, IL: Charles C Thomas; 2005.

27. ANSWER: B

The suprascapular nerve originates from the C5 and C6 nerves and is one of the most common peripheral nerve injuries in the upper limb in athletes. The nerve innervates the suprascapular muscle and passes through the spinoglenoid notch along the glenoid to innervate the infraspinatus muscle. This nerve is susceptible to injury in athletes who perform repetitive overhead activities and can be compressed at the suprascapular notch or spinoglenoid notch. Compression at the suprascapular notch is more common and can affect both the supraspinatus and the infraspinatus muscle, causing pain and weakness with both shoulder abduction and external rotation. Compression at the spinoglenoid notch affects only the infraspinatus muscle, thus affecting shoulder external rotation. Volleyball players in particular are susceptible to injury at this location due to the float serve, which causes rapid eccentric contraction of the infraspinatus muscle to slow internal rotation of the shoulder during follow through of the serve. This causes a traction injury of the nerve along the spinoglenoid notch.

FURTHER READING

Akuthota V, Herring S. Peripheral nerve injuries of the shoulder and upper arm. In: *Nerve and Vascular Injuries in Sports Medicine*. New York, NY: Springer; 2009.

28. ANSWER: E

Nerve conduction velocity has a direct relationship with the nerve fiber diameter, in which the larger diameter fibers have faster conduction velocities (Table 13.8). The large-diameter fibers have the most myelin and least electrical resistance, thus leading to faster conduction velocities. Small, unmyelinated fibers such as the C fibers have the slowest conduction velocity at 1 or 2 m/s.

Table 13.8 **NERVE TYPES, DIAMETER, AND CONDUCTION VELOCITY**

NERVE FIBER TYPE	DIAMETER (MM)	CONDUCTION VELOCITY (M/SEC)
Aα	10–20	50–120
Aβ	4–12	25–70
Aδ	1–5	5–30
C	<1	1–2

FURTHER READING

Freeman TL, Johnson EW, Freeman ED, et al. Electrodiagnostic medicine and clinical neuromuscular physiology. In: Cucurillo S (Ed.), *Physical Medicine and Rehabilitation Board Review*. 2nd ed. New York, NY: Demos; 2010.
Preston D, Shapiro B. Anatomy and neurophysiology. In: *Electromyography and Neuromuscular Disorders*. 3rd ed. Philadelphia, PA: Saunders; 2013.

29. ANSWER: B

The sciatic nerve—specifically the peroneal nerve fibers in the sciatic nerve—is the most commonly injured nerve following hip replacement surgery. The largest nerve in the human body, the sciatic nerve runs posterior to the hip joint and can be injured following a posterior hip dislocation in addition to being a complication following surgery due to stretch or retraction of the nerve or from methylmethacrylate cement eroding into the nerve months to years following surgery. The peroneal fibers are preferentially affected in most sciatic nerve lesions, and patients usually present with foot drop due to weak foot dorsiflexion.

FURTHER READING

Dumitru D, Zwarts MJ, Amato A. Lumbosacral plexopathies and proximal mononeuropathies. In: *Electrodiagnostic Medicine*. 2nd ed. Philadelphia, PA: Hanley & Belfus; 2002.

Freeman TL, Johnson EW, Freeman ED, et al. Electrodiagnostic medicine and clinical neuromuscular physiology. In: Cucurillo S (Ed.), *Physical Medicine and Rehabilitation Board Review*. 2nd ed. New York, NY: Demos; 2010.

Preston D, Shapiro B. Sciatic neuropathy. In: *Electromyography and Neuromuscular Disorders*. 3rd ed. Philadelphia, PA: Saunders; 2013.

30. ANSWER: D

The median innervated muscles of the hand can be remembered using the mnemonic "2LOAF." This includes the first and second *l*umbricals, *o*pponens pollicis, *a*bductor pollicis brevis, and *f*lexor pollicis brevis muscles. The flexor digitorum superficialis muscle is median innervated but at the level of the forearm and would not be affected by a median mononeuropathy at the wrist. Of note, the contents of the carpal tunnel include the median nerve, flexor pollicis longus tendon, four tendons of the flexor digitorum superficialis, and four tendons of the flexor digitorum profundus muscles.

KEY FACT: MEDIAN INNERVATED MUSCLES OF THE HAND

- 2LOAF = first and second *l*umbricals, *o*pponens pollicis, *a*bductor pollicis brevis, and *f*lexor pollicis brevis muscles.

FURTHER READING

Freeman TL, Johnson EW, Freeman ED, et al. Electrodiagnostic medicine and clinical neuromuscular physiology. In: Cucurillo S (Ed.), *Physical Medicine and Rehabilitation Board Review*. 2nd ed. New York, NY: Demos; 2010.

Preston D, Shapiro B. Median neuropathy at the wrist. In: *Electromyography and Neuromuscular Disorders*. 3rd ed. Philadelphia, PA: Saunders; 2013.

31. ANSWER: D

The lateral femoral cutaneous nerve originate from the L2 and L3 nerve roots through the posterior division of the lumbosacral plexus. Injury to this nerve, also known as meralgia paresthetica, presents as a pure sensory neuropathy with lateral thigh pain, numbness, or aching. This nerve can be injured from compression from tight clothing, trauma, or truncal obesity. It is of note that the femoral and obturator nerves originate from the L2, L3, and L4 nerve roots; the genitofemoral nerve originates from the L1 and L2 nerve roots; and the ilioinguinal and iliohypogastric nerves originate from the L1 and T12–L1 nerve roots, respectively.

FURTHER READING

Buschbacher R, Prahlow N. Lower limb motor nerve studies. In: *Manual of Nerve Conduction Studies*. 2nd ed. New York, NY: Demos; 2006.

Freeman TL, Johnson EW, Freeman ED, et al. Electrodiagnostic medicine and clinical neuromuscular physiology. In: Cucurillo S (Ed.), *Physical Medicine and Rehabilitation Board Review*. 2nd ed. New York, NY: Demos; 2010.

32. ANSWER: D

Upper trunk brachial plexopathy, also known as Erb's palsy, occurs when there is compression or nerve traction along the C5 and C6 nerve fibers (Table 13.9). In traumatic cases, this occurs when the head is pushed away from the shoulder, causing a traction injury. Patients classically present in the "waiter's tip" position, in which the arm is adducted, internally rotated, and extended, and the forearm pronated with the wrist in flexed position. This is also the most common type of plexopathy seen in newborn infants. On the other hand, Klumpke's palsy affects the C8 and T1 nerve fibers and occurs when the arm is pulled up, causing traction on the lower trunk of the brachial plexus. These patients have mostly intrinsic hand wasting with claw hand deformity, whereas the upper arm and shoulder girdle is preserved.

FURTHER READING

Freeman TL, Johnson EW, Freeman ED, et al. Electrodiagnostic medicine and clinical neuromuscular physiology. In: Cucurillo S

Table 13.9 COMMON BRACHIAL PLEXOPATHIES

	UPPER TRUNK/ERB'S PALSY	LOWER TRUNK/KLUMPKE'S PALSY
Nerve roots	C5–C6	C8–T1
Etiology	"Stinger," nerve traction as head is pushed away from the shoulder	Arm is pulled up and away from the body, causing traction to the lower trunk
Presentation	Waiter's tip Arm: Adducted, internally rotated, and extended Forearm: Pronated Wrist: Flexed	Intrinsic hand wasting and claw hand deformity Upper arm and shoulder girdle preserved

(Ed.), *Physical Medicine and Rehabilitation Board Review*. 2nd ed. New York, NY: Demos; 2010.

Preston D, Shapiro B. Brachial plexopathy. In: *Electromyography and Neuromuscular Disorders*. 3rd ed. Philadelphia, PA: Saunders; 2013.

33. ANSWER: C

Laser evoked potentials selectively stimulate Aδ and C fibers primarily using CO_2 lasers. This study can be used to assess patients with neuropathic pain and to demonstrate small fiber neuropathy. Prior studies used laser potentials to assess pain in diagnoses such as carpal tunnel syndrome, trigeminal neuralgia, diabetic polyneuropathy, and radiculopathy. In addition, diseases affecting the central nervous system, such as syringomyelia and multiple sclerosis, have demonstrated clinical utility for laser potentials. Syringomyelia may demonstrate the absence of laser evoked potentials, reduced amplitudes, and prolonged latencies. Superficial skin burns and pigmentation changes have been noted as a potential risk in performing this test.

FURTHER READING

Nishida T, Minieka MM. Neurophysiologic testing for pain. In: Benzon H, Raja H, Fishman S, et al. (Eds.), *Essentials of Pain Medicine*. 3rd ed. Philadelphia, PA: Saunders; 2011.

Valeriani M, Pazzaglia C, Cruccu G, et al. Clinical usefulness of laser evoked potentials. *Clin Neurophysiol*. 2012;42(5):345–353.

34. ANSWER: B

QST allows the ability to assess large and small sensory nerve fiber function, whereas conventional nerve conduction studies (NCSs) are limited to only large fibers. Stimulus is applied at different intensities on the patient's skin, and the patient is asked to state when he begins to feel the applied stimulus. Thresholds are determined based on when the patient feels the stimulus appear and disappear. Subsequently, QST lacks the objectivity of NCSs, and results of this test can be affected by patient distraction, drowsiness, confusion, and patient bias toward the testing. As a result, it is important that the interpreting clinician is aware of extraneous factors that may affect the test. QST does not localize a lesion to a specific part of the nervous system but does assess both peripheral and central nervous systems. Neuropathic pain can be characterized by a combination of positive (tingling) and negative (numbness) sensory symptoms, and QST has a distinct advantage of assessing both sensory disturbances.

FURTHER READING

Nishida T, Minieka MM. Neurophysiologic testing for pain. In: Benzon H, Raja H, Fishman S, et al. (Eds.), *Essentials of Pain Medicine*. 3rd ed. Philadelphia, PA: Saunders; 2011.

Yarnitsky D. Quantitative sensory testing. *Muscle Nerve*. 1997; 20(2):198–204.

35. ANSWER: A

The number of muscle fibers that belong to an axon is referred to as the innervation ratio. This ratio depends on the primary function of the motor unit, and muscles of gross movement have a larger amount of fibers innervated by an axon. Muscles of the leg have higher innervation ratios because greater force is generated by that motor unit. As a result, muscles such as the gastrocnemius may have a ratio of 600 muscle fibers to 1 axon, whereas smaller muscles that involve fine movement may have smaller ratios. Generally, compared to type 1 fibers, type 2 muscle fibers have higher innervation ratios because these muscle fibers generate more force.

FURTHER READING

Dumitru D, Andary M. Electrodiagnostic medicine I: Fundamental principles. In: Braddom R, et al. (Eds.), *Physical Medicine & Rehabilitation*. 3rd ed. Philadelphia, PA: Saunders; 2007.

Freeman TL, Johnson EW, Freeman ED, et al. Electrodiagnostic medicine and clinical neuromuscular physiology. In: Cucurillo S (Ed.), *Physical Medicine and Rehabilitation Board Review*. 2nd ed. New York, NY: Demos; 2010.

36. ANSWER: B

The sympathetic skin response is used to assess peripheral sympathetic nerve activity and is mediated by unmyelinated C fibers. The response is often a low-frequency potential and is recorded from the palm or sole of the foot, where there is a higher density of eccrine sweat glands. Recording at the forearm and axilla often fails to produce a response due to the lack of eccrine sweat glands. Appropriate stimuli can include an electric shock or a loud noise that the patient does not expect. The response can vary with multiple attempts, and it can be attenuated with decreasing temperatures, anti-cholinergic medications, and low levels of attention.

FURTHER READING

Kimura J. Other techniques to assess the peripheral nerve. In: *Electrodiagnosis in Diseases of Nerve and Muscle: Principles and Practice*. 3rd ed. New York, NY: Oxford University Press; 2013.

Nishida T, Minieka MM. Neurophysiologic testing for pain. In: Benzon H, Raja H, Fishman S, et al. (Eds.), *Essentials of Pain Medicine*. 3rd ed. Philadelphia, PA: Saunders; 2011.

14.

COMPLEMENTARY AND ALTERNATIVE MEDICINE

Elizabeth Huntoon

INTRODUCTION

Complementary and alternative medicine (CAM) is a broad area that has become popular with both patients and physicians. Most of the CAM practices are used together with conventional therapies and therefore have been called complementary to distinguish them from alternative practices, which are those used instead of standard care. CAM offers patients a variety of different nonconventional treatment options, especially when dealing with chronic illness and symptom alleviation. This category of medicine covers a wide range of topics, such as acupuncture, homeopathy, energy medicine, yoga, tai chi, magnet therapy, therapeutic touch, and herbal and vitamin supplements. It is important to note that this list is not exhaustive, and most of the therapies under the heading of CAM are considered safe as adjuncts or alternative treatments by the medical profession for a variety of pain problems. However, one area deserves special consideration: herbal and vitamin preparations. Herbal supplement use has increased in the past few years, and patients may fail to mention that they are taking these substances. This lack of disclosure (or our lack of inquiry about supplements) may put them at risk for herb–drug interaction.

The popularity of CAM therapies may be due largely to their presumed safety, efficacy, cultural acceptability, and lesser side effects compared with prescription medications.

QUESTIONS

1. Which of the following statements is most true?

A. Hypnosis is a state in which a patient is fully unconscious and not in control of his or her behavior.
B. The hypnotic state is a trance-like state in which patients are highly suggestible.
C. All people will respond to hypnosis.

D. The brains of highly hypnotizable patients are 20% smaller than those of moderately or slightly hypnotizable patients.

2. Osteopathy broadly refers to:

A. Diseases of the bone
B. Manipulation of the bones and ligaments
C. Pathology of osteoclasts and osteoblasts
D. A process of harvesting bone for grafting

3. Complementary and alternative medicine (CAM) refers to:

A. Acupuncture and herbal medicine
B. Homeopathy
C. Bee venom therapy
D. Energy medicine
E. All of the above

4. A 65-year-old female with back pain comes in for an initial evaluation. Her physical exam is significant for diffuse palpatory tenderness in the upper mid and lumbar spine, but the remainder of her exam, including the neurologic exam, is normal. You give her a presumptive diagnosis of myofacial pain and ask her to participate in physical therapy. You also request a serum 25-hydroxyvitamin D (25-(OH)D) level. The results of her lab work show a vitamin D level of 15 nmol/l. Your best recommendation to her is:

A. Continue with the current recommendation of participating in physical therapy but increase the number of sessions from twice to three times a week
B. Continue with normal diet; no need to supplement with vitamin D because the neurologic exam is normal
C. Supplement with Vitamin D
D. Urgent referral to an endocrinologist

5. The term *homeopathy* refers to which of the following?

A. A system of medical treatments that combines magnet therapy with reiki
B. A system of medical treatments that uses dilute medications to obtain a cure
C. A type of therapy performed at home, thus the term "home"-eopathy
D. A type of treatment that can involve herbal preparations
E. B and D

6. Low levels of vitamin D have been associated with:

A. Muscle pain
B. Cognitive dysfunction
C. Low bone mineral density
D. Inflammation
E. All of the above

7. The medical student working with you this month reports to you that the new patient she just examined has "fibromyalgia," and she wants to be allowed to do trigger point injections on the patient as part of the treatment plan that she devised. When questioned about this diagnosis, she explains that the patient has tender points "all over her low back." Your exam concurs that the patient indeed has tenderness in a diffuse region of her low back but no distinct trigger points. You do the following:

A. Allow the student to perform trigger point injections on this patient
B. Allow the patient to perform trigger point injections on this student
C. Educate the medical student regarding the difference between trigger points and tender points
D. Offer the patient medical marijuana

8. A 63-year-old female presents with complaints of back pain. You examine her and the results of her imaging studies, and you find evidence for the diagnosis of discogenic back pain. She has heard from her friends that CAM is not very popular with the traditional medical world, but she wants to try it anyway. You advise her:

A. It is not worth her time
B. It is not popular anywhere
C. She should consider it because the insurance will probably cover it
D. It is a natural approach to managing pain and therefore safe
E. None of the above

9. The same patient returns 1 month later; she has bruising all over her body. Her cardiologist has been adjusting her medications but cannot determine why there is a sudden increase in ecchymosis. She did not share with either of you that she has been taking an herbal supplement because:

A. She did not think it was any of your business
B. Neither you nor the cardiologist asked
C. She believed it was not important to know because the herbal preparation was natural and therefore safe
D. All of the above

10. All of the following are true except:

A. Interactions can exist between prescribed drugs and herbal medications.
B. Herbal medications are commonly being used in elderly adults.
C. Many patients neglect to tell their medical doctors that they use herbal medications.
D. All herbal products sold in the United States are required to include a list of potential side effects.

11. A 22-year-old female presents with benign abdominal pain. Her lab data, imaging studies, and physical exam are all normal. Which of the following suggestions would be most likely to be helpful for her pain?

A. Three weeks of opioids and tai chi
B. Physical therapy two times per week for 6 weeks
C. Hypnosis
D. Reiki

12. Which of the following statements is true regarding acupuncture in the perioperative period?

A. It reduces the anesthetic requirement during abdominal surgeries.
B. It is useful in the postoperative period for treating nausea and vomiting.
C. It has shown little value in the preoperative period for managing anxiety.
D. Acupuncture analgesia is not reversible with naloxone.
E. It is effective only in patients who believe it will work.

13. In traditional Chinese medicine, acupuncture can be helpful for managing which of the following conditions?

A. Peripheral joint pain
B. Low back pain
C. Neck pain
D. All of the above
E. B and C

14. An 85-year-old male with chronic hip and back pain has complained of decreased balance and strength. He has known osteoarthritis of the hips and spinal stenosis. His only athletic endeavor has been golf. He would like to get back to golfing but is afraid that he might fall. Which of the following could you recommend?

A. Tai chi
B. Weightlifting program at the local gym
C. Jogging 3 days per week
D. Brazilian jiu jitsu

15. Electroacupuncture is thought to produce analgesic effects through the peripheral nervous system by:

A. The placebo effect
B. The release of endogenous opioids
C. The accelerated uptake of exogenous opioids
D. Destruction of sensory receptors at the site of needle insertion
E. B and C

16. Which of the following statements about acupuncture is/are true?

A. Should never be used in children
B. Can be safely used in all stages of pregnancy
C. Has few associated side effects
D. Is covered by Medicare
E. B and C

17. When discussing chiropractic adjustment treatments with your patients who have chronic neck and low back, you must keep in mind which of the following?

A. Lumbar adjustments are associated with increased risk of dural damage with leakage of spinal fluid and subsequent development of postural headache.
B. High-velocity, low-amplitude adjustments are never used in current chiropractic medicine.
C. Due to the presence of spondylosis in the lumbar spine, there is more risk with adjustments of the low back compared to the neck in elderly patients.
D. The risk of injury to the patient increases with a concurrent use of long-term anticoagulant therapy.

18. Which of the following is the most significant reason for actively seeking an herbal medicine usage history from your patient?

A. The potential drug–herb interactions with conventional medications used in pain clinics
B. The lack of evaluation and safety reporting of herbal medications

C. The lack of efficacy of herbal medications
D. The improved insurance coverage offered for CAM

19. All of the following are true except:

A. Interactions can exist between prescribed drugs and herbal medications.
B. Herbal medications are commonly being used in elderly adults.
C. Many patients neglect to tell their medical doctors that they use herbal medications.
D. All herbal products sold in the United States are required to include a list of potential side effects.

20. When considering an epidural steroid injection for lumbar radiculopathy in a patient taking *Ginkgo biloba* to prevent dementia, one should:

A. Consider the increased risk of bleeding with concomitant use of fluoxetine
B. Advise the patient the he or she should discontinue the ginko because it does not increase blood flow to the brain
C. Consider complete blood count testing prior to epidural steroid injection
D. Advise the patient to switch to ginseng because it has been shown to be more effective in the prevention of dementia

21. Your established 34-year-old female fibromyalgia patient shows up in your clinic with increasing anxiety and shortness of breath. She reports that her fibromyalgia symptoms have been quiescent for several months despite her lack of follow-up with you since her last visit 1 year ago, when she was in severe pain. What should you do?

A. Consider that she might be experiencing a flare-up of her fibromyalgia symptoms.
B. Prescribe an antibiotic because she might be experiencing symptoms of an upper respiratory tract infection.
C. Consider ordering a chest X-ray.
D. Question her about other therapies she may be using to control her fibromyalgia symptoms.
E. C and D

22. A 55-year-old woman with metastatic breast cancer is having increasing back pain. She has tried multiple natural approaches to manage her pain and has increased her daily dose of herbal supplements, including garlic and bee pollen. A thorough workup finds metastatic lesions in several of her thoracic vertebrae. She has chosen you to place her intrathecal pain pump. When considering an invasive spinal intervention for

this patient, American Society of Regional Anesthesia and Pain Medicine (ASRA) guidelines recommend that the patient be advised to:

A. Discontinue her bee pollen supplements one week prior to her surgery.
B. Discontinue her garlic supplement 36 hours before surgery
C. Discontinue her garlic supplement 1 week prior to surgery
D. Supplement with vitamin K 1 week prior to surgery to counter the effects of the garlic

23. When designing a comprehensive multidisciplinary pain program, the inclusion of therapies such as relaxation and imagery can be helpful for which the following reasons?

A. Chronic pain patients are much more tense than acute pain patients and therefore would likely respond by reducing their narcotic usage.
B. Relaxation and imagery are usually part of a broader cognitive–behavioral treatment program.
C. There is no reason to include relaxation and imagery because there is often no change in a patient's function when used in the chronic pain population.
D. Relaxation and imagery have been shown to be effective for chronic low back pain as well as cancer pain.
E. B and D.

24. Concerning marijuana, all of the following are true except:

A. Cannabinoids inhibit the growth of different types of tumor cells.
B. Can reduce nausea and vomiting.
C. The legal oral forms are dronabinol and nabilone.
D. The main active ingredient in marijuana is Δ^5-tetrahydrocannabinol.

25. The term neutraceuticals refers most to:

A. All natural products.
B. Supplements that are prescribed by naturopathic practitioners
C. Herbal supplements that have been tested and found safe for human consumption
D. Products derived from food sources that are purported to provide extra health benefits

26. Pulsed electromagnetic field therapy and static magnetic therapy are touted as "safe and effective" methods of managing chronic pain. A vendor would like to sell you magnetic jewelry as well as electromagnetic mats so that you can offer them to your patients at your outpatient pain clinic. You consider your options and:

A. Decide that magnet/electromagnetic devises are a good investment because they are a safe alternative for managing pain
B. Decide to decline the request for a sale because magnet therapy and electricity therapy are two very different types of modalities
C. Realize that the benefits of this type of science are still unproven and potentially unsafe
D. Decide that the pulsed electromagnet field is much safer than the static magnetic field

ANSWERS

1. ANSWER: B

Clinical hypnosis is a highly relaxed state in which patients are in an altered state of awareness, perception, or consciousness. Patients are not unconscious, and they are aware of their surroundings. The hypnotized state bypasses critical thinking and therefore the hypnotized person may be more open to suggestion. Hypnosis helps patients to dissociate from pain, especially if they are considered highly hypnotizable. This group of patients has been found to be better able to inhibit pain from conscious awareness. Functional magnetic resonance imaging showed these patients to have a significantly larger corpus callosum area involved in transferring problem-solving information between the left and right hemispheres. In a hospitalized setting, hypnosis seems to be most effective when it can be applied to a predictable, discreet event such as burn wound care procedures.

FURTHER READING

Horton JE, Crawford HJ, Harrington G, et al. Increased anterior corpus callosum size associated positively with hypnotizability and the ability to control pain. *Brain*. 2004;127(8):1741–1747.

Simpson C. Complementary and alternative medicine. In: Fishman S, Ballantyne J, Rathmell J (Eds.), *Bonica's Management of Pain*. 4th ed. Philadelphia, PA: Lippincott Williams & Wilkins; 2010:1365–1374.

2. ANSWER B

Osteopathy/osteopathic medicine is based on the belief that most diseases are related to problems in the musculoskeletal system and that structure and function of the body are related to the well-being of an individual dependent on his or her bones, muscles, ligaments, and connective tissue functioning smoothly together. Oseopathic manipulation was once used to treat all types of diseases but now is used mostly for musculoskeletal dysfunction. There is little evidence that osteopathy is effective in treating any medical condition other than lower back pain, which is only weakly supported in the literature. Osteopathic physicians earn the degree of Doctor of Osteopathic Medicine (DO), a degree equivalent, although different in certain aspects, to that of Doctor of Medicine (MD). Serious complications have been linked to osteopathic adjustments/manipulation involving the cervical spine, including arterial damage leading to stroke.

FURTHER READING

Gevirtz C. Osteopathic manipulative therapy in pain management. *Topics Pain Manage*. 2014;30(1):1–6.

Wieting J, Andary M, Holmes T, et al. Manipulation, massage, and traction. In: Frontera W (Ed.), *Delisa's Physical Medicine & Rehabilitation: Principles and Practice*. Philadelphia, PA: Lippincott Williams & Wilkins; 2010:1713–1727.

3. ANSWER E

CAM is a broad category of alternative therapies whose origins range from ancient to modern; some of the most well known are acupuncture, tai chi, homeopathy, herbal medicine, and therapeutic touch. Other CAM therapies include ayurveda, meditation, reike, hypnosis, balneotherapy, qigong, yoga, relaxation with visualization, biofeedback, magnet therapy, bee venom, copper bracelets, Feldenkrais, and myofascial release therapy. This list is not exhaustive, but it indicates the wide range of CAM therapies that are available to patients. Many Americans use or have used CAM; however, most do not voluntarily disclose this information to their medical doctor. If not specifically queried about the use of CAM, particularly the herbal remedies readily available as "over-the-counter" preparations, patients may be exposed to unnecessary harm from side effects related to drug–herb interactions. In 2012, the National Institutes of Health estimated that 30% of adults and 12% of children use or have used CAM; "natural products" such as herbal or dietary supplements were the most popular CAM therapy in the 2012 survey, and fish oil supplements were reported as the most commonly used product.

FURTHER READING

Cooper KL, Harris PE, Relton C, et al. Prevalence of visits to five types of complementary and alternative medicine practitioners by the general population: A systematic review. *Complement Ther Clin Pract*. 2013;19(4):214–220.

National Center for Complementary and Alternative Health, National Institutes of Health. Complementary, alternative, or integrative health: What's in a name? Available at https://nccih.nih.gov/sites/nccam.nih.gov/files/CAM_Basics_What_Are_CAIHA_07–07–2014.2.pdf. Accessed October 16, 2015.

Simpson C. Complementary and alternative medicine. In: Fishman S, Ballantyne J, Rathmell J (Eds.), *Bonica's Management of Pain*. 4th ed. Philadelphia, PA: Lippincott Williams & Wilkins; 2010:1365–1374.

4. ANSWER: C

Lab values differ based on the assay method used to measure serum 25-(OH)D. Sufficient vitamin D, as defined by the Institute of Medicine, is a serum 25-(OH)D value of 50–125 nmol/l. Vitamin D inadequacy is a serum 25-(OH)D value of 30–49 nmol/l, and vitamin D deficiency is a serum 25-(OH)D less than 30 nmol/l; thus, your patient is deficient in vitamin D. Continuing with physical therapy is a good recommendation, but her diffuse muscle pain may not resolve until her vitamin D deficiency is corrected. Therefore, the best recommendation at this point is for supplementation. There is no need at this point for an urgent referral to endocrinology because vitamin D deficiency is not an uncommon cause of muscle pain. However, if she does not respond to vitamin D supplementation and has persistent myofacial symptoms, a referral is an option.

FURTHER READING

Looker AC, Johnson CL, Lacher DA, et al. Vitamin D status: United States 2001–2006. NCHS data brief, No 59. Hyattsville, MD: National Center for Health Statistics; 2011.

5. ANSWER: E

Homeopathy is defined as a system of medical treatments that evolved in the 1800s and is based on two basic principles: "the law of similar" and "the law of dilutions." The law of similar uses the premise that "like cures like," and the remedy given to the ill patient is based on what would cause the same symptoms in a healthy person. The law of dilution suggests that the more dilute a remedy is prepared, the more useful it becomes to treat the malady. Homeopaths believe that dilute remedies contain energy or biologic information that the patients' body then uses to heal symptoms. There is no clear consensus regarding the effect of placebo in the treatment outcomes with homeopathy. The major objection to homeopathic medicine is that the doses of medicine prescribed in some cases are too dilute for any active ingredient to be present. One of the most common tonics in homeopathy is *Arnica montana* for muscle bruises and soreness, although its effectiveness is controversial.

FURTHER READING

Boehm K, Raak C, Cramer H, et al. Homeopathy in the treatment of fibromyalgia—A comprehensive literature review and meta-analysis. *Complement Ther Med*. 2014;22(4):731–742.
Leskowitz E. Complementary and alternative medicine in pain management. In: Warfield C, Bajwa Z (Eds.), *Principles and Practice of Pain Medicine*. 2nd ed. New York, NY: McGraw-Hill; 2004;Chap. 77.
Shang A, Huwiler-Müntener K, Nartey L, et al. Are the clinical effects of homoeopathy placebo effects? Comparative study of placebo-controlled trials of homoeopathy and allopathy. *Lancet*. 2005;366(9487):726–732.

6. ANSWER: E

Low vitamin D (25-hydroxyvitamin D (25-(OH)D) has been associated with many disorders, including cognitive dysfunction in the elderly, inflammation, muscle pain, and low bone mineral density. In addition to these conditions, there is increasing evidence of an inverse association between weight gain, cardiovascular diseases, serum lipid concentrations, glucose metabolism disorders, infectious diseases, multiple sclerosis, and cancer. It is not clear from the limited research if low vitamin D levels are causing weight gain or are just reflecting it.

FURTHER READING

Autier P, Boniol M, Pizot C, et al. Vitamin D status and ill health: A systematic review. *Lancet Diabetes Endocrinol*. 2014;2(1):76–89.

7. ANSWER C

Myofascial trigger points (TrPs) were defined originally as "a hyperirritable spot in skeletal muscle that is associated with a hypersensitive palpable nodule in a taut band" (Travell and Simons, 1983, page 5). There is a characteristic pattern of referred pain that is elicited when the TrP is palpated; TrPs are diagnosed based on palpatory exam because there is no specific objective diagnostic testing available at this time. Tender points (TPs) are frequently as tender as TrPs but are different from TrPs because there should be an absence of a referred pain "triggered" elsewhere when TPs are palpated.

Treatment options for TrPs include acupuncture, massage, myofascial release, dry needling, injection, and ischemic compression, as well as gentle exercise.

FURTHER READING

Simpson C. Complementary and alternative medicine. In: Fishman S, Ballantyne J, Rathmell J (Eds.), *Bonica's Management of Pain*. 4th ed. Philadelphia, PA: Lippincott Williams & Wilkins; 2010:1365–1374.
Travell JG, Simons DG. *Myofascial Pain and Dysfunction—The Trigger Point Manual: The Upper Extremities*. Vol. 1. Baltimore, MD: Williams & Wilkins; 1983.

8. ANSWER: E

CAM is a growing field that is becoming increasingly popular with patients. It can be helpful for patients depending on their diagnosis, and when practiced by qualified professionals, the use of CAM offers a relatively safe alternative or adjunct to traditional medical options. It is generally not covered by Medicare, but it may be covered by some Medicare Advantage plans. Other insurance plans vary in coverage, but if offered as a benefit to the insured, the cost for acupuncture treatments is usually only partially covered. One should not advise patients to try CAM based on insurance coverage alone. CAM therapies do tend to be "more natural," but this does not imply absolute safety.

FURTHER READING

Simpson C. Complementary and alternative medicine. In: Fishman S, Ballantyne J, Rathmell J (Eds.), *Bonica's Management of Pain*. 4th ed. Philadelphia, PA: Lippincott Williams & Wilkins; 2010:1365–1374.

9. ANSWER: D

Patients usually have reasons for nondisclosure, some of which can be barriers to effective communication if not identified by the physician. On the other hand, physicians may assume that the medication list is complete and fail to inquire if a patient is taking other additional drugs/medications/supplements. In1993, the *New England Journal of Medicine* published the results of a 1990 national survey of more than 1500 adults in the United States. At that time, an estimated 34% of patients had used CAM in the prior year, and 72% of patient using CAM did not share this information with their medical doctors. A follow-up survey of 2055 adults published in 1998 showed an increase in the use of CAM to 42% of responders, and the expenditures of CAM therapies had increased by 45% with $12.2 billion estimated out-of-pocket cost to patients. The three top reasons cited by patients for nondisclosure about their CAM use were (1) "didn't feel it was important for the doctor to know," (2) the doctor did not ask, and (3) it was "none of the doctor's business." Because most CAM use is considered natural by patients, there is a belief of inherent safety in these therapies.

FURTHER READING

Eisenberg DM, Davis RB, Ettner SL, et al. Trends in alternative medicine use in the United States, 1990–1997: Results of a follow-up national survey. *JAMA*. 1998;280(18):1569–1575.
Eisenberg DM, Kessler RC, Foster C, et al. Unconventional medicine in the United States: Prevalence, costs, and patterns of use. *N Engl J Med*. 1993;328(4):246–252.
Simpson C. Complementary and alternative medicine. In: Fishman S, Ballantyne J, Rathmell J (Eds.), *Bonica's Management of Pain*. 4th ed. Philadelphia, PA: Lippincott Williams & Wilkins; 2010:1365–1374.

10. ANSWER: D

A 1990 survey of more than 1500 adults in the United States found that one in three had used CAM therapies in the past year and that 72% of CAM therapy users did not share their usage with their medical doctors. The use of CAM is not limited to the younger patient population; a study published in 2000 found that 30% of the respondents surveyed, aged 65 years or older, had used either herbal therapy or chiropractic care. Given the potential interaction between some of the types of therapies, namely the herbal therapies or supplements that could interact with conventional medications, it is important to be aware that patients may be using and not reporting the use of herbal medications. Herbal products are currently not regulated by the US Food and Drug Administration (FDA), the Drug Enforcement Administration (DEA), or any regulatory body, and manufacturers of these products are not required to include a list of potential side effects.

FURTHER READING

Eisenberg DM, Kessler RC, Foster C, et al. Unconventional medicine in the United States: Prevalence, costs, and patterns of use. *N Engl J Med*. 1993;328(4):246–252.
Foster DF, Phillips RS, Hamel MB, et al. Alternative medicine use in older Americans. *J Am Geriatr Soc*. 2000;48(12):1560–1565.
Simpson C. Complementary and alternative medicine. In: Fishman S, Ballantyne J, Rathmell J (Eds.), *Bonica's Management of Pain*. 4th ed. Philadelphia, PA: Lippincott Williams & Wilkins; 2010:1365–1374.

11. ANSWER: C

Hypnosis, also referred to as hypnotherapy, involves the induction of a state of mind in which a patient experiences relaxation, focus, and concentration and also a heightened receptivity to suggestions. Hypnosis influences the affective component of pain. Hypnosis also reduces the activity in the frontal cortex and may influence descending pathways that inhibit pain perception. Children are often receptive to hypnosis-guided imagery. Physical therapy can sometimes be effective, particularly if there is truncal weakness, but this patient's physical exam findings did not reveal weakness. Tai chi can help improve balance and endurance but does not specifically address abdominal pain. Reiki is a type of energy medicine based on the principle that the therapist can channel energy into the patient by means of touch to activate the natural healing processes of the patient's body and restore physical and emotional well-being. Reiki has not been clearly shown to be useful for any health-related purpose.

FURTHER READING

Drzymalski D, Gargarian M, Harrell G. Complementary and alternative medicine. In: *Clinical Anesthesia Procedures of the Massachusetts General Hospital*. 9th ed. Philadelphia: Lippincott Williams & Wilkins; 2015.

National Center for Complementary and Alternative Health, National Institutes of Health. Reiki: An introduction. Available at https://nccih.nih.gov/health/reiki/introduction.htm

Wobst AH. Hypnosis and surgery: Past, present, and future. *Anesth Analg.* 2007;104(5):1199–1208.

NIH Consensus Conference. Acupuncture. *JAMA* 1998;280:1518–1524.

Wang S, Kain ZN, White PF. Acupuncture analgesia: II. Clinical considerations. *Anesth Analg.* 2008;106(2):611–621.

12. ANSWER: B

The use of acupuncture to treat postoperative nausea and vomiting (PONV) has been well studied. It is very effective, even in children, who may be more tolerant of laser acupuncture. A 2009 Cochrane review of 40 trials involving more than 4800 patients showed that stimulation of the acupuncture point pericardium 6 (P6) on the volar aspect of the wrist was associated with reduced risk of PONV compared with sham treatment. This point is easy to access in both awake and sedated patients. Available data have shown that acupuncture does not change anesthetic requirements for any type of surgery and has been found to be useful for managing anxiety. Acupuncture analgesia is reversible with naloxone, a finding that suggests the involvement of mu opioid receptors.

FURTHER READING

Drzymalski D, Gargarian M, Harrell G. Complementary and alternative medicine. In: *Clinical Anesthesia Procedures of the Massachusetts General Hospital.* 9th ed. Philadelphia: Lippincott Williams & Wilkins; 2015.

Lee A, Fan LT. Stimulation of the wrist acupuncture point P6 for preventing postoperative nausea and vomiting. *Cochrane Database Syst Rev.* 2009;CD003281.

13. ANSWER: D

Multiple systematic reviews have shown benefit of acupuncture over control, placebo, or no-acupuncture groups for many medical conditions. Studies suggest that acupuncture analgesia can be used as an adjuvant in the treatment of conditions such as low back pain, osteoarthritis of the knee, and neck pain. The NIH consensus conference also supports the use of acupuncture as an adjuvant or alternative treatment for other conditions as well, showing efficacy of acupuncture in adult postoperative and chemotherapy nausea and vomiting, postoperative dental pain, addiction, stroke rehabilitation, headache, menstrual cramps, tennis elbow, fibromyalgia, myofascial pain, osteoarthritis, carpal tunnel syndrome, and asthma.

FURTHER READING

Lee MS, Ernst E. Acupuncture for pain: An overview of Cochrane reviews. *Chin J Integr Med.* 2011;17(3):187–189.

14. ANSWER: A

Tai chi can be safely added to a patient's treatment regimen because it is a slow, rhythmic, weight-bearing exercise that has been shown to promote strength and balance as well as cardiorespiratory function. It is usually performed in a group setting with supervision and can be performed safely by the elderly population. Weightlifting could be a good choice in a younger healthy adult; however, weightlifting in a gym setting is usually not supervised and would not be a good option for an elderly gentleman who has never lifted weights and may not know proper lift technique. Brazilian jiu jitsu is a martial art, combat sport, and a self-defense system that focuses on grappling and ground fighting. It would not be an appropriate first exercise program for an elderly individual.

FURTHER READING

Cramer H, Lauche R, Haller H, et al. A systematic review and meta-analysis of yoga for low back pain. *Clin J Pain.* 2013;29(5):450–460.

Lee MS, Pittler MH, Ernst E. Tai chi for osteoarthritis: A systematic review. *Clin Rheumatol.* 2008;27(2):211–218.

15. ANSWER: B

Endogenous opioids as well as other neurotransmitters have been shown to be released during activation of specific acupuncture points.

Electroacupuncture with low-frequency stimulation promotes the release of endorphins and enkephalin, whereas that of high-frequency selectively increases the release of dynorphin. A combination of the two frequencies has been reported to promote a simultaneous release of multiple opioid peptides. The analgesia that is produced at lower frequency has been found to be reversible with naloxone. It has been reported that mechanical and electrical acupuncture effects can be correlated to activation of a group of receptors in the skeletal muscles, which have both low and high threshold for mechanical stimulation, and are innervated by Aδ fibers and possibly C fibers but not by destruction of sensory receptors at the site of activation. Electroacupuncture also increases endogenous cannabinoid CB2 receptors.

FURTHER READING

Han JS. Acupuncture and endorphins. *Neurosci Lett.* 2004; 361(1–3):258–261.

Hsu ES, Criscuolo CM. Acupuncture. In: Benzon H, Raja S, Fishman S, et al. (Eds.), *Essentials of Pain Medicine*. 3rd ed. Philadelphia, PA: Saunders; 2011:175–179.

16. ANSWER C

There are few side effects or adverse events of acupuncture when applied by trained individuals. The most common side effects are dizziness; euphoria; relaxation; and, rarely, adverse events, including pneumothorax, infection, and bleeding/bruising. Various forms of acupuncture can be used in children, including laser acupuncture and acupressure, which is well tolerated by children and needle phobic adults. Because acupuncture energetics can induce labor, it should be used with caution in pregnant patients, especially in the third trimester. A few insurance companies cover some part of the cost of acupuncture treatments, but Medicare is not one of them.

FURTHER READING

Wolsko P, Eisenberg D, Davis R, et al. Insurance coverage, medical conditions, and visits to alternative medicine providers: Results of a national survey. *Arch Intern Med*. 2002;162(3):281–287.

17. ANSWER D

The two major osteopathic manipulation techniques used in patients with pain are high-velocity, low-amplitude (HVLA) and myofascial release. HVLA is used in modern chiropractic care. It is a technique that employs a rapid force of brief duration that travels a short distance within the anatomic range of motion of a joint. It is contraindicated in patients with Down syndrome because of instability of the atlantoaxial joint, fracture, metastatic bone fractures, osteomyelitis, osteoporosis, and severe cases of rheumatoid arthritis. It is also contraindicated with vascular disease such as aneurysms and in those with atherosclerotic disease of the carotid arteries or vertebral arteries. Risk of osteopathic manipulation is associated more with cervical adjustments; among subjects who visited a chiropractor, the likelihood of injury was increased in those with chronic coagulation defect, inflammatory spondylopathy, osteoporosis, aortic aneurysm and dissection, or long-term use of anticoagulant therapy. Dural damage is not considered a major risk in chiropractic adjustments.

FURTHER READING

Whedon JM, Mackenzie TA, Phillips RB, et al. Risk of traumatic injury associated with chiropractic spinal manipulation in Medicare Part B beneficiaries aged 66 to 99 years. *Spine*. 2015;40(4):264–270.

18. ANSWER: A

The potential for drug–drug interaction is an important aspect of patient care, and because the use of herbal medication is growing, the consequences of drug–herb interactions are becoming more significant. Clinical studies and case reports have identified a number of herb–drug interactions potentiated by the concurrent use of herbal medicines with prescription drugs. Many patients do not view herbal preparations as "medications" and thus may not report or will underreport their use. Common herbal medicines that interact with conventional drugs include St. John's wort (*Hypericum perforatum*), ginkgo (*Ginkgo biloba*), ginger (*Zingiber officinale*), ginseng (*Panax ginseng*), garlic (*Allium sativum*), dong quai, and danshen. St. John's wort is suspected to be a significant inducer of CYP3A4 isoenzyme activity and as such reduces the activity of cyclosporine, amitriptyline, tacrolimus, warfarin, digoxin, carisoprodol, and other medications that use the CYP3A4 enzymatic pathway. Ginkgo, ginger, ginseng, and garlic can potentiate the effects of anticoagulants, causing possible increased risk for bleeding.

FURTHER READING

Benzon H. Anticoagulants and neuraxial and peripheral nerve blocks. In: Benzon H, Raja S, Fishman S, et al. (Eds.) *Essentials of Pain Medicine*. 3rd ed. Philadelphia, PA: Saunders; 2011:635–638.

Narouze S, Benzon H, Provenzano D, et al. Interventional spine and pain procedures in patients on antiplatelet and anticoagulant medications: Guidelines from the American Society of Regional Anesthesia and Pain Medicine, the European Society of Regional Anaesthesia and Pain Therapy, the American Academy of Pain Medicine, the International Neuromodulation Society, the North American Neuromodulation Society, and the World Institute of Pain. *Reg Anesth Pain Med*. 2015;40(3):182–212.

19. ANSWER: D

A 1990 survey of more than 1500 adults in the United States found that one in three had used CAM therapies in the past year and that 72% of CAM therapy users did not share their usage with their medical doctors. The use of CAM is not limited to the younger patient population; a study published in 2000 found that 30% of the respondents surveyed, aged 65 years or older, had used either herbal therapy or chiropractic care. Given the potential interaction between some of the types of therapies, namely the herbal therapies or supplements that could interact with conventional medications, it is important to be aware that patients may be using and not reporting the use of herbal medications. Herbal products are currently not regulated by the FDA, DEA, or any regulatory body, and manufacturers of these products are not required to include a list of potential side effects.

FURTHER READING

Eisenberg DM, Kessler RC, Foster C, et al. Unconventional medicine in the United States: Prevalence, costs, and patterns of use. *N Engl J Med*. 1993;328(4):246–252.

Foster DF, Phillips RS, Hamel MB, et al. Alternative medicine use in older Americans. *J Am Geriatr Soc*. 2000;48(12):1560–1565.

Simpson C. Complementary and alternative medicine. In: Fishman S, Ballantyne J, Rathmell J (Eds.), *Bonica's Management of Pain*. 4th ed. Philadelphia, PA: Lippincott Williams & Wilkins; 2010:1365–1374.

20. ANSWER: A

Ginko biloba is commonly marketed as a treatment for dementia and memory improvement and is thought to exert it effects by inhibition of platelet activation factor. Ginseng is a popular herbal supplement that is proposed to improve physical and sexual function. It has not been proven to be superior to *Ginko biloba* for cognitive dysfunction. Fluoxetine is a selective serotonin reuptake inhibitor (SSRI). SSRIs are group of drugs known to cause increased bleeding risk especially when used in conjunction with nonsteroidal anti-inflammatory drugs (NSAIDs) and other antiplatelet drugs, as well as certain herbal supplements such as *Ginko biloba*. ASRA guidelines suggest that the patient be advised to discontinue *Ginko biloba* 1 week before spinal procedures and to perform antiplatelet testing.

FURTHER READING

Narouze S, Benzon H, Provenzano D, et al. Interventional spine and pain procedures in patients on antiplatelet and anticoagulant medications: Guidelines from the American Society of Regional Anesthesia and Pain Medicine, the European Society of Regional Anaesthesia and Pain Therapy, the American Academy of Pain Medicine, the International Neuromodulation Society, the North American Neuromodulation Society, and the World Institute of Pain. *Reg Anesth Pain Med*. 2015;40(3):182–212.

21. ANSWER: E

A flare-up of the patient's fibromyalgia syndrome is unlikely with only the two symptoms noted, and symptoms of an upper respiratory tract infection usually do not present with increasing anxiety. The fact that she has had her fibromyalgia symptoms under good control should prompt you to question her about other treatments that she might be seeking. A urine drug screen would rule out opioid use but would not help you determine the cause of her shortness of breath. Acupuncture may be effective in some fibromyalgia patients to reduce pain and stiffness and improve overall well-being. One of the major risks of acupuncture is pneumothorax, which may be asymptomatic or may present with shortness of breath and cough; if the pneumothorax is large enough, the patient may experience "air hunger," which might provoke anxiety. Acupuncture needles are typically placed only millimeters deep; however, in different Asian cultures, it is customary to place the acupuncture needles deeper or even break them off at the surface, which would allow them to migrate through the tissues, thus increasing the risk of pneumothorax.

FURTHER READING

White A. A cumulative review of the range and incidence of significant adverse events associated with acupuncture. *Acupunct Med*. 2004;22(3):122–133.

22. ANSWER C

The effects of dietary supplements on platelet function and coagulation are not well described, but it is known that garlic inhibits platelet aggregation, and its effect on hemostasis appears to last 7 days. The active compound in garlic (allicin) inhibits platelet aggregation by a variety of actions. The 2015 ASRA guidelines suggest that platelet function testing be done prior to high-risk procedures, especially in patients who are also using NSAIDs aspirin or SSRIs, and the garlic supplement be discontinued at least 7 days before the procedure. Bee pollen is considered a nutritious source of vitamins, minerals, proteins, and carbohydrates. Bee pollen is not the same as other substances derived from bees that are sometimes used as supplements, such as bee venom, royal jelly, and honey, and it has not been found to have effects on platelet function. Supplementing with vitamin K would not be necessary and may actually place the patient at increased risk for untoward events.

FURTHER READING

Narouze S, Benzon H, Provenzano D, et al. Interventional spine and pain procedures in patients on antiplatelet and anticoagulant medications: Guidelines from the American Society of Regional Anesthesia and Pain Medicine, the European Society of Regional Anaesthesia and Pain Therapy, the American Academy of Pain Medicine, the International Neuromodulation Society, the North American Neuromodulation Society, and the World Institute of Pain. *Reg Anesth Pain Med*. 2015;40(3):182–212.

23. ANSWER: E

Relaxation and imagery are one form of mind–body therapy that has been linked to reductions in pain in certain conditions, such as chronic low back pain, cancer pain, and rheumatoid arthritis. It is often included as part of cognitive–behavioral treatment programs. Relaxation and imagery exercises are similar to meditation but do not involve the use of repetitive words or phrases; more emphasis is placed on deep breathing techniques and release of tension, and guided imagery serves as a distraction by introducing alternative thoughts, images, or ways to perceive pain. Compared to hypnosis, relaxation and imagery appear to have a greater impact on physiologic changes such as heart rate, blood pressure, and alterations in blood flow.

FURTHER READING

Simpson C. Complementary and alternative medicine. In: Fishman S, Ballantyne J, Rathmell J (Eds.), *Bonica's Management of Pain*. 4th ed. Philadelphia, PA: Lippincott Williams & Wilkins; 2010:1365–1374.

24. ANSWER: D

The main active ingredient in marijuana is Δ^9-tetrahydrocannabinol. Cannabinoids inhibit the growth of different types of tumor cells, including glioma cells and pancreatic ductal adenocarcinoma. Two oral formulations of cannabinoids, dronabinol (Marinol) and nabilone (Cesamet), are approved by the FDA for use in chemotherapy-induced nausea and vomiting refractory to conventional antiemetic therapy. Cannabinoids also stimulate appetite and food intake, and they may have a role in the management of cancer-induced cachexia. Cannabinoids act in the body by mimicking endogenous substances (endocannabinoids) that activate specific cell surface receptors. There are two main cannabinoid receptors: CB1 and CB2.

The endocannabinoid system is widely distributed in the brain and spinal cord. CB1 receptors are concentrated in the basal ganglia, spinal cord/dorsal root ganglia, cerebellum, and hippocampus as well as peripheral nerves. CB2 receptors are found in the brain as well but at far less density than CB1 receptors. CB2 are also found in the gastrointestinal system and in various parts of the peripheral nervous system. It is interesting to note that electroacupuncture increases endogenous cannabinoid CB2 receptors.

FURTHER READING

Eisenberg E, Peterson D. Neuropathic pain pharmacotherapy. In: Fishman S, Ballantyne J, Rathmell J (Eds.), *Bonica's Management of Pain*. 4th ed. Philadelphia, PA: Lippincott Williams & Wilkins; 2010:1203–1204.

Koppel B, Brust J, Fife T, et al. Systematic review: Efficacy and safety of medical marijuana in selected neurologic disorders: Report of the Guideline Development Subcommittee of the American Academy of Neurology. *Neurology*. 2014;82(17):1556–1563.

25. ANSWER: D

Neutraceuticals is a relatively new term coined in 1989 that combines "nutrition" and "pharmaceutical." The term is applied to products derived from food sources that are purported to provide extra health benefits in addition to the basic nutritional value found in foods. They can be considered nonspecific biological therapies used to promote general well-being, control symptoms, and prevent malignant processes, although there are relatively few good-quality studies to strongly support such assumptions. Because of the potential nutritional and therapeutic effects and a presumed positive safety profile, nutraceuticals have attracted considerable interest in the past decade. They are considered helpful as antioxidants, as well as being supportive of immune function. Some studies have suggested that they also exhibit disease-modifying actions related to oxidative stress including allergy, Alzheimer's disease, cardiovascular diseases, cancer, eye conditions, Parkinson's diseases, and obesity.

FURTHER READING

Cotter A, Bartoli L, Rosenfeld J, et al. Complementary and alternative medicine. In: Frontera W (Ed.), *Delisa's Physical Medicine & Rehabilitation: Principles and Practice*. Philadelphia, PA: Lippincott Williams & Wilkins; 2010:2124–2127.

Huang HY, Caballero B, Chang S, et al. The efficacy and safety of multivitamin and mineral supplement use to prevent cancer and chronic disease in adults: A systematic review for a NIH state-of-the-science conference. *Ann Int Med*. 2006;145(5):372–385.

26. ANSWER C

Electricity and magnetism are two aspects of the same force. Moving electric charges generates magnetic fields, and varying magnetic fields will generate an electric current. Magnets and electromagnetic fields are used for a variety of different indications and have been around for centuries. Various strengths of magnets and electromagnetic devices have been studied for musculoskeletal and neuropathic pain and widely marketed for health purposes. The list of beneficial effects that have been claimed for magnetic field therapy is large, but there is little evidence to support its use. Pulsed magnetic field therapy (PMFT) mats are becoming popular along with the numerous magnetic jewelry products that are available. A recent study found that PMFT mats can exceed International Commission on Non-Ionizing Radiation Protection (ICNIRP) 1998 reference levels and ICNIRP 2010 basic restrictions. The 2010 reference levels are based on both central and peripheral nervous system effects. The evidence for the use of magnets and electromagnetic fields is inconsistent. Larger randomized controlled trials with consistent, statistically significant results are required before PMFT mats can be recommended as a valid pain therapy.

FURTHER READING

De Santis V, Douglas M, Nadakuduti J, et al. Human exposure from pulsed magnetic field therapy mats: A numerical case study with three commercial products. *Bioelectromagnetics*. 2015;36(2):149–161.

Lee FH, Raja SN. Complementary and alternative medicine in chronic pain. *Pain*. 2011;152:28–30.

Simpson C. C0omplementary and alternative medicine. In: Fishman S, Ballantyne J, Rathmell J (Eds.), *Bonica's Management of Pain*. 4th ed. Philadelphia, PA: Lippincott Williams & Wilkins; 2010:1365–1374.

15.

WORK REHABILITATION

Robert Yang

INTRODUCTION

Pain has wide-ranging effects on physical function, emotional well-being, and the ability to fulfill social roles. When pain affects a patient's ability to work, restoring the patient to his or her optimal function may require more than healing of the initial injury. Although a pain physician may not be managing a patient's work rehabilitation, understanding the importance of multidisciplinary treatment and rehabilitation optimizes comprehensive and integrated treatment.

Patients who are unable to work often become involved in disability or the workers' compensation systems. A pain physician should have an appreciation of medicolegal aspects of work rehabilitation because these issues can affect the treatment, and such understanding can help the physician advocate more effectively for patients in this system.

QUESTIONS

1. Each of the following is true regarding the flag system to identify risk factors in patients with low back pain except:

- A. Red flags are signs or symptoms that should prompt the health care provider to rule out serious and specific injury.
- B. Yellow flag symptoms were developed to address psychosocial disability determinants.
- C. An example of a yellow flag symptom is unhelpful beliefs about pain, such as an injury is uncontrollable and likely to worsen.
- D. Clinical depression is a yellow flag symptom that impacts psychosocial functioning.

2. Which of the following factors has not been associated with increased risk of chronic low back pain?

- A. Advanced age
- B. History of low back pain

- C. Job involving heavy labor
- D. Depression
- E. All of the above have been associated with increased risk of chronic pain.

3. A job that requires a patient to lift 20–50 pounds occasionally, 10–25 pounds frequently, and 10 pounds constantly is classified into which of the following categories according to the *Dictionary of Occupational Titles* standards?

- A. Sedentary
- B. Light
- C. Medium
- D. Heavy
- E. Very heavy

4. In general, with regard to economic analysis of disability management interventions, which of the following is not true?

- A. Given the overall poor quality of the economic analyses of disability management, no significant conclusions can be drawn about the effectiveness of these interventions.
- B. There is moderate evidence for interventions that include a physiotherapy component.
- C. There is moderate evidence for interventions that include a work/vocational rehabilitation component.
- D. There is moderate evidence to support improved patient–employer/workplace communication.

5. The following statements regarding return-to-work (RTW) expectations are true except:

- A. Patient RTW expectations are set early in the course of injury.
- B. Neither patients nor providers are accurate in their estimates of time to RTW.

C. Patients with negative RTW expectations prior to seeing a provider are less likely to have resumed work in 1–3 months.

D. Patient RTW expectations have a high predictive accuracy for length of time to RTW.

6. Which of the following is not true about RTW coordinators/case managers?

A. They are not required to undergo specific training and licensing requirements in medical and legal aspects of disability, social problem-solving, and workplace assessment.

B. Common activities of RTW coordinators include assessing workplace factors, developing plans for transitional duty, and facilitating communication and agreement among stakeholders.

C. They commonly have backgrounds in nursing or another health-related field and have knowledge of common disabling medical conditions.

D. Given that early RTW reduces the costs of an injury episode, RTW coordinators are usually employer-based.

7. The following statements about the Fear-Avoidance Belief Questionnaire are true except:

A. It is one of the most common instrument used to assess fear-avoidance beliefs.

B. It has a Physical Activity and Work subscale.

C. It has not been validated for chronic low back pain.

D. It requires that all items be completed because there is no procedure to adjust for incomplete items.

8. Which of the following is not true about fear-avoidance beliefs (FABs)?

A. FABs are generally associated with poorer RTW outcomes.

B. Clinician assessment of fear-avoidance behaviors correlates with patient self-reported FABs.

C. Pain intensity and FABs are difficult to evaluate independently.

D. The distribution of informational material addressing FABs has been shown to be effective for reducing them in patients with high FABs.

9. Successful RTW may be complicated by:

A. Preinjury problems with workplace relationships

B. Suspicious coworkers

C. Social dislocation with modified work

D. Challenging job modifications

E. All of the above

10. Which of the following is true regarding the epidemiology of work-related injuries?

A. The majority of patients will recover and return to work within a few months.

B. Although a small percentage of patients account for those with persistent pain and disability, litigation costs associated with such cases drive the majority of compensation costs.

C. Timing of return to work is best done after completion of healing from the initial injury.

D. The biomedical treatment approach should predominate in the acute phase of treatment, with biopsychosocial approaches reserved for cases in which recovery is delayed or slower than expected.

11. The rate of functional improvement of patients undergoing occupational rehabilitation is:

A. Worse for patients who are in shorter pain rehabilitation programs because gains do not have as much opportunity to compound

B. The same for older and younger patients

C. Directly proportional to the rate of pain reduction

D. Directly correlated with functional capacity evaluation (FCE) performance at program entry (i.e., a higher FCE performance is correlated with a greater rate of functional improvement)

E. Rapid for patients whose limitations are primarily physical in nature

12. Which of the following is true regarding the use of FCEs to reduce the risk of reinjury?

A. Because of the multifactorial nature of factors that affect RTW, longer FCEs are better at predicting reinjury rates than shorter evaluations.

B. FCEs may improve RTW times but do not appear to predict reinjury rates.

C. Rather than absolute performance on an FCE, performance as measured by the number of failed tests in the assessment is correlated with reinjury.

D. FCEs are ineffective in reducing reinjury rates because significant numbers of injured workers are asked to perform tasks that exceed their measured capabilities.

13. Which of the following is the most comprehensive type of FCE?

A. Functional goal setting

B. Work capacity evaluation

C. Occupational matching

D. Disability rating

E. Job matching

14. Which of the following is not one of the factors used to evaluate expert testimony in the Daubert criteria?

A. Whether the theory can be or has been tested—that is, whether it has been tested to determine if it can be falsified
B. Whether the theory or technique has been subjected to peer review and publication
C. The known or potential rate of error and the existence and maintenance of standards controlling the technique's operation
D. Whether the theory or technique has been generally accepted by the scientific community to which it belongs
E. Whether the theory or technique provides firm conclusions when applied to the issue at hand

15. For patients with low back pain of less than 6 months' duration, the following statements are true except:

A. Fear-avoidance behaviors are associated with greater pain, disability, and less RTW at 1-year follow-up.
B. Reducing fear-avoidance behaviors results in decreased pain, disability, and greater RTW.
C. Treatments aimed at reducing fear-avoidance behaviors are more effective than treatments based on the biomedical model.
D. The treatment of fear-avoidance behavior is more effective after physical healing is complete.

16. Which of the following is false regarding the use of medical factors as a predictive factor for outcomes in low back pain?

A. Research findings are difficult to interpret because most studies present findings as statistically significant odds ratio rather than as correct classification rates for the studied predictor variables.
B. Research findings are difficult to interpret because they have produced inconsistent and sometimes contradictory findings.
C. Medical factors are most predictive early in the course of injury and become steadily less so over time.
D. Medical factors are most predictive later in the course of injury once the recovery course has stabilized.

17. Which of the following is true regarding anatomic/biomedical predictive factors versus psychosocial factors in terms of disability?

A. Discography is more predictive than routine magnetic resonance imaging findings when determining future disability.

B. Although no single anatomic factor is predictive, a composite of physical examination, imaging studies, and discography has moderate predictive power for future disability events.
C. Psychosocial variables strongly predict both long- and short-term disability events.
D. A combination of anatomic and psychosocial variables are required to predict future disability events.

18. Which of the following statements is true regarding the timing of interdisciplinary functional rehabilitation programs for chronic disabling musculoskeletal disorders?

A. Patients who receive interdisciplinary rehabilitation earlier are more likely to return to their original job open.
B. Results are confounded by the non-inclusion of participants who did not complete the program, which potentially overestimates the benefits of early rehabilitation.
C. Patients who were treated within 4–8 months of onset of disability had comparable rates of success to patients who were seen more than 18 months after the onset of disability.
D. Overall early initiation of interdisciplinary rehabilitation results in significant reductions of the overall cost for patients.
E. All of the above are true.

19. Which of the following statements about fear of injury, disability, and aerobic fitness is true?

A. All three are significantly correlated with each other.
B. Fear of injury is correlated with aerobic fitness but not with disability.
C. Fear of injury is correlated with disability but not with aerobic fitness.
D. Disability is correlated with aerobic fitness but not with fear of injury.
E. None of these three are correlated with each other.

20. Which of the following scales is associated with better function with higher scores?

A. Pain Catastrophizing Scale
B. Tampa Scale of Kinesiophobia
C. Beck Depression Inventory II
D. Pain Self-Efficacy Questionnaire

21. Which of the following is not true regarding the amount of time out of work following a musculoskeletal injury?

A. The median number of days of absence from work for a low back injury is approximately 14 days and is shorter for other musculoskeletal injuries.

B. 80–90% of patients return to work within 1 or 2 months.

C. Of those out of work for at least 6 months, only 50% will return to work.

D. Of those out of work for at least 1 year, only 5% will return to work.

22. Which of the following pain scales is an adjunct to one of the other scales?

A. McGill Pain Questionnaire

B. Dartmouth Pain Questionnaire

C. Pain Disability Index

D. Pain Patient Profile

23. Which of the following statements is true regarding the biopsychosocial rehabilitation programs (BRPs) for the treatment of chronic low back pain?

A. BRPs are more effective than usual care in reducing pain but not disability.

B. BRPs are more effective than usual care in reducing disability but not pain.

C. BRPs are more effective than usual care in reducing pain and disability.

D. BRPs are more effective than usual care in reducing pain and disability as well as increasing the odds of being at work within 1 year.

E. BRPs are more effective than usual care at increasing the odds of being at work within 1 year but not reducing pain and disability at 12 months post-discharge from BRPs.

24. Which of the following statements is true about RTW notes and forms?

A. The person receiving the note may be a layperson who may not understand the information being conveyed.

B. Although these forms use plain English words, the terms used may have specific technical meanings that are meant to convey special meaning.

C. These forms frequently describe work-related activities, if any, that must be limited, modified, or avoided.

D. These forms frequently describe the consequences of failing to adhere to limitations of work-related activities.

25. The following illustrate different ways that work rehabilitation differs from traditional medical treatment except:

A. The patient is the rehabilitator.

B. The goals of treatment are functional.

C. The treatment modalities are psychosocial.

D. The approach to treatment involves the whole body.

26. Which of the following is not a component of work rehabilitation?

A. Musculoskeletal exercise

B. Aerobic training

C. Education

D. Work activity

E. All of the above are components of work rehabilitation.

27. Which of the following would be evidence that the patient is not complying with a work rehabilitation program?

A. A patient complains of muscle soreness with exercise progression.

B. In his last week in the program, a patient has a flare-up of pain, which limits progress.

C. A patient develops joint swelling and is unable to complete the rest of the program that day.

D. A patient takes extra breaks so she can perform better while exercising.

28. Maximal medical improvement (MMI) is:

A. The point at which a patient is no longer expected to improve within the next year with or without additional medical treatment

B. The point at which acute healing from the injury is complete and the patient can begin work rehabilitation

C. The maximum benefit expected from a specific medical treatment if rendered to the patient at the current time

D. A measurement of the disparity between the patient's current state and the theoretical optimal state given the patient's age and major preinjury comorbidities

29. Reasonable accommodations:

A. Require an employer to make adjustments to job structure, work space, work schedule, or tools to allow a person to perform a job successfully

B. Are typically determined by an administrative law judge and the person requesting it

C. Only cover physical limitations of individuals with disabilities

D. Are defined by the Americans with Disabilities Act

ANSWERS

1. ANSWER: D

Red flags are signs of symptoms of a potentially serious or specific condition that should be ruled out, such as spinal infection or cancer. Yellow flags were described by Kendall et al. in 1997 as an analogue to red flags in the area of psychosocial disability determinants rather than medical conditions. Yellow flags are centered around aspects of thoughts, feelings, and behaviors. Examples include catastrophizing; extreme pain disproportional to the injury; and unhelpful beliefs about pain and work, such as "If I go back to work, my pain will get worse."

Blue and black flags have also been defined in addition to red and yellow flags. Blue flags refer specifically to those issues related to perceptions about the relationship between work and health—for example, the belief that workplace supervisors and coworkers are unsupportive. Black flags refer to problems that are systemic or contextual in nature, such as conflict with the insurance carrier or a workplace that has little flexibility on work modifications.

Orange flags are typically psychiatric in nature, such as clinical depression or personality disorder. They differ from yellow flags in that they are more akin in severity to the red flags for medical injury alerting a clinician to serious problems that could be psychiatric and require referral to a specialist.

FURTHER READING

Kendall NA, Linton SJ, Main CJ. *Guide to Assessing Psychosocial Yellow Flags in Acute Low Back Pain: Risk Factors for Long-Term Disability and Work Loss*. Wellington, NZ: Accident Rehabilitation and Compensation Insurance Corporation of New Zealand and the National Health Committee; 1997.

Loisel P, Anema J. *Handbook of Work Disability—Prevention and Management*. New York, NY: Springer-Verlag; 2014.

Nicholas MK, Linton SJ, Watson PJ, et al. Early identification and management of psychological risk factors ("yellow flags") in patients with low back pain: A reappraisal. *Phys Ther*. 2011;91(5):737–753.

Shaw WS, van der Windt DA, Main CJ, et al.; Decade of the Flags Working Group. Early patient screening and intervention to address individual level occupational factors ("blue flags") in back disability. *J Occup Rehab*. 2009;19(1):64–80.

2. ANSWER: E

Because of the relatively high costs created by disability related to low back pain, there has been much interest in understanding what factors may be risk factors for the development of chronic pain. All of the factors listed in this question have been associated with the risk of developing low back pain. Other factors that have been associated with increased risk of chronic low back pain include workers in blue-collar jobs, low level of job satisfaction, and poor ratings from their supervisors. Overall, there is considerable heterogeneity (i.e., poor agreement between studies) in exactly which factors are associated with an increased risk of chronicity. Progression to chronic pain is more closely dependent on demographic, psychosocial, and occupational factors than on the medical characteristics of the spinal condition. Treatment should be prompt and comprehensive in these patients because the likelihood of a return to work decreases rapidly as sick leave duration increases.

FURTHER READING

Valat JP, Goupille P, Védere V. Low back pain: Risk factors for chronicity. *Rev Rhum Engl Ed*. 1997;64(3):189–194.

3. ANSWER: C

Because the work is often characterized by these terms, it is important to have a good understanding of these categories:

S—Sedentary work: Exerting up to 10 pounds of force occasionally and/or a negligible amount of force frequently to lift, carry, push, pull, or otherwise move objects. Sedentary work involves sitting most of the time, but it may involve walking or standing for brief periods of time. Jobs are sedentary if walking and standing are required only occasionally and all other sedentary criteria are met.

L—Light work: Exerting up to 20 pounds of force occasionally, and/or up to 10 pounds of force frequently, and/or a negligible amount of force constantly to move objects. Although the weight lifted may be only a negligible amount, a job should be rated light work (1) when it requires walking or standing to a significant degree; (2) when it requires sitting most of the time but entails pushing and/or pulling of arm or leg controls; and/or (3) when it requires working at a production rate pace entailing the constant pushing and/or pulling of materials even though the weight of those materials is negligible.

M—Medium work: Exerting 20–50 pounds of force occasionally, and/or 10–25 pounds of force frequently, and/or greater than negligible up to 10 pounds of force constantly to move objects.

H—Heavy work: Exerting 50–100 pounds of force occasionally, and/or 25–50 pounds of force frequently, and/or 10–20 pounds of force constantly to move objects.

V—Very heavy work: Exerting in excess of 100 pounds of force occasionally, and/or in excess of 50 pounds of force frequently, and/or in excess of 20 pounds of force constantly to move objects. Physical demand requirements are in excess of those for heavy work.

FURTHER READING

US Department of Labor. The dictionary of occupational titles. Appendix C: Components of the definition trailer: Physical demands–Strength rating. Available at http://www.oalj.dol.gov/PUBLIC/DOT/REFERENCES/DOTAPPC.HTM.

4. ANSWER: A

The cited study reviewed the literature and found many articles that did not meet the study criteria for inclusion. The authors were able to arrive at a number of conclusions regarding several components of disability management interventions. The study authors clustered the interventions into four groups to assess whether they were worth undertaking based on their financial merits. They found that there was moderate evidence to support studies that included an educational component, a physiotherapy component, and a work/vocational component. They found limited evidence for programs with behavioral components.

For the programs with work/vocational components, they found that key features of the intervention included (1) early contact with the worker by the workplace, (2) a work accommodation offer, (3) contact between the health care provider and the workplace, (4) ergonomic work site visit, and (5) RTW coordination.

As clinicians, the goal of health care treatment is the improvement of the patient's health and well-being. Being familiar with evidence that supports the economic benefits of pursuing comprehensive treatment can assist one to advocate effectively for patients.

FURTHER READING

Tompa E, de Oliveira C, Dolinschi R, et al. A systematic review of disability management interventions with economic evaluations. *Occup Rehabil.* 2008;18(1):16–26.

5. ANSWER: D

Patient RTW expectations are set relatively early in the course of injury for patients and play a significant role in the outcomes of patients after injury. Given that these expectations form earlier than the time when one would expect recovery in the biomedical model, it is important for practitioners to address patient concerns about return to work early in the course of treatment to alleviate uncertainty and educate about the possibility of spontaneous recovery. Interestingly, Kapoor et al. found that patients with a previous history of receiving medical care for low back pain had greater optimism about RTW.

FURTHER READING

Kapoor S, Shaw WS, Pransky G, et al. Initial patient and clinician expectations of return to work after acute onset of work-related low back pain. *J Occup Environ Med.* 2006;48(11):1173–1180.

6. ANSWER: D

The RTW process can involve complex communication between many parties, including clinicians, the patient, the employer, and the insurer. An RTW coordinator can facilitate such communication to prevent mistrust and disappointment that can lead to a failure of a patient to return to work. The person in this role can have many titles, including case manager, rehabilitation facilitator, or a qualified rehabilitation consultant.

Despite the finding in studies that an RTW coordinator can reduce costs and also the duration of disability, the role of an RTW coordinator is loosely defined. Although most RTW coordinators come from a clinical background (nursing, physical therapy, occupational therapy, psychology, case management, or vocational rehabilitation), there is no requirement that they must do so.

Activities of RTW coordinators include the assessment of worker and workplace circumstances; developing detailed plans for work modifications; and meeting on site with the worker, supervisor, and other stakeholders to facilitate agreement. Approaches that RTW coordinators can use include building rapport with workers and engaging them in collaborative problem-solving to overcome barriers to RTW or facilitating communication and mediating RTW arrangements between workers and employers. RTW coordinators can also facilitate the development of plans for transitional duty.

In most studies reviewed, the RTW coordinators were either independent or hospital based, not employer based.

FURTHER READING

Shaw W, Hong QN, Pransky G, et al. A literature review describing the role of return-to-work coordinators in trial programs and interventions designed to prevent workplace disability. *J Occup Rehabil.* 2008;18(1):2–15.

7. ANSWER: C

The Fear-Avoidance Belief Questionnaire (FABQ) was developed by Dr. Gordon Waddell to investigate FABs in patients with chronic low back pain. It is extremely important to ensure all items are completed because there is no procedure to adjust for incomplete items. The validity and reliability of the FABQ have been established for chronic low back pain. It also may be useful for other chronic pain conditions.

The FABQ questionnaire consists of 16 items, with each item scored from 0 to 6. Higher scores on the FABQ are indicative of greater fear and avoidance beliefs. The FABQ has two subscales, the Work Subscale (FABQ-W) and the Physical Activity Subscale (FABQ-PA), which facilitate the identification of the patient's beliefs about how work and physical activity affect pain. The scale is useful for patient assessment because a strong relationship exists between elevated FABs and chronic disability secondary to low back pain.

FURTHER READING

Lethem J, Slade PD, Troup JDG, et al. Outline of a fear avoidance model of exaggerated pain perceptions. *Behav Res Ther*. 1983;21:401–408.
Waddell C, Newton M, Henderson I, et al. A Fear-Avoidance Beliefs Questionnaire (FABQ) and the role of fear-avoidance beliefs in chronic low back pain and disability. *Pain*. 1993;52:157–168.

8. ANSWER: B

Fear avoidance beliefs and behaviors are generally correlated with worse outcomes in several areas, including RTW outcomes. Pain intensity and FABs often occur together, and sorting out the independent contribution of each factor is difficult.

Assessment of fear avoidance behaviors can be difficult for clinicians to gauge accurately, so a standardized instrument such as the FABQ is used.

FURTHER READING

Calley DQ, Jackson S, Collins H, et al. Identifying patient fear-avoidance beliefs by physical therapists managing patients with low back pain. *J Orthop Sports Phys Ther*. 2010;40:774–783.
Wertli MM, Rasmussen-Barr E, Held U, et al. Fear-avoidance beliefs— A moderator of treatment efficacy in patients with low back pain: A systematic review. *Spine J*. 2014;14:2658–2678.

9. ANSWER: E

Unfortunately, although by no means a comprehensive list, all these are potential challenges that may face an injured worker in returning to work. A physician should be aware of factors that may impede a patient's successful RTW. Difficulties with coworkers or with supervisors have been found in several studies to be a significant negative predictive factor for successful RTW. Coworkers who are suspicious about the patient malingering can also interfere with successful RTW.

Patients are sometimes moved into a different area and work at a different job with different coworkers. Thus, they are placed in an unfamiliar environment and job with different coworkers who may have a different work culture. Being outside of a familiar setting may make RTW more challenging.

Job modifications can be difficult to follow for many reasons. A patient may have difficultly trying to follow work restrictions/modified work in the work setting because they want to give full effort or find new ways of doing tasks that are too difficult or time-consuming. The restrictions might require the employer to provide equipment and modify the workplace to allow the patient to return to work. If too burdensome, employers may opt to delay RTW efforts until such restrictions can be lifted.

FURTHER READING

Berecki-Gisolf J, Clay FJ, Collie A, et al. Predictors of sustained return to work after work-related injury or disease: Insights from workers' compensation claims records. *J Occup Rehabil*. 2012;22(3):283–291.
MacEachen E, Clarke J, Franche RL, et al; Workplace-Based Return to Work Literature Review Group. Systematic review of the qualitative literature on return to work after injury. *Scand J Work Environ Health*. 2006;32(4):257–269.

10. ANSWER: A

Individuals who experience work-related injuries engage in a wide range of occupations and activities. Although the vast majority of patients with work-related injuries return to work quickly, the few who do not can be out of work for months or even years. The majority of costs associated with work-related injuries are time-loss and health care related, not litigation related.

Planning for early RTW, even if to a modified job/role, can occur prior to completion of healing and is associated with better outcomes.

Although biomedical treatment approaches need to be implemented early in the course of treatment, biopsychosocial approaches should not be delayed until the recovery course is delayed.

FURTHER READING

Nastasia I, Coutu MF, Tcaciuc R. Topics and trends in research on non-clinical interventions aimed at preventing prolonged work disability in workers compensated for work-related musculoskeletal disorders (WRMSDs): A systematic, comprehensive literature review. *Disabil Rehabil*. 2014;36(22):1841–1856.

11. ANSWER: E

The referenced study investigated the rate of functional change for 582 patients with workers' compensation claims for a variety of musculoskeletal complaints. The factors that affect the rate of functional change are multifactorial and include physical, demographic, clinical, and environmental factors. Some of the factors that were associated with a greater rate of functional improvement during occupational rehabilitation include younger age, male gender, lower reported disability on admission, and the absence of comorbidities.

Patients with specific conditions such as fractures typically displayed slow, steady improvement in function consistent with gains in physical strength and conditioning and healing of the underlying injury. For patients who displayed rapid improvements in function that were nonphysiologic, such improvements were attributed to behavioral changes due to altered beliefs and expectations about their condition. Patients limited primarily by psychosocial factors such as fear-avoidance behaviors have the potential to progress rapidly in such circumstances. This factor also potentially explains why a low FCE performance at program entry was found to be correlated with a greater rate of functional improvement.

Although there is a relationship between pain reduction and functional improvement in occupational programs, the relationship is not directly proportional. Improvements in function can occur in the absence of pain reduction, and generally improvements in function tend to be greater than reduction in pain.

FURTHER READING

Gross DP, Haws C, Niemelainen R. What is the rate of functional improvement during occupational rehabilitation in workers' compensation claimants? *J Occup Rehabil.* 2012;22:292–300.

12. ANSWER: B

The following is one of the key questions for employers after a worker has been injured: When can the employee return to work and under what conditions?

Although FCEs are often performed to answer this question, the supporting evidence for the predictive value of such testing for reinjury is fairly limited. Shortened forms of FCE evaluation as well as use of a single test, the floor-to-waist lift, were found to be just as predictive as the full evaluation. FCEs are found to be weakly associated with shorter RTW times but not with reinjury rates. Using the number of failed tests as a criteria has not been found to be predictive for outcomes.

FURTHER READING

Gross D, Battie M, Cassidy JD. The prognostic value of functional capacity evaluation in patients with chronic low back pain: Part 1. Spine. 29(8):914–919.
Gross D, Battie M. The prognostic value of functional capacity evaluation in patients with chronic low back pain: Part 2. *Spine.* 2004;29(8):920–924
Mahmud N, Schonstein E, Schaafsma F, et al. Functional capacity evaluations for the prevention of occupational re-injuries in injured workers. *Cochrane Database Syst Rev.* 2010;7(7):CD007290.

13. ANSWER: B

An FCE is a standardized battery of tests that is intended to assess a patient's ability to perform specific tasks safely. Depending on the circumstances of the patient, a physician may order an FCE for a variety of purposes. Understanding the nature and extent of the FCE evaluation aids a clinician in ordering and making use of the results.

Functional goal-setting measures the usual functional consequences of the impairment at the component level, such as joint range of motion or strength. This information can be used to set functional goals for therapy as well as provide objective performance measures to assess improvement.

When generating disability ratings, FCEs may provide additional information on the functional losses as a result of impairments. Such information is often used to support a treating physician's opinion regarding the patient's disability as well as work restrictions.

Job matching involves an assessment of a patient's ability to perform the essential functions of a job. The scope of type of FCE is determined using information from a job analysis to determine the physical demands of a job, whereas information about the impairment is from the medical examination.

Occupation matching is a more comprehensive evaluation because the patient's abilities are matched to the demands of an occupational group. The information on the demands of the occupation is typically defined in the US Department of Labor's *Dictionary of Occupational Titles* or the O*NET system. This testing is generally more complex and involved than job matching because it includes all job tasks for a variety of jobs rather than a single one.

Work capacity evaluation seeks to match the patient's abilities to the demands of all occupations in the competitive labor market and is the most comprehensive of the purposes listed in this explanation. It also may be the most demanding and lengthy of these tests.

FURTHER READING

Matheson LN. The functional capacity evaluation. In: Demeter SL, Andersson GBJ (Eds.), *Disability Evaluation.* St. Louis, MO: Mosby; 2003:748–768.

O*NET Resource Center. Available at https://www.onetcenter.org/overview.html. Accessed July 25, 2015.

14. ANSWER: E

Because cases involving injured workers often also involve administrative law or medicolegal settings, the evaluating clinician's opinions and conclusions may be subjected to additional scrutiny. An understanding of how evidence is evaluated may assist the clinician in choosing what tests to conduct.

Until the Supreme Court formulated the Daubert criteria in 1993, the previous standard had been that the theory or technique has been "generally accepted" by the scientific community. The Daubert criteria significantly raised the bar for evidence. Clinical observation and experience from clinical practice may be insufficient to address certain questions. Widely tested, highly structured tests may be favored because they more readily meet Daubert criteria.

Although ideally option E would be true, it is not one of the Daubert criteria.

FURTHER READING

Kulich RJ, Driscoll J, Prescott JC, et al. The Daubert standard: A primer for pain physicians. *Pain Med*. 2003;4(1):75–80.

15. ANSWER: C

In research studies, less effective treatment outcomes were associated with mixing of the study populations.

Fear-avoidance beliefs are one of the commonly used models to explain the impact of psychological factors on pain and disability. Negative beliefs about pain and illness can lead to dysfunctional or catastrophizing responses, which result in fear of activity.

FURTHER READING

Wertli MM, Rasmussen-Barr E, Held U, et al. Fear-avoidance beliefs—A moderator of treatment efficacy in patients with low back pain: A systematic review. *Spine J*. 2014;14:2658–2678.

16. ANSWER: D

In reviewing the literature regarding the role of medical assessment in predicting work disability, the medical literature was notable for the failure of research to consistently identify medical factors that predicted work disability. The analyses performed in studies to identify predictive factors were often done to demonstrate the differences between two tools but often not to demonstrate the ability of said factors to predict outcomes.

The importance of the medical examination in the acute phase of injury to detect serious pathology is widely recognized. Once such pathology has been addressed or in its absence, the role of medical factors is significantly diminished and psychosocial factors play an important role in patients with persistent pain and disability.

FURTHER READING

Hunt DG, Zuberbier OA, Kozlowski AJ, et al. Are components of a comprehensive medical assessment predictive of work disability after an episode of occupational low back trouble? *Spine*. 2002;27(23):2715–2719.

17. ANSWER: C

In the referenced article, a group of 100 patients with chronic mild low back pain had baseline measures taken of both physical findings and psychosocial factors. They were then followed for 5 years with regard to episodes of serious back pain, occupational disability, remission episodes, and medical treatment for low back pain.

The analysis of the data demonstrated that baseline psychosocial variables were strong predictive factors for the development of low back pain disability, whereas anatomic/structural variables were weakly associated with back pain episodes and demonstrated no association with disability or future medical care.

FURTHER READING

Carragee EJ, Alamin TF, Miller JL, et al. Discographic, MRI and psychosocial determinants of low back pain disability and remission: A prospective study in subjects with benign persistent back pain. *Spine J*. 2005;5:24–35.

18. ANSWER: E

The referenced article studied the cost-effectiveness of a biopsychosocial functional restoration program for patients with chronic disabling occupational musculoskeletal disorders. A cohort of 1119 patients who completed an interdisciplinary rehabilitation program were matched by age, sex, injured musculoskeletal region, and ethnicity and divided into three groups based on the elapsed time between their injury and the time when they started the interdisciplinary rehabilitation program: early, 4–8 months; intermediate, 9–18 months; and delayed, more than 18 months. Post-rehabilitation outcomes were assessed 1 year after program completion, and cost estimates included health care costs, lost productivity, indemnity costs, and RTW status.

Limitations of the study included the use of estimates for disability and medication costs. The design of the study was not a randomized controlled trial, so the ability to comment on causation is limited. The other limitation is a significant one that is seen in other studies of interdisciplinary treatment programs: The study included only those patients who completed the treatment program. The conclusions and findings do not apply to eligible patients who do not enroll or complete the program.

The findings of the study demonstrated that all groups demonstrated comparable rates of RTW, work retention, and additional health care utilization. There were significant improvements of 64% in medical costs and 80% in disability benefits for those in the early rehabilitations group compared to the other groups.

FURTHER READING

Theodore BR, Mayer TG, Gatchel RJ. Cost-effectiveness of early versus delayed functional restoration for chronic disabling occupational musculoskeletal disorders. *J Occup Rehabil*. 2015;25:303–315.

19. ANSWER: C

The findings in the two studies show that fear of injury and disability are correlated. They also found that disability was correlated to reduced aerobic fitness. However, the reduced aerobic fitness is not correlated to fear of injury. The study authors noted that the finding of the fear of injury being more strongly associated with disability than aerobic conditioning was not consistent with the theory that fear of injury led to physical deconditioning and subsequently disability. It suggests that another factor is the mechanism for the correlation between fear of injury and disability.

FURTHER READING

Smeets RJ, van Geel KD, Verbunt JA. Is the fear avoidance model associated with the reduced level of aerobic fitness in patients with chronic low back pain? *Arch Phys Med Rehabil*. 2009;90(1):109–117.

Verbunt JA, Seelen HA, Vlaeyen JW, et al. Fear of injury and physical deconditioning in patients with chronic low back pain. *Arch Phys Med Rehabil*. 2003;84(8):1227–1232.

20. ANSWER: D

The Pain Catastrophizing Scale (PCS) is a 13-item scale that quantifies the frequency of pain-related thoughts that are related to three subdimensions of catastrophizing: rumination, helplessness, and magnification. Total scores for the PCS range from 0 to 52; higher scores indicate a greater frequency of catastrophic thoughts.

The Tampa Scale of Kinesiophobia is a 17-item test that asks patients to rate their level of agreement to statements about pain, injury, and physical activity. Total scores range from 17 to 68, and higher scores indicate greater fear of movement.

The Beck Depression Inventory II is used to quantify the severity of depressive symptoms and instructs patients to endorse statements about their experience of depressive symptoms during the 2 weeks preceding assessment. Total scores range from 0 to 64, and higher scores indicate greater severity of depressive symptoms.

The Pain Self-Efficacy Questionnaire is used to measure participants' self-confidence in their ability to perform activities of daily living despite their pain. Patients rate their confidence on 10 items using a 7-point Likert-type scale (0–6). Total scores range from 0 to 60; low scores correspond to reduced pain self-efficacy, whereas higher scores are associated with greater RTW.

FURTHER READING

Wideman TH, Sullivan MJL. Differential predictors of the long-term levels of pain intensity, work disability, healthcare use, and medication use in a sample of workers' compensation claimants. *Pain*. 2011;152:376–383.

21. ANSWER: D

According to Bureau of Labor Statistics data from 2013, the median number of days of absence from work for a low back injury was 11 days, whereas it was 8 days for other causes of musculoskeletal injuries. Although 80–90% of patients return to work, a significant proportion of the total costs are incurred by the other 10–20%.

The duration of absence from work can be used to estimate the likelihood that someone will be able to return to work. For those out of work 6, 12, and 24 months, respectively, the chances of returning to work are 50%, 25%, and very unlikely to return to work.

FURTHER READING

US Department of Labor, Bureau of Labor Statistics. Injuries, illnesses, and fatalities. Available at http://www.bls.gov/iif/oshcdnew.htm.

22. ANSWER: B

Because there is no method for objectively determining pain through physical assessment, an understanding of pain rating instruments is helpful when considered detailed assessment of a patient's pain.

The McGill Pain Questionnaire measures pain as a multidimensional experience and examines intensity, sensory, and affective components of pain. It is scored on a scale from 0 to 78, with higher scores representing greater pain.

The Dartmouth Pain Questionnaire was developed as an adjunct to the McGill Pain Questionnaire. It adds assessment of objective measures of pain complaints, somatic interventions, impaired functioning, and remaining positive aspects of function and a subjective measure of changes in self-esteem since onset of pain.

The Pain Disability Index is a tool designed to help patients measure the degree to which their daily lives are disrupted by chronic pain. The tool measures categories of life activities, including family/home activity, recreation, social activity, occupation, sexual behavior, and life-support activities (eating, sleeping, and breathing). Higher scores represent greater levels of disruption by pain.

The Pain Patient Profile test is designed to measure the psychological distress from chronic pain and examines anxiety, depression, and somatization. It is based on patient self-report to specific items and also includes a validity scale.

FURTHER READING

Corson JA, Schneider MJ. The Dartmouth Pain Questionnaire: An adjunct to the McGill Pain Questionnaire. *Pain*. 1984;19(1):59–69.
Melzack R. The McGill Pain Questionnaire: Major Properties and Scoring Methods. *Pain*. 1975 Sep;1(3):277–99.
Pain Disability Index. Available at http://www.med.umich.edu/1info/FHP/practiceguides/pain/detpdi.pdf.
Willoughby SG, Hailey BJ, Wheeler LC. Pain Patient Profile: A scale to measure psychological distress. *Arch Phys Med Rehabil*. 1999;80(10):1300–1302.

23. ANSWER: C

The referenced article is a systematic review and random effects meta-analysis of randomized controlled trials to assess the long-term effects of multidisciplinary biopsychosocial rehabilitation for patients with chronic low back pain. The patients in this review had chronic low back pain, disability, and a generally poor prognosis. In many cases, they had already failed a course of conservative treatment. In these patients, BRPs resulted in better outcomes with respect to long-term pain and disability compared with usual care or physical treatments that included heat and electrostimulation modalities; aerobic, stretching, and strengthening exercises; manual therapies; and education intervention.

The results regarding BRPs on return to work were mixed. Several studies demonstrated increased likelihood of patients who received BRPs being at work in the long term compared to those who received physical treatments. However, other studies offering moderate quality evidence that BRPs did not improve the odds of being at work.

FURTHER READING

Kamper SJ, Apeldoorn AT, Chiarotto A, et al. Multidisciplinary biopsychosocial rehabilitation for chronic low back pain: Cochrane systematic review and meta-analysis. *Br Med J*. 2015;350:h444.

24. ANSWER: D

Writing good RTW forms requires an appreciation of the importance of good communication between the physician and the employer or third party. Recipients of these notes are often laypeople, so these notes should be written to such an audience. At the same time, one must also recognize that some terms have specific meanings other than their plain English meanings, so it is important that both the sender and the recipient have a common understanding of the language used in such notes.

For example, many forms use the US Department of Labor criteria. The term "sedentary work" might convey to someone that the employee should have a desk job and not be assigned manual labor duties. Although this scenario falls within the bounds of sedentary work, it could also mean that the patient must stand or walk up to 2 hours out of an 8-hour day or lift/carry objects weighing up to 10 pounds for 3 hours.

Such notes often describe the limitations of work-related activities, and conveying this information is the central purpose of such communication. These notes also often detail how long such restrictions are in place and whether such limitations are permanent or temporary. An employer may find it more helpful to understand what abilities a patient has when matching a patient to a job, so listing the capabilities of the patient may be as helpful as defining which activities should be avoided.

FURTHER READING

Demeter SL. How to fill out disability and return-to-work forms. In: Demeter SL, Andersson GBJ (Eds.), *Disability Evaluation*. St. Louis, MO: Mosby;2003:871–891.

25. ANSWER: C

The focus of work rehabilitation is different from that of traditional medical therapy, and work rehabilitation typically begins after the patient has healed to the point at which the musculoskeletal system can tolerate the activities associated with intensive rehabilitation progression. Work rehabilitation is typically considered when a patient's rate of recovery slows or plateaus and the patient is still unable to return to work.

In work rehabilitation, the focus of patient treatment is on self-management and self-rehabilitation rather than as a recipient of treatment. Although clinicians provide the overall parameters for a safe, effective program, the patient is responsible for engaging in therapy.

The focus of the rehabilitation program is on improving functional goals. Although most patients express a desire to "get back to where they were before the injury" or work pain-free, these goals may be neither realistic nor possible. If low back pain is a limiting factor in returning to work, working to improve spinal stability, improving ergonomics of work, or taking breaks will be strategies employed to improve a patient's ability to perform work.

Although work rehabilitation includes psychosocial treatment, this should not differentiate it from treatment rendered prior to work rehabilitation. Treatment modalities are not exclusively psychosocial in work rehabilitation.

Although a patient's injury may affect only a specific area, such as a knee injury, the patient as a whole has to function well at work. From a biomechanical perspective, an injury that began as a knee injury may end up involving the ankle or low back if the patient overloads those areas while protecting the knee. Also, in the course of injury, a patient's overall level of fitness and aerobic conditioning may decline and affect his or her ability to perform physical work and level of pain.

FURTHER READING

Isernhagen S. Work hardening. In: Demeter SL, Andersson GBJ (Eds.), *Disability Evaluation*. St. Louis, MO: Mosby; 2003:769–780.

26. ANSWER: E

Traditional components of musculoskeletal exercise address a number of key areas, such as stability/core strengthening, flexibility/mobility, strength, endurance, balance, and coordination. The work rehabilitation therapist should tailor a program to match the individualized needs of the patient.

Aerobic training can be performed any number of ways and does not require specialized equipment. It can be assessed by heart rate monitoring that patients perform on their own. In addition to producing a feeling of well-being in most people, it also has the benefit of increasing muscular strength and endurance.

The principles of safely performing work tasks and performing tasks in daily life are often the same as those of work-related tasks. In general, learning to problem-solve about how to adjust and modify tasks to accomplish goals is an important aspect of patient education.

The principle of specificity in exercise training suggests that training people on their specific work tasks would be an effective way to tailor therapy. Work tasks can either be simulated in the clinical environment or performed at the worksite. If equipment is required to perform work, it could be incorporated into a patient's work rehabilitation (e.g., protective gear for a firefighter or welding equipment).

FURTHER READING

Isernhagen S. Work hardening. In: Demeter SL, Andersson GBJ (Eds.), *Disability Evaluation*. St. Louis, MO: Mosby; 2003:769–780.

27. ANSWER: D

The correct answer is D, although the first three options are not uncommon complaints of patients in work rehabilitation programs and should be addressed by the patient and rehabilitation staff. In this scenario, the patient is modifying the program from what was recommended. Other examples of noncompliance that need to be addressed by staff include unauthorized absences, tardiness, submaximal effort, and negative behaviors such as talking back to staff or speaking negatively about other patients.

FURTHER READING

Isernhagen S. Work hardening. In: Demeter SL, Andersson GBJ (Eds.), *Disability Evaluation*. St. Louis, MO: Mosby; 2003:769–780.

28. ANSWER: A

MMI is a medicolegal concept that defines when the patient has reached a point at which no further improvement would be expected either with or without additional medical treatment. Work rehabilitation is treatment that may improve the patient's function or ability to work and therefore should be considered prior to placing a patient at MMI. Some states and jurisdictions may use alternative wording—for example, California uses the term *permanent and stationary* (P&S)—but the concepts are similar.

Although the other options represent interesting interpretations of the term maximum medical improvement, none are correct.

When patients are placed at MMI, a number of additional determinations may need to be made as well. The insurer and employer may be interested in obtaining statements about the degree of disability, such as partial versus total, as well as whether the patient's injury is permanent. A disability rating may be requested at this time as well, either from the treating physician or from a consulting physician via an independent medical examination. An insurer may be eager to have a patient placed at MMI because it may allow the insurer to release funds that have been held in reserve for a patient's treatment. The term "case closure" is sometimes used to indicate that a patient has reached MMI.

FURTHER READING

Rondinelli R, et al. *AMA Guides to the Evaluation of Permanent Impairment*. 6th ed. Chicago, IL: American Medical Association; 2007.

29. ANSWER: D

The Americans with Disabilities Act (ADA) requires that reasonable accommodations are provided to qualified individuals with a disability unless to do so presents an undue hardship to the employer. Such accommodations are typically discussed between an employer and the employee; the courts become involved if the employer and employee are unable to resolve the issue. ADA is not restricted to only physical limitations of individuals with disabilities.

An understanding of ADA is helpful to the physician who has a patient requiring modification of his or her work. Employers are not required to provide accommodations that would impose "significant difficulty or expense" on the employer in relation to its business and the resources available to provide the accommodation. A determination regarding whether an accommodation represents an undue hardship on an employer is based on an individualized assessment of the specific circumstances. Therefore, although ADA may require an employer to accommodate an employee as specified in answer A, such accommodation might also be an undue hardship to the employer.

FURTHER READING

US Equal Employment Opportunity Commission. Enforcement guidance: Reasonable accommodation and undue hardship under the Americans with Disabilities Act. Available at http://www.eeoc.gov/policy/docs/accommodation.html. Accessed July 25, 2015.

16.

ACUTE PAIN MANAGEMENT AND TISSUE PAIN

Ignacio Badiola

INTRODUCTION

This chapter examines the themes represented on the American Board of Anesthesiology's pain medicine certification exam. It covers Part 6 (tissue pain), Section 1 (acute pain). In detail, the epidemiology of acute pain, the current inadequacy of acute pain therapies, the physiology of acute pain, and both pharmacologic and nonpharmacologic aspects of acute pain treatment are discussed. Tools for assessing acute pain are reviewed, as well as the roles of both patient and family as they relate to adults and children in acute pain.

QUESTIONS

1. Which of the following exams tests for deficiencies in activities of daily living?

    A. Minnesota Multiphasic Personality Index (MMPI)
    B. Visual Analogue Scale
    C. Beck Depression Inventory
    D. Spielberger State Trait Anxiety Inventory
    E. Oswestry Low Back Pain Disability Questionnaire

2. Compared to COX-1 inhibitors and other nonsteroidal anti-inflammatory drugs (NSAIDs), COX-2 inhibitors are most likely to:

    A. Catalyze arachidonic acid conversion to prostaglandins, thromboxane, and levuloglandins
    B. Have more gastrointestinal (GI) side effects
    C. Protect against renal effects
    D. Not inhibit platelet aggregation
    E. Display greater cardiac protection

3. Opioids should be used cautiously in patients with which of the following conditions?

    A. Restrictive lung disease
    B. Chronic obstructive pulmonary disease (COPD)

    C. Obstructive sleep apnea (OSA)
    D. Scoliosis
    E. All of the above

4. Which of the following is changed in the elderly (compared to younger adults)?

    A. Clearance of a drug
    B. Volume of distribution
    C. Elimination half-life
    D. All of the above
    E. None of the above

5. Which of the following complications is the most common with acupuncture?

    A. Bleeding
    B. Infection
    C. Vasovagal reaction
    D. Pneumothorax
    E. None of the above

6. An orthopedic surgeon consults the acute pain service regarding a patient who is scheduled to undergo a below-the-knee amputation. The patient has heard of phantom limb pain (PLP) and wants to know the most likely time to expect it. You would tell him and the orthopedic surgeon:

    A. Within the first 2 weeks after the amputation
    B. Within the first month
    C. After 6 months
    D. More than 1 year after surgery
    E. None of the above

7. What percentage of sickle cell disease (SCD) patients have strokes by the time they are 20 years old?

    A. <1%
    B. Approximately 10%

C. Approximately 30%
D. Approximately 50%
E. None of the above

8. Mu (μ) opioid receptors mediate which of the following?

A. Respiratory depression
B. Nausea and vomiting
C. Bowel hypomobility
D. Miosis
E. All of the above

9. Which of the following are risk factors for chronic persistent postsurgical pain?

A. Female gender
B. Genetic predisposition
C. Acute pain
D. Younger age
E. All of the above

10. What is the main principle(s)/goal(s) of multimodal analgesic postoperative pain management?

A. Enable early mobilization
B. Allow early enteral nutrition
C. Decrease the perioperative stress response and its consequences
D. Give the patient a sense of control over his or her perioperative pain
E. All of the above

11. Which of the following is true regarding gender differences in pain?

A. Females report more severe pain than males with similar disease processes.
B. Females have a decreased prevalence of pain related to musculoskeletal origin.
C. Females have a lower prevalence of pain related to visceral origin.
D. None of the above are true.

12. Which of the following is classically considered to be the least painful?

A. First-degree burn
B. Second-degree burn
C. Third-degree burn
D. Fourth-degree burn

13. Hydroxyurea is a disease-modifying agent occasionally used in sickle cell disease. Which of the

following is thought to be its main mechanism of action?

A. Increasing normal hemoglobin A (Hb-A)
B. Increasing normal Hb-B
C. Increasing Hb-F
D. Decreasing Hb-F
E. None of the above

14. Which of the following is not typical of acute postoperative pain?

A. Increased heart rate
B. Decrease in circulating insulin
C. Hypoglycemia
D. Urinary retention
E. None of the above

15. Which of the following receptors are involved in analgesia from a transcutaneous electrical nerve stimulation (TENS) unit?

A. Peripheral α_2 receptors
B. Spinal opioid receptors
C. Spinal γ-aminobutyric acid (GABA) receptors
D. All of the above
E. None of the above

16. What percentage of patients following outpatient surgery continue to experience moderate to severe pain in the first 24 hour after discharge?

A. 10%
B. 25%
C. 40%
D. 75%

17. Ketamine decreases activation in which of the following?

A. Secondary somatosensory cortex
B. Thalamus
C. Anterior cingulate cortex
D. All of the above
E. None of the above

18. Which of the following increases the risk of respiratory depression due to a spinal administered opioid?

A. Patient older than 60 years
B. Placing the patient in the Trendelenburg position
C. Using spinal morphine
D. All of the above
E. None of the above

19. Which of the following surgeries are associated with a high (>10%) risk of persistent post-surgical pain?

A. Neuroma excision
B. Coronary artery bypass surgery (CABG)
C. Appendectomy
D. Hip arthroscopy and labral repair
E. None of the above

20. Preoperative education has been shown to:

A. Increase preoperative anxiety
B. Decrease length of hospital stay
C. Increase postoperative pain
D. Increase time to preoperative functional levels

21. Which of the following is associated with surgical trauma?

A. Decrease in catecholamines
B. Increase in angiotensin
C. Decreased platelet activation
D. Decreased platelet aggregation

22. A patient is scheduled for a total hip arthroplasty. A plan of general anesthesia for the case and a lumbar plexus block and catheter for postoperative pain management is formulated. Which of the following nerves does not originate from the lumbar plexus?

A. The femoral nerve
B. The ilioinguinal nerve
C. The lateral femoral cutaneous nerve
D. The genitofemoral nerve
E. The sural nerve

23. A patient is scheduled to undergo a rotator cuff repair and is asking you about his postoperative pain management options. You discuss an interscalene brachial plexus block. You also discuss the side effects associated with this block and tell him that the most common side effect is:

A. Pneumothorax
B. Horner's syndrome
C. Diaphragmatic paresis due to phrenic nerve block
D. Vertebral artery injection

24. Which of the following is true regarding family education about procedural pain?

A. A child will require greater use of restraints and will show higher levels of fear when parents provide reassurance during immunizations.
B. Parental distress has been shown to correlate with more pain and functional disability in children.
C. Parental anxiety has been shown to correlate with more pain and functional disability in children.
D. None of the above are true.
E. All of the above are true.

25. A 34-year-old woman is scheduled to undergo a right radial fracture repair. The orthopedic surgeon contacts the acute pain service because the patient is currently prescribed buprenorphine for a history of heroin abuse. He asks what is the best way to manage the buprenorphine prior to surgery:

A. Continue buprenorphine perioperatively
B. Divide the daily dose of buprenorphine to be taken every 6 hours in order to take advantage of its analgesic properties
C. If adequate time is available (i.e., surgery can be postponed for 7–10 days), convert the patient to a full agonist and allow sufficient time to metabolize and excrete all buprenorphine
D. None of the above
E. All of the above

ANSWERS

1. ANSWER: E

The Oswestry Low Back Pain Disability Questionnaire consists of 10 questions that cover nine aspects of activities of daily living. These include items evaluating personal care, lifting, walking, sitting, standing, sleeping, sex life, social life, and traveling. The Beck Depression Inventory is a 21-question multiple-choice inventory that measures severity of depression. The MMPI is a widely used test of adult personality and psychopathology. The Spielberger State Trait Anxiety Inventory is a 40-question test that measures state anxiety (anxiety about an event) versus trait anxiety (anxiety as a personal trait).

KEY FACTS

- There are four aspects of the acute pain experience: sensory, emotional, psychological, and cultural. All of these must be evaluated and treated in order to achieve optimal pain management.
- Most patients' expectations of pain following surgery tend to be unrealistic, and evaluating their expectations may prompt educational interventions such as preoperative instructional programs.

FURTHER READING

Cornell DJ. The measurement of pain: Objectifying the subjective. In: Waldman SD (Ed.), *Pain Management*. Philadelphia, PA: Saunders; 2007.

Mancuso CA, Graziano S, Briskie LM, et al. Randomized trials to modify patients' preoperative expectations of hip and knee arthroplasties. *Clin Orthop Relat Res*. 2008;466(2):424–431.

2. ANSWER: D

COX-2 inhibitors such as celecoxib preferentially bind to the COX-2 enzyme relative to the Cox-1 enzyme. COX-1 is involved in most body tissues including the GI system, in which it is involved in gastric mucosal protection. In platelets, it is involved in platelet aggregation. Thus, COX-2 inhibitors do not inhibit platelet aggregation and lead to less GI side effects. Both COX-1 and COX-2 catalyze arachidonic acid conversion to prostaglandins, thromboxane, and levuloglandins. Inhibition of COX-1 (and thus platelet aggregation) is known to lead to some cardioprotection. This is one reason why aspirin (inhibits COX-1) is given to some cardiac patients. It is possible that by inhibiting COX-2, but not COX-1, homeostasis is altered toward ill cardiac effects.

KEY FACT

- COX-2 inhibitors do not inhibit platelet aggregation.

FURTHER READING

Buvanendran A. Nonsteroidal anti-inflammatory drugs. In: Deer TR, Leong MS, Buvanendran A, et al. (Eds.), *Comprehensive Treatment of Chronic Pain by Medical, Interventional, and Integrative Approaches*. New York, NY: Springer; 2013.

3. ANSWER: E

Opioids are known respiratory depressants and can lead to hypoventilation and oxygen desaturation in patients with low respiratory reserve. They should be used with caution in patients with restrictive lung disease, COPD, OSA, and scoliosis.

KEY FACT

- Nausea and vomiting, constipation, respiratory depression, and pruritus are commonly seen side effects of opioids administered in the perioperative and acute pain setting.

FURTHER READING

Sharma S, Giampetro DM. Opioid adverse effects and opioid induced hypogonadism. In: Deer TR, Leong MS, Buvanendran A, et al. (Eds.), *Comprehensive Treatment of Chronic Pain by Medical, Interventional, and Integrative Approaches*. New York, NY: Springer; 2013.

Sinatra RS. Oral and parenteral opioid analgesics for acute pain Management. In: Sinatra RS, de Leon-Cassasola OA, Viscusi ER, et al. (Eds.), *Acute Pain Management*. New York, NY: Cambridge University Press; 2009.

4. ANSWER: D

Clearance of a drug refers to the rate at which the drug is removed from the blood, usually in the kidney or liver. The volume of distribution is the volume that the total amount of administered agent would have to occupy to result in the same concentration as it is currently in the blood. Lipid content increases as age increases (lean body mass decreases with age). Thus, lipid-soluble drugs that are used perioperatively, such as opioids and benzodiazepines, can have significant differences in volume of distribution and thus elimination. The elimination half-life refers to the time it takes for an agent to lose one-half of its pharmacological activity. Due to multiple factors, including changes in volume of distribution, the elimination half-life can change dramatically as age increases.

KEY FACTS

- Opioids in the elderly can lead to increased skeletal muscle rigidity, increased duration of both systemic and neuroaxial effects, as well as increased incidence of respiratory depression.
- Local anesthetics used in spinal/epidural perioperative pain management may have an increased duration of action in the elderly.

FURTHER READING

Barnett S. Elderly patients. In: Miller RD, Pardo M (Eds.), *Basics of Anesthesia*. 6th ed. Philadelphia, PA: Saunders; 2011.
Shafer SL. Basic pharmacologic principles. In: Miller RD, Pardo M (Eds.), *Basics of Anesthesia*. 6th ed. Philadelphia, PA: Saunders; 2011.

5. ANSWER: A

Complications from acupuncture are rare. The most commonly reported problem seen is usually mild bleeding. Vasovagal responses can also occur, and more severe complications such as pneumothorax are extremely uncommon.

KEY FACTS

- Acupuncture is safe and has minimal side effects/adverse effects.
- Proposed mechanisms of action include spinal inhibition, release of endorphins, stimulation of inhibitory descending pathways, and central modulation.
- Only a few studies have evaluated acupuncture in postoperative pain. The results are mixed, with some showing benefit and others not.

FURTHER READING

Ernst E. Acupuncture: A critical analysis. *J Intern Med.* 2006; 259:125–137.
Fitzgerald K, Buggy D. Nonconventional and adjunctive analgesia. In: Sorten G, Carr DB, Harmon D, et al. (Eds.), *Postoperative Pain Management: An Evidence-Based Guide to Practice*. Philadelphia, PA: Saunders; 2006.

6. ANSWER: A

PLP is most common within the first 1 or 2 weeks after amputation. However, it can occur from immediately after to many decades after the amputation. In some patients, the pain diminishes and ultimately resolves over time. Pain is usually described as intense with severe bouts of attack that vary from seconds to hours. It is usually felt distally in the amputated limb and usually corresponds in places where there are high levels of cortical representation.

KEY FACTS

- PLP is commonly considered a form of deafferentation pain with central sensitization as the sustaining pathophysiology.
- Predictors of phantom pain include pain prior to amputation and persistent stump pain.

FURTHER READING

Talbot RM, McCrory CR. Mechanisms of postoperative pain—Neuropathic. In: Sorten G, Carr DB, Harmon D, et al. (Eds.), *Postoperative Pain Management: An Evidence-Based Guide to Practice*. Philadelphia, PA: Saunders; 2006.

7. ANSWER: B

Approximately 10% of patients have evidence of a clinically relevant stroke by the time they are 20 years old. Approximately one-fourth of SCD patients will have evidence of a stroke by the time they are 45 years old.

KEY FACTS

- Multiple processes can lead to a painful crisis in SCD, including dehydration, infection, anxiety/stress, and oxygen deprivation from any cause. Some of the most common painful conditions seen in SCD are avascular necrosis (due to bone infarct), priapism (sickling in the vasculature of the penis), dactylitis (infarct of the metatarsals and metacarpals), and acute chest syndrome (occlusion of the pulmonary vasculature leading to lung infarcts).
- Some patients have baseline chronic pain with acute exacerbations, whereas others have no pain in between a painful crisis.

FURTHER READING

Smith K. Sickle cell pain. In: Waldman SD (Ed.), *Pain Management*. Philadelphia, PA: Saunders; 2007.
Wilson BH, Nelson J. Sickle cell disease pain management in adolescents: A literature review. *Pain Manage Nurs.* 2015; 16(2):146–151.

8. ANSWER: E

μ opioid receptors are also involved in euphoria and physical dependence. The other opioid receptors include κ receptors, which mediate spinal and visceral analgesia. They have negligible effects on respiration. Dynorphin is the primary endogenous ligand. δ opioid receptors may be involved in facilitating μ receptor activity.

KEY FACTS

• Once bound (opioid receptors are G-linked), there is a cascade of events ultimately leading to activation of ion channels influencing enzymes and gene transcription. Opioids also bind to presynaptic neurons, resulting in inhibition of neurotransmitter release (i.e., serotonin, substance P, and norepinephrine).

FURTHER READING

Koyyalagunta D. Opioid analgesics. In: Waldman SD (Ed.), *Pain Management*. Philadelphia, PA: Saunders; 2007.

Trescott A. Clinical use of opioids. In: Deer TR, Leong MS, Buvanendran A, et al. (Eds.), *Comprehensive Treatment of Chronic Pain by Medical, Interventional, and Integrative Approaches*. New York, NY: Springer; 2013.

9. ANSWER: E

Many factors contribute to and are risk factors for the development of persistent pain after surgery. Female gender, acute pain at the surgical site (and, in some studies, pain at other sites), a younger age, and genetic predisposition all increase the risk of developing chronic pain after surgery.

KEY FACT

• Amputation, breast surgery, thoracotomy, inguinal hernia repair, CABG, and cesarean (C)sections are

Table 16.1 INCIDENCE OF CHRONIC POSTSURGICAL PAIN

PROCEDURE	INCIDENCE (%)
Amputation	30–50
Breast surgery	20–30
Thoracotomy	30–40
Inguinal hernia repair	10
CABG	30–50
C-section	10

SOURCE: Data from Kelhet H, Jensen T, Woolf C. Persistent postsurgical pain: Risk factors and prevention. *Lancet*. 2006;367:1618–1625.

common procedures with a high incidence of chronic postsurgical pain (Table 16.1).

FURTHER READING

Katz J, Setzer Z. Transition from acute to chronic postsurgical pain: Risk factors and protective factors. *Expert Rev Neurother*. 2009;9(5):723–744.

Kelhet H, Jensen T, Woolf C. Persistent postsurgical pain: Risk factors and prevention. *Lancet*. 2006;367:1618–1625.

10. ANSWER: E

One of the main principles/goals of multimodal analgesia is providing analgesia using various agents/modalities that are synergistic and lead to less adverse effects. Early mobilization, early enteral nutrition, as well as decreasing the perioperative stress response are important goals. Multimodal analgesia usually includes a combination of opioids, NSAIDs, acetaminophen, and adjuncts such as gabapentin/pregabalin. Regional anesthesia including peripheral nerve blocks and epidural analgesia can also play a role.

KEY FACTS

• Multimodal analgesia uses lower doses of individual drugs (drug sparing) in combination, which helps lower the severity of each drug's side effects, achieving equianalgesia with that of single agents.

FURTHER READING

Pergolizzi J, Wills LM. Multimodal analgesic therapy. In: Sorten G, Carr DB, Harmon D, et al. (Eds.), *Postoperative Pain Management: An Evidence-Based Guide to Practice*. Philadelphia, PA: Saunders; 2006.

11. ANSWER: A

Females may experience pain differently than men. Although there is bias in the literature, women tend to report more severe pain for a similar disease process. Compared to men, they also tend to report more anatomically diffuse pain and pain that lasts longer. Although somewhat controversial, females tend to have a higher prevalence than males with regard to musculoskeletal and visceral pain.

KEY FACTS

• Gender differences may be involved in acute pain presentation.
• Hormonal differences may be involved in how a patient perceives pain.

FURTHER READING

Wellington J, Chia Y. Patient variables influencing acute pain management. In: Sinatra RS, de Leon-Cassasola OA, Viscusi ER, et al. (Eds.), *Acute Pain Management*. New York, NY: Cambridge University Press; 2009.

12. ANSWER: C

First-degree burns involve the epidermal skin layer, leading to inflammation, erythema, and hyperalgesia. Second-degree burns are also known as partial-thickness burns and involve the dermis. They can be subdivided into superficial second-degree burns (the upper dermis is involved) and deep second-degree burns with involvement of the reticular dermis. This area is rich in sensory receptors, leading to marked pain and hyperalgesia. Third-degree burns involve destruction of the epidermis and dermis, including sensory structures. Although classically described as less painful, pain and hyperalgesia can still be present. Fourth-degree burns extend through the skin and involve deeper structures, such as muscle and bone.

KEY FACTS

- Pain in burn patients can be classified as constant pain at rest and motion (background pain), aggravated by episodes of intense and sudden pain (breakthrough pain).
- Background pain is constant and is best treated by around-the-clock/scheduled analgesics. This can include continuous intravenous infusions (e.g., patient-controlled analgesia) or scheduled oral long-acting opioids. Scheduled adjuncts such as NSAIDs can also be added. Background pain will usually decrease with time, so these medications can be tapered over time. Breakthrough pain is a transitory increase in pain from background pain. This can be due to multiple causes from changes in the wound (i.e., during healing or from new-onset infection) to patient movement and activity. It is important to recognize this and treat the underlying cause. Analgesia can be provided by short-acting/rapid-onset opioids and adjuncts (i.e., NSAIDs or acetaminophen).
- Procedural pain is extremely difficult to manage due to multiple factors. In burn patients, procedural pain is usually from dressing changes. Depending on the situation, only an extra dose of a short-acting/rapid-onset opioids may be required. In more involved cases (i.e., more extensive burns), moderate and even deep sedation may be required. Procedural pain tends to be intense and usually of short duration. Strategies vary by institution, however; typical management involves using highly potent opioids with short duration of action along with adjuncts such as anxiolytics (i.e., midazolam). Agents such as ketamine and dexmedetomidine can also be used. Other nonpharmacologic therapy can also be used, such as distraction and imagery.

FURTHER READING

Sharar SR, Patterson DR, Askay SW. Burn pain. In: Waldman SD (Ed.), *Pain Management*. Philadelphia, PA: Saunders; 2007.

13. ANSWER: C

Although the exact mechanism of hydroxyurea is debatable, its efficacy is usually attributed to its ability to increase the amount of circulating hemoglobin F (fetal hemoglobin). This decreases the amount of sickle cell hemoglobin (HbS), leading to less polymerization of HbS. The exact mechanism by which it does this is currently under debate, with some believing that hydroxyurea is cytotoxic to the rapidly dividing late-stage red cell precursors. This may lead to an increase in production of earlier stage red cell precursors that produce HbF. Others believe that it may interfere with the red cell precursor machinery, reprogramming them to produce more HbF.

KEY FACTS

- Sickle cell anemia (in which only hemoglobin S is produced) is the most severe form. Hemoglobin S tends to aggregate under low oxygen tensions, causing sickling of hemoglobin with occlusion of vessels and thus leading to ischemia and pain.
- Pain is the hallmark of SCD and is one of the most common reasons for emergency room visits by these patients. These painful crises may be unpredictable and can occur anywhere in the body. Multiple processes can lead to a painful crisis, including dehydration, infection, anxiety/stress, and oxygen deprivation from any cause. Some of the most common painful conditions seen in SCD include avascular necrosis (due to bone infarct), priapism (sickling in the vasculature of the penis), dactylitis (infarct of the metatarsals and metacarpals), and acute chest syndrome (occlusion of the pulmonary vasculature leading to lung infarcts). Box 16.1 presents treatment options.

FURTHER READING

Smith K. Sickle cell pain. In: Waldman SD (Ed.), *Pain Management*. Philadelphia, PA: Saunders; 2007.
Varadarajan JL, Weisman SJ. Acute pain management in sickle cell disease patients. In: Sinatra RS, de Leon-Cassasola OA, Viscusi ER,

Box 16.1 TREATMENT OPTIONS FOR SICKLE CELL PAIN CRISES

Aggressive hydration
    Limits sludging of cells in the vasculature
Oxygen
    May help limit the number of sickled red blood cells
Blood transfusion
    Usually avoided due to adverse effects of repeated blood transfusion; may also worsen occlusion from increased red blood cells
Exchange transfusion may be used to lower HbS levels
Opioids
    Codeine
    Hydrocodone
    Merperidine
    Hydromorphone
    Morphine
    Fentanyl
Adjuvants
    Antihistamines
    Antidepressants
    Anticonvulsants
    α agonis

FURTHER READING

Prabhakar A, Mancuso KF, Owen CP, et al. Perioperative analgesia outcomes and strategies. *Best Pract Res Clin Anaesthesiol.* 2014;28(2):105–115.

15. ANSWER: D

Multiple mechanisms of TENS-induced analgesia have been proposed, including activation of peripheral α_2 receptors, spinal opioid receptors, and spinal GABA receptors.

KEY FACTS

- A TENS unit uses electric pulses via electrodes placed on the skin near the surgical site. Its mechanism of action is believed to be via activation of GABA and opioid receptors at the spinal level reducing antegrade nociceptive transmission. It may possibly release endorphins as well.
- Although there does appear to be evidence that TENS may be useful in some patients with postoperative pain, not all studies have reached this conclusion. However, given that some benefit may be possible and the low risk associated with this technique, this may be used as part of a multimodal analgesic plan.

FURTHER READING

Fitzgerald K, Buggy D. Nonconventional and adjunctive analgesia In: Sorten G, Carr DB, Harmon D, et al. (Eds.), *Postoperative Pain Management: An Evidence-Based Guide to Practice.* Philadelphia, PA: Saunders; 2006.
Meissner W. The role of acupuncture and transcutaneous electrical nerve stimulation for postoperative pain control. *Curr Opin Anaesthesiol.* 2009;22(5):623–626.

16. ANSWER: C

Approximately 40% of patients will complain of moderate to severe pain in the first 24 hours following surgery. Better

et al. (Eds.), *Acute Pain Management.* New York, NY: Cambridge University Press; 2009.
Williams H, Tanabe P. Sickle cell disease. A review of non-pharmacological approaches for pain. *J Pain Symptom Manage.* 2016;51(2):163–177.

14. ANSWER: C

Acute pain and acute postoperative pain can lead to a multitude of physiologic changes, including hyperglycemia. Table 16.2 summarizes some of these changes.

Table 16.2 PHYSIOLOGIC CHANGES CAUSED BY ACUTE PAIN AND ACUTE POSTOPERATIVE PAIN

SYSTEM	PHYSIOLOGIC CHANGES
Central nervous system	Persistent pain, primary and secondary hyperalgesia, peripheral and central sensitization
Psychological	Fear, anxiety, depression, insomnia, fatigue
Cardiovascular	Hypertension, tachycardia, increased oxygen consumption, myocardial ischemia, myocardial infarct, dysrhythmia
Pulmonary	V/Q mismatch, hypoxemia, atelectasis, hypercapnia, decreased pulmonary toilet

analgesic regimens (including peripheral nerve catheters) and acute pain medicine consultation may help reduce this percentage.

KEY FACTS

- More than 51.4 million inpatient surgical procedures were performed in 2010 in the United States alone, according to the Centers for Disease Control and Prevention.
- 80% of patients experienced pain after surgery, with 86% of these patients noting moderate to severe pain.

FURTHER READING

Apfelbaum JL, Chen C, Mehta SS, et al. Postoperative pain experience: Results from a national survey suggest postoperative pain continues to be undermanaged. *Anesth Analg*. 2003;97:534–540.

Beauregard L, Pomp A, Choiniere M. Severity and impact of pain after day-surgery. *Can J Anaesth*. 1998;45(4):304–311.

US Department of Health and Human Services, National Center for Health Statistics. National hospital discharge survey 2010. Available at http://www.cdc.gov/nchs/nhds.htm.

17. ANSWER: D

Ketamine acts on various regions in the central nervous system, including the secondary somatosensory cortex, insula, thalamus, and anterior cingulate cortex. Ketamine was shown to be involved in reducing the connectivity in the locations of the brain that are responsible for the sensing of pain as well as affective processing.

KEY FACTS

- Ketamine acts on NMDA receptors as well as sodium channels and opioid receptors.
- Ketamine reduces pain intensity and possibly improves patient satisfaction, rehabilitation, and prevents chronic postsurgical pain syndromes.

FURTHER READING

Lui F, Kwok-Fu J. Adjuvant analgesics in acute pain. *Expert Opin Pharmacother*. 2011;12(3):363–385.

Radvansky BM, Shah K, Parikh A, et al. Role of ketamine in acute postoperative pain management: A narrative review. *BioMed Res Int*. 2015;2015:749837.

18. ANSWER: D

Respiratory depression is one of the most feared complications from epidural or intrathecal opioids. It is usually seen many hours (up to 12 hours) after administration. Risk factors include using large volumes of opioid injectate, use of simultaneous parenteral opioids, age older than 60 years, coexisting pulmonary/respiratory disease, elevated intrathoracic pressure, and Trendelenberg position.

KEY FACTS

- Respiratory depression following epidural morphine is described as biphasic, with an early phase (<2 hours) and a delayed phase (>12 hours).
- Delayed respiratory depression is due to rostral spread via the cerebrospinal fluid with penetration into the ventral medulla, specifically the pre-Botzinger complex.

FURTHER READING

Dabu-Bondoc, Franco SA, Sinatra RS. Neuroaxial analgesia with hydromorphone, morphine, and fentanyl: Dosing and safety guidelines. In: Sinatra RS, de Leon-Cassasola OA, Viscusi ER, et al. (Eds.), *Acute Pain Management*. New York, NY: Cambridge University Press; 2009.

Sultan P, Gutierrez MC, Carvalho B. Neuraxial morphine and respiratory depression: Finding the right balance. *Drugs*. 2011;71(14):1807–1819.

19. ANSWER: B

Inadequate acute pain management can have devastating long-term consequences and poor outcomes. This includes worse outcomes in the immediate postoperative period as well as in the long term (i.e., chronic postsurgical pain). It is a consequence of many types of surgeries, with prevalence estimates as high as 50%. Up to 10% of these patients are left with severe pain. Amputation, breast surgery, thoracotomy, inguinal hernia repair, CABG, and C-sections are common procedures with a high incidence of chronic postsurgical pain.

KEY FACTS

- Long-term pain following surgery is a complex process that involves biological, social, psychological, and environmental factors.
- A common factor seen in many surgical procedures associated with persistent pain is surgical nerve injury. However, not all patients with demonstrated nerve injury develop persistent postsurgical pain.

FURTHER READING

Akkaya T, Ozkan D. Chronic post-surgical pain. *Agri*. 2009;21(1):1–9.

Katz J, Seltzer Z. Transition from acute to chronic postsurgical pain: Risk factors and protective factors. *Expert Rev Neurother*. 2009;9(5):723–744.

20. ANSWER: B

Isolated studies examining various surgical procedures have shown that for many types of surgical procedures, but not all, preoperative education increases knowledge of surgical procedures, reduces anxiety and postoperative pain, decreases length of hospital stay, and reduces the time to return to preoperative functional levels.

KEY FACT

- Many types of preoperative education have been described. Table 16.3 provides a summary of some of them.

Table 16.3 **TYPES OF PREOPERATIVE EDUCATION**

EDUCATION TECHNIQUE	DESCRIPTION
One on one (physician/nurse and patient)	• Most common technique • Must consider time, knowing what and how to teach, documentation of what you teach
Group education (physician/nurse and group of patients)	• Must consider time, knowing what and how to teach, documentation of what you teach • Educator must have knowledge about the group process to be effective • More cost-effective than one on one
Structured education	• Based on objectives and outlines • Allows for preparation, identification of patient goals, and development of educational resources
Unstructured education	• Teaching materials with no objective/outlines and instead relies on teacher discretion • More patient focused than structured and allows for spontaneity because it usually occurs based on patient questions
Verbal education	• Preferred by most patients • Teacher must be aware of patient's intellectual level and interest in hearing the information • Supplement verbal with written information to make it easier to retain
Written material	• Should be understandable, up-to-date, accurate, unambiguous with short words and no jargon

FURTHER READING

Louw A, Diener I, Butler DS, et al. Preoperative education addressing postoperative pain in total joint arthroplasty: Review of content and educational delivery methods. *Physiother Theory Pract.* 29(3):175–194.
Oshodi TO. The impact of preoperative education on postoperative pain: Part 1. *Br J Nurs.* 2007;16(12):706–710.

21. ANSWER: B

Surgical trauma results in multiple physiological changes that can be detrimental. These include an increase in circulating catecholamines (norepinephrine and epinephrine), which can lead to increases in sympathetic tone and altered local perfusion. Decreases in renal perfusion lead to increases in the renin–angiotensin–aldosterone system, resulting in elevated angiotensin. The increases in catecholamine and angiotensin along with various other pathophysiological changes lead to an increase in platelet activation, resulting in platelet aggregation.

KEY FACT

- Refer to Table 16.2 for a summary of how surgical stress/trauma affect various organ systems and physiology.

FURTHER READING

Ghori MK, Zhang Y, Sinatra RS. Pathophysiology of acute pain. In: Sinatra RS, de Leon-Cassasola OA, Viscusi ER, et al. (Eds.), *Acute Pain Management.* New York, NY: Cambridge University Press; 2009.
Prabhakar A, Mancuso KF, Owen CP, et al. Perioperative analgesia outcomes and strategies. *Best Pract Res Clin Anaesthesiol.* 2014;28(2):105–115.

22. ANSWER: E

The lumbar plexus is a collection of nerves that originate from L1–L4 (occasionally also T12) and pass through the psoas muscle on their way to innervate the lower extremity. Nerves from the lumbar plexus include illiohypogastric (T12–L1), illioinguinal (L1), genitofemoral (L1 and L2), lateral femoral cutaneous (L2 and L3), femoral (L2–L4), obturator (L2–L4), and saphenous (L2–L4). The sural nerve is a branch of the sciatic nerve, a nerve of the sacral plexus.

- Innervation to the lower extremity consists of nerves from the lumbar plexus and nerves from the sacral plexus.

FURTHER READING

Dilberovic F, Kapur E, Wong C, et al. Functional regional anesthesia anatomy. In: Hadzic A (Ed.), *Textbook of Regional Anesthesia and Acute Pain Management*. New York, NY: McGraw-Hill; 2007.

Waldman SD. Ultrasound guided lumbar plexus nerve block. In: *Comprehensive Atlas of Ultrasound Guided Pain Management Injection Techniques*. Philadelphia, PA: Lippincott Williams & Wilkins; 2014.

23. ANSWER: C

An interscalene brachial plexus block attempts to block the brachial plexus at the root/trunk level as it lies in between the middle and anterior scalene muscles. It is frequently performed for procedures involving the shoulder, lateral clavicle, proximal portion of the humerus, and shoulder joint. Side effects are common and include hemidiaphragm paresis due to spread of local anesthetic near the phrenic nerve. This occurs in almost 100% of interscalene blocks. Horner's syndrome (ptosis, miosis, and anhydrosis) is also commonly seen. Vertebral artery injection and pneumothorax are less common but more devastating complications.

KEY FACT

- Hematoma, vascular puncture/injury, local anesthetic toxicity, Horner's syndrome, nerve injury, total spinal anesthesia, and diaphragmatic paresis are possible complications associated with interscalane blocks.

FURTHER READING

Borgeat A, Blumenthal S. Interscalene brachial plexus block. In: Hadzic A (Ed.), *Textbook of Regional Anesthesia and Acute Pain Management*. New York, NY: McGraw-Hill; 2007.

Waldman SD. Ultrasound guided brachial plexus block: Interscalene approach. In: *Comprehensive Atlas of Ultrasound Guided Pain Management Injection Techniques*. Philadelphia, PA: Lippincott Williams & Wilkins; 2014.

24. ANSWER: E

It is important to address both the patient and the parents in pediatric pain management. Both parent and child play a role in the child's perception of pain. Research has shown that a child will require more restraints and will show higher levels of fear when parents provide reassurance during immunizations. Although counterintuitive, this may be related to tone and pitch used during reassurance. Parental distress, parental anxiety, and pain-specific catastrophizing have been shown to correlate with more pain and functional disability in children.

KEY FACTS

- The more a parent responds with distress in response to his or her child's pain, leading to more protective behavior, the more functional disability a child experiences.
- A parent's anxiety can lead to distress and catastrophizing during procedures, thus leading to more fear on the child's part.

FURTHER READING

Sieberg CB, Manganella J. Family beliefs and interventions in pediatric pain management. *Child Adolesc Psychiatric Clin North Am.* 2015;24:631–645.

Vervoot T, Goubert L. Child's and parents' catastrophizing about pain is associated with procedural fear in children: A study in children with diabetes and their mothers. *Psychol Rep.* 2011;109(3):879–895.

25. ANSWER: E

Perioperative management/acute pain management of patients on buprenorphine poses a significant challenge. All of the options can be correct. One option is to continue buprenorphine—aware that a significant amount of full opioid agonist may be needed for postoperative analgesia. Another option is to split the daily dose of the buprenorphine to be taken every 6 hours. This helps take advantage of its analgesic properties. However, most patients who are not opioid naive will still need full agonists due to both tolerance and the partial agonist properties of buprenorphine. If adequate time is available, the patient can be converted to a full agonist prior to surgery to allow sufficient metabolism and excretion of buprenorphine. No studies have been performed to determine which option is best.

KEY FACTS

- Buprenorphine is an opioid agonist up to 50 times more potent than morphine.

- Buprenorphine is considered a partial agonist with limited effect on the μ receptor and can act as an antagonist when used along with a full agonist.
- Buprenorphine has a slow dissociation from μ receptors, contributing to its long half-life.

FURTHER READING

Alford DP, Compton P, Samet JH. Acute pain management for patients receiving maintenance methadone or buprenorphine therapy. *Ann Intern Med*. 2006;144:127–134.

Chern SY, Isserman R, Chen L, et al. Perioperative pain management for patients on chronic buprenorphine: A case report. *J Anesth Clin Res*. 2013;3(250):1000250.

17.

CANCER PAIN

Amitabh Gulati and Joseph C. Hung

INTRODUCTION

Cancer pain treatment is complex and requires a different and more encompassing focus than many pain processes. Not only can tumor or metastatic lesions cause various types of pain but also the medical, radiological, and surgical treatments of the cancer may eclipse the original cause in some cases. Although treatment is often palliative, the transition from curative to palliative therapies is rarely straightforward, and the influence of patient and family beliefs and sources of meaning may have implications for treatment. This chapter focuses on differentiation of various situations that a pain physician might encounter in clinical practice.

QUESTIONS

1. Which is not an axis (criteria) used in the International Association for the Study of Pain (IASP) published classification of chronic pain patients?

A. Region of the body affected
B. Level of physical impairment and activity restrictions
C. Temporal characteristics of pain and pattern of occurrence
D. Intensity and time since onset of pain
E. Presumed etiology

2. A 76-year-old male with a history of metastatic prostate cancer is considering entering a palliative and hospice care center for continued care. He is most likely to continue which of the following treatments?

A. Chemotherapy and hormonal therapy for his prostate cancer
B. Radiation therapy for curative intent
C. Continued spiritual support

D. Regular visits with his oncologist to discuss further therapeutic options
E. Surgical consultations for prostate resection

3. Which of the following statements is true regarding hospice care as defined by Medicare in the United States?

A. Respite care for primary caregivers is supported by Medicare services.
B. Patients with a terminal illness may have unlimited stay in hospice care after an initial evaluation by a hospice team.
C. Patients must have a primary diagnosis of terminal cancer to qualify for hospice-related care.
D. Life expectancy for qualification for a patient considering hospice care is 3 months or less.
E. Although hospice care is geared toward "comfort care" including physical, emotional, social, and spiritual needs, a patient may continue treatment for curative intent if indicated by the hospice doctor.

4. A 50-year-old male is seen in clinic complaining of weight loss and significant back pain when lying flat. He tells you that sometimes he has to sleep in a recliner. He may have pathology involving which of the following?

A. Retroperitoneum
B. Abdominal wall
C. Lumbosacral disc
D. Cervical disc
E. Lumbar paraspinal muscles

5. How does leptomeningeal metastatic disease most commonly present?

A. Nuchal rigidity
B. Headache

C. Multiple areas of back pain associated with neurologic symptoms
D. Incontinence
E. Seizures

6. A 40-year-old female is seen in clinic complaining of severe and unrelenting pain in the lower extremities associated with paresthesias, weakness, and leg edema. She most likely has what kind of cancer?

A. Sarcoma
B. Colorectal
C. Lymphoma
D. Cervical
E. Lung

7. A 35-year-old female with a history of breast cancer treated with radiation and mastectomy 6 months ago is seen in clinic complaining of episodes of sharp and severe axillary pain radiating to the chest. Her arm on the same side is swollen and edematous. Her presentation is most consistent with:

A. Cancer recurrence
B. Postherpetic neuralgia
C. T1–T2 neuropathy
D. Paraneoplastic syndrome
E. Radiation-induced brachial plexopathy

8. A 40-year-old male is admitted to the hospital with nausea, confusion, and intractable muscle cramps. These symptoms are likely a sequelae of which type of cancer?

A. Small cell lung cancer
B. Non-small cell lung cancer
C. Pancreatic cancer
D. Thyroid cancer
E. Leukemia

9. A referral is made to a pain clinic regarding a patient with hepatocellular carcinoma with cirrhosis and complaints of severe constant abdominal pain. He has a past history of alcohol abuse and a family history of cardiac disease. He states that the pain does not improve with nonsteroidal anti-inflammatory drugs (NSAID) therapy. The appropriate next step is:

A. Consultation with a palliative service for consideration of hospice care
B. Initiation of morphine therapy to treat the patient's severe abdominal pain
C. Blood work to determine the extent of liver function

D. Assessment with a pain scale and symptom scale such as the Memorial Symptom Assessment Scale (MSAS)
E. Surgical consultation to address esophageal varices

10. A 57-year-old male has recently been diagnosed with adenocarcinoma of the pancreas. He has begun having left upper quadrant abdominal pain. Which of the following is the most accurate description of his disease course and treatment of his pain?

A. Because the tumor involves the head of the pancreas, primarily visceral pain is expected during the treatment course.
B. A medical pain treatment model targeting his tumor is most appropriate to treat underlying pain complaints.
C. He most likely will suffer from back pain that is worse with sitting and standing.
D. Because of the solitary nature of pancreatic cancer, he is unlikely to have associated suffering and depressive symptoms.
E. Invasion of the tumor by macrophages contributes significantly to the presentation of pain for pancreatic cancer patients.

11. A 51-year-old male has recently been diagnosed with head and neck cancer. He begins having oral mucositis, with pain worse when swallowing, after his chemotherapy and radiation treatments. Which of the following is true regarding his oral pain?

A. His chemotherapy regimen is far more likely to cause his symptoms of oral mucositis than his radiation therapy.
B. Topical anesthetics is the primary option for his oral mucositis.
C. Antimicrobial therapy may be considered in some causes of oral mucositis.
D. Changes in chemotherapy dose are unlikely to mitigate symptoms.
E. Regardless of the cause, oral mucositis is a rare complication of treatments related to head and neck cancer.

12. Which of the following cancer therapies is not directly associated with peripheral neuropathy?

A. Vinca alkaloids
B. Cisplatin
C. Taxanes
D. Bisphosphonates
E. Interferon

13. A patient with which of the following malignancies is most likely to receive tumor-related pain relief and symptom palliation with chemotherapy?

A. Lung cancer
B. Colorectal cancer
C. Pancreatic cancer
D. Testicular cancer
E. Sarcoma

14. What is the most common time course in terms of onset and resolution of oral mucositis after induction of autologous stem cell transplantation cytotoxic therapy?

A. Onset 1 or 2 days after marrow infusion with resolution by day 5
B. Onset 2–5 days after marrow infusion with resolution by day 15
C. Onset 5–10 days after marrow infusion with resolution by day 21
D. Onset 2 or 3 weeks after marrow infusion with resolution after day 30
E. The time course of oral mucositis after induction therapy for autologous stem cell transplantation is highly variable and not predictable.

15. A 74-year-old male diagnosed with end-stage respiratory failure from chronic obstructive sleep apnea chooses to enter hospice care. During his care, he begins gasping for air. The appropriate next step in his management is:

A. Discharge from hospice and consultation with an available pulmonary service for treatment
B. Use of morphine in small doses intravenously
C. Preparation for airway management and intubation
D. Intravenous injection of midazolam
E. Initiation of albuterol nebulizer treatment

16. A 40-year-old patient with metastatic melanoma is admitted to the hospital for spinal cord compression. After starting a multimodal analgesic regimen, he starts to complain of worsening burning pain in his groin area. This adverse side effect is likely secondary to which of the following?

A. NSAIDs
B. Corticosteroids
C. Bisphosphonates
D. Opiates
E. Pregabalin

17. The majority of cognitive impairment resulting from opioid use occurs during which time frame?

A. First few hours
B. First few days
C. First few weeks
D. First few months
E. Persists indefinitely

18. Tramadol is a part of which level of the World Health Organization (WHO) analgesic ladder?

A. Step 0
B. Step 1
C. Step 2
D. Step 3
E. It is not a part of the WHO analgesic ladder.

19. Which is true regarding opioid-related gastrointestinal side effects?

A. Constipation is universal, and laxatives should be prophylactically given.
B. If constipation occurs, then opioid rotation should be considered.
C. Nausea is uncommon, and prophylactic prescriptions are unwarranted.
D. If nausea occurs, then opioid rotation should be considered.
E. A single class of laxative should be prescribed at one time.

20. Which is true regarding opioid-related myoclonic jerks?

A. Extensor muscles are affected more so than flexor muscle groups.
B. The legs are usually affected more commonly compared to the arms.
C. Muscle relaxants rarely help to reduce the degree of myoclonus.
D. Myoclonus is usually persistent and does not abate over time.
E. Myoclonus usually improves along with opioid dose reduction.

21. A patient with metastatic colon cancer presents with an intractable headache and right upper quadrant abdominal pain refractory to parenteral opioids. What is the next best treatment?

A. Bisphosphonates
B. Muscle relaxants
C. Ketamine
D. Corticosteroids
E. Surgical intervention

22. An 85-year-old male admitted to a cancer hospital is started on a new analgesic protocol for metastatic prostate cancer. He becomes agitated overnight and eventually needs to be chemically restrained. What is the most likely cause?

A. Patient-controlled analgesia with fentanyl
B. Prednisolone
C. Dexamethasone
D. Haldol
E. Zyprexa

23. A 72-year-old male is newly diagnosed with prostate cancer and presents with mild (Visual Analogue Scale (VAS) 2/10) pelvic pain that is intermittent and sharp in nature and not related to movement. His creatinine is 1.3 mg/dl. What is the most appropriate medication for improving his pain symptoms?

A. Morphine
B. Hydrocodone
C. Ibuprofen
D. Fentanyl
E. Cyclobenzaprine

24. A 48-year-old female with a history of lung cancer presents to the emergency room with severe sharp (VAS 8/10) anterior chest wall pain. A chest X-ray and computed tomography (CT) of the chest are obtained showing metastatic bone lesion at the anterior seventh rib with no signs of infection or infusion. What is the most appropriate next treatment for her pain?

A. Intravenous meperidine
B. Radiation therapy
C. Sublingual buprenorphine
D. Intravenous hydromorphone
E. Surgical consultation for rib resection

25. A 61-year-old female with a history of renal cell cancer status post surgical resection of her right kidney is currently using hydrocodone immediate release for her pain. She states that her pain is sharp and achy and has become more severe (VAS 7/10) and constant. She has a history of low creatinine clearance, with a current creatinine of 1.9 mg/dl. Which is the most appropriate treatment for her pain symptoms?

A. Fentanyl transdermal system
B. Morphine extended release
C. Hydromorphone immediate release
D. Gabapentin
E. Methadone

26. A 68-year-old female with a history of chronic low back pain and end-stage renal disease has decided to enter palliative treatment with hospice care. During her care, she begins having severe back pain (VAS 8/10), which is treated with intravenous morphine. She begins having myoclonus and increasing pain. An appropriate next step is:

A. Increasing the morphine dosage to improve her pain symptoms
B. Initiation of phenytoin intravenously
C. Opioid rotation to hydrocodone orally
D. Consultation with the anesthesiology service for propofol infusion therapy
E. Begin oral clonazepam therapy

27. A 65-year-old female with a history of breast cancer is beginning to have low back and axial pain of the back. Upon examination, she complains of midline tenderness of the lumbar spine to palpation with worsening pain when standing. Metastatic disease to the vertebral body is suspected. Which of the following is true regarding her disease process?

A. Bone metastatic disease is primarily an osteolytic process involving increased osteoclast activity.
B. Radiographic studies such as bone scan, X-ray, and magnetic resonance imaging are indicated for evaluation of the extent of metastasis.
C. Opioids such as morphine are most important in treating the patient's bone-related pain.
D. Bisphosphonate therapy has become a tertiary treatment option since the addition of radionucleotides for the treatment of bone-related pain.
E. Interventional therapies such as kyphoplasty offer little benefit for this patient.

28. When attempting spinal chemoneurolysis, what is the most appropriate patient position when using alcohol as a neurolytic agent?

A. Painful side up, tilted away from the operator standing on the patient's dorsal side
B. Painful side down, tilted away from the operator standing on the patient's dorsal side
C. Painful side up, tilted toward the operator standing on the patient's dorsal side
D. Painful side down, tilted toward the operator standing on the patient's dorsal side

29. A 46-year-old female continues to have severe unremitting right leg pain from malignancy. She has failed multiple pain modalities and is considering neurolysis

as a treatment option. Which of the following is an accurate description of neurolytic agents?

A. Alcohol will be less painful than phenol in the intrathecal space.
B. Positioning herself semiprone with her right side down is appropriate for alcohol neurolysis.
C. Both epidural and intrathecal neurolysis may be considered with phenol.
D. A local anesthetic diagnostic block may not be necessary prior to injection of alcohol.
E. With proper positioning, the C fibers can be selectively neurolyzed without risk to motor fibers with intrathecal alcohol and phenol injections.

30. Radiation-induced fibrosis as a cause of brachial plexopathy may be differentiated from reversible radiation injury by which of the following factors?

A. Radiation fibrosis causes pain more frequently compared to reversible radiation injury.
B. Myokymia is commonly seen in electromyography (EMG) testing with reversible radiation injury.
C. CT imaging of the brachial plexus is often normal with radiation-induced fibrosis.
D. Pain is often more severe with reversible radiation injury.
E. Neurologic symptoms tend to be progressive with radiation fibrosis.

31. Radiation therapy is typically not associated with which of the following?

A. Eradication of bone-based tumors
B. Increased risk of fracture
C. Connective tissue fibrosis
D. Enteritis
E. Secondary malignancy

32. Which is true regarding localized external beam radiotherapy?

A. Pain relief is immediate.
B. Pain relief tends to evolve over a period of weeks after treatment.
C. Toxicity is common, and 4- to 6-week intervals are often needed in between treatments to allow recovery of bone marrow.
D. Prolonged high-dose schedules are more efficacious compared to single doses of 8–10 Gy.
E. Pain relief is unreliable.

33. Which of the following is true regarding pain related to cryosurgical techniques?

A. The severity of pain is not related to the duration of the freeze period.
B. The pain is mitigated with prophylactic NSAID administration.
C. Pain is usually localized and decreases in severity within 7 days.
D. Diffuse myalgias and arthralgias are commonly associated with cryosurgery.
E. Pain is uncommon because local nociceptor endings are frozen with this technique.

34. A 46-year-old female complains of diffuse sharp epigastric pain with radiation to her mid back. A recent abdominal CT scan showed a pancreatic head mass, and she is undergoing chemotherapy. Her pain does not seem to respond to opioid and adjuvant medications. The most appropriate next step is:

A. Superior hypogastric plexus blockade
B. Dorsal column stimulation of the thoracic spine
C. Surgical consultation for Whipple procedure
D. Evaluation for radiation therapy to target the pancreatic mass
E. Thoracic splanchnic nerve neurolysis

35. A 63-year-old male with a history of pancreatic mass and abdominal pain decides to undergo a celiac plexus neurolysis. The patient requests a discussion of the risks and benefits of the procedure. Which of the following statements is the most accurate to make during the discussion?

A. The retrocrural approach to the celiac plexus (targeting the splanchnic nerves) is associated with less orthostatic hypotension than the anterocrural approach.
B. The retrocrural approach to the celiac plexus (targeting the splanchnic nerves) is more likely to cause transient diarrhea than the anterocrural approach.
C. Transient backache with orthostatic hypotension are expected side effects and can be safely monitored at home after discharge.
D. Chemical neurolysis of the celiac plexus may result in paraplegia.
E. Choosing CT guidance for the celiac plexus block significantly reduces risks of side effects.

36. A 37-year-old male with a history of rectal cancer, treated with chemotherapy and subsequent radiation, presents with burning pain in the perineal area. A CT/positron emission tomography (PET) scan is obtained, showing no progression of disease, but his pain persists

despite opioid therapy. The most appropriate intervention at this time is:

A. Ganglion impar neurolysis
B. Surgical resection of the rectum
C. Superior hypogastric plexus blockade
D. Stellate ganglion block
E. Bilateral pudendal nerve ablation

37. A 63-year-old male has a history of metastatic non-small cell lung cancer and presents with right leg pain. A metastatic lesion is discovered in the right femoral shaft. He is considering radiation therapy for the treatment of his pain. Which of the following is the most appropriate statement?

A. Radiation can be delivered at any dose because the focus of the field only involves the shape of the metastatic lesion.
B. Radiation dosing schedules are determined by tumor type.
C. Radiopharmaceuticals such as strontium-89 may be an option if the patient has diffuse bone metastasis.
D. Surgery has no role in patients with femur lesions.
E. Palliative chemotherapy should be considered prior to radiation therapy.

38. Damage to which of the following is a common cause of functional impairment after radical neck dissection?

A. Spinal accessory nerve
B. Sympathetic chain
C. Thyroid
D. Baroreceptors
E. Carotid bodies

39. Which of the following is not an appropriate recommendation when treating an addict with cancer-related pain?

A. Transdermal fentanyl patches are often useful in this circumstance and may require replacement under direct observation.
B. Co-management with an addiction specialist is highly recommended if the prescribing clinician is not well trained in addiction medicine.
C. Long-acting oral or transdermal opioids are preferred treatment options.
D. If the patient is in active recovery and/or maintenance therapy, the prescribing clinician should remain in constant communication with the patient's counselor/therapist.
E. Opioid medications should be avoided at all costs when treating an addict with cancer pain.

40. A 31-year-old female with a history of rectal cancer presents for the first time to the pain clinic with burning sensation of the rectum. Which of the following is the most appropriate assessment during the initial pain history?

A. Given her cancer diagnosis, the patient's pain and suffering are indistinguishable and need not be assessed independently.
B. Because her pain has an organic cause, her emotional experience is unlikely to influence her symptoms.
C. Validated assessment tools such as the Edmonton Symptom Assessment Scale are helpful in distinguishing pain associated with cancer from other chronic pain syndromes.
D. Distinguishing types of pain, such as somatic or neuropathic pain, in the cancer patient may help determine pain management strategies.
E. Because pain is a subjective experience, family caregivers may be more effective in estimating a patient's pain complaint.

41. Which of the following cancer types is more highly associated with depression?

A. Colon
B. Lymphoma
C. Uterine
D. Breast
E. Ovarian

42. A 22-year-old male with a history of substance abuse and stage IV germ cell cancer frequently makes trips to various emergency departments seeking opioid medications. What is the most likely cause?

A. Opioid pseudo-addiction
B. Opioid addiction
C. Opioid tolerance
D. Anxiety
E. Malingering

43. Which of the following is a true statement regarding the perception of pain in the pediatric population?

A. Pain management can be completely disregarded in infants and neonates because their immature nervous systems cannot process nociception.
B. The majority of children are used to recurrent episodes of pain secondary to vaccinations, rough play, and childhood injuries.
C. The psychological and social domains of cancer pain management in children can be more complex compared to those of adults.

D. The psychologic aspects of pain do not have to be considered in the pediatric population due to the paucity of anxiety disorders in this population.
E. This issue remains largely uninvestigated given the low incidence of pediatric malignancies and high mortality rates.

44. A 2-year-old female has recently been diagnosed with a neuroblastoma of the abdomen. She is beginning to rub her abdomen and is crying more regularly. Which of the following statements correctly affects her pain management strategy?

A. Because of her age, her developmental stage significantly affects her pain assessment by a pain physician.
B. She is unlikely to suffer from fear and anxiety because her emotional development is not complete at her age.
C. Her parents are unlikely to be helpful, and the physician may have to depend on physical exam to assess her pain.
D. Her primary source of pain will be related to treatment of the tumor.
E. Opioid management should be considered first-line treatment in most of her painful situations.

45. Which of the following stimuli is most likely to evoke pain from a visceral structure?

A. Cutting
B. Burning
C. Pinching
D. Stretching
E. Slow distention

46. Which of the following is not a feature of visceral pain?

A. Less emotional and autonomic components compared with somatic pain
B. Difficult to localize by physical examination
C. Migratory
D. May induce the perception of pain in another organ
E. Discourages movement and physical activity

47. What is the most common mechanism by which fractures occur in tumor-bearing bone?

A. Primary invasion of stroma by cancer cells
B. Osteoclast-mediated bone resorption in an acidic environment
C. Osteoclast hypertrophy and invasion of stroma
D. Alterations in bone calcium bone metabolism that drive accelerated osteopenia
E. Tumor-mediated inflammatory factors stimulate innate macrophages and T cells to destroy bone stroma

48. Which of the following correctly characterizes chronic tumor-related pain?

A. Insidious, increases progressively with tumor growth, and may improve with tumor shrinkage
B. Insidious, increases progressively with tumor growth, and is often persistent despite tumor shrinkage
C. Acute onset, increases progressively with tumor growth, and may improve with tumor shrinkage
D. Acute onset, increases progressively with tumor growth, and is often persistent despite tumor shrinkage
E. Highly variable and does not have common characteristics

ANSWERS

1. ANSWER: B

The IASP expert-based multiaxial taxonomy of chronic pain classifies patients according to the following:

Region of the body (Axis I)

System whose abnormal functioning could conceivably produce pain (Axis II)

Temporal characteristics of pain and pattern of occurrence (Axis III)

Statement of intensity and time since onset of pain (Axis IV)

Presumed etiology (Axis V)

All of the listed answers correspond to one of these axis except for choice B, which deals with functional capacity. The International Classification of Functioning Disability and Health (ICF) incorporates functional outcomes more for patient evaluation and treatment, with less importance on classification.

FURTHER READING

Fishman S, Ballantyne J, Rathmell JP, et al. (Eds.). *Bonica's Management of Pain*. 4th ed. Baltimore, MD: Lippincott Williams & Wilkins; 2010:18–19.

2. ANSWER: C

Palliative and hospice care involves the management of pain and symptoms of end-of-life diseases. Physicians may recommend palliative services to provide "active total care of patients to disease that is not responsive to curative treatment." Hospice care will address pain, psychological, social, and spiritual support during the end-of-life process (usually defined as <90 days). Medicare supports palliative services for both inpatient and home usage. Patients will decide to give up treatments for curative intent, such as chemotherapy, radiation, and surgery; however, treatments for palliation of symptoms can be continued and/or considered. Most hospices will have staff available to treat a patient's symptoms, so regular visits with an oncologist will likely not be necessary.

FURTHER READING

Benzon HT (Ed.). *Essentials of Pain Medicine*. 3rd ed. Philadelphia, PA: Saunders; 2011:520.

3. ANSWER: A

Medicare hospice benefits in the United States are defined by the Centers for Medicare and Medicaid Services (CMS).

Patients considering hospice and palliative services have to be accepted by a hospice team (and physician). Patients must be diagnosed with a terminal disease, which includes both cancer and noncancer diagnosis (e.g., refractory congestive heart failure). A patient considering hospice care must not seek treatment for curative intent. Life expectancy is defined as 6 months or less, although this can be renewed by the hospice physician with a re-evaluation of the patients disease state. Although most hospice care is delivered in the home environment, a request may be made by the patient's primary caregiver for respite care. CMS supports respite care up to 5 days of inpatient stay for the patient.

FURTHER READING

US Department of Health and Human Services, Centers for Medicare & Medicaid Services. Medicare hospice benefits. Available at https:// www.medicare.gov/Pubs/pdf/02154.pdf.

4. ANSWER: A

The retroperitoneal pain stretch maneuver can reproduce this pain-exacerbating condition. It is performed with the patient sitting upright in bed with knees flexed, a pillow in the small of the back to exaggerate throttle lumbar lordosis, and the legs stretched out. Back pain with lowering the back of the bed (and subsequent back extension) may suggest a retroperitoneal source of back pain such as a retroperitoneal tumor. It may take several minutes for this pain to fully manifest itself.

Abdominal wall pain may be elicited using Carnett's maneuver, which consists of palpating the abdominal wall while the patient tenses the abdominal wall musculature. Creating abdominal wall muscle tension is most easily accomplished by having the patient lie flat while lifting both legs a few centimeters in the air or having him or her lift both shoulders off the bed. The straight leg raise or crossed straight leg raise is commonly used to provoke pain secondary to a herniated disc affecting the lumbosacral nerve roots. Spurling's test may be used to detect cervical nerve root compression. Dysfunction in the lumbar paraspinal muscles may be uncovered with back flexion, lateral flexion, and/or rotation. It is unlikely that lying flat would exacerbate pain from the lumbar paraspinal muscles because they are relaxed when the spine is straight.

FURTHER READING

Fishman S, Ballantyne J, Rathmell JP, et al. (Eds.). *Bonica's Management of Pain*. 4th ed. Baltimore, MD: Lippincott Williams & Wilkins; 2010:552–553.

5. ANSWER: C

Tumor cells may spread to the meninges through direct hematogenous spread, direct extension, venous transport, extension along neural structures, the lymphatic system, or iatrogenic causes. Patients most commonly present with multiple signs and symptoms involving more than one area of the neuraxis. These include headache, back pain, radiculopathy, cranial nerve dysfunction, spinal nerve involvement, and mental status alterations. Pain is the most common symptom and occurs in 30–76% of cases.

FURTHER READING

Fishman S, Ballantyne J, Rathmell JP, et al. (Eds.). *Bonica's Management of Pain*. 4th ed. Baltimore, MD: Lippincott Williams & Wilkins; 2010:570.

6. ANSWER: B

A hallmark feature of direct tumor infiltration into the lumbosacral plexus is a severe and unrelenting pain affecting the pelvis, low back, hip, and/or lower extremities. With progressive disease, sensory changes, weakness, lower extremity sympathetic dysfunction, and lower extremity edema often develop in conjunction with pain. Most lumbosacral plexopathy occurs secondary to local extension from colorectal malignancies but may also result from other pelvic tumors, melanoma, lymphoma, breast, or lung cancer.

FURTHER READING

Fishman S, Ballantyne J, Rathmell JP, et al. (Eds.). *Bonica's Management of Pain*. 4th ed. Baltimore, MD: Lippincott Williams & Wilkins; 2010:571.

7. ANSWER: C

The intercostobrachial nerve is a sensory nerve arising from T1 and T2. Its anatomic course is highly variable, making it difficult to avoid during surgeries that involve axillary dissection. Damage to the nerve after breast surgery often presents with lancinating axillary pain, chest tightness, and/or burning in the axilla/upper arm soon after the procedure or even months afterwards. Intercostobrachial neuropathy is seen as part of the postmastectomy pain syndrome and can be differentiated from radiation plexopathy by the anatomic location of symptoms, the presence of lymphedema, and usually more severe pain. Although cancer recurrence

should always be in the differential diagnosis of any patient with previous cancer presenting with pain, worsening pain from cancer recurrence is typically seen after a longer time course. Although paraneoplastic syndromes may also present with sensory changes, there are often other neurologic sequelae, including ataxia, dizziness, dysphasia, autonomic dysfunction, and weakness.

FURTHER READING

Fishman S, Ballantyne J, Rathmell JP, et al. (Eds.). *Bonica's Management of Pain*. 4th ed. Baltimore, MD: Lippincott Williams & Wilkins; 2010:572–573.

8. ANSWER: A

Clinical paraneoplastic syndromes can be classified into endocrine, neurological, mucocutaneous, and hematological categories. Lung cancers are often the cause, with small cell lung cancers most commonly implicated. A large fraction of hyponatremia secondary to the syndrome of inappropriate antidiuretic hormone secretion (SIADH) is seen in elderly smokers due to small cell lung cancer. This metabolic derangement is the result of excessive production of arginine vasopressin by tumor cells. Hypercalcemia is more common with non-small cell lung cancer, especially with squamous cell carcinomas. Neurologic paraneoplastic syndromes are more rare and can include cerebellar degeneration, optic neuritis, retinopathy, necrotizing myelopathy, and peripheral neuropathy.

FURTHER READING

Fishman S, Ballantyne J, Rathmell JP, et al. (Eds.). *Bonica's Management of Pain*. 4th ed. Baltimore, MD: Lippincott Williams & Wilkins; 2010:567.

9. ANSWER: D

When a patient is referred to a pain clinic, an appropriate history and physical should be performed. In addition, pain and symptom assessments are indicated for further evaluation prior to decision for a treatment plan. The VAS is a simple tool to assess symptom severity. Assessment scales such as the MSAS or MD Anderson Symptom Inventory (MDASI) are indicated for end-of-life cases. This would be done prior to a decision of palliative care consultation or hospice discussion. For an end-of-life disease, it is likely that surgical consultation would be a less appropriate action during an end-of-life discussion. Although the treatment of the patient's pain with morphine may be appropriate, this should be done after complete evaluation and assessment of the patient's pain and symptoms is completed.

FURTHER READING

Benzon HT (Ed.). *Essentials of Pain Medicine*. 3rd ed. Philadelphia, PA: Saunders; 2011:521–524.

10. ANSWER: E

Left upper quadrant pain is more likely associated with tumor of the pancreatic tail. Furthermore, during the disease course, although visceral pain is common, treatment and tumor extension-related pain may occur as well. Both surgery and radiation therapy may cause neuropathic pain syndromes, and direct tumor invasion of bony structures and muscle may cause somatic pain. As such, medical models treating the tumor may improve pain; however, anesthetic, palliative, and rehabilitative models for pain control may be administered jointly. The back pain associated with pancreatic cancer is usually in the distribution of T10–L2 and worse with lying flat. Both suffering and depression are common with the diagnosis of pancreatic cancer. This may be associated with nausea and fatigue, and these symptoms need to be treated appropriately. Macrophages are involved initially in starting the inflammatory process that is related to pancreatic pain. Macrophages may induce increased levels of calcitonin gene-related peptide, which in turn cause neuronal sprouting and pain syndromes.

FURTHER READING

Fishman S, Ballantyne J, Rathmell JP, et al. (Eds.). *Bonica's Management of Pain*. 4th ed. Baltimore, MD: Lippincott Williams & Wilkins; 2010:760–764.

11. ANSWER: C

Both radiation and chemotherapy can cause oral mucositis. Various chemotherapeutic treatments can lead to different presentations of oral mucositis. Although topical anesthetics are part of the paradigm of treatment for mucositis, basic oral care, oral rinse, systemic analgesics, and, in some cases, oral antibiotics may be indicated for treatment of the painful condition. It is likely that if oral mucositis is persistently severe, a reduction in chemotherapy dosage may lessen the symptom burden. Depending on the treatment of the cancer, oral mucositis may be a very common presentation, for example, in myeloablative chemotherapy regiments during hematopoietic cell transplants.

FURTHER READING

Fishman S, Ballantyne J, Rathmell JP, et al. (Eds.). *Bonica's Management of Pain*. 4th ed. Baltimore, MD: Lippincott Williams & Wilkins; 2010:835–838.

12. ANSWER: D

Peripheral neurotoxicity is common with a number of chemotherapy agents, including the vinca alkaloids, platinum agents, and taxanes. Platinum agents cause neuronal apoptosis and can damage large myelinated sensory fibers. Taxanes aggregate microtubules and have an increased neurotoxic effect when combined with platinum agents. Non-chemotherapy agents used in cancer therapy, such as interferons, thalidomide, and amphotericin-B, are also frequently implicated as neurotoxic agents. Bisphosphonates are commonly used agents in cancer patients for the treatment of malignant disease involving bony structures. They may acutely cause bone pain and osteonecrosis, with the mandible being frequently involved. Chronic bisphosphonate-induced osteonecrosis may eventually involve neural structures to cause pain and sensory changes, but the drug itself is not thought to be neurotoxic.

FURTHER READING

Fishman S, Ballantyne J, Rathmell JP, et al. (Eds.). *Bonica's Management of Pain*. 4th ed. Baltimore, MD: Lippincott Williams & Wilkins; 2010:619.

13. ANSWER: D

Many of the adenocarcinomas (lung, colorectal, esophageal, pancreatic, and prostate), brain tumors, melanomas, and sarcomas are poorly responsive to chemotherapy agents. As a result, anticancer medications are rarely effective in shrinking the size of the tumor or in offering significant analgesia or symptom relief secondary to tumor-associated mass effects. Choriocarcinomas, certain types of leukemia, lymphomas, and testicular cancer are among the few malignancies that have very high chemotherapy response rates.

FURTHER READING

Fishman S, Ballantyne J, Rathmell JP, et al. (Eds.). *Bonica's Management of Pain*. 4th ed. Baltimore, MD: Lippincott Williams & Wilkins; 2010:658–659.

14. ANSWER: B

Oral mucositis following marrow induction therapy for autologous stem cell transplantation usually becomes evident 2–5 days after marrow infusion, with resolution in 90% of patients by day 15. Mucosal damage usually presents in a bilateral pattern primarily involving the cheeks, lateral/ventral tongue, floor of the mouth, soft palate, and labial mucosa. Induction therapy for allogenic stem cell transplantation follows a slightly delayed time course: It presents with a slightly slower onset with a slower resolution of symptoms. Patients additionally conditioned for transplantation with total body irradiation are at risk for increased mucosal insult.

FURTHER READING

Fishman S, Ballantyne J, Rathmell JP, et al. (Eds.). *Bonica's Management of Pain*. 4th ed. Baltimore, MD: Lippincott Williams & Wilkins; 2010:621.

15. ANSWER: B

Dyspnea (among other symptoms, such as pain, constipation, sedation, anxiety, and depression) is common among patients at the end of life. The mainstay of treatment for "air hunger" is opioid therapy with short duration of action. Morphine or hydromorphone intravenously would be a common regimen used to ameliorate the symptoms of dyspnea. Hospice care systems are expected to manage these symptoms, and it is unlikely that a transfer out of the hospice system is needed. Both anxiolytics and symptomatic treatments (e.g., albuterol) may be indicated as secondary options for symptom control. When a patient is in hospice care, usually he or she has a "do not resuscitate" order that would preclude airway management with intubation.

FURTHER READING

Benzon HT (Ed.). *Essentials of Pain Medicine*. 3rd ed. Philadelphia, PA: Saunders; 2011:523.

16. ANSWER: B

Dexamethasone is a commonly used agent to treat inflammation secondary to spinal cord compression and malignancy-related bone pain. The standard dose ranges from 12 to 24 mg daily and can be administered once daily due to the long half-life of the drug. Some patients receiving high-dose corticosteroids may report burning perineal pain.

Of note, cancer patients may also develop perineal discomfort 6–18 months after receiving pelvic radiotherapy. Lyrica is associated with sedation, ataxia, cognitive dysfunction, and peripheral edema. Bisphosphonates are associated with gastrointestinal (GI) upset, flu-like symptoms, and, uncommonly, osteonecrosis of the mandible. NSAIDs can cause GI upset, platelet dysfunction, and renal dysfunction as a result of COX inhibition. Although patients on high-dose and rapidly escalated opioids may report opioid-induced hyperalgesia, allodynia isolated to the groin area would be uncommon. In addition, opioid-induced hyperalgesia is typically associated with other signs and symptoms, including myoclonus.

FURTHER READING

Fishman S, Ballantyne J, Rathmell JP, et al. (Eds.). *Bonica's Management of Pain*. 4th ed. Baltimore, MD: Lippincott Williams & Wilkins; 2010:640–641.

17. ANSWER: B

The majority of research has found that most cognitive impairment from opioid use occurs during the first several days. Chronic pain patients who have been on opioid therapy for more than 3 days have been shown to exhibit few differences in cognitive performance compared with matched patients not using opioid medications. However, there still remain many unanswered questions related to specific mechanisms of opiate-related cognitive impairment, risk factors for impairment, and interpatient variability. The influence of opioids on driving ability remains a contentious issue due to the increasing number of patients taking opioids who continue to drive.

FURTHER READING

Fishman S, Ballantyne J, Rathmell JP, et al. (Eds.). *Bonica's Management of Pain*. 4th ed. Baltimore, MD: Lippincott Williams & Wilkins; 2010:598.

18. ANSWER: C

The WHO analgesic ladder suggests a stepwise escalation of analgesic medications through a hierarchy of increasingly potent drugs. Tramadol is currently a step 2 analgesic. Medications on this step qualify as "weak opioids" that should be added should a patient fail to achieve pain control with paracetamol and/or NSAID derivatives. Other WHO step 2 analgesics include codeine and dihydrocodeine.

However, some physicians choose to avoid WHO step 2 analgesics altogether because there is some evidence that these medications may delay patients from receiving stronger opioids and thus remain in pain. In addition, the analgesic efficacy of CYP2D6-metabolized drugs, including codeine, hydrocodone, and dihydrocodeine, is very unpredictable given genetic factors that result in a wide range of CYP2D6 action.

FURTHER READING

McMahon SB (Ed.). *Wall and Melzack's Textbook of Pain*. 6th ed. Philadelphia, PA: Saunders; 2013:1077.
Smith HS. Opioid metabolism. *Mayo Clin Proc*. 2009;84(7): 613–624.

19. ANSWER: A

Constipation is ubiquitous among patients taking opioid medications and among all classes of opioid medications. Prophylactic regular administration of both stimulant and softening laxatives is warranted to maintain regular bowel function. Nausea also occurs very frequently (~30–50%) among patients using opioid medications. Prophylactic antiemetic medications should be prescribed along with opioid medications so that they are readily available.

FURTHER READING

McMahon SB (Ed.). *Wall and Melzack's Textbook of Pain*. 6th ed. Philadelphia, PA: Saunders; 2013:1078.

20. ANSWER: E

Myoclonic jerks are a manifestation of flexor group myoclonus and represent a form of opioid toxicity. They usually occur in the arms but can also occur in the legs. Patients should be cautioned to walk and handle hazards such as sharp objects and hot drinks with care. Myoclonic jerks usually improve with time and with opioid dose reduction. If still persistent, benzodiazepine administration may also help to reduce the degree of myoclonic jerks.

FURTHER READING

McMahon SB (Ed.). *Wall and Melzack's Textbook of Pain*. 6th ed. Philadelphia, PA: Saunders; 2013:1079.

21. ANSWER: D

Corticosteroids are very useful in cancer patients for several reasons. They improve well-being, appetite, and have indications for pain relief in certain situations. For example, they are very beneficial in treating pain associated with increased intracranial pressure from cerebral metastatic disease and also upper abdominal pain from hepatic distention. In this case, the likely etiology is capsular distention. Corticosteroids also can relieve pain from tumors causing compressive symptoms in other areas of the body, such as the abdomen, pelvis, head, and neck.

FURTHER READING

McMahon SB (Ed.). *Wall and Melzack's Textbook of Pain*. 6th ed. Philadelphia, PA: Saunders; 2013:1079.

22. ANSWER: C

Although cognitive impairment is a known side effect from opioid therapy, it is unlikely that this particular patient would have persistent opioid toxicity from patient-controlled analgesia using a medication with a short half-life such as fentanyl. Acute psychotomimetic effects such as psychosis, depression, and insomnia are well-known side effects from steroid therapy. Compared to prednisolone, which more commonly causes fluid retention, dexamethasone is more likely to cause psychosis. Antipsychotic medications such as Haldol or Zyprexa may be useful for treating acute delirium.

FURTHER READING

McMahon SB (Ed.). *Wall and Melzack's Textbook of Pain*. 6th ed. Philadelphia, PA: Saunders; 2013:1079, 1085.

23. ANSWER: C

The World Health Organization released an analgesic treatment ladder for pain in 1986 for cancer and palliative patients. The treatment algorithm is based on severity of pain (mild, VAS 1–3/10; moderate, VAS 4–6/10; and severe, VAS 7–10/10). Patients who have mild pain are started on NSAIDs or acetaminophen. Should the pain escalate to moderate, "weak opioids" are initiated (e.g., hydrocodone and tramadol), with severe pain treated with "strong" opioids (e.g., morphine and fentanyl). Adjuvants such as cyclobenzaprine can be added at any time if indicated. The described patient does not seem to have muscle spasms; thus, cyclobenzaprine is less likely to be helpful.

neuropathic pain symptoms (this patient's pain seems to be somatic in nature).

FURTHER READING

Benzon HT (Ed.). *Essentials of Pain Medicine*. 3rd ed. Philadelphia, PA: Saunders; 2011:512.

FURTHER READING

Benzon HT (Ed.). *Essentials of Pain Medicine*. 3rd ed. Philadelphia, PA: Saunders; 2011:515–516.

24. ANSWER: D

The patient presents with severe pain that is usually initially treated with "strong opioids" such as morphine or hydromorphone. This follows the WHO ladder treatment for severity of cancer pain. Meperidine is rarely indicated because of severity of side effects secondary to metabolites. Although buprenorphine has been shown to be effective in some cancers, such as head and neck cancer, partial agonists are usually not first-line opioids for severe cancer-related pain. Radiation therapy would be a long-term solution to the patient's disease, but it would be considered after better pain control. Usually, surgical resection would be an option should other strategies not be effective. Although not a listed option for this question, intravenous corticosteroids may be an option, especially with metastatic disease near the spinal cord.

FURTHER READING

Benzon HT (Ed.). *Essentials of Pain Medicine*. 3rd ed. Philadelphia, PA: Saunders; 2011:512–514.

25. ANSWER: A

Immediate-release formulations of medications (NSAIDs and immediate-release opioids) are indicated for intermittent pain. However, if pain becomes constant, and remains severe, sustained-release formulations are considered as therapeutic options. The patient would benefit from a sustained-release opioid such as the fentanyl transdermal system. Morphine is not indicated given the patient's poor creatinine clearance, which would likely cause a buildup of metabolites of morphine (specifically morphine 3-gluconoride), possibly leading to central nervous system excitation. Although hydromorphone immediate release may help her pain symptoms, it is better indicated for severe intermittent or breakthrough pain. Methadone is usually not considered first line in patients who are relatively opioid naive, especially given its long and variable half-life. Gabapentin is an adjuvant that may be more effective for

26. ANSWER: E

Myoclonus and hyperalgesia may be resultant from metabolites of morphine and hydromorphone (the 3-gluconoride metabolites). These metabolites may increase in the setting of renal failure and decrease in renal clearance. A usual course for treatment of mild myoclonus is the addition of benzodiazepines. Both myoclonus and hyperalgesia may be treated with reduction of opioid dose or rotation to another similar opioid (e.g., fentanyl). Hydrocodone would be indicated in moderate pain states (VAS 4–7/10). Should the neurotoxicity progress to seizures, faster infusions such as propofol and intravenous benzodiazepines are indicated. Phenytoin may be used to treat acute seizures. Naloxone has not been shown to reverse neurotoxicity from opioid metabolites.

FURTHER READING

Benzon HT (Ed.). *Essentials of Pain Medicine*. 3rd ed. Philadelphia, PA: Saunders; 2011:523.

27. ANSWER: B

Metastatic disease of the bone is a complex process that may be both osteoblastic and osteolytic depending on the pathophysiology of the cancer. Osteoclast activity is only a part of the overall disease process. Radiologic studies are crucial to the diagnosis and treatment options for metastatic disease. Depending on radiographic location, radiation therapy may be used for focal disease treatment. Opioids are useful in pain control; however, NSAIDs and steroid formulations are also instrumental in pain relief. Morphine is also associated with increased progression of disease in animal models of bone cancer. Bisphosphonate therapy is critical in a patient's care, and significant research supports its inclusion in therapies for bone metastasis. Calcitonin may have some marginal benefit for the treatment of metastatic bone-related pain. Kyphoplasty for metastatic bone-related vertebral body pain has been shown to be helpful for pain relief. This can be offered in conjunction or after chemo or radiation treatment of metastatic bone disease to the spine without neurologic compromise.

Fishman S, Ballantyne J, Rathmell JP, et al. (Eds.). *Bonica's Management of Pain*. 4th ed. Baltimore, MD: Lippincott Williams & Wilkins; 2010:853–857.

28. ANSWER: A

Compared to cerebrospinal fluid (CSF), alcohol is hypobaric and will "float," whereas phenol is hyperbaric and will "sink." Ideally, the patient should be positioned so that the neurolytic substance in the CSF is targeting the sensory dorsal roots in the dorsolateral subarachnoid space. Therefore, the painful side should be facing up for alcohol neurolysis and facing down for phenol neurolysis. An operator standing on the dorsal side of the patient should rotate away for alcohol neurolysis and rotate toward for phenol neurolysis. Very small aliquots of the neurolytic agent are then incrementally injected through a small spinal needle at the appropriate nerve root level while monitoring the patient for sensory and dermatomal changes. Because patients may be more uncomfortable lying on their painful side, alcohol neurolysis has traditionally been preferred.

Fishman S, Ballantyne J, Rathmell JP, et al. (Eds.). *Bonica's Management of Pain*. 4th ed. Baltimore, MD: Lippincott Williams & Wilkins; 2010:610–611.

29. ANSWER: C

Epidural and intrathecal neurolysis of both the epidural and the intrathecal space with alcohol or phenol could be considered primarily during end-of-life discussions for patients in pain that is refractory to multiple other treatments. In general, alcohol is painful (initial burning pain), whereas phenol acts initially as a local anesthetic when placed near neural tissue. Positioning is critical when considering intrathecal neurolysis. Alcohol is less dense than CSF; thus, the positioning requires both the patient to be semiprone and the painful side to be superior from the dependent side. Phenol intrathecal neurolysis requires the patient to be semisupine and the painful side to be dependent. Because alcohol is a painful injection, prior local anesthetic use is recommended. The local anesthetic injection can also help determine the location of the neurolytic target that may help with pain relief. Unfortunately, although positioning can help limit the spread of the neurolytic to the dorsal root entry zone (the target for pain transmission), spread to the anterior rootlets and the spinal cord is possible and difficult to control. This may lead to significant complications, such as paraplegia, and this should be discussed with patients prior to considering this intervention.

Benzon HT (Ed.). *Essentials of Pain Medicine*. 3rd ed. Philadelphia, PA: Saunders; 2011:531–533.

30. ANSWER: E

Compared with transient weakness affecting the distal nerve roots (C6–T1) as seen with reversible radiation injury, neurologic sequelae from radiation fibrosis tend to be progressive and have a tendency to affect more proximal nerve roots (C5–C6). Pain from reversible radiation-induced plexopathy has an incidence (40%) more than twice that of radiation fibrosis (18%). However, when it does occur, pain from radiation fibrosis tends to be more intense and may be severe in up to 35% of affected patients. Reversible radiation injury may lack any pathologic appearance on CT imaging compared to diffuse tissue infiltration of the plexus as seen with radiation fibrosis. The presence of myokymia in EMG testing is a distinguishing characteristic of radiation fibrosis-induced plexopathy.

Fishman S, Ballantyne J, Rathmell JP, et al. (Eds.). *Bonica's Management of Pain*. 4th ed. Baltimore, MD: Lippincott Williams & Wilkins; 2010:571.

31. ANSWER: A

Radiation therapy often has a ceiling due to its effect primarily because of potential damage to surrounding tissues around the metastatic lesion. As a result, it is very difficult to administer large enough doses of radiation to completely eliminate most tumors. Side effects from radiation therapy include an increased lifetime bone fracture rate, enteritis, cystitis, connective tissue fibrosis, neural damage, proctitis, bowel stricture formation, fistula formation, chronic pain, and even secondary malignancies. Onset of these symptoms may occur as late as years after radiation therapy.

Fishman S, Ballantyne J, Rathmell JP, et al. (Eds.). *Bonica's Management of Pain*. 4th ed. Baltimore, MD: Lippincott Williams & Wilkins; 2010:641, 646.

32. ANSWER: B

Localized external beam radiotherapy has been shown to be a very effective treatment for pain related to metastatic bone disease. A large number of controlled trials and Cochrane reviews suggest a number needed to treat of approximately 3.6 (95% confidence interval, 3.2–3.9) to achieve at least 50% pain relief. The current literature suggests that single doses of 8–10 Gy are just as effective as prolonged high-dose treatment courses. Because of modern technology that can localize the radiation field, toxicity is mild and related to the site of treatment. The pattern of pain relief usually evolves over a period of 4–6 weeks after treatment. This is in contrast to the pattern of pain relief following widefield external beam radiotherapy. Pain relief tends to occur more rapidly but radiation-related toxicity is much more common when treating larger volumes with radiation. Interestingly, the underlying primary tumor histology is not thought to influence response to radiotherapy.

FURTHER READING

McMahon SB (Ed.). *Wall and Melzack's Textbook of Pain*. 6th ed. Philadelphia, PA: Saunders; 2013:1079.

33. ANSWER: C

Cryosurgical techniques are often used to manage skin and pelvic tumors, including cervical and prostate cancers. Pain is often localized, which decreases over a period of 2–7 days. The severity of pain is related to the freeze period duration and is not alleviated with prophylactic NSAID administration.

FURTHER READING

McMahon SB (Ed.). *Wall and Melzack's Textbook of Pain*. 6th ed. Philadelphia, PA: Saunders; 2013:1040–1042.

34. ANSWER: E

Classic pain from pancreatic cancer includes epigastric pain with radiation to the mid-thoracic spine, usually worse with lying flat. Initial strategies to control the pain include opioids and adjuvant therapy, although if ineffective, interventional pain procedures may be considered. Surgeries, such as the Whipple procedure, are usually considered a treatment option depending on the tumor progression. The patient is undergoing chemotherapy, likely precluding surgical options. Radiation therapy may be used for palliative treatment in this setting. Dorsal column stimulation may be of benefit, although this is likely a secondary option. Sympathetic blockade of the abdominal viscera, via either the splanchnic nerves or celiac plexus, has been well established as a procedure to treat pancreatic-related pain. The superior hypogastric plexus innervates hindgut viscera such as the bladder and other organs in the pelvis.

FURTHER READING

Benzon HT (Ed.). *Essentials of Pain Medicine*. 3rd ed. Philadelphia, PA: Saunders; 2011:525.

35. ANSWER: D

Targeting the splanchnic nerves at the retrocrural space has been shown to increase the incidence of orthostatic hypotension but decrease the risk of diarrhea compared to the transcrural approach. Both techniques are associated with a risk of neurologic compromise when considering chemical neurolysis with either phenol or alcohol. Although paraplegia is rare, it is thought that chemical irritants may cause ischemic effects to the spinal cord, more so in patients with atherosclerotic disease. Should patients complain of post-procedure backache and have orthostatic hypotension, retroperitoneal hematoma should be considered. Serial monitoring of hematocrit is recommended. Finally, although image guidance for a celiac plexus block may be helpful, no image-guided modality has been shown to be superior in reducing potential complications.

FURTHER READING

Benzon HT (Ed.). *Essentials of Pain Medicine*. 3rd ed. Philadelphia, PA: Saunders; 2011:526–527.

36. ANSWER: A

The patient is suffering neuropathic pain in the rectum, which may be secondary to the malignancy or treatment. The most likely intervention would be the ganglion impar block and neurolysis. The ganglion is the terminal ganglion of the sympathetic chain and sits anteriorly at the sacrococcygeal junction. Surgical resection may not improve the pain. A pudendal nerve block would be indicated for somatic pain in the perineum; however, bowel and bladder innervation would be interrupted. Table 17.1 presents common sympathetic blocks and associated visceral pain targets.

Table 17.1 **COMMON SYMPATHETIC TARGETS FOR ASSOCIATED VISCERAL PAIN SYNDROMES**

SYMPATHETIC CHAIN	ASSOCIATED TARGET AFTER BLOCKADE
Stellate ganglion (C7–T1)	Ipsilateral arm and face
Esophageal plexus (T5–T6)	Esophagus and gastroesophageal junction
Celiac plexus (T12–L1)	Organs of the foregut (pancreas, liver, kidney, adrenal glands)
Lumbar splanchnics (L3–L4)	Ipsilateral lower extremity
Superior hypogastric plexus (L5–S1)	Pelvic organs of the hindgut (bladder, cervix, uterus, genitalia)
Ganglion of impar	Rectum and coccyx

FURTHER READING

Benzon HT (Ed.). *Essentials of Pain Medicine.* 3rd ed. Philadelphia, PA: Saunders; 2011:529–530.

37. ANSWER: C

The primary limitation to increased radiation dosage applied to a tumor is the effect of radiation on surrounding healthy tissue. Radiation dosing schedules are determined by multiple variables, including tumor type, location of surrounding critical normal structures (e.g., the spinal cord), patient's ability to tolerate treatment, and type of radiation used (e.g., conventional electrons or protons). Surgery may be considered if there is an impeding fracture or pathologic fracture present at the location of the metastatic disease. Palliative chemotherapy and radiation therapy are part of the treatment options for pain control in the palliative patient and are considered independently for each patient's case. In diffuse metastatic disease, radiopharmaceuticals such as radium and strontium have been used with some efficacy in improving metastatic bone-related pain.

FURTHER READING

Fishman S, Ballantyne J, Rathmell JP, et al. (Eds.). *Bonica's Management of Pain.* 4th ed. Baltimore, MD: Lippincott Williams & Wilkins; 2010:875–882.

38. ANSWER: A

Neck dissection is often performed for the treatment of cervical lymph nodes. Damage to the spinal accessory nerve during neck dissection results in denervation of the upper trapezius muscle. Patients often present with a "shoulder syndrome" consisting of pain, limited abduction of the shoulder, and anatomic deformities including protraction or drooping of the shoulder. Sternoclavicular joint hypertrophy and stress fractures involving the middle third of the clavicle can result from strain as a result of abnormal shoulder positioning. Extensive dissections involving the posterior triangle of the neck may be more responsible for postoperative neck and shoulder pain.

FURTHER READING

Fishman S, Ballantyne J, Rathmell JP, et al. (Eds.). *Bonica's Management of Pain.* 4th ed. Baltimore, MD: Lippincott Williams & Wilkins; 2010:573, 620.

39. ANSWER: E

All patients deserve adequate pain control, and it is unethical to withhold appropriate analgesia even in an addict with cancer-related pain. All the other answer choices are appropriate pain management recommendations when treating patients with substance abuse issues.

FURTHER READING

Fishman S, Ballantyne J, Rathmell JP, et al. (Eds.). *Bonica's Management of Pain.* 4th ed. Baltimore, MD: Lippincott Williams & Wilkins; 2010:539, 556–557.

40. ANSWER: D

Cancer patients often have suffering and pain, which may need to be independently assessed to optimize treatment. Understanding a patient's suffering as it relates to a his or her pain is incumbent upon a pain physician for successful treatment. Regardless of the cause of pain, emotional and subjective experience as it relates to physical damage is the definition of pain and thus individuals may interpret similar organic pain symptoms differently. Valid assessment tools for pain help gauge pain and symptoms, but they are not designed to separate cancer from noncancer symptoms. In general, because pain is a subjective experience, the patient tends to be the most accurate in assessing his or her pain. Family and physicians typically overestimate pain that the patient is suffering. During a patient history, determining the type of pain, whether somatic or neuropathic, may help in the decision of treatment options.

Fishman S, Ballantyne J, Rathmell JP, et al. (Eds.). *Bonica's Management of Pain*. 4th ed. Baltimore, MD: Lippincott Williams & Wilkins; 2010:739–745.

41. ANSWER: D

Psychologic factors play an important role in exacerbating chronic pain. Severity of depression has been correlated with pain, anxiety, disease type, and numerous other factors affecting patient quality of life. Certain cancer types are highly associated with depression, including oropharyngeal, pancreatic, breast, and lung cancer. For reasons unknown, prevalence of depression among patients with colon, gynecological, and lymphoma malignancies is not as high.

FURTHER READING

Fishman S, Ballantyne J, Rathmell JP, et al. (Eds.). *Bonica's Management of Pain*. 4th ed. Baltimore, MD: Lippincott Williams & Wilkins; 2010:562.

42. ANSWER: A

Addiction even within the setting of high-dose morphine in the cancer population is uncommon. It is a complex psychological, behavioral, and physical phenomenon characterized by drug craving and social changes to enable continuation and stockpiling supplies of the relevant drug. Physical dependence or tolerance is a universal physiologic occurrence in all patients in response to opioid receptor stimulation. Abrupt cessation of opioids in any opioid-tolerant patient may result in withdrawal symptoms. Opioid pseudo-addiction describes the situation in which inadequate analgesia is provided to a patient suffering from severe pain (which in this case represents a patient with stage IV cancer). Such patients will sometimes go to extreme lengths to seek medical attention in order to obtain adequate supplies of opioid medications. Unfortunately, this scenario still occurs in modern health care settings and can be misinterpreted as addiction.

FURTHER READING

McMahon SB (Ed.). *Wall and Melzack's Textbook of Pain*. 6th ed. Philadelphia, PA: Saunders; 2013:1079.

43. ANSWER: C

The biopsychosocial model of pain is more complex in children because the pediatric stage of development needs special attention compared to adults. Major neurodevelopmental changes in childhood occur rapidly until young adulthood. Pain perception in neonates has been extensively studied. Although it was previously thought that newborns could not experience pain, this assumption has largely been disproved. In fact, noxious stimuli may cause a more severe perception of pain due to immature nociceptive inhibitory systems. Inability to properly communicate feelings and painful symptoms and the lack of experience with chronic medical conditions and health care systems may result in amplified anxiety, fear responses, and discomfort among children. Studies have even shown that childhood cancer survivors can develop a form of post-traumatic stress disorder due to memories of invasive cancer treatment-related procedures.

FURTHER READING

Fishman S, Ballantyne J, Rathmell JP, et al. (Eds.). *Bonica's Management of Pain*. 4th ed. Baltimore, MD: Lippincott Williams & Wilkins; 2010:669–671.

44. ANSWER: A

In the pediatric population, developmental stages significantly affect pain assessment. At age 2 years, the lack of communication may make this patient's pain presentation difficult to determine. Although she is young, she is very likely to suffer from fear and anxiety, especially because of procedures and unknown surroundings. Physicians will have to rely on physical exam as well as family and parental assessments to determine her pain level. During her treatment, she is as likely to suffer pain from treatment as from diagnostic procedures such as intravenous placements. Furthermore, she will likely have pain related to psychologic stressors. As a result, although opioids may be helpful for pain management, a comprehensive pain program including psychological treatment involving cognitive–behavioral therapy and multiple strategies is needed.

FURTHER READING

Fishman S, Ballantyne J, Rathmell JP, et al. (Eds.). *Bonica's Management of Pain*. 4th ed. Baltimore, MD: Lippincott Williams & Wilkins; 2010:906–908.

45. ANSWER: D

Normal stimuli that activate somatic nociceptors may not consistently cause reports of pain when applied to visceral structures. Visceral pain is most likely elicited by stretching or distention of visceral structures, ischemia, inflammation, and/or insult to the neural structures supplying a particular organ. Although organ distention may cause visceral pain, gentle or slow progressive distention/obstruction may not manifest discomfort until ischemia or rupture result.

FURTHER READING

Fishman S, Ballantyne J, Rathmell JP, et al. (Eds.). *Bonica's Management of Pain*. 4th ed. Baltimore, MD: Lippincott Williams & Wilkins; 2010:636.

46. ANSWER: A

Visceral pain is often migratory in nature, difficult to reproduce using physical examination techniques, and vague in character. Visceral pain is represented throughout the limbic system in the anterior cingulate gyrus, insular cortex, and amygdala, which may contribute to the strong emotional component often seen with visceral pain. Decreased patient activity, nausea, gastroparesis, and hypotension are common, whereas agitation, reactivity, and hypertension are more commonly seen with somatic pain. Visceral hypersensitivity can cause the perception of pain coming from another organ receiving innervation from the same spinal segment as the affected organ.

FURTHER READING

Fishman S, Ballantyne J, Rathmell JP, et al. (Eds.). *Bonica's Management of Pain*. 4th ed. Baltimore, MD: Lippincott Williams & Wilkins; 2010:647–648.

47. ANSWER: B

Cancer cells are not primarily responsible for bone destruction. Rather, they commonly express the receptor activator of nuclear κB ligand (RANKL), which activates RANK receptors on osteoclasts. Once activated, proliferation and hypertrophy of osteoclast cells occurs through formation of acidic "pits" around each osteoclast and bone. Research has repeatedly suggested that medications that inhibit osteoclast function significantly reduce bone cancer-mediated pain.

FURTHER READING

McMahon SB (Ed.). *Wall and Melzack's Textbook of Pain*. 6th ed. Philadelphia, PA: Saunders; 2013:1034.

48. ANSWER: A

Chronic tumor-related pain is often insidious, increases progressively with tumor growth, and usually improves with tumor shrinkage. A few exceptions exist, such as acute pain secondary to a pathologic fracture. Pain behaviors and sympathetic responses are often blunted or absent. However, chronic tumor-related pain is often associated with affective disturbances such as anxiety, depression, anorexia, and insomnia.

FURTHER READING

McMahon SB (Ed.). *Wall and Melzack's Textbook of Pain*. 6th ed. Philadelphia, PA: Saunders; 2013:1040–1041.

CERVICAL RADICULAR PAIN

Joshua Horowitz

INTRODUCTION

Cervical radicular pain is a common reason for patients in pain to seek care from a pain physician. Differing from low back pain and lumbar radiculopathy, cervical radicular pain is often not related to disc protrusion alone but, rather, a combination of disc and degenerative pathologies, such as uncovertebral hypertrophy and spondylosis. Likewise, the natural history is quite favorable if no treatments are applied, mandating greater safety for the treatments applied. Indeed, the most recent American Society of Anesthesiologists closed claims database report suggests that adverse occurrences from procedural therapies for cervical radicular pain are increasing. This chapter broadly discusses the anatomy, pathophysiology, and various approaches to treatment of these disorders.

QUESTIONS

1. In the sagittal plane, which direction best describes the location of the vertebral artery in relation to the exiting nerve roots of the cervical spine?

    A. Dorsal
    B. Lateral
    C. Ventral
    D. Medial

2. Uncovertebral joints exist in all of the following spinal segments except

    A. C3–C4
    B. C6–C7
    C. C2–C3
    D. C7–T1

3. The nerve root passing through the intervertebral foramen at the C5–C6 interspace provides sensory innervation to the:

    A. Ulnar forearm
    B. Lateral forearm
    C. Upper shoulder
    D. Lateral arm

4. A 23-year-old male with a history of T7 traumatic spinal cord injury from a motor vehicle accident that resulted in paraplegia presents to the pain clinic with complaints of bilateral upper extremity and shoulder pain. He describes it as a throbbing, dull, aching pain that originates between his shoulders and radiates bilaterally. He denies allodynia, hyperesthesia, and dysesthesia. Spurling's text is negative on exam. The most likely diagnosis is:

    A. Myofascial pain
    B. Transition "end zone" pain
    C. Cervical spondylosis with radiculopathy
    D. Central pain syndrome

5. A 79-year-old male presents to the pain clinic reporting 8 weeks of neck pain and stiffness. What finding on physical exam would be least concerning for spoldylotic myelopathy?

    A. Unsteady gait
    B. Lhermitte's sign
    C. Hyporeflexia
    D. Atrophy of the hand musculature

6. A 53-year-old female presents to the pain clinic with a 3-month history of right neck, shoulder, and arm pain. She describes her pain as sharp/shooting and from her neck into her thumb and forefinger in the right hand. The most appropriate intervention to perform at this time would be:

    A. Cervical flexion and extension radiographs
    B. Computed tomography (CT) myelogram of the cervical spine

C. Cervical interlaminar epidural steroid injection
D. T_1- and T_2-weighted magnetic resonance imaging (MRI) of the cervical spine

7. The 53-year-old patient described in the previous question underwent T_1- and T_2-weighted MRI of the cervical spine. The following was noted: "At the C5–6 interspace, the disc is narrow. A broad-based disc–osteophyte complex effaces the ventral thecal sac without compressing the cord. Uncovertebral spurring and facet degeneration contribute to severe neuroforaminal stenosis on the right." What intervention would be considered the most appropriate for treatment of the described pathology?

A. C6 selective nerve root block with 10 mg of Depo-Medrol
B. C7–T1 cervical interlaminar epidural steroid injection with 10 mg of dexamethasone
C. C6 transforaminal epidural steroid injection with 4 mg of dexamethasone
D. C5, C6, and C7 diagnostic cervical medial branch blocks

8. Recent data on anatomical variation of the arterial supply in the cervical intervertebral foramen suggest that the following area is the "safest" location for needle placement:

A. Needle tip extending just beyond the midsaggital plane of the articular pillar in the anteroposterior (AP) midsaggital view
B. No area of the intervertebral foramen appears to be safer than another
C. Dorsal midpoint of the intervertebral foramen
D. Needle tip remaining slightly outside the intervertebral foramen

9. Which of the following tests remains the "gold standard" for electrodiagnostic evaluation of radiculopathies?

A. Electromyography
B. Needle electrode examination
C. Magnetic resonance imaging
D. Somatosensory evoked potentials

10. A 76-year-old Caucasian male presents with symptoms of slowly progressive myelopathy on clinical examination. Lateral radiographs demonstrate ossification in the posterior longitudinal ligament of the upper cervical spine. A recent postgadolinium sagittal T_1-weighted image with fat saturation shows a C6–C7 level of hyperintensity of the spinal cord. What is the most appropriate next step in management?

A. Interlaminar epidural steroid injection
B. Conservative management with physical therapy and myofascial release
C. Refer for evaluation of surgical decompression
D. Acupuncture therapy

11. The structure in Figure 18.1 identified by the number 6 corresponds to which of the following structures?

A. Joint of Luschka
B. Facet joint
C. Lateral mass
D. C4 transverse process

12. The condition depicted by Figure 18.2 correlates least with which of the following clinical presentations?

A. Hyperesthesia, allodynia, and trophic changes of the lateral forearm
B. Progressive upper extremity weakness
C. Cauda equina syndrome
D. Neck and shoulder stiffness

13. The cardinal neurologic complication of cervical interlaminar epidural steroid injections is:

A. Infarction of the spinal cord
B. Vasospasm of the radicular artery
C. Arachnoiditis
D. Direct needle injury to the spinal cord

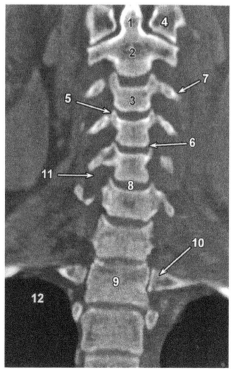

Figure 18.1 Coronal CT.

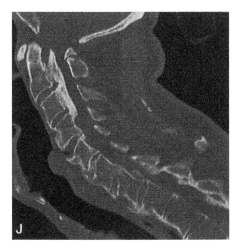

Figure 18.2 Sagittal CT reconstruction of the cervical spine.

14. The cardinal neurologic complication associated with cervical transforaminal epidural steroid injections is:

A. Infarction of the spinal cord
B. Direct needle injury to the spinal cord
C. Vasospasm of the radicular artery
D. Indirect injury resulting in cord ischemia

15. Which technique has been shown to have the least impact on safety during a cervical epidural steroid injection?

A. The use of nonparticulate steroid
B. The use of digital subtraction imaging
C. The use of a local anesthetic test dose
D. The use of extension tubing

16. The most common intervertebral space of the cervical spine to develop pathology resulting in cervicobrachialgia is:

A. C4–C5 interspace
B. C7–T1 interspace
C. C5–C6 interspace
D. C2–C3 interspace

17. Which of the following is not a prognostic factor for surgical decompression of the cervical spine in patients with cervical spondylotic myelopathy?

A. Intramedullary T2 hyperintensity
B. Extramedullary uptake of gadolinium
C. Intramedullary T1 hypointensity
D. Recovery of cross-sectional area after decompression

18. Which finding on MRI of patients with cervical spondylotic myelopathy correlates best with the severity of myelopathy?

A. The presence of diffuse idiopathic skeletal hyperostosis
B. Degree of ossification of posterior longitudinal ligament
C. Transverse area of the spinal cord
D. Degree of lateral recess stenosis

ANSWERS

1. ANSWER: C

In the cervical spine (Figure 18.3), the intervertebral foramen runs obliquely anterolaterally from C1 to C7. The pedicle, uncinate process, vertebral body, and superior articular process define the borders of the intervertebral foramen. The vertebral artery enters the foramen at C6, but it can enter as high as C3. The vertebral artery lies only a few millimeters ventral to the exiting nerve roots of the cervical spine. Reported complications of cervical transforaminal epidural steroid injections, such as anterior spinal artery syndrome, have been attributed to inadvertent vertebral artery cannulation.

FURTHER READING

Rozin L, Rozin R, Koehler SA, et al. Death during a transforaminal epidural steroid nerve root block (C7) due to perforation of the left vertebral artery. *Am J Forensic Med Pathol*. 2003;24:351–355.

2. ANSWER: D

The uncovertebral joints (joints of Luschka) exist only in the cervical spine (Figure 18.4). They are formed by the osseous processes of the superior end plates of the vertebral bodies of C2–C7, and they articulate with the inferior end plate of the superior corresponding vertebral body. These joints possess characteristics of both a synovial joint and a cartilaginous joint and are susceptible to degenerative changes resulting in foraminal and central canal stenosis. Because these joints are only present in the cervical spine, the superior end plate of T1 does not possess uncinate processes: as a result, there is no uncovertebral joint at the C7–T1 interspace. Radiculopathies result from herniated nucleus pulposus in only approximately 25% of cases; the majority of them are caused by cervical spondylosis.

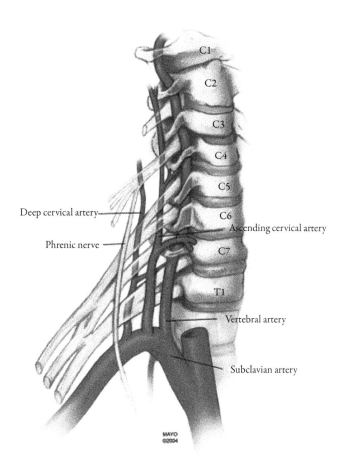

Figure 18.3 Illustration of the cervical spine.
SOURCE: Reprinted with permission from Huntoon MA. Anatomy of the cervical intervertebral foramina: Vulnerable arteries and ischemic neurologic injuries after transforaminal epidural injections. *Pain*. 2005;117(1–2):104–111

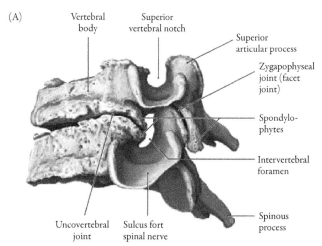

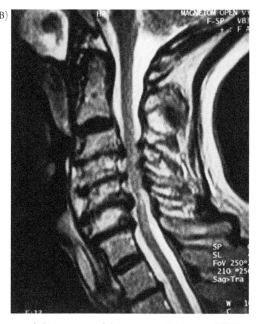

Figure 18.4 (A) Anatomy of the uncovertebral joint. (B) Uncovertebral joint hypertrophy (spondylosis) resulting in central spinal canal narrowing.

Radhakrishnan K, Litchy WJ, O'Fallon WM, et al. Epidemiology of cervical radiculopathy: A population-based study from Rochester, Minnesota, 1976 through 1990. *Brain*. 1994;11:325–335.

3. ANSWER: B

In the cervical spine, there are eight paired cervical nerve roots; thus, there is one more nerve root than cervical vertebrae. The first cervical nerve root (C1) exits the spinal canal between the base of the skull and first cervical vertebrae. Therefore, the nerve root exiting at the level of the C3–C4 interspace is the C4 nerve root. The nerve roots correlate with specific sensory dermatomes (Table 18.1). The C5–C6 interspace corresponds to the C6 nerve root, which provides sensation over the lateral forearm.

Table 18.1 NERVE ROOTS AND SENSORY DERMATOMES

INTERSPACE	NERVE ROOT	SENSORY	REFLEX
C3–C4	C4	Lower neck	n/a
		Upper shoulder	
C4–C5	C5	Lateral arm	Biceps
C5–C6	C6	Lateral arm	Brachioradialis
		Thumb	
C6–C7	C7	Dorsal forearm	Triceps
		Third digit	
C7–T1	C8	Medial forearm	n/a
		Fifth digit	

N/A, not applicable.

4. ANSWER: A

Myofascial pain syndrome is a chronic pain syndrome related to muscular trigger points. Trigger points are painful areas of soft tissue in which skeletal muscle forms taut, hypercontracted bands, and they are exquisitely tender to palpation. The pathophysiology of myofascial pain seems to be multifactorial, with neurologic (radicular), psychosocial, and nutritional factors, as well as depression and anxiety. It has been characterized as an autonomic dysregulation resulting in a centralized pain state. Multiple chemical mediators have been implicated in the transmission of myofascial pain, including norepinephrine, bradykinin, serotonin, substance P, tumor necrosis factors, and interleukins.

A careful history and physical exam remain paramount in the diagnosis of myofascial pain syndrome. The most common presentation of myofascial pain syndrome includes the following criteria: regional body pain and stiffness, limited range of motion of the affected muscle, referred pain from a trigger point to a zone of reference, and resolution of the symptoms with local anesthesia applied to the trigger point. Trigger points may be identified by feeling the taut band with gentle palpation directed perpendicular to the muscle fibers.

Central pain syndrome is a broad term used to describe pain states associated with pain disorders of the central nervous system, including both neuropathic and nociceptive pain states. Central pain associated with traumatic spinal cord injury occurs with a very high prevalence. This pain tends to be refractory to many medical therapies, and it can consist of both neuropathic and nociceptive qualities, such as burning, stabbing, aching, and throbbing. Allodynia, hyperesthesia, and dysthesia are also very common features of central pain. Pain in patients with incomplete spinal cord transections that is central in nature tends to be worse at the level of injury, and it is known as "transition zone" or "end zone" pain. It is important to keep in mind that although patients with spinal cord injuries are prone to developing centralized pain, they can just as commonly develop ailments not directly related to their spinal cord trauma.

Cervical spondylosis describes the degenerative changes of the spine seen most commonly in the elderly population. This can result in central and transforaminal stenosis, with radicular symptoms along a specific nerve root distribution.

5. ANSWER: C

Cervical spondylotic myelopathy (CSM) is the most common cause of spinal cord dysfunction in patients older than age 55 years. CSM refers to clinically evident spinal cord dysfunction with the presence of upper motor neuron signs secondary to compression of the spinal cord. Clumsiness of the hands, weakness or stiffness in the legs, and unsteady gait when seen concomitantly are pathognomonic of CSM.

Patients with CSM typically present with neck pain, neck stiffness, and shoulder pain. These patients may also present with pain in the arm, elbow, wrist, or hand. The pain may be described as stabbing, aching, or dull, and it may or may not have a dermatomal distribution. Pain that conforms to a dermatomal distribution is referred to as a radiculopathy rather than a myelopathy. Symptoms of both myelopathy and radiculopathy may be present simultaneously. Radiculopathies result from herniated nucleus pulposus in only approximately 25% of cases; the majority of them are caused by cervical spondylosis.

Physical exam findings include positive Lhermitte's sign (flexion of the neck eliciting electrical shooting pain down the back of the legs), unsteady gait, atrophy of intrinsic hand musculature, and abnormal sensory perception that may or may not be in the distribution of a dermatome. Compression of the spinal cord elicits upper motor neuron symptoms such as hyperreflexia below the level of injury and hyporeflexia at or above the level of injury. Hoffman's and Babinski's signs are often seen in patients with moderate to severe CSM.

MRI of the cervical spine is the imaging modality of choice when screening a patient suspected to have CSM. CT may also be utilized and offers improved delineation of bony structures. Imaging studies showing spinal stenosis and cord compression as a result of disc herniation, uncinate process or ligamentum hypertrophy, and osteophytic growth are diagnostic for CSM.

FURTHER READING

Radhakrishnan, K, Litchy WJ, O'Fallon WM, et al. Epidemiology of cervical radiculopathy: A population-based study from Rochester, Minnesota, 1976 through 1990. *Brain* 1994;11:325–335.

6. ANSWER: D

Evaluation of the cervical spine requires a thorough history and physical exam, directed to differentiate nonradicular etiologies from radicular pathology. Pain described in the distribution of a specific cervical dermatome is suggestive of nerve root pathology, particularly if reproducible on provocatory testing, such as with the Spurling's test.

Regarding cases in which pain is suspected to be due to impingement of a cervical nerve root, and the patients may benefit from an epidural steroid intervention, a recent consensus paper consisting of 13 multispecialty groups concluded that cervical interlaminar injections should not be undertaken unless inspection of imaging taken before the procedure demonstrates that the epidural space at the segmental level at which the injection will be undertaken is sufficient in size to admit a needle safely. Imaging should also be used to exclude absolute contraindications to cervical epidural injection if suspected, such as metastases and infection.

7. ANSWER: C

Conservative care of cervical radiculopathy may include epidural administration of corticosteroids and local anesthetics. Techniques include interlaminar and transforaminal epidural injections. Recent case reports of neurologic deficits such as anterior spinal artery syndrome and cerebellar injury after these injections have raised concerns regarding their safety.

In 2015, a consensus group of 13 multispecialty organizations presented the following recommendations for performing cervical interlaminar and tranforaminal epidural steroid injections:

1. The use of image guidance for all cervical interlaminar injections to avoid penetration of the spinal cord.
2. Cervical interlaminar injections should not be undertaken unless inspection of imaging taken before the procedure demonstrates that the epidural space at the segmental level at which the injection will take place is sufficient in size to admit a needle safely.
3. Appropriate lateral or oblique views to gauge depth of needle insertion.
4. Reliance on loss-of-resistance or anterior–posterior views alone does not protect from penetration of the spinal cord due to excessive needle depth.
5. Heavy sedation or a patient being unresponsive during the procedure is associated with a significantly higher risk of spinal cord injury during cervical procedures.
6. During transforaminal injections of both the cervical and lumbar spine, a test dose of contrast medium is essential to identify unintended arterial cannulation prior to other agents being injected.
7. Dexamethasone is recommended as the first-line agent for transforaminal injections to avoid inadvertent intra-arterial injection of particulate steroid, resulting in catastrophic neurologic consequences.
8. Digital subtraction imaging was endorsed for tranforaminal injections because it significantly increases the sensitivity of vascular uptake of contrast medium.
9. Extension tubing is recommended to be used such that once the needle is positioned, it is no longer touched, and the risk of dislodgement is minimized.

FURTHER READING

Bush K, Hillier S. Outcome of cervical radiculopathy treated with periradicular/epidural corticosteroid injections: A prospective study with independent clinical review. *Eur Spine J.* 1996;5(5):319–325.

Rathmell JP, Benzon HT, Dreyfuss P, et al. Safeguards to prevent neurologic complications after epidural steroid injections: Consensus opinions from a multidisciplinary working group and national organizations. *Anesthesiology.* 2015;5(122):974–984.

Rowlingson JC, Kirschenbaum LP. Epidural analgesic techniques in the management of cervical pain. *Anesth Analg.* 1986;65:938.

Slipman CW, Lipetz JS, Jackson HB, et al. Therapeutic selective nerve root blocks in the nonsurgical management of atraumatic cervical spondylotic radicular pain: A retrospective analysis with independent clinical review. *Arch Phys Med Rehabil.* 2000;81:741–746.

Vallée JN, Feydy A, Carlier RY, et al. Chronic cervical radiculopathy: Lateral-approach periradicular corticosteroid injection. *Radiology.* 2001;218(3):886–892.

8. ANSWER: B

Several recent reports of anterior spinal artery syndrome have raised concerns about the safety of cervical tranforaminal epidural steroid injections. The conventional technique involves introducing the needle laterally in the neck and directing it toward the superior articular process at the posterior aspect of the intervertebral foramen (Figure 18.5). The needle tip is then redirected to enter the dorsal midpoint of the foramen, and confirmation of the needle not extending beyond the midsaggital plane of the cervical articular pillar is performed with an AP view.

A cadaveric study examining the anatomy of the intervertebral foramina and the relationship of the ascending or deep cervical arteries and their susceptibility to injection or needle trauma during transforaminal epidural injections demonstrated the location of these critical arteries in the posterior aspect of the intervertebral foramen. These ascending and deep cervical arterial branches were noted to enter at the external opening of the intervertebral foramen in the "classic" posterior triangle described in the conventional technique. It was also found that these critical arteries are contributors to the anterior spinal artery, and thus cannulation or injury has the potential to result in catastrophic neurologic injury.

Some physicians may not completely advance the needle into the foramen because of the fear of cannulating a segmental vessel. However, the vessels for those supplying the anterior spinal cord are more likely to be cannulated at the external foraminal opening because of their larger size in this location.

Therefore, it is highly recommended that during transforaminal epidural steroid injections, one should consider the use of digital subtraction imagery, nonparticulate steroids, and perhaps avoidance of needle placement inferiorly to the intervertebral foramen to help prevent cannulation of critical vessels of the anterior spinal cord.

FURTHER READING

Huntoon MA. Anatomy of the cervical intervertebral foramina: Vulnerable arteries and ischemic neurologic injuries after transforaminal epidural injections. *Pain.* 2005;117(1–2):104–111.

Rathmell JP, Aprill C, Bogduk N. Cervical transforaminal injection of steroids. *Anesthesiology.* 2004;100:1595–1600.

9. ANSWER: A

Despite the controversy, some consensus exists regarding the usefulness of somatosensory evoked potentials in diagnosing

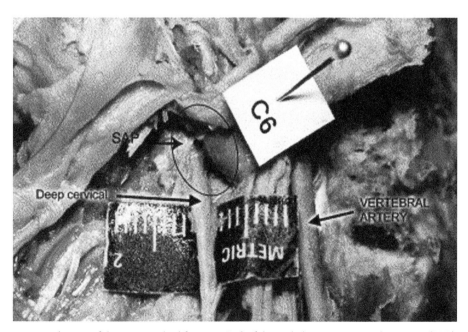

Figure 18.5 An oval approximates the area of the intervertebral foramen. Left of the oval, the superior articular process (SAP) is shown. Inferior to the oval, the right deep cervical artery (large arrow) is shown entering the posterior aspect of the C5–C6 foramen. At top middle, the C6 ventral ramus is retracted cephalad. The vertebral artery, only marginally larger than the deep cervical artery, is shown at right.

SOURCE: Reprinted with permission from Huntoon MA. Anatomy of the cervical intervertebral foramina: Vulnerable arteries and ischemic neurologic injuries after transforaminal epidural injections. *Pain.* 2005;117(1–2):104–111.

radiculopathies. They are purportedly useful for radiculopathies in which sensory symptoms predominate and diagnosis by other techniques such as electromyography (EMG) is difficult. However, EMG remains the gold standard for the electrodiagnostic evaluation of radiculopathies.

EMG is a method of testing both the physiologic state and the anatomic integrity of lower motor neuron structures, their sensory components, and some spinal and brainstem reflex pathways. EMG is the stimulation of a motor nerve with subsequent measured motor response. Lesions resulting in radiculopathy of the spine typically are located proximal to the dorsal root ganglion. Because of this, motor and sensory nerve conduction studies are commonly found to be normal due to most muscles of the limbs being supplied by more than one nerve root. A normal study does not exclude the diagnosis of radiculopathy; however, when findings on EMG are abnormal, they provide objective evidence of functional impairment in the nerve root and localize the lesion to one or more roots.

Needle electrode examination is a broad term describing the process of electrodiagnosis, and it includes modalities such as nerve conduction studies, EMG, and evoked potentials.

10. ANSWER: C

Cervical spondylotic myelopathy is the most common cause of spinal cord dysfunction in patients older than age 55 years. The surgical treatment for patients with cervical radiculopathy or myelopathy is indicated when symptoms persist despite approximately 6 weeks of conservative nonsurgical treatment or a progressive motor deficit is present with correlating radiographic evidence. There are several surgical approaches for addressing cervical radiculopathy due to either a herniated nucleus pulposus or spondylosis. These surgeries include:

1. Anterior cervical discectomy with or without fusion
2. Posterior laminoforaminotomy

In patients presenting with symptoms consistent with myelopathy of the spinal cord, requiring decompression; the following surgical approaches may include:

1. Anterior cervical discectomy
2. Anterior cervical corpectomy with fusion
3. Laminectomy with or without fusion
4. Laminoplasty

11. ANSWER: A

Figure 18.1 is a coronal CT identifying the following structures:

1. Odontoid process
2. C2 vertebral body
3. C3 vertebral body
4. C1 lateral mass
5. Uncinate process
6. Uncovertebral joint (joint of Luschka) of C4–C5
7. C3 transverse process
8. C5–C6 intervertebral disc
9. T2 vertebral body
10. First rib
11. Nerve root
12. Lung apex

12. ANSWER: A

The sagittal CT reconstruction of the cervical spine demonstrates thick bone density to the vertebral body extending from C2 to C4 causing moderate to severe narrowing of the central spinal canal. The posterior longitudinal ligament is a band of collagen and elastin fibers that extends along the posterior margins of the vertebral bodies from the atlas to the sacrum. Ossification of the posterior longitudinal ligament (OPLL) is a result of hypertrophy of the ligament with progressive mineralization and ossification. OPLL typically occurs in patients older than age 40 years and can result in narrowing of the central spinal canal.

Most often, OPLL is found in the upper cervical spine (70%, C2–C4) and less often in the upper thoracic spine (15%, T1–T4). Cervical OPLL occurs twice as often in males as in females.

FURTHER READING

Czervionke LF, Fenton DS. *Imaging Painful Spine Disorders.* Philadelphia, PA: Saunders; 2011.

13. ANSWER: D

The evidence of neurologic injuries with interlaminar epidural steroid injections is limited to case reports and closed claim analyses, and although they do occur, they occur so infrequently that there is not sufficient data to report incidence.

The cardinal neurologic complication of cervical interlaminar injections is direct needle injury to the spinal cord. In a review of malpractice claims involving chronic pain management between 2005 and 2008, 294 cases were identified; of these, 20 cases of direct spinal cord injury occurred. There has been one report of indirect spinal cord injury with regard to cervical epidural steroid injections, presumed to be due to a transient increase in pressure within the epidural space during injection, causing ischemia to the spinal cord.

Representatives of the US Food and Drug Administration Safe Use Initiative, in conjunction with an expert multidisciplinary working group and 13 specialty stakeholder societies, concluded in 2015 that image guidance for all cervical interlaminar injections was recommended to avoid penetration of the spinal cord as a result of improper insertion of the needle.

Infarction of the spinal cord during cervical epidural steroid injections is postulated to be the result of direct microvascular embolization as a consequence of particulate steroid injection. As such the use of particulate steroids during cervical transforaminal epidural steroid injections is not advised due to the higher incidence of inadvertent cannulation of critical vessels during needle placement.

Arachnoiditis is a rare, although recognized, complication of epidural steroid injections of the spine, usually due to contamination of injectate. Adhesive arachnoiditis may result from the solvent of depo-steroid polyethylene glycol. In the setting of febrile episodes or new symptoms concerning for infectious etiology, an urgent MRI is indicated. Abnormal conglomeration of nerve roots or clumping on MRI are signs concerning for arachnoiditis.

FURTHER READING

Rathmell JP, Benzon HT, Dreyfuss P, et al. Safeguards to prevent neurologic complications after epidural steroid injections: Consensus opinions from a multidisciplinary working group and national organizations. *Anesthesiology*. 2015;5(122):974–984.

14. ANSWER: A

The evidence of neurologic injury with cervical transforaminal epidural steroid injections is limited to case reports and malpractice claims. A review of closed claims identified nine instances of spinal cord infarction during cervical tranforaminal epidural steroid injection; in all cases, particulate steroids were used. This injury is hypothesized to be the result of particulate steroid injection into either the vertebral artery or the radicular artery, causing compromise of vascular flow and subsequently spinal cord infarction. Thus, digital subtraction imaging is endorsed for transforaminal epidural steroid injections to aid in the detection of vascular uptake of contrast medium.

The evidence of neurologic injury with cervical interlaminar epidural steroid injections is limited to case reports

and closed claim analyses, and although they do occur, they occur so infrequently that there is not sufficient data to report incidence.

FURTHER READING

Rathmell JP, Benzon HT, Dreyfuss P, et al. Safeguards to prevent neurologic complications after epidural steroid injections: Consensus opinions from a multidisciplinary working group and national organizations. *Anesthesiology*. 2015;5(122):974–984.

15. ANSWER: C

Representatives of the US Food and Drug Administration Safe Use Initiative, in conjunction with an expert multi- disciplinary working group and 13 specialty stakeholder societies, concluded in 2015 that the following prac- tices, when performed, should lead to a reduction in the incidence of neurologic injury during epidural steroid injection: Similar to the answer for question 7, use of non-particulate steroids, low volume extension tubing and digital subtraction imaging were all felt to be reasonable safety measures to prevent neurological events.

1. The use of image guidance for all cervical interlaminar injections to avoid penetration of the spinal cord.
2. Cervical interlaminar injections should not be undertaken unless inspection of imaging taken before the procedure demonstrates that the epidural space at the segmental level at which the injection will take place is sufficient in size to admit a needle safely.
3. Appropriate lateral or oblique views to gauge depth of needle insertion.
4. Reliance on loss-of-resistance or anterior–posterior views alone does not protect from penetration of the spinal cord due to excessive needle depth.
5. Heavy sedation or a patient being unresponsive during the procedure are associated with a significantly higher risk of spinal cord injury during cervical procedures.
6. During transforaminal injections of both the cervical and lumbar spine, a test dose of contrast medium is essential to identify unintended arterial cannulation prior to other agents being injected.
7. Dexamethasone is recommended as the first-line agent for transforaminal injections to avoid the consequence of inadvertent intra-arterial injection

of particulate steroid resulting in catastrophic neurologic consequences.

8. Digital subtraction imaging was endorsed for tranforaminal injections because it significantly increases the sensitivity of vascular uptake of contrast medium.

9. Extension tubing is recommended to be used such that once the needle is positioned, it is no longer touched, and the risk of dislodgement is minimized.

FURTHER READING

Rathmell JP, Benzon HT, Dreyfuss P, et al. Safeguards to prevent neurologic complications after epidural steroid injections: Consensus opinions from a multidisciplinary working group and national organizations. *Anesthesiology*. 2015;5(122):974–984.

16. ANSWER: C

Cervicobrachialgia is defined as pain from a particular cervical nerve root, commonly is localized in the mid and lower cervical area, and radiates beyond the shoulder into the arm in a dermatomal distribution. This pathology can be a cervical disc protrusion with irritation of a spinal nerve, central spinal canal stenosis, or spondylosis resulting in narrowing of the intervertebral foramen.

The most common cervical nerve roots to be involved are C6, C7, and, to a lesser degree, C5. The corresponding intervertebral spaces are C5–C6, C6–C7, and C4–C5, respectively.

The diagnosis of cervical radiculopathy requires a detailed history and physical exam and also the use of appropriate clinical diagnostic modalities to confirm the involvement of a suspected nerve root.

FURTHER READING

Benzon HT, Srinivasa R, Fishman SE, et al. (Eds.). *Essentials of Pain Medicine*. 3rd ed. Philadelphia, PA: Saunders; 2011.

17. ANSWER: B

Patients with progressive neurologic symptoms concerning for cervical spondylotic myelopathy require a timely and appropriate workup so that therapeutic interventions, primarily surgical decompression, can be considered. The ultimate goal of imaging is to improve the clinical outcome in patients with CSM. A large body of literature has examined the role of imaging in predicting clinical response to surgical decompression. The following have been determined to be poor prognostic factors for surgical decompression:

1. Intramedullary T1 hypointensity (Figure 18.6A)
2. Intramedullary T2 hyperintensity (Figure 18.6B)
3. Intramedullary gadolinium enhancement

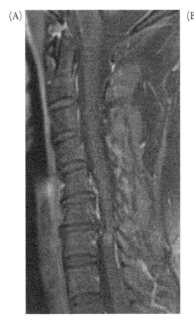 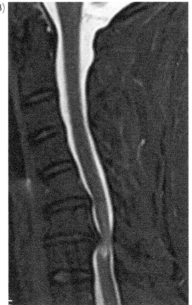

Figure 18.6 (A) T1 hypointensity and (B) T2 hyperintensity.

4. No increase in metabolic activity at the site of compression on ^{18}F-fluorodeoxyglucose positron emission tomography (^{18}F-FDG PET)
5. Residual postoperative compression and failure of re-expansion of the cord

FURTHER READING

Maus TP. Imaging of spinal stenosis. *Radiol Clin North Am.* 2012;50:651–679.

18. ANSWER: C

The transverse area of the spinal cord as measured by MRI correlates well with the severity of myelopathy and the pathologic changes observed in the spinal cord in CSM.

FURTHER READING

Benzon HT, Srinivasa R, Fishman SE, et al. (Eds.). *Essentials of Pain Medicine.* 3rd ed. Philadelphia, PA: Saunders; 2011.

19.

LOW BACK PAIN AND RADICULAR PAIN

Marc A. Huntoon

INTRODUCTION

Low back pain is one of the most common pain syndromes in the world and a leading cause of disability and physician visits. Although degenerative disc disease and zygapophyseal joint spondylotic changes are common and lead to more permanent problems such as spinal stenosis, the interplay of biological and psychosocial factors is largely key to the chronification of many back pain disorders.

QUESTIONS

1. A 78-year-old male is experiencing chronic low back and leg pain and notices that while pushing a shopping cart he can tolerate longer periods of painless movement without rest. Which of the following is most correct regarding spinal stenosis?

A. Spine exercise programs focus on neutral or flexion exercises.
B. Ligamentum flavum hypertrophy, disc degeneration, and spondylosis are key anatomical features.
C. Epidural corticosteroid injections are evidence based for spinal stenosis.
D. All of the above.
E. A and B only.

2. Which of the following is true regarding the structure of the intervertebral disc?

A. The vertebral end plates, containing proteoglycans and collagen fibers, resemble the disc structure.
B. Proteolytic enzymes or metalloproteinases are secreted in the intervertebral disc.
C. The principal component of both the annulus fibrosis and the nucleus pulposus is water.
D. All of the above.

3. A patient with moderate to severe spondylosis (facet arthropathy) has a large zygopophyseal cyst at the right L4–L5 level and leg pain radiating to the foot. Which of the following is the most likely next step in management?

A. Surgical referral for cyst decompression
B. A short-term oral steroid dose pack and gabapentin trial
C. Dynamic lumbar stabilization exercises with extension bias
D. Medial branch blocks
E. Cyst needle drainage and periradicular steroid

4. A 69-year-old female presents to clinic for increased pain in the back and left leg. She finds that she easily trips on uneven surfaces, and on exam she has sensory change in her plantar foot and weakness of her plantar flexors. The procedure depicted in Figure 19.1 would be expected to improve which problem?

A. No improvement expected because the needle is at the wrong level
B. Possibly improved pain with less clear effects on weakness
C. No improvement because the pain is clearly caused by her instrumentation
D. Likely improved sensation on the anterior lower leg

5. Characteristics of the intervertebral disc include?

A. Investment by vertebral end plate vessels and calcitonin gene-related peptide-containing neurons with advancing degeneration
B. Increasing likelihood of ipsilateral disc degeneration after discography
C. Increased interleukin-8 (IL-8) in periradicular fat samples at discectomy
D. A and B only
E. All of the above

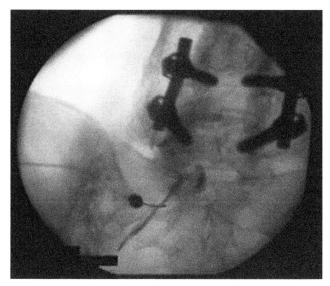

Figure 19.1 A procedure performed on a 69-year-old female with increased pain in the back and left leg. The patient trips easily on uneven surfaces and, on exam, has sensory change in her plantar foot and weakness of her plantar flexors.

6. During performance of an ultrasound (US)-guided left intra-articular hip injection, the innervation to consider is:

A. The anterior branch of the obturator nerve
B. The posterior branch of the accessory obturator nerve
C. The nerve to the quadratus femoris
D. A and C
E. All of the above

7. A 46-year-old female status post L4–S1 spinal fusion with iliac crest bone graft presents for evaluation and management of a chronic right buttock pain with allodynia near the posterior superior iliac spine. The most likely cause of her pain is:

A. Postsurgical piriformis syndrome
B. Quadratus lumborum syndrome
C. Injury to the cluneal nerve
D. Sacroiliitis

8. A 46-year-old female presents with significant buttock and radiating leg pain after a hard fall on her buttock area from slipping on ice. A US-guided piriformis muscle injection is contemplated. Characteristics of piriformis syndrome include:

A. The sciatic nerve passing anterior to the muscle in approximately 85% of patients
B. A divided sciatic nerve passing through the piriformis muscle approximately 25% of the time

C. Lasegue's sign positive with pain on voluntary flexion, adduction, and hip internal rotation
D. Pain on Freiberg test (forceful external rotation of hip)
E. A and C

9. A 53-year-old obese female presents with symptoms of fatigue, waking poorly refreshed, poor sleep hygiene, "spastic colon," and multisite tenderness including both upper and lower extremities, trunk, and abdomen. For the past 3 months, her worst pain is an aching pain in the lateral hip and thigh. Which of the following is the most likely cause?

A. Somatization disorder
B. Hip osteoarthritis
C. Meralgia paresthetica due to nerve entrapment
D. Fibromyalgia

10. A 62-year-old male custodian experiences low back pain when running a floor polishing machine. Which of the following statements is true regarding discogenic pain?

A. Disc disease is primarily due to genetic factors with little effect from smoking.
B. Discogenic pain is infrequent because the nucleus pulposus (NP) is not innervated.
C. Disc dehydration varies directly with age.
D. There is no relationship to disc disease with previous ipsilateral discography.
E. Disc vascularity increases in proximity to the NP.

11. Fibromyalgia can be a source of low back pain. This disease is characterized by which sequence of findings?

A. Increased secondary hyperalgesia, increased response to exogenous opioids, and decreased descending inhibition
B. Decreased secondary hyperalgesia, increased response to exogenous opioids, and decreased descending inhibition
C. Increased secondary hyperalgesia, decreased response to exogenous opioids, and decreased descending inhibition
D. Decreased secondary hyperalgesia, decreased response to exogenous opioids, and increased descending facilitation

12. A 65-year-old male is involved in a rear-end car collision in which he was restrained by his seat belt. He complains of new back and leg pain. On exam, he has a positive reverse straight leg raise sign. This corresponds to:

A. Sciatica
B. S1 deceleration neuropraxia

C. Sacral insufficiency fracture
D. Upper lumbar nerve root involvement

13. A 75-year-old female has pain with testing of both the Fortin finger test and Gaenslen's test. Her findings are most consistent with:

A. A lumbar facet syndrome, which is highly concordant with these tests
B. A piriformis syndrome, which is highly concordant with these tests
C. Sacroiliac pain, which is poorly concordant with these tests
D. Maigne's syndrome, for which these tests are poorly concordant

14. A 22-year-old male reports new pain in his left foot and new-onset back pain after doing a dead lift exercise with 400 pounds. When examining the patient, which findings would be concordant for an L5 radiculopathy?

A. Weak anterior tibialis, absent Achilles tendon reflex, and allodynia in the lateral plantar area
B. Weak flexor hallucis, hyperreflexia at Achilles tendon, and hypoesthesia in the dorsum of foot
C. Weak soleus muscle, absent Achilles tendon reflex, and lateral plantar allodynia
D. Weak extensor hallucis longus, decreased Achilles tendon reflex, and hypoesthesia of dorsum of foot

15. A 23-year-old female patient who developed severe pain in her lower back and gluteal region after falling off her horse 12 days ago is referred by her primary care physician for epidural corticosteroid injections. She has been at near bed rest since the accident. She describes pain solely in the buttock on the right side and states she "has been passing out from the pain." X-rays show no fracture. Her lumbosacral magnetic resonance imaging (MRI) shows a broad-based disc bulge mildly effacing the ventral thecal sac at L4–L5 but is otherwise normal. Your next best step is to:

A. Not do the injection because you will need an electromyogram (EMG) to verify the L5 radiculopathy
B. Do the injection because any MRI abnormality in a younger person is likely pathological
C. Not do the injection because MRI findings are often abnormal, even in asymptomatic patients
D. Do the injection because the level of pain suggests that the pathology is serious

16. A 35-year-old obese male presents with pain 6 months after a recent discectomy and instrumented

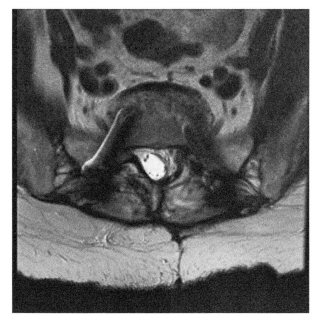

Figure 19.2 T_2-weighted axial MRI image at L5.

fusion for radiculopathy. The T_2-weighted axial MRI image (Figure 19.2) at L5 is obtained. This demonstrates:

A. The left pedicle screw is malpositioned.
B. There is an urgent need for decompression at this level due to mass effect.
C. There is apparent epidural fibrosis surrounding the nerve root sleeve.
D. A pseudomeningocoele is present.

17. A 38-year-old female requests that you send her to a surgeon because she has been suffering with right L4 radicular pain without red flag symptoms (progressive neurological changes, weight loss, urinary incontinence, etc.) for more than 8 months. You advise her that the natural history of radicular pain over time suggests:

A. Matrix metalloproteinase-induced macrophage disc resorption may cause improvement over time.
B. The majority of disc herniations viewed by MRI decrease in size over the first 2 years.
C. Aspects of size, type of disc pathology, and cytokine release and activity play key roles in the process of disc resorption.
D. All of the above.

18. A 52-year-old female with new-onset radiculopathy and radicular pain in an L4 distribution presents for evaluation. She desires immediate surgery despite lack of neurological findings on exam but with MRI evidence of a right paracentral disc protrusion at

L3–L4. **You advise that evidence-based treatment supports:**

A. Surgical instrumented fusion
B. Lumbar traction at 30 pounds
C. Oral corticosteroids for short term
D. Oral gabapentin for long term
E. All of the above

19. A 70-year-old female presents to your clinic with upper buttock and groin pain on the left that also radiated down her leg almost to the knee. The flexion abduction and external rotation (FABER) and Gaenslen's tests are positive. The injection seen in Figure 19.3 is performed. What is the evidence for treatments aimed at this area at this time?

A. Zygapophyseal joint injections of corticosteroid show substantial efficacy versus placebo.
B. Sacrolateral branch radiofrequency ablation was more efficacious with strip lesions.
C. Intra-articular sacroiliac joint injections are more effective than exercise.
D. Sacroiliac arthrodesis has shown long-term efficacy in trials.

20. A 72-year-old male has MRI evidence of a small L5–S1 paracentral disc herniation and a grade 2 spondylolisthesis. He complains of moderately severe low back pain, but he denies leg pain. He has not improved with oral corticosteroids or gabapentin. Which of the following statements about surgery in this setting is true?

A. The patient will likely have a poor early response but at 2 years will unequivocally be improved compared to conservative treatment.

B. The patient will likely have early improvement that will be sustained and superior to conservative care at 2 years.
C. The patient will likely have little improvement because spondylolisthesis is largely unrelated to low back pain without radiculopathy.
D. The patient is unlikely to improve after surgical care due to his failure to respond to other treatments to date.

21. A 69-year-old patient with discectomy and fusion for radicular pain is not helped by her surgery. The most likely extraspinal source of pain is:

A. Pirifromis syndrome
B. Hip osteoarthritis
C. Greater trochanter syndrome
D. Nerve entrapment
E. All of the above

22. Of the following structures, which defines the borders of what constitutes lumbar back pain?

A. The 12th thoracic spinous process
B. The first sacral spinous process
C. The erector spinae musculature
D. A and B only
E. All of the above

23. A 25-year-old male presents with leg pain after a weightlifting injury. When considering the cause, the quality of pain is most likely?

A. Radicular pain; lancinating or electrical and follows a narrow band
B. Somatic referred pain; dull and aching or pressure-like

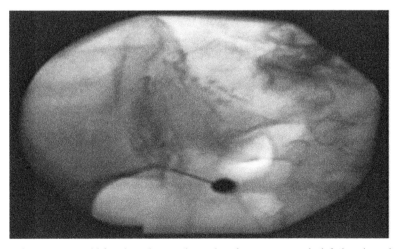

Figure 19.3 An injection performed on a 70-year-old female with upper buttock and groin pain on the left that also radiated down her leg almost to the knee.

C. Both of the above
D. Neither of the above

24. Which of the following statements regarding fractures of the pars interarticularis is true?

A. They are most common in obese sedentary individuals.
B. They are more common in patients with back pain, linking them with causation.
C. They are concerning for an infectious process.
D. Athletes with lumbar extension and rotation are most susceptible.

25. A 22-year-old female presents with low back pain. Indications for plain X-rays to determine the cause include?

A. Participation in gymnastics intramural events
B. History of previous cancer
C. History of previous disc herniation
D. Complex regional pain syndrome

26. A 47-year-old male presents with chronic low back pain and is thought to have pain emanating from the zygopophyseal joints in the lumbar spine. Well-controlled diagnostic medial branch blocks requiring complete pain relief suggest a prevalence of back pain from this cause is likely:

A. 5%
B. 40%
C. 1–2%
D. 25%

27. Internal disc disruption is characterized by nuclear degradation and development of annular fissures that are graded 1–4. Which of the following answers is correct?

A. Grade 1 fissures are confined to the nucleus.
B. Grade 2 fissures extend circumferentially in the middle third of the annulus.
C. Grade 3 fissures reach the outer third of the annulus.
D. Grade 4 fissures extend into the neural foramina.

28. Concerning discogenic pain, MRI, and discography, which of the following statements is true?

A. Annular fissures do not correlate with pain on discography.

B. The majority of patients with annular fissures of grade 3 or 4 have a high-intensity zone (HIZ) on MRI.
C. The majority of patients with concordant pain on discography have MRI evidence of annular tearing.
D. Both B and C.

29. A 24-year-old woman presents to your clinic with pain in her low back since falling at home. She complains of multiple sites of pain dating back to her early teens, but her exam is normal. On questioning, she is dramatic and inconsistent. She may most likely have:

A. Somatization disorder
B. Malingering
C. Factitious disorder
D. Myofascial pain syndrome

30. High-frequency spinal cord stimulation for chronic low back pain will most likely result in which outcome?

A. Improved back pain relief relative to conventional spinal stimulation
B. Return to work in the majority of patients
C. Cessation of opioids in most patients
D. Less insertional complications compared to conventional stimulation

31. Regarding interventional pain procedures for lumbar radiculopathy, which is most representative of current evidence?

A. Enhanced outcome for thermal radiofrequency compared to sham
B. Enhanced long-term relief from caudal epidural corticosteroids
C. Decreased spine surgery when receiving epidural corticosteroid
D. Short-term improvement from epidural corticosteroids

32. Regarding surgical treatment for lumbar spondylolisthesis, which of the following is true?

A. Spondylolithesis is consistently correlated with painful movement.
B. Spondylolisthesis with radiculopathy may require decompression.
C. Spondylolisthesis is indicative of spinal instability.
D. Both B and C.
E. All of the above.

33. The injectate(s) that may enhance lesion size most during conventional thermal radiofrequency procedures is most likely:

A. Normal saline
B. Hypertonic saline
C. Local anesthetics
D. Dextrose
E. All of the above

34. Considering functional restoration and rehabilitation programs, the following statement is true:

A. Attempting to "carve out" various aspects of interdisciplinary care leads to declining psychological and vocational outcomes.
B. The number of functional team-based restoration programs is declining relative to population needs.
C. Functional restoration programs have found little evidence that they can fully solve the characterological defects inherent to many chronic pain patients.
D. All of the above.

ANSWERS

1. ANSWER: E

In general, gentle strengthening and stretching exercises (lumbar flexion) and core abdominal strengthening are beneficial for spinal stenosis patients, whereas extension-based exercises may exacerbate symptoms. Specifically, activities such as bicycling may be better tolerated than walking. Core strengthening of abdominal musculature may also aid in avoidance of excessive extension. Narrowing of the spinal canal, caused by degeneration of discs and facets, leads to buckling of the ligamentum flavum, osteophyte formation, and spondylolisthesis. Physical examination should search for extension-based involvement of proprioceptive fibers (Romberg test), with altered gait and instability. Patients may show evidence of neurogenic claudication and have bilateral motor and sensory changes. Epidural steroid injections, although commonly used, have fallen into disfavor for spinal stenosis because a recent trial suggested that the local anesthetic group fared just as well as the steroid group.

KEY FACTS

- Spinal stenosis patients should preferentially be prescribed flexion-based exercises.
- The process of spinal stenosis is the culmination of several processes, including ligamentum flavum thickening, spondylosis, and other degenerative processes.
- Although still performed, epidural injections may not be as useful for this condition as they are for radicular pain.

FURTHER READING

Friedly JL, Comstock BA, Turner JA, et al. A randomized trial of epidural glucocorticoid injections for spinal stenosis. *N Engl J Med.* 2014;371:11–21.

Katz JN, Harris MB. Spinal stenosis. *N Engl J Med.* 2008;358:818–825.

2. ANSWER: D

The nucleus pulposus is approximately 70–90% water, with the proportion varying by age. The intervertebral disc generally "dries out" as one ages. Proteoglycans (65% of dry weight) and collagen fibrils (25% of dry weight) are other major components. The annulus fibrosis is also approximately 65% water, with collagen fibers and a proteoglycan gel that fills the spaces between the lamellae to prevent shearing. Because the vertebral end plate is similar to the disc, it has similar diffusion characteristics, allowing small molecules to pass unimpeded. The repair functions of the proteolytic enzymes (matrix metalloproteinases 1–3) allow old components of the matrix to be replaced. Activators and inhibitors of this enzymatic process are normally in a tight balance, but they can be disrupted in certain cases to degrade the matrix. The disc is a remarkable organ capable of handling various pressure loads with dispersal across a broad surface area.

KEY FACTS

- Human intervertebral discs desiccate as one ages.
- The vertebral end plate is an important structure that invests the disc with blood vessels and pain-sensitive neuronal structures.
- Proteolytic enzymes are important in repair processes.

FURTHER READING

Bogduk N. *Clinical Anatomy of the Lumbar Spine and Sacrum.* 4th ed. New York: Churchill Livingstone; 2005:12–20.

3. ANSWER: B

Lumbar facet synovial cysts are uncommon but can project either anteriorly into the neural foramen or posteriorly. They appear to be most common at the L4–L5 level. Multiple treatments have been tried, including oral agents, facet joint aspiration and injection, and surgery to remove the cyst and potentially spinal fusion to prevent instability. Although often performed for recalcitrant degenerative conditions, surgery is not well supported for this, and complications can be significant. Generally, the progression of treatments should be from simple to more advanced; thus, it is not unreasonable to try other accepted treatments for joint and radicular pain, including nonsteroidal anti-inflammatory drugs (NSAIDs), gabapentinoids, and oral steroids. If conservative treatments are unsuccessful, attempted needle decompression of the facet, facet joint steroids, and perineural steroids are reasonable prior to surgery unless there is a compelling neurological reason to progress directly to surgery. Medial branch blocks might be temporarily effective but do not aspirate the facet joint directly. Extension-based physical therapy might exacerbate the pain and would be unlikely to directly treat the pathology, although exercise is a reasonable addition.

KEY FACTS

- Degenerative facet cysts may cause pain, and their management is somewhat controversial.
- Generally, conservative treatments should be trialed prior to consideration of surgery unless neurological findings are advancing.

FURTHER READING

Allen TL, Tatli Y, Lutz GE. Fluoroscopic percutaneous lumbar zygapohyseal joint cyst rupture: A clinical outcome study. *Spine J.* 2009;9:387–395.

Brummett CM, Cohen SP. Benzon H, et al. Pathogenesis, diagnosis and treatment of zygapophyseal (facet) joint pain. In: Benzon HT, Rathmell JP, Wu CL, et al. (Eds.), *Practical Management of Pain.* 5th ed. Philadelphia, PA: Mosby; 2014:816–845.

4. ANSWER: B

The depicted procedure is an S1 transforaminal epidural injection with contrast tracing the exiting spinal nerve and into the epidural space. Although the procedure is commonly applied for radicular pain (a narrow band of lancinating, sharp, or burning neuropathic pain) with success for up to a few weeks, improvement of radiculopathy is less certain. Patients may manifest decreased ability to toe walk, with antalgic gait. With S1 involvement and radiculopathy, one might also expect weakness of the plantar flexors of the foot, a diminished Achilles reflex, and plantar sensory disturbance.

KEY FACTS

- Radicular pain and radiculitis may be present simultaneously or may be exclusive of one another.
- Epidural injections may not be as successful for neurological findings such as numbness and/or weakness.

FURTHER READING

Malik K, Benzon HT. Low back pain. In: Benzon HT, Rathmell JP, Wu CL, et al. (Eds.), *Practical Management of Pain.* 5th ed. Philadelphia, PA: Mosby; 2014:312–327.

5. ANSWER: A

The intervertebral disc is made up of an annulus fibrosus (AF) and nucleus pulposus (NP) and is invested by the vertebral end plates. Both the AF and the NP are primarily water. The disc is largely avascular, with nutritional supply via passive diffusion. Innervation is via anterior plexi from gray rami communicantes and a posterior plexus of fibers, both somatic and sympathetic, from the sinuvertebral nerves. Release of pro-inflammatory cytokines, including tumor necrosis factor-α (TNF-α), IL-1β, IL-6, IL-8, and others, contributes to disc pain. These cytokines have been recovered from herniated disc at the time of discectomy.

Ipsilateral provocative discography may be associated with an increased risk for future herniation.

KEY FACTS

- The intervertebral disc is innervated anteriorly by gray rami communicantes and posteriorly by the sinuvertebral nerves.
- Inflammatory cytokines have been recovered from herniated discs.
- Ipsilateral discography has been associated with an increased rate of future herniation.

FURTHER READING

Bottros MM, Cohen SP. Lumbar discogenic pain and diskography. In: Benzon HT, Rathmell JP, Wu CL, et al. (Eds.), *Practical Management of Pain.* 5th ed. Philadelphia, PA: Mosby; 2014:885–914.

Burke JG, Watson RW, McCormack D, et al. Intervertebral discs which cause low back pain secrete high levels of proinflammatory mediators. *J Bone Joint Surg Br.* 2002;84:196–201.

Carragee EJ, Don AS, Hurwitz EL, et al. Does discography cause accelerated progression of degeneration changes in the lumbar disc: A ten year matched cohort study. *Spine.* 2009;34:2338–2345.

6. ANSWER: D

The articular innervation of the hip is complex and is largely from the anterior division of the obturator nerve, the sciatic nerve, the femoral nerve, the superior gluteal nerve, and the nerve to the quadratus femoris. The posterior hip joint is supplied by nerve to quadratus femoris, superior gluteal nerve, and sciatic nerve. The anterior and medial aspects of the joint are innervated by the articular branches from the anterior division of the obturator nerve and the femoral nerve. Although some studies have suggested some involvement of an accessory obturator branch, this was not seen in the study by Birnbaum et al.

KEY FACT

- Multiple nerves contribute to the innervation of the hip, including the obturator nerve, sciatic nerve, femoral nerve, nerve to the quadratus femoris, and superior gluteal nerve.

FURTHER READING

Birnbaum K, Prescher A, Hepler S, et al. The sensory innervation of the hip joint—An anatomical study. *Surg Radiol Anat.* 1997;19:371–375.

7. ANSWER: C

Maigne and colleagues have previously described the cutaneous nerves derived from the thoracolumbar junction (T12–L3). Of these, the most important are the cluneal nerves. The medial superior cluneal nerve branch was found to arise from L1 approximately 60% of the time and from L2 20% of the time, with an occasional branch from L3. The medial cluneal nerve can be part of a painful syndrome that has been termed Maigne's syndrome. The nerve can become entrapped in an osseo fibrous tunnel between the posterior iliac crest and the superior thoracolumbar fascia, causing what appears to be an entrapment neuropathy. Likewise, the nerve is also vulnerable to injury from spinal fusion procedures wherein the nerve is cut or injured or from too medial placements of spinal cord stimulation pulse generator packs. Patients afflicted will present with burning, hyperalgesic, or allodynic pain over the area. Maigne originally posited that the syndrome could be diagnosed by (1) pain in the distribution of the nerve, (2) a trigger point 7 cm from the midline near the iliac crest, and (3) relief by perineural injection (nerve block).

KEY FACT

- Maigne's syndrome describes a neuropathic pain in the iliac crest area related to entrapment of the medial cluneal nerve.

FURTHER READING

Maigne JY, Doursounian L. Entrapment neuropathy of the medial superior cluneal nerve: Nineteen cases surgically treated with a minimum of two years follow up. *Spine*. 1997;22:1156–1159.
Maigne JY, Lazareth JP, Guérin-Surville H, et al. The lateral cutaneous branches of the dorsal rami of the thoracolumbar junction: A study on 37 dissections. *Surg Radiol Anat*. 1989;11:289–293.
Tubbs RS, Levin MR, Loukas M, et al. Anatomy and landmarks for the superior and middle cluneal nerves: Application to posterior iliac crest harvest and entrapment syndromes. Laboratory investigation. *J Neurosurg Spine*. 2010;13:356–359.

8. ANSWER: E

Piriformis syndrome is an underdiagnosed condition that may mimic sciatica caused by other pathology (e.g., disc). Common associations have been noted, including previous trauma, female gender, pregnancy, obesity, leg length discrepancies, and hypertrophy/spasm of the piriformis or surrounding muscles. Dissections have characterized that the undivided sciatic nerve passing anterior/below the muscle is most common 84–98% of the time. Multiple other configurations are possible, but the divided nerve passing through the muscle is far less common than 25%. Testing for piriformis syndrome often includes the following

> Pace sign: The patient is seated, and the examiner asks the patient to flex and abduct the hip against resistance.
>
> Lasegue's sign: The patient attempts to adduct, internally rotate, and flex the hip without examiner resistance.
>
> Freiberg sign: Pain with patient extending thigh and the examiner's internal rotation of the hip.

KEY FACTS

- Previous trauma, female gender, pregnancy, leg-length discrepancy, obesity, and hypertrophy of the piriformis muscle may be commonly noted in patients with piriformis syndrome.
- Most of the anatomical findings show a sciatic nerve that is undivided and passing anteriorly to the muscle.

FURTHER READING

Cohen SP, Benzon HT. Pain originating in the buttock: Sacroiliac joint syndrome and piriformis syndrome. In: Benzon H, Raja S, Fishman S, et al. (Eds.), *Essentials of Pain Medicine*. 3rd ed. Philadelphia, PA: Saunders; 2011:337–339.

9. ANSWER: D

Fibromyalgia (FM) is thought to be the presence of chronic widespread pain and symptoms of cognitive slowing, waking unrefreshed, and fatigue. Patients meet diagnostic criteria if they have a symptom severity (SS) scale and widespread pain index (WPI) as follows from Wolfe's criteria:

- WPI score >7 and SS scale score >5 or WPI score of 3–6 and SS scale score >9
- Symptoms present at a similar level for at least 3 months
- No disorder present that would otherwise explain the pain

Although the patient discussed in this question is also obese and probably does have some hip osteoarthritis, it is less likely that this is her main diagnosis given the constellation of other findings. Likewise, although meralgia paresthetica is more common in obese patients, the other features are more consistent with FM. Indeed, as many as 50% of patients with FM may have gastrointestinal findings such as dyspepsia, irritable bowel, interstitial cystitis, or other pelvic and bladder pains. Although patients with fibromyalgia may seem to be having so many complaints that one might consider a somatoform diagnosis in the differential, somatization disorder is less likely unless the patient has concomitant anxiety/ panic disorder, depression, disproportionate thoughts about his or her health condition, persistent pains since the age of 30 years, and perseveration/fixation regarding his or her health matters.

KEY FACTS

- Patients with FM can be diagnosed using Wolfe's criteria.
- FM likely involves central sensitization leading to widespread pain and other symptoms that are seen with great prevalence.
- Patients with FM may present with features of other processes, such as facet joint pain, that may lead to poorer outcomes of interventional treatments.

FURTHER READING

Adams MCB, Clauw D. Chronic widespread pain. In: Benzon HT, Rathmell JP, Wu CL, et al. (Eds.), *Practical Management of Pain.* 5th ed. Philadelphia, PA: Mosby; 2014:392–407.
Wolfe F, Clauw DJ, Fitzcharles M-A, et al. The American College of Rheumatology preliminary diagnostic criteria for fibromyalgia and measurement of symptom severity. *Arthritis Care Res.* 2010;62:600–610.

10. ANSWER: C

The intervertebral disc is largely avascular except at the outer annulus fibrosis and is high in water content. With normal aging, the disc dessicates, and in the process, some of the high resistance to compressive force is reduced. Although genetic factors play some role in the development of disc degeneration, patient factors such as obesity, vascular insufficiency as exacerbated by smoking, frequent heavy lifting, and other modifiable lifestyle factors are also important. A study by Carragee and colleagues demonstrated increased propensity for future disc herniation on the side ipsilateral to disc puncture for discography. Also see answer to Question 5.

KEY FACTS

- The intervertebral disc is mostly avascular.
- Certain environmental factors, such as obesity, frequent heavy lifting, and smoking, may accelerate degeneration.

FURTHER READING

Carragee EJ, Don AS, Hurwitz EL, et al. Does discography cause accelerated progression of degenerative changes in the lumbar disc: A ten year matched cohort study. *Spine.* 2009:34:2338–2345.

Malik K, Benzon HT. Low back pain. In: Benzon HT, Rathmell JP, Wu CL, et al. (Eds.), *Practical Management of Pain.* 5th ed. Philadelphia, PA: Mosby; 2014:312–327.

11. ANSWER: C

FM presents with enhanced sensory perception, not just of touch pressure pain but also of other senses such as hearing. This is evidence that central sensitization or sensory amplification is occurring. In addition to secondary hyperalgesia, FM patients also demonstrate decreased descending inhibition. In a classic study, Julien and colleagues compared FM patients to low back pain patients using a cold stimulus and while the back pain patients changed their responses to a spatial summation testing protocol, the FM patients had a deficit in their descending inhibition. Patients with FM may have increased endogenous opioids but a decreased effect from exogenous opioids. Opioid therapy for FM, although common, is largely ineffective, and side effects such as tolerance, induced hyperalgesia, constipation, and addiction need to be considered.

KEY FACTS

- FM patients display enhanced sensory perception.
- Descending inhibition may be impaired.
- Opioid response to exogenous treatment may be suboptimal.

FURTHER READING

Adams MCB, Clauw D. Chronic widespread pain. In: Benzon HT, Rathmell JP, Wu CL, et al. (Eds.), *Practical Management of Pain.* 5th ed. Philadelphia, PA: Mosby; 2014:392–407.
Julien N, Goffaux P, Arsenault P, et al. Widespread pain in fibromyalgia is related to a deficit of endogenous pain inhibition. *Pain.* 2005;114:295–302.

12. ANSWER: D

Nerve root tension signs are one way of delineating the involved level of injury when radicular pain/radiculopathy is considered in the differential diagnosis. The straight leg raise (SLR) stretches the lower lumbar spinal roots and exacerbates radicular pain in those distributions. The crossed straight leg test may be even more specific for lumbar nerve irritation. A femoral stretch test is performed with the patient lying prone with knee bent and preferentially places tension on the upper lumbar (L2 and L3) nerve roots, indicating the pathology is originating from those roots.

Table 19.1 NEURAL TENSION TESTS FOR THE
LUMBAR SPINE

SEATED SLUMP TEST	STRAIGHT LEG RAISE	FEMORAL STRETCH TEST
• Provocative test for lower lumbar disc herniation • May help differentiate hamstring tightness from lumbosacral radicular pain • Found to be more sensitive than the straight leg raise	• Provocative test for lower lumbar disc herniation • Positive test considered if pain reproduced between 30° and 70° of flexion • Found to be more specific than the seated slump test	• Provocative test for upper lumbar disc herniation • May have false positives from other etiologies, such as a femoral neuropathy, quadriceps tightness, or hip pathology

KEY FACTS

- See Table 19.1 for the neural tension tests for the lumbar spine.
- SLR testing is often performed as a test for sciatica.
- Femoral stretch testing more appropriately tests upper lumbar roots.
- False-positive tests are not uncommon due to various other conditions.
- The seated slump test may be more sensitive but less specific for sciatica compared to the SLR.

FURTHER READING

Malik K, Benzon HT. Low back pain. In: Benzon HT, Rathmell JP, Wu CL, et al. (Eds.), *Practical Management of Pain*. 5th ed. Philadelphia, PA: Mosby; 2014:312–327.

13. ANSWER: C

The sacroiliac joint is a diarthrodial synovial fluid-filled joint with articular surfaces formed between the sacrum and ilium bilaterally. The joint is capable of motion and transfers weight from the trunk to the pelvis and lower extremities. With aging, the joint surface becomes more irregular. The joint is a relatively frequent cause of lower back, buttock, groin, and hip/thigh pain and can mimic other causes. A variety of physical examination tests have been developed; unfortunately, however, they have poor sensitivity and specificity. Thus, some call for at least three positive tests and diagnostic blockade to confirm the diagnosis. These provocative tests included FABER, Gaenslen's test, Patrick's test, Gillett's test, the sacroiliac shear test, the Fortin finger test, and Yeoman's test. The Fortin finger test

is performed by simply placing one's finger on the exact spot of the pain times two. This should correspond to an area just inferomedial to the posterior superior iliac spine. These tests are designed to stress the joint and/or distract the joint to cause pain. With Maigne's syndrome, as in the previous question, the patient may have neural irritation from the medial superior cluneal nerve causing localized pain, allodynia, and hyperalgesia. Piriformis syndrome is tested as in the answer to Question 8. Finally, facet joint pain can be tested by extension and ipsilateral twisting to "load" the zygopohyseal (facet) joints causing pain.

KEY FACTS

- Multiple physical exam tests exist for diagnosing the sacroiliac joint as the etiology of pain, but they are poorly sensitive and specific in corroborating the diagnosis without other confirmatory testing.
- Facet joint pain can be tested by "facet loading" with a similar lack of sensitivity/specificity.

FURTHER READING

Agerson A, Benzon HT, Malik K. Sacroiliac joint syndrome. In: Benzon HT, Rathmell JP, Wu CL, et al. (Eds.), *Practical Management of Pain*. 5th ed. Philadelphia, PA: Mosby; 2014:866–875.

14. ANSWER D

An L5 radiculopathy can be diagnosed based on concordant physical exam findings. L5 innervated muscles include parts of the tibialis anterior (L4 and L5) and, specifically, the extensor hallicus longus (great toe extension) and peroneus longus (foot eversion). Although the Achilles reflex is more specific for S1 lesions, it may be decreased or absent in patients with an L5 radiculopathy. Sensory testing should be more than just light touch, specifically to include temperature, vibration sense, pin prick, and proprioception. Generally, a systematic dermatomal-specific testing process can be followed to test each lumbar root.

KEY FACT

- L5 innervated muscles include the extensor hallicus longus and peroneus longus.

FURTHER READING

Dubin A, Lalani I, Argoff CE. History and physical examination of the pain patient. In: Benzon HT, Rathmell JP, Wu CL, et al. (Eds.), *Practical Management of Pain*. 5th ed. Philadelphia, PA: Mosby; 2014:151–161.

15. ANSWER: C

The patient in this scenario is young and probably had a significant fall, but her imaging is not indicative of neural impingement, nor of any other significant findings save the bulging disc. Studies by Boden and colleagues and others have shown that MRI is often abnormal, even in asymptomatic patients who had never had sciatica or other back symptoms. Whereas patients older than 60 years in this study had findings such as herniated discs and spinal stenosis greater than 50% of the time (37% disc herniation and 21% spinal stenosis), the findings in patients the 20- to 39-year age range were even more surprising, with 35% of these younger individuals having a bulging or degenerated disc. Regarding the patient discussed in this question, her pain does not exhibit a radicular pattern in a narrow band going down her leg, so the MRI scan is not indicated. Likewise, an EMG is not indicated unless one suspects a radiculopathy, which would certainly not be the case only 12 days after the start of the pain. The pain at this early juncture qualifies as acute by definition because it has not persisted past 12 weeks. Bed rest is not helpful, and the patient needs reassurance and coaching to begin to resume normal activities because this is demonstrated to be more helpful to ultimate recovery. Although it is tempting to prescribe oral agents such as NSAIDs, muscle relaxants, and opioids, their use is, at best, minimally helpful with very small effect sizes. Natural history is favorable for most acute back pain incidents.

KEY FACTS

- Acute low back pain is defined as pain in the back that does not persist beyond 12 weeks from injury.
- EMG at too early of a time is not indicated; see section on electrodiagnosis.
- Up to one-third of all young people may have radiologic changes on MRI while asymptomatic, signaling the importance of closely correlating imaging with neurological exam and history when assessing patients.

FURTHER READING

Boden SD, Davis DO, Dina TS, et al. Abnormal magnetic resonance scans in asymptomatic subjects: A prospective investigation. *JBJS Am.* 1990;72:403–408.

McGuirk BA, Bogduk N. Acute low back pain. In: Fishman SM, Ballantyne JC, Rathmell JC (Eds.), *Bonica's Management of Pain*. 4th ed. Philadelphia, PA: Lippincott Williams & Wilkins; 2009.

16. ANSWER: C

Pseudomeningocoeles can occur after spinal surgery when cerebrospinal fluid escapes into the soft tissues but not through the skin closure. Pseudomeningocoeles can eventually form a fibrous capsule and a spongy benign enlargement if close to the surface. Pseudomeningocoeles sometimes occur after spinal catheter placements. No fluid is seen that is consistent with a pseudomeningocoele in this T_2-weighted image. There is evidence of pedicle screws placed bilaterally, but there is insufficient detail to determine any malplacement. There does appear to be some epidural fibrosis that surrounds the dilated nerve root sleeve (cicratrization) with concomitant mass effect on the thecal sac, making choice C the correct answer. The importance of epidural fibrosis is arguable. Most spinal surgeries result in the formation of some scarring near the site of previous surgical pathology. Several studies and systematic reviews suggest no difference in patients who are aymptomatic and those with significant back and recurrent leg pain simply based on whether they had imaging evidence of fibrosis or not. The evidence for adhesiolysis in these settings also remains controversial, with some studies suggesting a short to intermediate effect in patients with fibrosis.

KEY FACTS

- Epidural fibrosis occurs after essentially all back surgeries to varying degrees.
- Studies in which imaging is correlated with pain and neurological symptoms and signs suggest that the mere presence of epidural fibrosis may not be causative of chronification of symptoms.

FURTHER READING

Schofferman J. Failed back surgery syndrome. In: Fishman SM, Ballantyne JC, Rathmell JP (Eds.), *Bonica's Management of Pain*. 4th ed. Philadelphia, PA: Lippincott Williams & Wilkins; 2009.

17. ANSWER: D

All of the processes discussed can lead to disc resorption over time with gradual clinical improvement. If a weakened annulus is stressed, disc material can remain contained, herniate, extrude, or be sequestered. One of the larger studies by Bush and colleagues, with computed tomography confirmation, suggested that the majority of cases of patients with herniation or sequestration of disc material (64 of 84) were either partially or completely resolved at 1 year with conservative treatment. The action of macrophages and specific matrix metalloproteinases in disc resorption has been elucidated. In animal models, activated macrophages release TNF-α in the presence of matrix metalloproteinase 7 (MMP-7) and TNF-α is rendered soluble. The soluble TNF-α allows MMP-3 production by chondrocytes, which leads to macrophage infiltration of the disc material for resorption. Exposure to vascular structures is an important feature of this process.

KEY FACTS

- Disc resorption is possible and part of the natural history of sciatica caused by disc herniation.
- A vascular environment and key processes involving macrophages, MMP, and TNF-α are necessary elements of the "cleanup" of the disc material.

SUGGESTED READING

Bush K, Cowan N, Katz DE, et al. The natural history of sciatica associated with disc pathology. *Spine.* 1992;17:1205–1212.
Haro H, Crawford HC, Fingleton B, et al. Matrix metalloproteinase-7-dependent release of tumor necrosis factor-α in a model of herniated disc resorption. *J Clin Invest.* 2000;105:143–150.
Saal JA. Natural history and non-operative treatment of lumbar disc herniation. *Spine.* 1996;21:2S–9S.

18. ANSWER: C

Lumbar traction requires a much greater force application than that for cervical spine. Thus, for an average adult male or female, 30 pounds would be insufficient to offer meaningful spinal distraction. Newer techniques of traction, such as vertebral axial decompression or nonsurgical spinal decompression, have been touted but remain understudied, with the latter having no prospective, blinded, randomized trials. A single-level disc protrusion would be unlikely to require instrumented fusion, unless there were other factors present that would destabilize the spine. Both oral corticosteroids and gabapentinoids have been partially validated for short-term use only. Thus, answer C is correct. Neither agent appears to affect leg pain significantly in the immediate term.

KEY FACTS

- Currently, there is a lack of good evidence for traction for lumbar radiculopathy.
- Oral corticosteroids and gabapentinoids appear to have some effect on leg pain, but only for the short term.

FURTHER READING

Pinto RZ, Maher CG, Ferreira ML, et al. Drugs for relief of pain in patients with sciatica: Systematic review and meta-analysis. *Br Med J.* 2012;344:e497.
Wolf CJ, Brault JS. Manipulation, traction, and massage. In: Cifu DX (Ed.), *Braddom's Physical Medicine & Rehabilitation.* 5th ed. Philadelphia, PA: Elsevier; 2016:347–367.

19. ANSWER: B

The sacroiliac joint is pictured after a fluoroscopically guided injection. Sacroiliac joint injections of corticosteroids are commonly performed but are short-lasting, and evidence-based studies have been equivocal. The sacroiliac joints are innervated by the L5 dorsal rami and sacral lateral branches of S1–S3, with contributions from L4 less commonly. Although conventional radiofrequency (RF) ablation is performed, the need for multiple lesions, the disparities and depths of the sacral lateral branches, and other technical factors confound this treatment.

KEY FACT

- The posterior innervation of the sacroiliac joint is derived from the L5 dorsal ramus, the sacral lateral branches of S1–S3, and possibly (variably) fourth sacral nerve.

FURTHER READING

Agerson A, Benzon HT, Malik K. Sacroiliac joint syndrome. In: Benzon HT, Rathmell JP, Wu CL, et al. (Eds.), *Practical Management of Pain.* 5th ed. Philadelphia, PA: Mosby; 2014:866–875.

20. ANSWER: C

Spondylolisthesis is present when one vertebral body subluxates relative to another. This is usually L5 relative to the sacrum or, less commonly, L3 or L4. Although this would seem to be unstable, radiographic studies have not corroborated instability in most patients. Similar to nonconcordant MRI and back pain, although some patients with spondylolisthesis have back pain, there is no proven causal relationship. Indeed, spondylolisthesis occurs at similar frequency in patients having or not having back pain. Thus, surgery for back pain alone, regardless of the small disc herniation in the patient in question, is probably not indicated. If the patient had radicular pain and also signs/symptoms of radiculopathy on exam, surgery to decompress the involved area may be indicated but would likely require spinal fusion due to the amount of bony lamina and periforaminal bone requiring removal. The fact that the patient in question did not respond to oral steroids or gabapentin is not unusual because these agents are only evidence-based treatments for short term use in patients with radicular pain/sciatica.

KEY FACTS

- Spondylolisthesis is subluxation of one vertebra relative to another and can be graded as to degree.

- Spondylolisthesis by itself is not an indication for surgery.
- Spondylolisthesis with radiculopathy is likely the best indication for surgery.

FURTHER READING

Ghabrial Y, Bogduk N. Surgery for low back pain. In: Fishman SM, Ballentyne JC, Rathmell JC (Eds.), *Bonica's Management of Pain*. 4th ed. Philadelphia, PA: Lippincott Williams & Wilkins; 2009.

21. ANSWER: E

Low back pain is a diffuse, nonspecific diagnosis with many etiologies. The answer choices listed for this question are but a few of the possible syndromes that have a referral pattern that mimics disc-based radicular pain. In piriformis syndrome, the *piriformis muscle* can either irritate or compress the proximal sciatic nerve due to spasm and/or contracture (nerve entrapment). *Piriformis syndrome* is also referred to as pseudosciatica, wallet sciatica, and hip socket neuropathy. Hip osteoarthritis may or may not present with pain, either within the hip joint with weight-bearing activities or as a radiating pain to the posterior part of the thigh and may extend below the knee but not to the ankle or foot. The pain is considered less specific than sciatica pain. As many as three trochanteric bursae have been described around the greater trochanter, the largest of which is the subgluteus maximus bursa, which is located lateral to the greater trochanter and deep in the fibers of the tensor fascia latea and gluteus maximus muscle. Because of the location of all of these bursae, irritation within or around these structures can cause a pattern of pain referred down the leg.

KEY FACTS

- Due to the complexity of bursae and gluteal region muscular attachments, greater trochanteric bursitis is also known as greater trochanteric pain syndrome.
- Various syndromes can mimic radiculopathy and occasionally send referred pain below the knee.

FURTHER READING

Benzon H, Nader A. Hip, sacroiliac joint, and piriformis injections. In: Benzon H, Rathmell J, Wu C, et al. (Eds.), *Raj's Practical Management of Pain*. 4th ed. Philadelphia, PA: Mosby; 2008:1063–1064.

Malik K, Benzon H. Low back pain. In: Benzon H, Rathmell J, Wu C, et al. (Eds.), *Raj's Practical Management of Pain*. 4th ed. Philadelphia, PA: Mosby; 2008:367–368.

22. ANSWER: E

Low back pain is generally described as pain between the costal margin and the gluteal folds—that is, from the 12th thoracic spinous process down to the first sacral spinous process. The musculature of the lumbar spine can be divided anatomically into posterior and anterior muscles. The posterior muscles include the latissimus dorsi and the paraspinals. The lumbar paraspinals consist of the erector spinae (iliocostalis, longissimus, and spinalis), which act as the chief extensors of the spine, and the deep layer (rotators and multifidi), which are stabilizers to limit flexion of the lumbar spine. The anterior muscles of the lumbar spine include the psoas and quadratus lumborum. The hip joints, lumbar facet joints, as well as sacroiliac joints are also anatomic locations that can be a source of low back pain.

KEY FACT

- The boundaries of the low back include the areas between the gluteal fold and the costal margin, from the 12th spinous process to the first sacral process.

FURTHER READING

Barr K, Concannon L, Harrast M. Low back pain. In: Cifu DX, Kaelin D, Kowalske K, et al. (Eds.), *Braddom's Physical Medicine and Rehabilitation*. 5th ed. Philadelphia, PA: Elsevier; 2016:711–745.

23. ANSWER: A

The etiology of this patient's pain is likely from a herniated intervertebral disc, and the presentation of pain most likely represents a radicular pain pattern that is described as lancinating and traveling in a narrow band down the leg. Somatic referred pain is carried along the sensory fibers and is described as intense, particularly centrally, not dull and aching. It is not the most likely type of pain that this weightlifter is experiencing given the mechanism of injury inferred by his activity. Somatic referred pain is poorly focused and broadly distributed. The patients may note boundaries are indistinct but well maintained.

KEY FACT

- Radicular pain differs from somatic referred pain due to the narrow band-like, lancinating pattern as opposed to a more diffuse, broadly focused type of pain.

FURTHER READING

Chekka K, Benzon H, and Jabri R. Taxonomy: Definition of pain terms and chronic pain syndromes. In: Benzon H, Raja S, Fishman S, et al. (Eds.), *Essentials of Pain Medicine.* 3rd ed. Philadelphia, PA: Saunders; 2011:17–18.

24. ANSWER: D

Spondylolysis is a defect or fracture of the pars interarticularis and is a common cause of back pain in athletic youth and young adults. Young athletes have a higher prevalence of spondylolysis than nonathletes, and the mechanism of injury appears to be repetitive chronic, low-grade stress through extension and rotation movements such as seen with certain sports (e.g., gymnastics). Low back pain is a common finding in obese sedentary patients, but it is not necessarily linked with pars interarticularis fractures in this group of patients. The finding of a pars fracture in an otherwise healthy young athlete with a history appropriate for this type of pain presentation should not cause one to suspect an infectious etiology. However, in nonathletic children complaining of back pain without trauma, an infectious etiology should remain in the differential diagnosis.

FURTHER READING

Barr K, Concannon L, Harrast M. Low back pain In: Cifu DX, Kaelin D, Kowalske K, et al. (Eds.), *Braddom's Physical Medicine and Rehabilitation.* 5th ed. Philadelphia, PA: Elsevier; 2016:711–745.

25. ANSWER: A

As per the preceding question, the fact that the patient in this question participated in gymnastics intramural events suggests that she may have been exposed to typical extension and rotation forces that could result in pars fracture. The best indication for plain X-rays of the spine is ruling out post-traumatic fracture. In patients who are presenting with suspected stress fracture such as a pars fracture, bone scan or X-ray may be useful; however, an MRI, which can detect stress reactions and actual fractures with high sensitivity and specificity, is better. Other conditions, such as a history of cancer, unexplained weight loss, night sweats, severe osteoporosis, or other red flag symptoms, may warrant other imaging and/or serum testing. Of the detractors, it is unlikely that a history of previous disc herniation would be enhanced by plain X-rays. Complex regional pain syndrome may be associated with osteopenia, but three-phase bone scanning is more useful. For history of cancer, bone scan or MRI may be sensitive in detecting pathology, but greater specificity is seen with MRI.

KEY FACTS

- Fractures of the pars interarticularis may be diagnosed with bone scan, MRI, or X-ray, but MRI is the better test.
- Other than post-traumatic fracture, there are few low back pain conditions for which X-ray is useful.
- Previous cancer history is less commonly a cause of back pain in the younger patient, but if a history is present in those younger than age 50 years, MRI is likely warranted.

FURTHER READING

McGuirk BE, Bogduk N. Acute low back pain. In: In: Fishman SM, Ballantyne JC, Rathmell JP (Eds.), *Bonica's Management of Pain.* 4th ed. Philadelphia, PA: Lippincott Williams & Wilkins; 2009.

26. ANSWER: A

Chronic low back pain can be multifactorial, and the zygapophyseal (facet) joints have been implicated as being causative in 15–45% of cases. Commonly used criteria for medial branch blocks to temporarily denervate the joints have been set at 50% or 80%, thus allowing for some degree of false-positive results. When criteria are set at complete relief of pain for medial branch blocks, the number of positive responses is far closer to 5%. Even when small volumes of injectate are used (0.3–0.5 ml), local anesthetic can spread to other neural or soft tissue structures. When considering an elderly population, the true incidence of facet joint as the cause of low back pain may be approximately one in three.

KEY FACTS

- Facet joint pain may be overrepresented as the primary cause of low back pain in non-elderly groups.
- Controlled diagnostic medial branch blocks suggest that the true incidence of facet joint pain may be as low as 5%.

FURTHER READING

McGuirk BE, Bogduk N. Chronic low back pain. In: Fishman SM, Ballantyne JC, Rathmell JP (Eds.), *Bonica's Management of Pain.* 4th ed. Philadelphia, PA: Lippincott Williams & Wilkins; 2009.

27. ANSWER: C

Internal disc disruptions are generally graded from 1 to 4 based on their specific pattern. As a result of severe compression force-related fatigue injury or a small fracture of the vertebral end plate, nuclear degradation extends as a radial fissure into the annulus fibrosus. Grade 1 describes a fissure that reaches to the inner third of the annulus, grade 2 reaches the middle third of the annulus, grade 3 extends to the outer third of the annulus, and grade 4 describes the extension of the fissure circumferentially. Thus, answer C is correct.

KEY FACTS

- Internal disc disruptions are caused by fatigue-related forces or small end plate fractures,
- Fissures may extend all the way through the annulus and can be progressively graded.

FURTHER READING

McGuirk BE, Bogduk N. Acute low back pain. In: Fishman SM, Ballantyne JC, Rathmell JP (Eds.), *Bonica's Management of Pain.* 4th ed. Philadelphia, PA: Lippincott Williams & Wilkins; 2009.

28. ANSWER: C

High-intensity zones are bright signals seen in T_2-weighted MRI in the posterior annulus. They likely represent vascularized granulation tissue in annular tears. They have a high correlation with that disc being the source of the patient's pain and a high specificity. However, not all painful discs demonstrate a HIZ. Therefore, choice B is incorrect. Most concordantly, painful discs do show evidence of degeneration and annular fissuring; thus, choice C is correct. Discography is a provocative test whereby the presumed painful disc is pressurized with manometry and compared with normal level(s). Disc pain at pressures between 30 and 50 psi and pain scores 4–6/10 can be utilized to help prevent false-positive interpretations. Research suggests that when pressures are painful at a level of 4/10 at ≥30 psi or at a level of 6/10 at ≥50 psi, the false-positive ratios are nearly zero. Somatization and behavioral issues may cause false-positive results.

KEY FACTS

- Although not common, high-intensity zones, when present, are highly correlated with the painful disc.
- Discography is controversial, but when performed with strict manometric control, it has a low likelihood of false-positive results.

FURTHER READING

Bottros MM, Cohen SP. Lumbar discogenic pain and discography. In: Benzon HT, Rathmell JP, Wu CL, et al. (Eds.), *Practical Management of Pain.* 5th ed. Philadelphia, PA: Mosby; 2014:885–914.
McGuirk BE, Bogduk N. Acute low back pain. In: Fishman SM, Ballantyne JC, Rathmell JP (Eds.), *Bonica's Management of Pain.* 4th ed. Philadelphia, PA: Lippincott Williams & Wilkins; 2009.

29. ANSWER: C

Somatization disorder is a psychiatric disorder that requires at least 4 symptoms of pain, two symptoms of gastrointestinal symptoms, one sexual symptom and at least one pseudoneurological symptom (seizure, aphonia, swallowing disorder, loss of sensation,paralysis, hallucinations, blindness, etc.). These pains must start before age 30 and are present over a period of many years. Sexual abuse history is common.

Myofascial pain syndrome is unlikely because the complaints are widespread and no trigger points are found. Malingering is not a psychiatric disorder. Presence of external incentives for the pain symptoms distinguishes factitious disorder from malingering, thus factitious disorder is an intentional feigning of symptoms but there is no external reward other than assuming the sick role. Patients are dramatic and inconsistent, thus C is correct.

FURTHER READING

Wasan AD, Sullivan MD, Clark MR. Psychiatric illness, depression, anxiety, and somatiform disorders, Chapter 31. In: Fishman SM, Ballantyne JC, Rathmell JC (Eds.), *Bonica's Management of Pain.* 4th ed. Philadelphia, PA: Lippincott Williams & Wilkins; 2009.p 409.
McGuirk BA, Bogduk N. Acute low back pain. In: Fishman SM, Ballantyne JC, Rathmell JC (Eds.), *Bonica's Management of Pain.* 4th ed. Philadelphia, PA: Lippincott Williams & Wilkins; 2009. p 1109.

30. ANSWER: A

High-frequency spinal cord stimulation is different from conventional spinal cord stimulation (SCS) in that 10-kHz frequencies are utilized, as opposed to normal SCS frequencies of approximately 40–80 Hz. These high frequencies result in a nodal/conduction block. A large multicenter study demonstrated better back pain coverage compared to conventional SCS; thus, answer A is correct. A preponderance of patients were significantly improved with respect to both pain scores and function. Despite these good outcomes, most patients continued to utilize opioids for their pain, although some were able to reduce or eliminate them. This was not a primary or secondary outcome of the major study. Return-to-work rates were not specifically studied compared to other treatments. Insertion of SCS leads is very similar to existing techniques, so complications of insertional activity were similar.

KEY FACTS

- Stimulation of 10 kHz produces a paresthesia-free conduction block that may be superior to conventional spinal stimulation.
- Opioid usage declined relative to conventional frequency SCS, but an active management style was not utilized, nor was this a specific study outcome.
- Functionality and remission rates were superior in the largest prospective trial.

FURTHER READING

Kapural L, Yu C, Doust MW, et al. Novel 10-kHz high-frequency therapy (HF-10 therapy) is superior to traditional low-frequency spinal cord stimulation for the treatment of chronic back and leg pain: The SENZA RCT randomized controlled trial. *Anesthesiology.* 2015;123:851–860.

31. ANSWER: C

Recent large meta-analyses have examined the various interventional treatments for radicular pain. Although epidural corticosteroid injections are likely helpful in the short term, there is little evidence for long-term improvement and no evidence for long-term success in avoiding surgery. Both conventional (thermal) RF ablation and pulsed RF have also been studied. Although pulsed RF has had some success in small prospective studies, much more evidence is necessary to determine its efficacy. The best trials to date suggest that thermal RF ablation is not helpful.

KEY FACTS

- Meta-analyses of key studies suggest that epidural steroid injections do not affect incidence of surgery.
- Although pulsed RF treatments appear to have blocking effects on pro-inflammatory cytokine levels and also decrease central sensitization, more studies are necessary to quantitate efficacy.

FURTHER READING

Dworkin RH, O'Connor AB, Kent J, et al. Interventional management of neuropathic pain: NeuPSIG recommendations. *Pain.* 2013;154:2249–2261.
Van Boxem K, Huntoon M, van Zundert J, et al. Pulsed radiofrequency: A review of the basic science as applied to the pathophysiology of radicular pain: A call for clinical translation. *Reg Anesth Pain Med.* 2014;39:149–159.

32. ANSWER: B

While appearing to be indicative of instability, spondylolisthesis may in fact confer greater stability, both radiographically and clinically. Thus, its occurrence or an incidental finding of spondylolisthesis on imaging studies is not an indication for surgical repair. Spondylolisthesis occurrence does not seem to be any more common in patients with pain than in those who are asymptomatic. If radicular pain occurs, however, the spinal nerve can be affected by the narrowing or dynamic compression caused by subluxation. Decompressive surgery may then be indicated for radiculopathy in the presence of spondylolisthesis. Thus, answer B is the best answer. In terms of surgery for the combination of surgical decompression for radicular pain in the setting of spondylolisthesis, laminectomy, foraminotomy, and fusion may all be required.

KEY FACTS

- Spondylolisthesis is a subluxation of one vertebra upon another.
- Spondylolisthesis alone is usually not a surgically remediable condition unless associated with radiculopathy/radicular pain due to dynamic compression with movement.

FURTHER READING

Ghabrial Y, Bogduk N. Surgery for low back pain. In: Fishman SM, Ballantyne JC, Rathmell JP (Eds.), *Bonica's Management of Pain.* 4th ed. Philadelphia, PA: Lippincott Williams & Wilkins; 2009.

33. ANSWER: B

The use of preinjectates to enhance RF lesion size has been studied in ex vivo preparations. Non-ionic injections of sterile water and dextrose had no appreciable effect on lesion size. Gradual increases in the tonicity of saline preparations from 0.7% to greater than 23% resulted in increased energy, enhanced lesion size, and lowered impedance.

FURTHER READING

Provenzano DA, Liebert MA, Somers DL. Increasing the NaCl concentration of the preinjected solution enhances monopolar radiofrequency lesion size. *Regional Anesth Pain Med.* 2013;38:112–123.

34. ANSWER: D

True interdisciplinary chronic pain management programs have been declining relative to population needs. Insurance-based care does not reward interdisciplinary care because of the high upfront costs for the program and the need for multiple types of therapy and therapists (physicians for medication management, opioid weaning, oversight; physical and occupational therapists for functional restoration programming; psychologists trained in group therapy, mindfulness training, and cognitive–behavioral therapies; and coaches for active ongoing care). Studies have shown that patients with severe characterological defects cannot be remedied by these types of programs, and often patients may need to be split off from core groups due to their destructive effects on group dynamics. Attempts to carve out specific aspects of the program, such as physical therapy, to the exclusion of other aspects (e.g., mindfulness training or active coping instruction) are not as successful.

FURTHER READING

Schatman ME. Interdisciplinary chronic pain management: Perspectives on history, current status, and future viability. In: Fishman SM, Ballantyne JC, Rathmell JP (Eds.), *Bonica's Management of Pain*. 4th ed. Philadelphia, PA: Lippincott Williams & Wilkins; 2009.

CHRONIC PELVIC PAIN

Martha J. Smith

INTRODUCTION

Chronic pelvic pain is a debilitating and frustrating medical condition for both the patient and the provider. Often, a source cannot be determined, which makes guiding a treatment plan more difficult. This chapter focuses primarily on nonmalignant chronic pelvic pain, which is defined as nonmenstrual pain below the level of the umbilicus that has continued for at least 6 months or more and is severe enough to seek medical or surgical treatment. In chronic pelvic pain, the pain and disability may often appear out of proportion to physical abnormalities, and this pain is often refractory to medical and surgical therapies. It is estimated that in the United States, chronic pelvic pain will affect one in seven women of reproductive age (18–50 years old). Chronic pelvic pain complaints comprise 10% of all gynecologic referrals. There are significant psychiatric comorbidities and many medical comorbidities that often accompany pelvic pain. Among these are concomitant depression, anxiety, and often a history of physical or sexual abuse. Approximately 30–50% of patients with chronic pelvic pain report a history of abuse, with a higher incidence of developing chronic pelvic pain if the abuse was experienced before age 15 years. The international prevalence of chronic pelvic pain is estimated to be equal to that of migraines, asthma, and back pain. Although the majority of pelvic pain patients are female, there are several conditions that can also cause chronic pelvic pain in males. Among the most common are chronic prostatitis, prostatodynia, orchialgia, inguinal neuralgia, and interstitial cystitis. When evaluating and diagnosing various pelvic pain conditions, it is imperative to rule out malignancy and other organic causes first. Pelvic floor dysfunction, sacroiliac joint instability, and other mechanical issues are often partially involved in the process of chronic pelvic pain, if not the primary source. As a clinician, all of these variables must be taken into consideration when evaluating and treating the chronic pelvic pain patient.

QUESTIONS

1. Vulvodynia is commonly associated with all of the following chronic pain conditions except:

A. Fibromyalgia
B. Irritable bowel syndrome
C. Bacterial vaginosis infection
D. Interstitial cystitis
E. Endometriosis

2. The most common level for approaching a celiac plexus block is:

A. T9 to T10
B. T10 to T11
C. T11 to T12
D. T12 to L1
E. L1 to L2

3. Which of the following statements best defines the syndrome of proctalgia fugax?

A. Proctalgia fugax is a nonmalignant pain syndrome characterized by constant anorectal pain and the urge to defecate.
B. Proctalgia fugax presents more commonly in males, often with characteristic neurotic, perfectionist, and hypochondriac personality traits.
C. Proctalgia fugax is often seen in patients who also have diverticulitis.
D. Proctalgia fugax is associated with a higher lifetime risk of squamous cell carcinoma of the colon.
E. Proctalgia fugax attacks may be relieved or aborted by ingesting food or drink at the onset, Valsalva or defecation, digital rectal stimulation, and enemas.

4. A male patient underwent a second celiac plexus block for treatment of his chronic pancreatitis. He contacted the pain clinic the following day reporting symptoms of diarrhea, dizziness upon standing, and back pain. You advise him:

A. Go to the emergency department for further evaluation.
B. His symptoms are normal side effects for routine celiac plexus blocks and will resolve in a few days.
C. Present to the clinic for orthostatic blood pressure testing and a prescription to help manage his diarrhea.
D. His symptoms are unrelated and likely consistent with an unrelated viral illness.

5. All of the following conditions are associated with hypertonic pelvic floor dysfunction except:

A. Vulvodynia
B. Stress urinary incontinence
C. Coccygodynia
D. Piriformis syndrome
E. Proctalgia fugax

6. Which of the following statements regarding sympathetic innervations is correct?

A. The celiac plexus provides sympathetic innervation from the distal third of the esophagus to the ascending colon, including liver, pancreas, gallbladder, stomach, spleen, kidneys, small intestine, large intestine, and adrenal glands.
B. The lumbar sympathetic chain provides innervation from the descending colon, proximal sigmoid colon, and kidneys.
C. The superior hypogastric plexus provides innervation to the distal sigmoid colon, kidneys, rectum, testes, and ovaries.
D. The terminal end of the sympathetic chain, or ganglion impar, innervates the distal rectum, distal urethra, uterus, vulva, and distal third of the vagina.

7. All of the following are techniques used for celiac plexus blockade except:

A. Transesophageal approach
B. Transaortic approach
C. Transdiscal approach
D. Retrocrural approach
E. Splanchnic nerve approach

8. The percentage of diagnostic laparoscopies performed for complaints associated with chronic pelvic pain is approximately:

A. <10%
B. 20%
C. 40%
D. 75%

9. Psychological comorbidities and history of preexisting physical and sexual abuse are common in patients with chronic pelvic pain (CPP). All of the following statements regarding these associations are true except:

A. CPP patients have higher incidence rates of depression, anxiety, somatization, and hostility.
B. There is no distinct demographic group that presents with higher incidence rates of chronic pelvic pain.
C. Approximately 25% of all patients presenting with CPP symptoms have a history of physical or sexual abuse.
D. Patients with coexisting depression are more refractory to therapeutic treatment strategies.

10. A 39-year-old female undergoes an uneventful superior hypogastric plexus block with conscious sedation. During her recovery in the post-anesthesia care unit, she complains of some dermatomal numbness, decreased temperature sensation to ice, and concordant weakness in the right lower extremity. Which of the following is the most likely explanation?

A. Antegrade spread of local anesthetic to the right L5 nerve root
B. Retrograde spread of local anesthetic to the right L5 nerve root
C. Antegrade spread of local anesthetic to the right S1 nerve root
D. Retrograde spread of local anesthetic to the right S1 nerve root

11. Pelvic floor hypertonic muscle dysfunction is noted in the majority of patients with vulvodynia. Which muscle is most involved in this process?

A. Pubococcygeus
B. Obturator internus
C. Piriformis
D. Coccygeus

12. All of the following are true statements regarding ilioinguinal neuralgia except:

A. Ilioinguinal pain is worsened with lumbar extension.
B. Ilioinguinal neuralgia may present with ipsilateral abdominal wall weakness.
C. The most common cause of ilioinguinal neuralgia is congenital spermatic cord defects.
D. The ilioinguinal nerve is a branch of the L1 nerve root in most individuals.

13. The most common vascular structure encountered during a fluoroscopic-guided superior hypogastric plexus block is:

A. Inferior mesenteric artery
B. Inferior vena cava
C. Aorta
D. Common iliac vein
E. Renal vein

14. The following diagnostic test is useful in evaluating interstitial cystitis:

A. Urinary tumor necrosis factor (nerve growth factor)
B. Urinary sodium
C. Urinary myoglobin
D. Urinary potassium

15. Pain in the labia majora and minora would be addressed by blockade of which peripheral nerve?

A. Iliohypogastric nerve
B. Genitofemoral nerve
C. Superficial clitoral nerve
D. Obturator nerve

16. All of the following are common causes of nonmalignant chronic pelvic pain in men except:

A. Orchialgia
B. Epididymal congestion
C. Interstitial cystitis
D. Prostatodynia
E. Aseptic prostatitis

17. Chemical neurolysis can be adequately achieved with which one of the following agents?

A. 70% ethyl alcohol
B. 50% glycerol
C. 5% hypertonic saline
D. 3% phenol

18. The most commonly associated comorbid medical condition associated with interstitial cystitis is:

A. Fibromyalgia
B. Inflammatory bowel disease
C. Systemic lupus erythematosus
D. Atopic allergies

19. All of the following statements regarding pudendal neuralgia are true except:

A. The pudendal nerve travels through Alcock's canal between the sacrospinous and sacrotuberous ligaments.
B. The pudendal nerve is derived from S2–S4 of the sacral plexus.
C. Hip adduction and internal rotation exacerbate pain symptoms in the buttock. There is often associated sciatica on the ipsilateral extremity.
D. Urinary incontinence, fecal incontinence, and sexual dysfunction may also accompany the pain symptoms of pudendal neuralgia.

20. When performing an ilioinguinal nerve block, the following statement is correct:

A. The ilioinguinal nerve is blocked in the fascial plane between the internal oblique and transversus abdominis muscles.
B. The ilioinguinal nerve is derived from the T10–T12 nerve roots.
C. The ilioinguinal nerve is usually blocked approximately 2 inches superior and medial to the anterior superior iliac spine.
D. The genitofemoral nerve is often blocked simultaneously as the ilioinguinal nerve due to its close proximity.

21. All of the following statements regarding interstitial cystitis (IC) are true except:

A. The majority of women diagnosed with IC have a history of prior pelvic surgery.
B. The pathophysiology of IC is hypothesized to be due to a dysfunctional and leaky glycosaminoglycan barrier in the bladder wall.
C. Hunner's ulcers in the bladder wall are a pathologic feature found in nearly all patients with IC.
D. Low-frequency sacral stimulation of the S3 nerve root is an effective treatment modality for IC.

22. Which of the following statements regarding chemical neurolysis agents is correct?

A. Axonal regeneration occurs at a faster rate following chemical neurolysis with phenol versus ethyl alcohol.
B. When performing neurolysis, phenol must be mixed with local anesthetic or administered following local anesthetic to minimize burning pain and dysesthesias along the nerve.
C. 50–70% ethyl alcohol is not frequently utilized for neurloysis due to its poor shelf life, requirement of refrigeration, and rapid oxidation.
D. 50–70% ethyl alcohol can be mixed with glycerin to aide administration at the desired location.

23. Which of the following statements concerning medication management of chronic pelvic pain is correct?

A. A short course of opioids at presentation is considered first-line therapy to treat somatic pain sources.

B. Tricyclic antidepressant (TCA) therapy has been shown to be more effective alone or in a combination therapy than anticonvulsant therapy alone.

C. Combination therapy with nonsteroidal anti-inflammatory drugs (NSAIDs) and oral contraceptives has been shown to be more efficacious than either drug used alone.

D. TCAs alone are more efficacious agents in most chronic pain conditions compared to selective serotonin reuptake inhibitors (SSRIs) alone.

24. Sacroiliac joint dysfunction may be a mechanical source of chronic pelvic pain. All of the following statements concerning the sacroiliac joint are correct except:

A. Sacroiliac joint pain rarely refers above the L5 area of the low back.

B. Sacroiliac joint pain is often related to asymmetry or oblique rotation of the bony pelvis.

C. The sacroiliac joint is a true synovial joint that extends from ilium to the inferior edge of the sacrum.

D. The sacroiliac is an articulating joint that allows movement and rotation.

25. Which of the following statements regarding treatment modalities for nonmalignant chronic pelvic pain is correct?

A. Excision of the superior hypogastric plexus is considered a surgical treatment option for chronic pelvic pain.

B. Laparoscopic uterine nerve ablation remains the gold standard for surgical treatment of refractory chronic pelvic pain.

C. Chemical neurolysis of the superior hypogastric plexus is a common nonsurgical treatment option for chronic pelvic pain.

D. In neuromodulation trials for chronic pelvic pain, retrograde placement of sacral leads has provided more effective pain relief than thoracic lead placement.

ANSWERS

1. ANSWER: C

Vulvodynia is a neuropathic pain condition associated with a chronic inflammatory process. Histologic samples have shown that all the other listed conditions share three common findings: significant increase in mast cell numbers, increased amounts of degranulated mast cells, and significantly increased numbers of mast cells close to pain nerve fibers. Recurrent *Candida albicans* infections have been linked to an increased incidence of vulvodynia. The findings of multiple case–control studies of provoked vulvodynia suggest that these women have more frequent *Candida* infections. A gene polymorphism that reduces the ability to control the growth of *C. albicans* has been associated with vestibulodynia, and it may play a central role in the triggering of this painful condition.

FURTHER READING

Graziottin A, Murina F. *Clinical Management of Vulvodynia: Tips and Tricks*. Milan, Italy: Springer-Verlag Italia, 2011:7–14, 39–52.

2. ANSWER: D

A celiac plexus is located at the level of T12 to L1 in the retroperitoneal space. It is anterior and caudal to the crura of the diaphragm. The celiac plexus receives sympathetic fibers from the greater (T9–T10), lesser (T10–T11), and least (T12) splanchnic nerves. It receives parasympathetic fibers from the vagus nerve.

FURTHER READING

Montgomery K, Hurley R. Nerve destruction for the alleviation of visceral pain. In: Huntoon M, Benzon H, Nauroze S, et al. (Eds.), *Spinal Injections & Peripheral Nerve Blocks*. Philadelphia, PA: Saunders; 2011:88–100.

3. ANSWER: E

Proctalgia fugax is a nonmalignant pain syndrome with no known cause. It is characterized by paroxysmal (not constant) anorectal pain with pain-free periods between episodes. Spontaneous remission of these attacks may occur for weeks to years. It is more common in females, and it is often associated with irritable bowel syndrome (not diverticulitis). Personality traits of perfectionism, hypochondriasis, and neurosis are often associated in patients with proctalgia fugax. Abortive methods reported to help relieve the pain of an attack include ingesting food or drink at the immediate onset of an attack, rectal suppositories or enemas, attempting defecation or Valsalva, and perineal pressure. Proctalgia fugax is a diagnosis of exclusion, and it is imperative that malignancy be excluded. However, there is no associated increased risk of colon cancers in patients with proctalgia fugax.

FURTHER READING

Waldman S, Waldman J. Proctalgia fugax. In: Waldman S (Ed.), *Pain Management*. 2nd ed. Philadelphia, PA: Saunders; 2011:687–692.

4. ANSWER: A

The development of new back pain following a celiac plexus block is concerning for the development of a retroperitoneal hematoma. This is considered an emergency and should be ruled out with at minimum two serial hematocrits an hour apart and/or imaging. The presence of orthostatic hypotension in the setting of back pain is concerning for retroperitoneal hematoma and should not be ignored as a routine side effect or procedural pain from a celiac plexus block because the consequences can be devastating. Orthostatic hypotension is most common with the splanchnic approach (52%) and retrocrural approach (50%) compared to the antecrural approach (10%). Orthostatic hypotension may persist for approximately 5 days following the procedure. Other side effects and complications of a celiac plexus block include diarrhea, pneumothorax, abdominal aortic dissection, dysesthesia, interscapular pain, pleurisy, hiccups, and hematuria.

FURTHER READING

Montgomery K, Hurley R. Nerve destruction for the alleviation of visceral pain. In: Huntoon M, Benzon H, Narouze S, et al. (Eds.), *Spinal Injections & Peripheral Nerve Blocks*. Philadelphia, PA: Saunders; 2011:88–100.

5. ANSWER: B

Stress urinary incontinence is associated with hypotonic pelvic floor dysfunction. Conditions associated with hypertonic pelvic floor dysfunction include overactive bladder, vulvodynia, coccygodynia, proctalgia fugax, levator ani syndrome, vaginismus, piriformis syndrome, pelvic floor spasm, and tension myalgia of the pelvic floor.

FURTHER READING

Cervigni M, Natale F. Pelvic floor dysfunction in bladder pain syndrome. In: Nordling J, Wyndaele J, vand de Merwe J, et al. (Eds.), *Bladder Pain Syndrome: A Guide for Clinicians*. New York, NY: Springer; 2013:125–141.

6. ANSWER: B

This is the correct sympathetic innervation of the lumbar sympathetic chain. The celiac plexus innervates the distal third of the esophagus to the descending colon. The rest of the statement is correct. The superior hypogastric plexus does not innervate the kidneys. This is covered by the lumbar sympathetic chain. The uterus receives sympathetic innervation from the superior hypogastric plexus, not the ganglion impar.

FURTHER READING

Montgomery K, Hurley R. Nerve destruction for the alleviation of visceral pain. In: Huntoon M, Benzon H, Narouze S, et al. (Eds.), *Spinal Injections & Peripheral Nerve Blocks*. Philadelphia, PA: Saunders; 2011:88–100.

7. ANSWER: A

A transesophageal approach has not been described. However, endoscopic guidance can be used for a transgastric approach. The most common approach is computed tomography or the fluoro-guided posterior retrocrural approach. The antecrural approach does utilize a transaortic technique. Although not commonly performed because of concern for discitis, a transdiscal approach has also been described. The splanchnic nerve approach is also described.

FURTHER READING

Montgomery K, Hurley R. Nerve destruction for the alleviation of visceral pain. In: Huntoon M, Benzon H, Nauroze S, et al. (Eds.), *Spinal Injections & Peripheral Nerve Blocks*. Philadelphia, PA: Saunders; 2011:88–100.

8. ANSWER: C

Approximately 40% of diagnostic laparoscopies are performed for pelvic pain complaints. Chronic pelvic pain comprises approximately 10% of all gynecologic referrals. The lifetime incidence of chronic pelvic pain is estimated as high as 33%, with approximately 15–20% of women aged 18–50 years reporting pelvic pain more than 1 year in duration.

9. ANSWER: C

CPP is associated with higher incidences of psychological conditions including depression, anxiety, somatic complaints, and hostility. CPP patients with depression are more likely to have higher pain scores and be less responsive to treatment modalities.

Demographic data of age, ethnicity, socioeconomic status, education, and employment status have not revealed an increased incidence in any particular group. There are occurrence factors that can increase the risk of developing CPP, such as a history of pelvic inflammatory disease, endometriosis, and pregnancy risk factors (large fetal birth weight, pelvic muscle weakness, lumbar lordosis, etc.).

History of previous physical or sexual abuse is a significant predisposing factor for developing subsequent CPP. At least 50% of patients with CPP report a history of abuse. Obtaining a thorough history of abuse is important in the assessment of CPP.

FURTHER READING

Christo P, Hobelmann G. Pelvic pain. In: Smith H (Eds.), *Current Therapy in Pain*. Philadelphia, PA: Saunders; 2009:216–227.

10. ANSWER: B

Retrograde spread of local anesthetic to the L5 nerve root can occur, especially with higher volume blocks. This is often a result of needle placement more lateral than anterolateral with respect to the L5 disc.

FURTHER READING

Montgomery K, Hurley R. Nerve destruction for the alleviation of visceral pain. In: Huntoon M, Benzon H, Narouze S, et al. (Eds.), *Spinal Injections & Peripheral Nerve Blocks*. Philadelphia, PA: Saunders; 2011:88–100.

11. ANSWER: A

The pubococcygeus and iliococcygeus muscles make up the levator ani. Hypertonicity of the levator ani is found in 80–90% of women with vulvodynia. The other structures also support the pelvic floor but are less involved in this mechanism. It is unclear whether this hypertonic pelvic floor dysfunction is a primary mechanism from painful trigger points or neuropathic pain from pelvic nerves. It is likely a combination of both sources. The levator ani muscles are innervated by the levator ani nerve, with no evidence of pudendal nerve innervation. However, both the levator ani motor neurons and pudendal motor neurons contain primary afferent fibers that terminate in the sacral spinal cord. Thus, there is a great deal of overlap between them. Vulvodynia is considered a neuropathic pain condition, so there is obvious neural involvement in this disorder. The leading opinion is that neuropathic vulvar pain can cause levator ani spasm, and this hypertonicity perpetuates the pain into a chronic process.

FURTHER READING

Brookoff D. Genitourinary pain syndromes: Interstitial cystitis, chronic pancreatitis, pelvic floor dysfunction, and related disorders. In: Smith H (Ed.), *Current Therapy in Pain*. Philadelphia, PA: Saunders; 2009:205–215.

12. ANSWER: C

Ilioinguinal neuralgia rarely occurs spontaneously. It is usually caused by compression of the nerve along its course as it passes through the transverse abdominis muscle in proximity to the anterior superior iliac spine. Common causes of ilioinguinal neuralgia or compression include trauma, traction, or direct trauma during inguinal hernia surgery or other pelvic surgeries. The ilioinguinal nerve is a branch of the L1 nerve root in most people; however, there is occasionally a T12 source or overlap in some individuals. Chronic neuralgia can result in weakening of the ipsilateral abdominal wall musculature, which can protrude asymmetrically and be mistaken for an inguinal hernia. Lumbar extension puts traction on the ilioinguinal nerve and reproduces the pain. A classic finding is patients preferring a "bent skier's" posture of lumbar flexion to relieve this traction.

FURTHER READING

Waldman S. Ilioinguinal, iliohypogastric, and genitofemoral neuralgia. In: Waldman S. (Ed.), *Pain Management*. 2nd ed. Philadelphia, PA: Saunders; 2011:687–692.

13. ANSWER: D

The common iliac vessels are in the trajectory of the typical L5–S1 approach of superior hypogastric plexus block, making those the most common vascular structures encountered.

FURTHER READING

Montgomery K, Hurley R. Nerve destruction for the alleviation of visceral pain. In: Huntoon M, Benzon H, Narouze S, et al. (Eds.), *Spinal Injections & Peripheral Nerve Blocks*. Philadelphia, PA: Saunders; 2011:88–100.

14. ANSWER: D

Increased urinary potassium levels are associated with interstitial cystitis. Potassium instillation testing using an intravesicular solution of 0.4 M KCl has been described, but it is generally avoided due to significant patient discomfort in the setting of interstitial cystitis and prostatitis. Typically, a food history revealing recent ingestion of high-potassium-containing foods is sufficient. It is hypothesized that patients with interstitial cystitis have increased bladder permeability and the bladder is "leaky," so these high-potassium-containing foods (alcohol, tomatoes, oranges, leafy greens, etc.) are able to cross the bladder epithelium, causing irritation, pain, and an inflammatory cascade.

FURTHER READING

Brookoff D. Genitourinary pain syndromes: Interstitial cystitis, chronic pancreatitis, pelvic floor dysfunction, and related disorders. In: Smith H (Ed.), *Current Therapy in Pain*. Philadelphia, PA: Saunders; 2009:205–215.

15. ANSWER: B

In women, the genital branch of the genitofemoral nerve innervates the round ligament, labia majora, and labia minora. It arises from the L1 and L2 nerve roots. It divides into a genital and femoral branch as it passes through the psoas muscle. The femoral branch passes under the inguinal ligament with the femoral vessels and provides cutaneous innervation to a small patch on the inner thigh.

In men, the genitofemoral nerve passes along with the spermatic cord to innervate the bottom of the scrotum and the cremaster muscles.

FURTHER READING

Christo P, Hobelmann G. Pelvic pain. In: Smith H (Eds.), *Current Therapy in Pain*. Philadelphia, PA: Saunders; 2009:216–227.

16. ANSWER: B

Chronic male pelvic pain accounts for approximately 2 million urologic visits per year. Common causes include interstitial cystitis, prostatodynia, aseptic prostatitis, orchialgia, and post-surgical pain (inguinal hernias, vasectomy, orchiectomy, etc.). Epididymal congestion, epididymal hypertension ("blue balls"), and epididymitis are typically acute issues related to sexual arousal, venous congestion, semen drainage, or infection in the case of the latter.

FURTHER READING

Bal R, Diwan S, Gritsenko K. Pelvic pain. In: Benzon H, Raja S, Fishman S, et al. (Eds.), *Essentials of Pain Medicine.* 3rd ed. Philadelphia, PA: Saunders; 2011:378–385.

17. ANSWER: A

The most common agents for chemical neurolysis are 4–10% phenol and 50–70% ethyl alcohol. Various concentrations of hypertonic saline and glycerol have also reportedly been used. Glycerol was used most frequently for trigeminal neurolysis.

FURTHER READING

Montgomery K, Hurley R. Nerve destruction for the alleviation of visceral pain. In: Huntoon M, Benzon H, Narouze S, et al. (Eds.), *Spinal Injections & Peripheral Nerve Blocks.* Philadelphia, PA: Saunders; 2011:88–100.

18. ANSWER: B

Of the conditions listed, irritable bowel syndrome has the strongest association with interstitial cystitis. Compared with normal controls, persons with interstitial cystitis are 100 times more likely to have irritable bowel syndrome and 30 times more likely to have systemic lupus erythematosus. Atopic allergy conditions, fibromyalgia, and migraines were also found to have increased incidences among interstitial cystitis patients, likely due to central pain processing disorders (central sensitization).

FURTHER READING

Brookoff D. Genitourinary pain syndromes: Interstitial cystitis, chronic pancreatitis, pelvic floor dysfunction, and related disorders. In: Smith H (Ed.), *Current Therapy in Pain.* Philadelphia, PA: Saunders; 2009:205–215.

19. ANSWER: C

Pudendal neuralgia is typically exacerbated by sitting and hip flexion, and it is relieved with standing or lying down.

The pudendal nerve divides into three branches after it passes through the sacrospinous and sacrotuberous ligaments in Alcock's canal at the ischial spine: anal/rectal, perineal, and clitoral/penile.

The condition described in answer C is more suggestive of piriformis syndrome. The piriformis muscle functions to abduct, externally rotate, and extend the hip. Although the sciatic nerve may have a variable course behind, through, or in front of the piriformis muscle, patients with piriformis syndrome will often present with a concordant sciatica.

FURTHER READING

Fitzgerald C, Hynes C. Female perineal/pelvic pain: The rehabilitation approach. In: Smith H (Ed.), *Current Therapy in Pain.* Philadelphia, PA: Saunders; 2009:227–233.

20. ANSWER: A

The ilioinguinal nerve is derived from the T12–L1 nerve roots. The anatomic landmarks for blockade are approximately 2 inches inferior and medial to the anterior superior iliac spine. The iliohypogastric nerve runs in close proximity at this level and is often blocked along with the ilioinguinal nerve. The ilioinguinal nerve is usually blocked under ultrasound guidance in the fascial plane between the internal oblique and the transversus abdominis muscles.

FURTHER READING

Waldman S. Ilioinguinal, iliohypogastric, and genitofemoral neuralgia. In: Waldman S. (Ed.), *Pain Management.* 2nd ed. Philadelphia, PA: Saunders; 2011:687–692.

21. ANSWER: C

Urothelial ulcers, known as Hunner's ulcers, are a pathologic finding most commonly associated with interstitial cystitis. However, they are found in only approximately 5–10% of patients diagnosed with interstitial cystitis.

Most women diagnosed with IC have a history of prior pelvic surgery, most commonly hysterectomy.

The glycosaminoglycan layer in the bladder epithelium maintains the permeability barrier of the bladder wall. Dysfunction of this layer can render it "leaky" and allow solutes, water, potassium, and other irritants of urine to diffuse back through, thus leading to pain and irritation.

The S3 nerve root is generally targeted for low-frequency (5–50 Hz) neurostimulation because the majority of the somatic fibers that control the closing pressure of the external urethral sphincter are derived from this level.

FURTHER READING

Brookoff D. Genitourinary pain syndromes: Interstitial cystitis, chronic pancreatitis, pelvic floor dysfunction, and related disorders. In: Smith H (Ed.), *Current Therapy in Pain*. Philadelphia, PA: Saunders; 2009:205–215.

22. ANSWER: A

Phenol seems to allow faster axonal regeneration following a neurolytic block compared to ethyl alcohol.

Concentrations of 50–100% ethyl alcohol are sufficient for neurolysis. However, ethyl alcohol injection perineurally causes significant discomfort and dysesthesias along the nerve when injected. This may last minutes or weeks. For this reason, it is recommended to inject local anesthetic first to anesthetize the nerve or to mix local anesthetic with the ethyl alcohol for the neurolytic procedure.

Phenol is poorly soluble in water and only forms a 6.7% aqueous solution at room temperature. It is often constituted with contrast dyes, saline, glycerin, or sterile water. Phenol will rapidly oxidize when exposed to room air, discoloring it to red-brown. However, it can be stored up to 1 year if protected from light in a refrigerated environment.

FURTHER READING

Montgomery K, Hurley R. Nerve destruction for the alleviation of visceral pain. In: Huntoon M, Benzon H, Narouze S, et al. (Eds.), *Spinal Injections & Peripheral Nerve Blocks*. Philadelphia, PA: Saunders; 2011:88–100.

23. ANSWER: D

In meta-analyses comparing TCAs and SSRIs in chronic pain conditions, TCAs generally show better efficacy.

Anticonvulsant agents either alone or in combination therapy have been shown to be more efficacious than antidepressant drugs alone.

Oral contraceptives and NSAIDs have a synergistic effect compared with either agent alone for chronic pelvic pain.

FURTHER READING

Bal R, Diwan S, Gritsenko K. Pelvic pain. In: Benzon H, Raja S, Fishman S, et al. (Eds.), *Essentials of Pain Medicine*. 3rd ed. Philadelphia, PA: Saunders; 2011:378–385.

24. ANSWER: C

The sacroiliac joint is a true joint with a synovial space only on the inferior portion. This is the target area for sacroiliac joint injections. The sacroiliac joint has been shown to have true movement of approximately 1–3° rotationally. It is a common generator of low back pain; however, it rarely refers above the L5 region of the pelvis. It may also radiate to the posterior legs and mimic radiculopathy. It is the most common source of pregnancy-related pelvic pain.

FURTHER READING

Fitzgerald C, Hynes C. Female perineal/pelvic pain: The rehabilitation approach. In: Smith H (Ed.), *Current Therapy in Pain*. Philadelphia, PA: Saunders; 2009:227–233.

25. ANSWER: A

Laparoscopic presacral neurectomy, or excision of the superior hypogastric plexus, was shown to be more effective than exploratory laparoscopy in the treatment of chronic pelvic pain in a double-blind randomized controlled trial. The presacral neurectomy group was found to have statistically significant lower pain intensity compared to controls. Potential risks of this procedure include vena cava injury, which could be catastrophic or fatal.

Laparoscopic uterine nerve ablation (LUNA) is a surgical technique that has had mixed results. Initial data appeared to be promising; however, a recent randomized control trial found no significant differences in several pain variables at 69 months. Currently, there is no gold standard for surgical treatment of chronic pelvic pain, especially given that more often than not, the etiology cannot be defined and is often influenced by psychologic factors.

Chemical neurolysis is generally reserved for palliative treatment of malignant pain conditions. Complications of neurolysis can include permanent motor or sensory deficits, deafferentation pain, sexual dysfunction, bowel or bladder incontinence, neuritis, or neuroma formation.

Neuromodulation trials have shown more efficacy with thoracic lead placement at T11–L1 versus retrograde S2–S3 lead placement.

FURTHER READING

Bal R, Diwan S, Gritsenko K. Pelvic pain. In: Benzon H, Raja S, Fishman S, et al. (Eds.), *Essentials of Pain Medicine*. 3rd ed. Philadelphia, PA: Saunders; 2011:378–385.

OBSTETRIC PAIN

Hans P. Sviggum and Adam K. Jacob

INTRODUCTION

This chapter reviews the complex pathophysiologic processes of pain transmission and perception experienced by women throughout pregnancy, management of pain in the peripartum period, and how preexisting chronic pain or opiate use affects the care of parturients. It discusses mechanisms of pain; common pain pathways; and factors influencing the perception of pain during pregnancy, labor, and delivery. It compares the benefits and adverse effects of current strategies for managing maternal pain during labor and after delivery. Finally, it reviews maternal and fetal effects of peripartum pain management in opiate- and non-opiate-dependent mothers.

QUESTIONS

1. Which of the following patients would experience the greatest benefit of a transversus abdominis plane block for analgesia following cesarean delivery?

A. A patient undergoing her fourth cesarean delivery
B. A patient with a body mass index of 45
C. A patient with a strong visceral component to her pain
D. A patient with an allergy to nonsteroidal anti-inflammatory drugs (NSAIDs)
E. A patient not receiving neuraxial morphine or hydromorphone

2. A 34-year-old G3P1 at 39 weeks of gestation is admitted after 2 hours of painful uterine contractions that have caused a change in her cervical dilation from 2 to 4 cm. Which of the following is true about first-stage labor pain?

A. It is primarily visceral in origin.
B. It is primarily somatic in origin.

C. It is nearly equal parts visceral and somatic in origin.
D. It can be treated by a pudendal nerve block.
E. Intrathecal fentanyl is ineffective as a treatment.

3. Which parturient would be expected to have the highest level of acute pain in the first 2 days following delivery?

A. 34-year-old after delivery of twins without epidural analgesia
B. 18-year-old with second-degree vaginal laceration after spontaneous delivery of 9-pound infant
C. 28-year-old who underwent cesarean delivery under spinal anesthesia for breech presentation
D. 41-year-old after delivery of her eighth child with epidural analgesia
E. 34-year-old who delivered 28 hours after being induced for preeclampsia with epidural analgesia

4. Which of the following oral medications is least likely to provide analgesic benefit for patients undergoing cesarean delivery?

A. Acetaminophen
B. Ibuprofen
C. Gabapentin
D. Oxycodone
E. All of the above have unequivocally been shown to significantly improve post-cesarean analgesia.

5. Which of the following statements regarding labor pain is most accurate?

A. The intensity of pain is consistent between individuals.
B. The majority of women experience pain classified as minimal or mild.
C. Multiparous women rate pain as more severe compared to nulliparous women.

D. Severe pain is unlikely to occur until the second stage of labor.

E. Rated severity of pain correlates closely with degree of cervical dilation.

6. A 31-year-old G2P1 is admitted for induction of labor at 41 weeks of gestation. She desires epidural analgesia. Which of the following statements about epidural analgesia is most true?

A. There is no association between epidural analgesia and rates of instrumented delivery (e.g., forceps and vacuum).

B. Epidural analgesia prolongs the first stage of labor.

C. Epidural analgesia causes a small, but significant, increase in cesarean delivery rate compared with systemic analgesia.

D. Epidural analgesia increases the risk for perineal tears and/or anal sphincter injury.

E. Effective epidural analgesia prolongs the second stage of labor.

7. A 27-year-old G1P0 presents to obstetric triage with painful regular uterine contractions that started 4 hours ago. She is found to have a cervical dilation of 6 cm and is admitted to the obstetric ward in active labor. Compared to prelabor, which of the following is least likely to be seen?

A. Periods of intermittent hyperventilation

B. Increased plasma levels of norepinephrine and epinephrine

C. Increased gastrointestinal and urinary motility

D. Increased maternal cardiac output

E. Enhanced oxytocin release

8. A 32-year-old woman presents to the emergency room 2 days after delivering her first child under neuraxial analgesia. She is complaining of a severe frontal–occipital headache that is worse when standing and completely relieved while lying down. Which of the following about postdural puncture headaches is most true?

A. The incidence is not related to the experience of the anesthesia provider.

B. Cutting bevel needle designs decrease the risk compared to pencil-point needle designs.

C. The majority start within 48 hours of the procedure.

D. Epidural analgesia decreases the risk compared to combined spinal–epidural analgesia.

E. A loss-of-resistance to saline technique decreases the risk compared to loss-of-resistance to air technique.

9. A 35-year-old G4P3 presents to the obstetric ward in active labor. Her cervical exam reveals 9-cm dilation

and appears to be progressing rapidly. She has a history of rapid deliveries. Which of the following most accurately reflects the obstetric pain pathways in the late first stage and second stage of labor?

A. Afferent nerve fibers in the cervix and lower uterine segment no longer play a role in transmission of pain.

B. The dermatomal level of analgesia required is similar to that of a cesarean delivery anesthesia.

C. Second-stage labor pain can be effectively treated with neuraxial opioids alone.

D. Pelvic pain is transmitted by visceral afferent nerve fibers that accompany sympathetic nerve fibers.

E. Pelvic pain is transmitted by somatic nerve fibers that enter the spinal cord at the S2–S4 segments.

10. A woman who receives standard epidural analgesia is more likely to experience which adverse event compared to a woman who receives combined spinal–epidural analgesia?

A. Pruritus

B. Meningitis

C. Fetal bradycardia

D. Postdural puncture headache

E. None of the above

11. A 30-year-old G1P0 presents with spontaneous labor. Cervical exam reveals 4-cm dilation, 50% effacement, –2 station. An epidural is placed, and an infusion of 0.075% bupivacaine + 2 μg/ml of fentanyl is started at 8 ml/hour. Eight hours later, she is having increasing pelvic pain, and repeat cervical exam reveals complete cervical dilation, 100% effacement, and +1 station. What treatment will be most effective for managing her increased pain?

A. Increasing the epidural infusion rate to 12 ml/hour

B. Providing a 6-ml epidural bolus of 0.25% bupivacaine

C. Providing a 100-μg epidural bolus of fentanyl

D. Switching the epidural infusion to 0.5% lidocaine + fentanyl 2 μg/ml at 8 ml/hour

E. Having the obstetrician perform a paracervical block with 2% lidocaine and increasing epidural infusion rate to 12 ml/hour

12. When considering substitution therapy in opiate-dependent parturients, which statement is most correct comparing the use of methadone to buprenorphine?

A. Women treated with buprenorphine are more likely to have abnormal presentation and delivery via cesarean section compared to women treated with methadone.

B. Buprenorphine crosses the placenta, whereas methadone does not.

C. Mothers who receive buprenorphine are equally likely to discontinue treatment as mothers treated with methadone.

D. The incidence of medical complications at the time of delivery is similar between women treated with buprenorphine and those treated with methadone.

E. Infants whose mothers were exposed to buprenorphine are more likely to have decreased head circumference compared to infants whose mothers received methadone.

13. When considering the administration of neuraxial opioids for post-cesarean analgesia, which of the following plays the key role in determining the onset of analgesia, dermatomal spread, and duration of activity?

A. Lipid solubility
B. Volume of injectate
C. Degree of ionization
D. Molecular weight
E. Drug concentration

14. A 21-year-old G2P2 woman presents 2 days after a vaginal delivery during which she had an epidural placement that was complicated by a dural puncture. Subsequent epidural placement was successful, and the rest of her labor and delivery was uneventful. The day after delivery, she developed a frontal headache associated with neck stiffness. The headache is worse when upright and has continued to be disabling despite the use of acetaminophen, ibuprofen, and oxycodone. She has no other complaints. What would be the most appropriate next step?

A. Obtain an magnetic resonance imaging (MRI) scan of her head
B. Perform an epidural blood patch
C. Obtain a computed tomography (CT) scan of her head
D. Continue current conservative management for another 48 hours
E. Administer 500 mg caffeine sodium benzoate over 30–60 minutes intravenously

15. Which of the following statements about parturients suffering from chronic pain syndromes is most true?

A. Buprenorphine has been associated with neonatal respiratory depression.
B. Patients on methadone should not receive neuraxial morphine for cesarean delivery.
C. Women who abuse illegal drugs have similar postpartum pain to that of women who do not.

D. Anxiety is a predictor of labor pain.
E. NSAIDs are of little benefit in the immediate postpartum period.

16. Which of the following statements about local anesthetic administration in pregnancy is most true?

A. Chloroprocaine should be avoided in patients less than 34 weeks' gestational age because the high doses necessary for its use can create ion trapping in the fetus.
B. Pregnant women exhibit a more rapid onset and a longer duration of spinal anesthesia than do nonpregnant women.
C. Pregnancy increases the susceptibility to cardiac toxicity of bupivacaine.
D. Decreased local anesthetic dose requirements during pregnancy typically begin to manifest in the mid-to-late third trimester
E. Increased spinal cerebral spinal fluid (CSF) volume during pregnancy creates a dilutional effect necessitating a 20–30% increase in local anesthetic doses for spinal anesthesia.

17. Which of the following will result in the most effective pain relief while minimizing side effects for a woman receiving an epidural infusion of 0.075% bupivacaine at 8 ml/hour who experiences breakthrough pain in first stage of labor?

A. 100 μg fentanyl via lumbar epidural
B. 100 μg fentanyl intravenously
C. 50 μg fentanyl single injection into caudal space
D. 50 μg fentanyl intravenously
E. 50 μg fentanyl via lumbar epidural

18. A 27-year-old G3P2 woman presents in active labor. Combined spinal–epidural labor analgesia is provided with 25 μg intrathecal fentanyl followed by initiation of an epidural infusion of 0.125% bupivacaine at 10 ml/hour. What is the most common side effect expected in this woman?

A. Hives
B. Sedation
C. Pruritus
D. Fetal tachycardia
E. Headache

19. You have been asked to consult on a 30-year-old G2P0 woman with chronic back pain and long-standing daily opiate use in which the dose has been escalating. She denies any other recent illicit drug use, although she has experimented with multiple substances in the past. She is now 8 weeks pregnant, and her obstetric

provider recommended that she begin methadone. She is concerned about what effect methadone might have on her pregnancy and her baby. Which of the following statements regarding methadone use in pregnancy is most likely true?

A. She should undergo a rapid detoxification program to eliminate her use of all opiates during pregnancy.
B. There is no apparent risk for preterm delivery with maintenance use of methadone.
C. She would not be a candidate for labor epidural analgesia at the time of delivery.
D. Her infant is at risk for abnormal ophthalmologic development if she continues methadone use during pregnancy.
E. Methadone pharmacokinetics will not change significantly during the course of her pregnancy.

20. A 26-year-old G2P0 woman at 41 weeks of gestation presents in active labor. She is interested in exploring all of her options for labor analgesia. Which of the following statements is most accurate?

A. Sterile water papules are contraindicated in active labor.
B. Hydrotherapy is not an option for her due to her gestation age being greater than 40 weeks.
C. There is no evidence of analgesic benefit of hydrotherapy during labor.
D. Acupuncture has been abandoned as a labor analgesic technique due to concerns of fetal bradycardia leading to emergent delivery.
E. Hypnosis can be used in conjunction with continuous labor analgesia for treatment of labor pain.

21. Which statement about pain during pregnancy is most accurate?

A. Pregnancy and labor are associated with an increase in the threshold to pain.
B. A reduction in cerebral blood flow during pregnancy leads to deactivation of μ opioid receptors.
C. Patients with chronic low back pain are likely to experience remission of symptoms in late pregnancy.
D. Although actual pain thresholds do not change, most women develop hyperalgesia in late pregnancy.
E. Pregnancy is associated with decreased plasma levels of β-endorphins.

22. A 19-year-old G1P0 desires pharmacologic treatment of labor pain but declines epidural placement. Which statement about the use of intravenous remifentanil for labor analgesia is true?

A. Nausea is a significant limiting side effect.
B. Intravenous remifentanil provides less effective pain relief compared to epidural techniques.
C. Neonates are more likely to require admission to an intensive care unit after birth.
D. Maternal oxygen saturations are similar to those of epidural analgesia.
E. Patient-controlled intravenous analgesia is less effective than a continuous infusion.

23. Which of the following statements about chronic pain after childbirth is true?

A. The incidence of persistent pain is higher 6 months after delivery compared to 2 months after delivery.
B. Women are more likely to experience chronic pain after vaginal delivery compared to cesarean delivery.
C. The incidence of chronic pain after childbirth is comparable to that after general abdominal surgery.
D. The incidence of new-onset pelvic and/or abdominal pain from delivery at 1 year after childbirth is less than 1%.
E. Perioperative administration of 600 mg gabapentin at the time of cesarean delivery has been shown to reduce the incidence of chronic pain.

24. Which of the following is a risk factor for persistent pain and depression following delivery?

A. Induction of labor versus spontaneous labor
B. Two or more doses of nalbuphine in the first 24 hours following delivery
C. Less than 200 μg morphine as part of spinal anesthesia
D. Cesarean delivery performed for twin gestation
E. The presence of severe acute pain within 36 hours postpartum

25. When comparing the efficacy of epidural to combined spinal–epidural for initiation of labor analgesia, which of the following statements is correct?

A. Onset of analgesia is similar between epidural and combined spinal–epidural techniques.
B. Catheters placed with a plain epidural technique have a greater failure rate for labor analgesia compared to catheters placed using a combined spinal–epidural technique.
C. Successful conversion to epidural anesthesia for cesarean delivery is more likely with catheters placed using a combined spinal–epidural technique compared to a plain epidural technique.
D. Maternal satisfaction with labor analgesia is higher after combined spinal–epidural than after plain epidural placement.

E. The average duration of the second stage of labor is shorter in women who received combined spinal–epidural analgesia compared to women who received plain epidural analgesia.

26. A 32-year-old G1P0 woman presents for a scheduled induction of labor at 41 weeks of gestation. During your discussion with her about options for labor analgesia, she inquires about the use of inhaled nitrous oxide. Which of the following statements is most accurate?

A. Nitrous oxide provides as effective relief of labor pain as epidural analgesia.
B. The most common maternal side effect of inhaled nitrous oxide is drowsiness.
C. Nitrous oxide is most commonly administered as a 70:30 mix with air.
D. For maximum analgesia benefit, inhalation of nitrous oxide should begin 30 seconds before the next anticipated contraction.
E. There is no association of nitrous oxide use and neurodegeneration in developing animals.

27. A 20-year-old G3P0 at 33 2/7 weeks of gestation with no prenatal care presents to the labor and delivery triage area with vaginal bleeding. She is confused and lethargic, and she is observed to have constricted pupils. Upon questioning, she admitted to recent heroin use, and an empty bottle of oxycodone is found in her purse. Thirty minutes after presentation, she precipitously delivers a viable 1500-g male infant. Which of

the following statements regarding chronic opioid use during pregnancy and neonatal abstinence syndrome (NAS) is true?

A. NAS scoring should start at birth and be repeated every 3 or 4 hours for the infant's entire birth hospitalization.
B. Among infants with prenatal exposure to opioids, the reported rate of NAS requiring pharmacotherapy ranges from 5% to 10%.
C. Premature infants are at a higher risk for developing NAS compared to term infants.
D. Onset of NAS most commonly develops within 1 hour of delivery.
E. Diazepam should be considered the first-line pharmacologic treatment.

28. A 33-year-old G1P1 suffers a back injury while falling down stairs 2 weeks after delivering her infant at term gestation. She questions which medication, if any, she can take to treat her pain while continuing to breast-feed her infant. Which parameter is most clinically relevant for determining the safety of a medication prescribed to a mother who is breast-feeding her infant?

A. Lactation chemical coefficient
B. Fetal birth weight
C. Relative infant dose
D. Degree of ionization
E. None; she needs to stop lactation before taking any medication

ANSWERS

1. ANSWER: E

Analgesia following cesarean delivery (CD) is best achieved by a multimodal approach. The cornerstone of this multimodal approach is neuraxial opioids. Morphine is the most widely used and studied in this regard, although hydromorphone is also used. Typical dosing of 1.5–3 mg epidural or 100–200 μg intrathecal morphine provides good analgesia for 16–36 hours. In addition, scheduled acetaminophen, NSAIDs, and oral opioids are used concomitantly.

The transversus abdominis plane (TAP) block provides somatic pain relief to the lower thoracic dermatomes. Compared to controls, TAP blocks provide significant analgesic benefit for women undergoing CD. However, TAP blocks have been shown to be inferior to neuraxial opioids with regard to reported pain scores and opioid consumption following CD. The role of the TAP block for CD appears to be (1) for patients allergic or having previous bad reactions to intrathecal opioids; (2) as a rescue technique for patients having pain in the recovery room despite standard multimodal therapy; and (3) for patients who do not receive neuraxial opioids (e.g., general anesthesia for emergency CD).

KEY FACTS

- Neuraxial opioids are the cornerstone of a multimodal analgesic approach to post-cesarean analgesia.
- Transversus abdominis plane blocks are inferior to neuraxial opioids in terms of analgesic benefit, but they can be useful in cases in which neuraxial opioids are not used.

FURTHER READING

Petersen PL, Mathiesen O, Torup H, et al. The transversus abdominis plane block: A valuable option for postoperative analgesia? A topical review. *Acta Anaesthesiol Scand*. 2010;54:529–535.
Verstraete S, Van de Velde M. Post-cesarean section analgesia. *Acta Anaesth Belg*. 2012;63:147–167.

2. ANSWER: A

Pain during the first stage of labor arises from uterine contractions and cervical dilation. These pain signals are transmitted through afferent (sympathetic) nerves entering the spinal cord from T10–L1. This first-stage labor pain is mostly visceral in origin. This pain likely increases over time as a result of the sensitization of peripheral and central pain-signaling pathways. During the second stage of labor (after complete cervical dilation has been achieved), stretching of perineal structures and the physical movement of the fetus through the birth canal transmit pain signals through the pudendal nerve and S2–S4 sacral nerves. This adds a significant somatic pain on top of the visceral pain from uterine contractions.

Neuraxial opioids are very effective in treating visceral pain, but local anesthetics are needed to adequately alleviate pain of somatic origin. Thus, intrathecal fentanyl or epidural fentanyl would likely be effective when used to treat first-stage labor pain. For second-stage labor pain, epidural or intrathecal local anesthetics or a pudendal nerve block would be needed to provide adequate pain relief.

KEY FACTS

- Pain during the first stage of labor is primary visceral in origin, whereas second-stage labor pain has a strong somatic component as well.
- Often, pain during the first stage of labor can be effectively treated by neuraxial opioids.

FURTHER READING

Eltzschig HK, Lieberman ES, Camann WR. Regional anesthesia and analgesia for labor and delivery. *N Engl J Med*. 2003;348:319–332.
Hawkins JL. Epidural analgesia for labor and delivery. *N Engl J Med*. 2010;362:1503–1510.

3. ANSWER: C

Post-delivery pain results from direct trauma to tissue and subsequent inflammation. Generally, more trauma occurs during a cesarean delivery than during a vaginal delivery. The severity of acute pain after vaginal delivery is highly variable and less predictable than that of pain after cesarean delivery. Patients undergoing an episiotomy or suffering a perineal laceration can experience severe pain but not usually to the extent of cesarean delivery, especially for first- and second-degree lacerations. Age and parity are not known to be significant contributors to the severity of acute post-delivery pain. Although epidural analgesia is highly effective for treating labor pain, no difference in acute post-delivery pain between women delivering with versus those delivering without epidural analgesia has been shown.

KEY FACTS

- Regardless of indication, women generally experience higher acute pain following cesarean delivery compared to vaginal delivery.

- No relationship between epidural use for vaginal delivery and severity of acute pain has been shown.

FURTHER READING

Flood P, Aleshi P. Postoperative and chronic pain: Systemic and regional analgesic techniques. In: Chestnut DH, Wong CA, Tsen LC, et al. (Eds.), *Chestnut's Obstetric Anesthesia*. 5th ed. Philadelphia, PA: Saunders; 2014.

4. ANSWER: C

Gabapentin has been shown to reduce acute postoperative pain and opioid consumption after a variety of surgical procedures. However, in a randomized study of the cesarean delivery population, a single preoperative dose did not improve post-cesarean analgesia or maternal satisfaction in the context of a multimodal analgesic regimen.

Gabapentin has been assigned a pregnancy category C drug. Animal studies have revealed evidence of abnormal bone development and hydronephrosis in fetuses. There are no reports of fetotoxicity in humans when given as a single preoperative dose. The effects of maternal gabapentin use on breast-feeding infants are unknown.

KEY FACT

- The addition of preoperative gabapentin to a multimodal analgesic regimen does not improve patient analgesia following cesarean delivery.

FURTHER READING

Short J, Downey K, Bernstein P, et al. A single preoperative dose of gabapentin does not improve postcesarean delivery pain management: A randomized, double-blind, placebo-controlled dose-finding trial. *Anesth Analg*. 2012;115:1336–1342.

5. ANSWER: E

Labor pain is a complex, subjective, multifactorial, dynamic entity that is influenced by a number of physical, emotional, and psychosocial factors. There is considerable variability in the rated intensity of pain during labor. Women who have not experienced childbirth previously (nulliparous) are more likely to rate labor pain as being severe than are women who have delivered previously (multiparous), although this difference is minor and may not be clinically relevant.

Cervical distension is the primary cause of pain during the first stage of labor. The likelihood of severe pain increases as labor progresses, and this is closely associated with the degree of cervical dilation. This correlation implies the existence of a causal relationship between cervical dilation and pain severity. The majority of women will report severe pain during the latter part of the first stage of labor. This increases the likelihood that a woman will request analgesic intervention as labor progresses.

KEY FACTS

- There is a large amount of interindividual variability when rating the severity of labor pain.
- The likelihood of severe pain increases as labor progresses, and this is linked to cervical dilation.

FURTHER READING

Pan P, Eisenach J. The pain of childbirth and its effect on the mother and the fetus. In: Chestnut DH, Wong CA, Tsen LC, et al. (Eds.), *Chestnut's Obstetric Anesthesia*. 5th ed. Philadelphia, PA: Saunders; 2014.

6. ANSWER: E

After controlling for confounding factors, a literature review and large cohort study by Lowwenberg-Weisband et al. showed that epidural analgesia was not associated with severe perineal tears. In contrast, many speculate that epidural analgesia allows for patient comfort and timely repair of perineal tears when they do occur, limiting morbidity in these cases.

Epidural analgesia has variable effects on the progress of labor. It does not have a consistent impact on the first stage of labor, with some evidence that it may shorten this time period compared to systemic analgesia. There is evidence that epidural analgesia prolongs the second stage of labor by approximately 45 minutes on average, but this is also variable. Although epidural analgesia is associated with higher rates of instrumented vaginal delivery, it has not been shown to increase the rate of cesarean delivery performance.

KEY FACTS

- Epidural analgesia is associated with increased rates of instrumented vaginal delivery, but it does not increase the risk for cesarean delivery.
- Epidural analgesia has a variable impact on the length of labor, but it consistently prolongs the second stage of labor.
- Epidural analgesia is not associated with higher rates of severe perineal tears.

Cambic CR, Wong CA. Labour analgesic and obstetric outcomes. *Br J Anaesth*. 2010;105:i50–i60.

Cheng YW, Shaffer BL, Nicholson JM, et al. Second stage of labor and epidural use: A larger effect than previously suggested. *Obstet Gynecol*. 2014;123:527–535.

Loewenberg-Weisband Y, Grisaru-Granovsky S, Loscovich A, et al. Epidural analgesia and severe perineal tears: A literature review and large cohort study. *J Matern Fetal Neonatal Med*. 2014;27:1864–1869.

Wong CA, Scavone BM, Peaceman AM, et al. The risk of cesarean delivery in neuraxial analgesia given early versus late in labor. *N Engl J Med*. 2005;352:655–665.

7. ANSWER: C

Labor pain has a number of physiologic effects on the mother. Neural input from ascending spinal tracts leads to increased oxytocin release from the pituitary (Ferguson's reflex). It is controversial as to whether or not neuraxial analgesia interferes with plasma oxytocin concentrations and the progress of labor. Labor pain leads to increased sympathetic nervous system activity, resulting in higher plasma catecholamine concentrations, particularly norepinephrine and epinephrine. This can increase maternal cardiac output and peripheral vascular resistance. Effective neuraxial analgesia significantly reduces maternal catecholamine concentrations. Labor pain stimulates the respiratory system, leading to periods of intermittent hyperventilation and an overall increase in minute ventilation. Periods of compensatory hypoventilation can be seen between uterine contractions.

Labor pain, along with anxiety and stress, leads to an increase in the release of gastrin and an inhibition of gastrointestinal and urinary motility. The recumbent position and exogenous medication (e.g., opioids) can further decrease gastric motility. These changes theoretically increase the risk of pulmonary aspiration of gastric contents for laboring women.

KEY FACT

- Labor pain activates the sympathetic nervous system, leading to cardiovascular (increased cardiac output), respiratory (increased minute ventilation), and gastrointestinal (reduced motility) effects.

FURTHER READING

Pan P, Eisenach J. The pain of childbirth and its effect on the mother and the fetus. In: Chestnut DH, Wong CA, Tsen LC, et al. (Eds.), *Chestnut's Obstetric Anesthesia*. 5th ed. Philadelphia, PA: Saunders; 2014.

8. ANSWER: C

Postdural puncture headache is the most common risk after labor neuraxial block performance, with an incidence of 1% or 2% after labor epidurals performed at teaching hospitals. A number of factors increase the risk for developing a postdural puncture headache, including increasing needle size, cutting bevel needle designs, vaginal delivery, younger patient age, and block performance by inexperienced (trainee) anesthesia providers. Large studies have failed to show a significant difference in headache incidence between combined spinal–epidural blocks and epidural blocks. Similarly, no study has shown a difference in headache incidence between loss-of-resistance to air and loss-of-resistance to saline techniques, provided anesthesiologists are allowed to use the technique with which they are most comfortable.

Classically, postdural puncture headaches are experienced in the frontal and/or occipital regions, develop 24–48 hours after the dural puncture, and often very debilitating. They are positional in nature, worsening in the upright position and nearly completely relieved by lying down. They may be associated with nausea, vomiting, neck stiffness, altered hearing, and visual disturbances such as photophobia. Rare associated complications can include cranial nerve palsies and subdural hemorrhage. The majority start within 48 hours of the dural puncture occurrence, although some can present a number of days later.

KEY FACTS

- Postdural puncture headaches are the most common complication following epidural placement in a laboring patient (1% or 2% incidence).
- Most postdural puncture headaches manifest within 48 hours of dural puncture.

FURTHER READING

Hendricks M, Stocks GM. Post-dural puncture headache in the parturient. *Anaesth Intens Care Med*. 2007;8:309–311.

Turnbull DK, Shepard DB. Post-dural puncture headache: Pathogenesis, prevention and treatment. *Br J Anaesth*. 2003;91:718–729.

9. ANSWER: E

Pain during the first stage of labor primarily results from uterine contractions causing physical changes in the cervix and lower uterine segment. However, during the late first stage and the second stage of labor, the pattern of pain changes. Distention of the perineum, vagina, and pelvic floor structures creates a different pain pathway. This pelvic pain is transmitted by somatic nerve fibers that enter the spinal cord at the S2–S4 segments. In addition, visceral pain from uterine contractions is still present.

Unlike first-stage labor pain, which is primarily visceral in origin, second-stage labor pain cannot be treated effectively by neuraxial opioids alone. The somatic pain from the lower sacral nerve roots requires the action of local anesthetics for effective analgesia. Successful analgesia for cesarean delivery also requires effective treatment of both visceral and somatic pain, but a much higher dermatomal level (T4) is needed compared to that for labor analgesia.

KEY FACTS

- Late first-stage and second-stage labor pain is transmitted by somatic nerve fibers that enter the spinal cord at the S2–S4 segments.
- Neuraxial local anesthetics are effective in treating second-stage somatic labor pain.

FURTHER READING

Hawkins JL. Epidural analgesia for labor and delivery. *N Engl J Med.* 2010;362:1503–1510.

Naveen N, Wong CA. Spinal, epidural, and caudal anesthesia: Anatomy, physiology, and technique. In: Chestnut DH, Wong CA, Tsen LC, et al. (Eds.), *Chestnut's Obstetric Anesthesia.* 5th ed. Philadelphia, PA: Saunders; 2014.

10. ANSWER: E

The use of combined spinal–epidural (CSE) techniques became popular in the 1990s as an alternative technique for labor analgesia due to perceived benefit of more rapid onset of analgesia and potential for decreased motor blockade compared to traditional epidural techniques. However, differences in procedure-related adverse effects for CSE and epidural techniques have been debated.

Women who receive CSE labor analgesia are more likely to experience generalized, transient pruritus secondary to intrathecal opiate administration. In addition, the incidence of fetal bradycardia is significantly increased (relative risk = 1.81) among women who receive intrathecal opiates compared to women who do not. Despite the increased risk for spinal opiate-related pruritus and fetal bradycardia, there is no significant difference in meningitis or postdural puncture headache that might be expected from the dural puncture of a CSE compared to an epidural-only technique.

KEY FACTS

- The risk for pruritus and fetal bradycardia is greater among women who receive intrathecal opiates as part of a CSE compared to women who receive epidural analgesia alone.

- There is no difference in the risk for meningitis or postdural puncture headache between CSE and epidural techniques.

FURTHER READING

Mardirosoff C, Dumont L, Boulvain M, et al. Fetal bradycardia due to intrathecal opioids for labour analgesia: A systematic review. *BJOG.* 2002;109:274–281.

Niesen AD, Jacob AK. Combined spinal–epidural versus epidural analgesia for labor and delivery. *Clin Perinatol.* 2013;40(3):373–384.

11. ANSWER: B

Pain during the late first stage and second stage of labor is primarily transmitted by somatic nerve fibers that enter the spinal cord at the S2–S4 segments. It is common for patients to report increased pelvic pain despite a functional epidural that is producing an apparently adequate dermatomal level of analgesia. The sacral nerve roots are relatively large and may require a relatively higher concentration of local anesthetic to adequately anesthetize. Breakthrough pelvic pain in the second stage of labor has been termed "sacral sparing." This sacral sparing phenomenon has led some anesthesiologists to prefer a CSE technique when delivery is imminent.

Paracervical blocks have questionable efficacy for first-stage labor pain and are rarely performed for this indication. They would have minimal benefit for a woman with significant sacral pain in the second stage of labor. Although a 100 μg bolus of epidural fentanyl would provide analgesia (mainly visceral analgesia), the patient in this case would most benefit from 0.25% bupivacaine (a higher concentration relative to that of typical labor epidural infusions). Combining the 0.25% bupivacaine bolus with epidural fentanyl may work synergistically. Moderate increases in the rate of epidural infusions can be an effective strategy to manage first-stage labor pain with inadequate dermatomal coverage, but they would be unlikely to provide significant pain relief in this case.

KEY FACTS

- Breakthrough pelvic pain in the second stage of labor ("sacral sparing") is most effectively treated by increased concentration of local anesthetics.

FURTHER READING

Arendt K, Segal S. Why epidurals do not always work. *Obstet Gynecol.* 2008;1:49–55.

12. ANSWER: D

Although methadone has been used since the 1960s, in 2012 the American College of Obstetricians and Gynecologists concluded that the available evidence supported the use of buprenorphine as a first-line medication for pregnant opioid-dependent women who are new to treatment. To date, comparative data of these agents on maternal and fetal outcomes have been limited to a few observational and randomized controlled studies.

Other than a lower incidence of treatment retention among women treated with buprenorphine compared to methadone, there are no apparent differences in maternal outcomes between these opiate agonists (including overall medical complications, fetal presentation, or mode of delivery). Methadone and buprenorphine both cross the placenta, and fetuses exposed to methadone exhibit greater motor activity suppression as well as greater suppression of fetal heart rate and fetal heart rate reactivity during nonstress testing compared to buprenorphine-exposed fetuses.

Regarding neonatal outcomes, no significant differences have been demonstrated in abnormal fetal/birth outcomes, birth weight, length, or head circumference between the two medications. Although NAS may develop after exposure to either medication, NAS after methadone may be more severe and require treatment with larger doses of opioids compared to NAS after buprenorphine exposure.

KEY FACTS

- Methadone and buprenorphine are both considered first-line treatments for pregnant opioid-dependent women.
- Other than a larger proportion of women stopping treatment with buprenorphine compared to methadone, maternal outcomes are similar.
- Fetuses exposed to methadone are generally less reactive during nonstress testing and biophysical profile testing.
- Neonatal outcomes are generally similar except for more severe NAS among methadone-exposed newborns.

FURTHER READING

Jones HE, Heil SH, Baewert A, et al. Buprenorphine treatment of opioid-dependent pregnant women: A comprehensive review. *Addiction*. 2012;107:5–27.

Mozurkewich EL, Rayburn WF. Buprenorphine and methadone for opioid addiction during pregnancy. *Obstet Gynecol Clin*. 2014;41(2):241–253.

13. ANSWER: A

Many factors affect the distribution and movement of opioids within the central nervous system. The major portion of epidural opioids is absorbed by blood vessels or dissolved in epidural fat. Of the opioid that does enter the CSF, a small fraction of molecules bind to and activate opioid receptors. Whereas lipophilic opioids quickly leave the CSF and penetrate into spinal tissue, hydrophilic opioids largely remain sequestered in CSF and are slowly transported rostrally. This accumulation in CSF allows gradual spinal uptake, larger dermatomal spread, and a longer duration of effect.

Opioid dose, volume of injectate, and degree of ionization also affect analgesia onset, dermatomal spread, and activity duration. However, it is the degree of lipid solubility that is the key determining factor. Opioids with high lipid solubility (e.g., sufentanil) have a quick onset of action. Opioids with low lipid solubility (e.g., morphine) are not as rapidly absorbed and remain in the CSF and spinal tissues for a longer time and exhibit greater dermatomal spread.

KEY FACTS

- Lipid solubility is the opioid property that largely dictates onset of analgesia, degree of dermatomal spread, and duration of activity.
- Opioids with low lipid solubility exhibit larger degrees of dermatomal spread and longer duration of activity.
- Opioids with high lipid solubility exhibit quicker onset of analgesia.

FURTHER READING

Carvalho B, Butwick A. Postoperative analgesia: Epidural and spinal techniques. In: Chestnut DH, Wong CA, Tsen LC, et al. (Eds.), *Chestnut's Obstetric Anesthesia*. 5th ed. Philadelphia, PA: Saunders; 2014.

Dahl JB, Jeppesen IS, Jorgensen H, et al. Intraoperative and postoperative analgesic efficacy and adverse effects of intrathecal opioids in patients undergoing cesarean section with spinal anesthesia. *Anesthesiology*. 1999;91:1919–1927.

14. ANSWER: B

Although the diagnosis of postdural puncture headache (PDPH) is usually clear from history and physical examination, more serious neurologic problems may present as what appears to be a PDPH. The differential diagnosis of a severe postpartum headache can include migraine, cortical vein thrombosis, subarachnoid hemorrhage, subdural hematoma, and meningitis. Indications for further workup (e.g., CT scan and MRI) of the headache include focal neurologic signs, seizures, altered consciousness, fever, and lack of other explainable causes. The woman described in this question is displaying classic signs and symptoms of a PDPH.

Epidural blood patches are the gold standard for PDPH. The parturient with a PDPH should be actively managed with scheduled analgesics. Although so-called "conservative" management (e.g., rest, hydration, social support, acetaminophen, and NSAIDs) often makes symptoms manageable until the headache resolves, this patient has failed such management and an epidural blood patch is the next appropriate treatment step. In some cases of PDPH, it may be prudent to proceed directly to epidural blood patch. Some studies have shown that caffeine (oral or intravenous) can diminish the severity of PDPH, but its effect is largely transient and minor. It is most effective in patients who usually ingest large amounts of caffeine and have been unable to do so due to their pregnancy.

KEY FACTS

• Epidural blood patches are the gold standard treatment for PDPH.
• Although it is acceptable to proceed directly to epidural blood patch in cases of PDPH, initial therapy usually consists of psychological support, oral analgesics, and rest.

FURTHER READING

Boonmak P, Boonmak S. Epidural blood patching for preventing and treating post-dural puncture headache. *Cochrane Database Syst Rev.* 2010;CD001791.
Camann WR, Murray RS, Mushlin PS, et al. Effects of oral caffeine on postdural puncture headache: A double-blind, placebo-controlled trial. *Anesth Analg.* 1990;70:181–184.
Hendricks M, Stocks GM. Post-dural puncture headache in the parturient. *Anaesth Intens Care Med.* 2007;8:309–311.

15. ANSWER: D

Parturients experiencing chronic pain can be difficult to manage during labor and in the postpartum period. Often, women with preexisting pain syndromes can display significant anxiety in regard to labor pain. Regardless of etiology, anxiety itself is a predictor of labor pain. Higher levels of anxiety are associated with higher levels of pain during labor.

Women who abuse illegal drugs are more likely to have poorly controlled labor pain and postpartum pain compared to those who do not. Buprenorphine and methadone are common medications that pregnant patients use to treat opioid addiction. Although infants of these mothers may experience symptoms of opioid withdrawal, they do not experience significant respiratory depression. In the event of cesarean delivery, these women receive analgesic benefits of long-acting neuraxial opioids and of postpartum nonsteroidal drug therapy.

KEY FACTS

• Patient anxiety level is a predictor of the degree of labor pain women experience.
• Patients with chronic pain syndromes should be maintained on their normal analgesic regimen throughout the peripartum period. Additional mediation will likely be necessary to treat postpartum pain, especially in the event of cesarean delivery.

FURTHER READING

Bell J, Harvey-Dodds L. Pregnancy and injecting drug use. *Br Med J.* 2008;336:1303–1305.
Jones HE, Finnegan LP, Kaltenbach K. Methadone and buprenorphine for the management of opioid dependence in pregnancy. *Drugs.* 2012;72:747–757.
Lang AJ, Sorrell JT, Rodgers CS, et al. Anxiety sensitivity as a predictor of labor pain. *Eur J Pain.* 2006;10:263–270.

16. ANSWER: B

There are several anesthetic implications of physiologic changes that occur during pregnancy. In general, pregnant women require lower doses of anesthetic drugs (volatile, intravenous, and local anesthetics) compared to a nonpregnant state. When specifically evaluating spinal anesthesia, pregnant women exhibit a more rapid onset and a longer duration of spinal anesthesia compared to nonpregnant women receiving the same dose of local anesthetic. This is due to a combination of factors, including (but not limited to) a reduction in CSF volume and an increased neural sensitivity to local anesthetics. The increased sensitivity to local anesthetics may occur by direct action on the nerve tissue, by indirect action through hormone effects, or a combination of the two.

Although one should always be cognizant of the amount of local anesthetic used and should administer epidural local anesthetics in fractionated doses after a test dose, there is not consistent evidence that pregnancy itself increases the risk of cardiac toxicity of bupivacaine. Chloroprocaine is rapidly hydrolyzed by plasma pseudocholinesterase and has not been found to cause significant ion trapping in the fetus, even when fetal acidosis or prematurity is present.

KEY FACTS

• Compared to nonpregnant women, parturients experience a more rapid onset and longer duration of spinal anesthesia at the same dose of local anesthetic.
• Parturients have a reduced CSF volume compared to their nonpregnant state.

- There is not convincing evidence that pregnant women are more susceptible to the cardiotoxic effects of bupivacaine.

FURTHER READING

Datta S, Lamber DH, Gregus J, et al. Differential sensitivities of mammalian nerve fibers during pregnancy. *Anesth Analg.* 1983;62:107–112.

Gaiser R. Physiologic changes of pregnancy. In: Chestnut DH, Wong CA, Tsen LC, et al. (Eds.), *Chestnut's Obstetric Anesthesia.* 5th ed. Philadelphia, PA: Saunders; 2014.

17. ANSWER: A

Epidural fentanyl is used frequently to provide labor analgesia, in both continuous infusions and bolus doses. Fentanyl administered in the epidural space is more than three times as potent as when administered intravenously. The increase in potency is due to a predominantly spinal mechanism of action for epidural fentanyl. The presence of local anesthetics may enhance the spinal analgesic effect in a synergistic interaction. In addition to this spinal effect, epidurally administered fentanyl also produces analgesia via systemic redistribution to the brain. In a study evaluating heat pain tolerance thresholds, a dose of 100 μg epidural fentanyl produced analgesia to heat stimulation, but a 50-μg dose and a placebo did not. The patient would be expected to have more analgesic benefit from epidural administration of 100 μg than 50 μg. Often, epidural fentanyl is administered in conjunction with a local anesthetic (e.g., 0.25% bupivacaine) to enhance the benefits of each medication.

KEY FACTS

- For abdominal pain, fentanyl is more potent when administered epidurally than intravenously, reflecting a significant spinal mechanism of action for epidural fentanyl.
- This analgesia is enhanced by the presence of local anesthetics, and bolus doses of 100 μg are more efficacious than doses of 50 μg.

FURTHER READING

Eichenberger U, Giani C, Petersen-Felix S, et al. Lumbar epidural fentanyl: Segmental spread and effect on temporal summation and muscle pain. *Br J Anaesth.* 2003;90:467–473.

Ginosar Y, Columb MO, Cohen SE, et al. The site of action of epidural fentanyl infusions in the presence of local anesthetics: A minimum local analgesic concentration infusion study in nulliparous labor. *Anesth Analg.* 2003;97:1439–1445.

18. ANSWER: C

CSE analgesia produces a faster onset of labor analgesia than epidural techniques. CSE analgesia can be accomplished by administering intrathecal local anesthetic, opioid, or the two in combination. Opioids (typically fentanyl or sufentanil) in the intrathecal space are very effective in relieving visceral pain associated with uterine contractions and cervical dilation. Typical doses are 10–25 μg for fentanyl and 5–10 μg for sufentanil.

Intrathecal fentanyl is associated with possible side effects. The most common of these is pruritus. The incidence of pruritus after 25 μg of intrathecal fentanyl has been reported to be as high as 90–100%. Although controversial, a number of studies have shown an increased incidence of fetal bradycardia after the administration of intrathecal fentanyl or sufentanil for labor analgesia. Headache is rare after CSE analgesia, with approximately a 1% or 2% incidence. Sedation is an uncommon side effect after normal intrathecal doses of lipophilic opioids. In the absence of patient allergy, intrathecal opioids very rarely cause hives.

KEY FACT

- The most common side effect of intrathecal fentanyl is pruritus, and the severity is dose dependent.

FURTHER READING

Dahl JB, Jeppesen IS, Jorgensen H, et al. Intraoperative and postoperative analgesic efficacy and adverse effects of intrathecal opioids in patients undergoing cesarean section with spinal anesthesia: A qualitative and quantitative systematic review of randomized controlled trials. *Anesthesiology.* 1999;98:1919–1927.

Simmons SW, Taghizadeh N, Dennis AT, et al. Combined spinal–epidural versus epidural analgesia in labour. *Cochrane Database Syst Rev.* 2012:CD003401.

Wells J, Paech MJ, Evans SF. Intrathecal fentanyl-induced pruritus during labour: The effect of prophylactic ondansetron. *Int J Obstet Anesth.* 2004;13:35–39.

19. ANSWER: D

Methadone has been used for decades for treatment of opioid dependency during pregnancy. In general, pregnant women who are physiologically dependent on heroin or other opioids are potential candidates for methadone treatment. Perinatal methadone substitution treatment provides numerous maternal, obstetrical, and neonatal benefits, including (but not limited to) reduction in illegal opiate use and high-risk behavior to obtain opiates, fluctuation in maternal drug level, greater likelihood that the mother will seek prenatal care, more stable intrauterine environment, lower risk of preeclampsia, and closer monitoring of fetal and maternal well-being. It is generally recommended that opiate-dependent and opiate-addicted mothers not undergo detoxification during pregnancy.

If started or maintained on methadone, it is important to note that normal pregnancy-related physiologic changes will result in significant changes in methadone pharmacokinetics as the pregnancy progresses. The half-life of methadone will decrease from an average of 22–24 hours in nonpregnant women to as low as 8 hours in pregnant women, potentially requiring escalating doses over the course of the pregnancy. Peripartum management should not deviate significantly from that of non-opioid-dependent patients. Other than opioid tolerance, pain control during labor and postpartum in opioid-dependent pregnant women should be similar to that in non-substance abusing women. Assuming no other contraindications, women on methadone would be candidates for regional anesthesia techniques during labor and delivery.

Neonatal effects associated with chronic methadone use include premature delivery, low birth weight, microcephaly, jaundice, thrombocytosis, arrhythmias including prolonged QTc interval, and NAS. There is also growing concern about the effects of methadone on the developing eyes, including reduced visual acuity, nystagmus, strabismus, delayed visual maturation, and cerebral impairment.

KEY FACTS

- Methadone is commonly used to treat opiate-dependent women during pregnancy, and it may have significant maternal and fetal benefits compared to continuing short-acting or illicit opiate use.
- Peripartum management of women on chronic methadone should not be significantly different from that of non-opiate-dependent women.
- Several adverse effects have been described in infants born to mothers using methadone, including prematurity, low birth weight, abnormal visual development, and NAS.

FURTHER READING

Jones HE, Finnegan LP, Kaltenbach K. Methadone and buprenorphine for the management of opioid dependence in pregnancy. *Drugs.* 2012;72(6):747–757.

Mozurkewich EL, Rayburn WF. Buprenorphine and methadone for opioid addiction during pregnancy. *Obstet Gynecol Clin.* 2014;41(2):241–253.

20. ANSWER: E

Despite its association with significant pain, not every woman in labor desires or needs pharmacologic pain relief and/or neuraxial analgesic techniques. Many alternative methods of labor analgesia are used throughout the United States. There is scientific evidence to support the pain-relieving benefits of techniques such as hydrotherapy, hypnosis, acupuncture, acupressure, and the injection of sterile water papules. Specifically, sterile water papules are often effective at treating severe back pain or "back labor," which can sometimes be difficult to manage effectively with epidural analgesia. There is no association between acupuncture during labor and fetal bradycardia or rates of cesarean delivery. One of the most effective nonpharmacologic methods of labor analgesia may be the presence of a person (e.g., husband, friend, and doula) who can provide emotional and physical support, advice, and decrease levels of anxiety.

One of the most appealing aspects about nonpharmacologic methods is that nearly all of them are entirely compatible with receiving epidural analgesia. They do not need to be mutually exclusive, and women can often experience the benefits of both. Physicians should be aware of the nonpharmacologic methods used to treat labor pain so that they can accurately discuss options and provide guidance to patients.

KEY FACTS

- There is some scientific evidence to support the analgesic efficacy of hypnosis, acupressure, acupuncture, hydrotherapy, and sterile water injections in the treatment of labor pain.
- Virtually all nonpharmacologic analgesic techniques can be used in conjunction with neuraxial analgesia during labor.

FURTHER READING

Arendt KW, Camann W. Alternative (non-pharmacologic) methods of labor analgesia. In: Suresh M et al. (Eds.), *Shnider and Levinson's Anesthesia for Obstetrics.* 5th ed. Philadelphia, PA: Lippincott Williams & Wilkins; 2013.

Hodnett ED, Gates S, Hofmeyr GJ, et al. Continuous support for women during childbirth. *Cochrane Database Syst Rev.* 2011:CD003766.

21. ANSWER: A

Pain thresholds are increased during pregnancy and labor. This is largely the result of an increase in circulating β-endorphins and activated spinal cord κ opioid receptors. Circulating progesterone may also play a mechanistic role in elevating the pain threshold. Increased endorphin and enkephalins levels are found in the plasma and CSF of pregnant patients.

Factors such as weight gain, posture and hormone changes, and increased stress tend to worsen back pain in pregnant patients with preexisting back pain. Cerebral blood flow increases during pregnancy, and this does not have an appreciable effect on opioid receptor activation.

- Higher levels of circulating β-endorphins contribute to increased pain thresholds during pregnancy and labor.

FURTHER READING

Cogan R, Spinnato JA. Pain and discomfort thresholds in late pregnancy. *Pain*. 1986;27:63–68.

Ohel I, Walfisch A, Shitenberg D, et al. A rise in pain threshold during labor; A prospective clinical trial. *Pain*. 2007;132:S104–108.

22. ANSWER: B

Remifentanil is a short-acting opioid with rapid onset of action and rapid metabolism by plasma and tissue esterases. Its context-sensitive half-life of approximately 3.5 minutes is independent of the duration of infusion. Its quick onset and elimination have made it appealing for use as an intravenous route for labor anesthesia. When used for labor analgesia, a patient-controlled intravenous analgesia (PCIA) technique is used, with or without a continuous background infusion.

Although the analgesic efficacy of remifentanil has been clearly demonstrated, it is not equivalent to neuraxial blockade. Compared to parturients employing epidural analgesia, those using remifentanil PCIA report higher pain scores throughout labor. Although nausea is rarely a significant side effect, patients using remifentanil PCIA demonstrate increased drowsiness and lower oxygen saturations compared to patients using epidural analgesia. To date, studies have reported a good maternal and neonatal safety profile, but the potential for adverse events warrants close supervision and continuous monitoring for parturients using remifentanil for labor analgesia.

KEY FACTS

- The analgesic efficacy of intravenous remifentanil is less than that of neuraxial blockade.
- Recent studies have shown intravenous remifentanil to have a good safety profile for both mothers and neonates, but careful monitoring and continuous supervision of women using remifentanil for labor analgesia are strongly recommended.

FURTHER READING

Douma MR, Middeldrop JM, Verwey RA, et al. A randomized comparison of intravenous remifentanil patient-controlled analgesia with epidural ropivacaine/sufentanil during labour. *Int J Obstet Anesth*. 2011;20:118–123.

Liu ZQ, Chen XB, Li HB, et al. A comparison of remifentanil parturient-controlled intravenous analgesia with epidural analgesia: A meta-analysis of randomized controlled trials. *Anesth Analg*. 118:598–603.

Schnabel A, Hahn N, Broscheit A, et al. Remifentanil for labour analgesia: A meta-analysis of randomized controlled trials. *Eur J Anaesthesiol*. 2012;29:177–185.

Wilson SJ, Fernando R. Systemic and inhalational agents for labor analgesia. In: Suresh M et al. (Eds.), *Shnider and Levinson's Anesthesia for Obstetrics*. 5th ed. Philadelphia, PA: Lippincott Williams & Wilkins; 2013.

23. ANSWER: D

The reported incidence of chronic pain after childbirth varies widely due to differences in its definition. Some reports include all types of chronic pain, whereas others strictly delineate new pain after delivery from preexisting pain. Recent studies have shown that the incidence of chronic pain after childbirth is lower than previously thought. When focusing on *new-onset* (as opposed to preexisting) pelvic/abdominal/perineal pain, the incidence is less than 1% at 1 year after delivery. This incidence is approximately 10% at 2 months after delivery and decreases as time progresses. There is conflicting evidence regarding whether or not cesarean delivery is associated with higher rates of chronic pain compared to vaginal delivery. The degree of acute pain immediately after delivery likely influences the incidence of chronic pain. The use of gabapentin at the time of cesarean delivery has not been shown to decrease the severity or incidence of acute or chronic pain.

Emerging evidence suggests that chronic pain after childbirth is more rare than would be expected from the degree of physical trauma. The incidence of chronic pain after cesarean delivery is significantly less than that observed after similar abdominal procedures such as abdominal hysterectomies in nonpregnant women. Although not proven, the low incidence of new chronic pain after childbirth points toward a potential protective effect of pregnancy and/or delivery on the response to physical injury.

KEY FACTS

- The incidence of new-onset pain from delivery is less than 1% at 12 months after childbirth.
- The incidence of chronic pain after childbirth is lower than that after general surgery.

FURTHER READING

Eisenach JC, Pan P, Smiley R, et al. Resolution of pain after childbirth. *Anesthesiology*. 2013;118:143–151.

Flood P, Wong CA. Chronic pain secondary to childbirth. *Anesthesiology*. 2013;118:16–18.

Lavand'homme P. Postcesarean analgesia: Effective strategies and association with chronic pain. *Curr Opin Anaesthesiol.* 2006;19:244–248.

Short J, Downey K, Bernstein P, et al. A single preoperative dose of gabapentin does not improve postcesarean delivery pain management: A randomized, double-blind, placebo-controlled dose-finding trial. *Anesth Analg.* 2012;115:1336–1342.

24. ANSWER: E

Although most recover from the process of labor and delivery without any significant impact to their health, some develop persistent postpartum pain. In a study of more than 1000 patients, Eisenach et al. tested whether mode of delivery had an independent role in persistent pain and depression at 8 weeks postpartum. They found that although mode of delivery (cesarean vs. vaginal) was not related to the risk for persistent pain or depression, the severity of acute postpartum pain was related to this risk. Women with severe acute postpartum pain had nearly a threefold increased risk for persistent pain and depression compared to those with mild acute postpartum pain. The authors suggested that persistent pain may not be related to degrees of physical tissue trauma but, rather, may be related to an individual's pain response to that injury.

Although there is evidence that induction of labor is associated with higher degrees of labor pain compared to spontaneous labor, neither have been associated with a higher incidence of persistent postpartum pain. Similarly, the use of postoperative nalbuphine, dose of intrathecal morphine, or indication for cesarean delivery have not been shown to increase the risk of persistent or chronic pain.

KEY FACTS

- The severity of postpartum pain is independently related to the risk for persistent pain and depression when measured 8 weeks postpartum.
- Although there is conflicting evidence, mode of delivery does not appear to be an independent risk factor for the development of persistent pain after delivery.

FURTHER READING

Eisenach JC, Pan PH, Smiley RM, et al. Severity of acute pain after childbirth, but not type of delivery, predicts persistent pain and postpartum depression. *Pain.* 2008;140:87–94.

25. ANSWER B

Epidural and CSE techniques are both safe, effective methods of analgesia in the laboring patient. There appears to be no difference between epidural and CSE techniques for progress of labor or instrumented or cesarean delivery. CSE exhibits a significantly more rapid onset of analgesia. Despite a shorter time to onset of effective analgesia and greater initial mobility, there is no apparent difference in overall satisfaction between CSE and low-dose epidural techniques. Catheters placed using a plain epidural technique appear to have a greater failure rate for labor analgesia but similar intervention rates for rescue analgesia and similar failure rates for conversion to anesthesia for cesarean delivery.

KEY FACTS

- CSE produces more rapid onset of effective analgesia compared to plain epidural.
- Catheters placed using a plain epidural technique versus CSE have a greater failure rate for labor analgesia but similar failure rates for conversion to anesthesia for cesarean delivery.

FURTHER READING

Niesen AD, Jacob AK. Combined spinal–epidural versus epidural analgesia for labor and delivery. *Clin Perinatol.* 2013;40(3):373–384.

Simmons SW, Taghizadeh N, Dennis AT, et al. Combined spinal–epidural versus epidural analgesia in labour. *Cochrane Database Syst Rev.* 2012;10:CD003401.

26. ANSWER: D

Inhaled nitrous oxide (typically a blend of 50% nitrous oxide and 50% oxygen or air) for labor pain management has been used for decades in several European countries as well as Australia, New Zealand, and Canada, in part due to lack of availability of epidural labor analgesia. However, its use in the United States has been limited to a few medical centers. It is usually self-administered via a facemask or mouthpiece intermittently, with inhalation beginning approximately 30 seconds before each contraction in order for the analgesic efficacy to peak (up to 50 seconds) at the time of contraction. The safety of the technique is that the parturient will be unable to hold the mask if she becomes too drowsy and thus will cease to inhale the anesthetic.

The exact mechanism of analgesia is unclear, but it is likely due to transient release of endogenous opioids and NMDA receptor inhibition. The degree of pain relief is variable, but it is generally less effective than with neuraxial analgesia. Reported side effects are nausea, vomiting, dizziness, and drowsiness, with nausea and dizziness being the most common. Although animal studies have demonstrated an association between nitrous oxide exposure and neurodegeneration, no human studies have suggested this association and nitrous oxide use in countries such as the United Kingdom has a record of safe outcomes for both mother and child.

KEY FACTS

- The analgesic efficacy of inhaled nitrous oxide in labor is variable, but it is less effective than traditional neuraxial techniques.
- There is no known safety risk to fetuses in women who use nitrous oxide for labor analgesia.

FURTHER READING

Collins MR, Starr SA, Bishop JT, et al. Nitrous oxide for labor analgesia: Expanding analgesic options for women in the United States. *Rev Obstet Gynecol*. 2012;5(3–4):e126–e131.

Klomp T, van Poppel M, Jones L, et al. Inhaled analgesia for pain management in labour. *Cochrane Database Syst Rev*. 2012;9:CD009351.

Likis FE, Andrews JC, Collins MR, et al. Nitrous oxide for the management of labor pain: A systematic review. *Anesth Analg*. 2014;118(1):153–167.

27. ANSWER: A

NAS is a variable, complex, and incompletely understood spectrum of neonatal signs and symptoms resulting from sudden cessation of drug exposure after interruption of the fetoplacental circulation at time of delivery. Most commonly, NAS results from opioid withdrawal, but it can also result from cessation of numerous other sedative–hypnotic and antidepressant drugs. With the growing problem of opioid abuse in the United States, the incidence of NAS has increased during the past decade from 1.2 to 5.8 cases per 1000 hospital births per year. The incidence of NAS requiring treatment ranges from 42% to 94% among infants with chronic prenatal exposure to opioids.

NAS is more likely to develop among term infants of normal birth weight born to mothers with polysubstance abuse. The onset, duration, and severity of NAS depend on several characteristics of the drug(s) abused by the mother, but typical onset after opioid use is within the first 24–48 hours after delivery, with symptoms lasting up to 30 days. There are numerous scoring systems available to assess the severity of NAS, but the modified Finnegan scoring system is the most common, particularly for opiate withdrawal. Assessment should begin immediately after birth and be performed after feeds, at 3- or 4-hour intervals, when the infant is awake. Nonpharmacologic management may be sufficient for mild withdrawal symptoms, but opioid therapy (typically morphine) is considered first-line treatment if pharmacotherapy is needed.

KEY FACTS

- The incidence of NAS is increasing with the growing abuse of and addiction to opioids in the United States.
- Early and regular newborn assessment for NAS immediately after birth is important to prevent potential life-threatening withdrawal.
- Mild withdrawal symptoms may be treated with nonpharmacologic therapy, but often the infant may require pharmacologic treatment with opioids (or additional medications) to prevent or treat symptoms.

FURTHER READING

Kocherlakota P. Neonatal abstinence syndrome. *Pediatrics*. 2014;134:e547–e561.

Patrick SW, Davis MM, Lehmann CU, et al. Increasing incidence and geographic distribution of neonatal abstinence syndrome: United States 2009 to 2012. *J Perinatol*. 2015;35(8):650–655.

Stanhope TJ, Gill LA, Rose C. Chronic opioid use during pregnancy. *Clin Perinatol*. 2013;40(3):337–350.

28. ANSWER: C

The rate of breast-feeding worldwide has been increasing during the past four decades. The large majority of these women take one or more medications regularly, and analgesic medications (prescription and nonprescription) are among the most frequently used medications in this time period. Because all medications taken by the mother are transferred into breast milk to some degree, some women discontinue breast-feeding for fear of exposing their infant to the medication. Although nearly all medication package inserts suggest discontinuing breast-feeding while taking medication, this is not always the correct decision. Most mothers could easily continue to breast-feed and take the medication without risk to the infant.

The ability of a medication to transfer into breast milk is determined by the physiochemical properties of that drug—mainly the molecular weight, pKa, degree of protein binding, and lipophilicity. The most clinically relevant method for determining the safety of the medication is to relate the weight-normalized dose received by the infant via milk. This is termed the relative infant dose (RID), and it is generally expressed as a percentage of the mother's dose present in the mother's milk. It provides a standardized method of relating the infant's dose to the maternal dose. If the RID is less than 10%, most medications are sufficiently safe to use. The RID of the vast majority of drugs is less than 1%. Ultimately, each situation should be individually evaluated and heed given according to the overall toxicity of the medication and the ability of the infant to handle small amounts of the medication, in addition to the RID.

KEY FACTS

- The RID is the best clinical parameter to use when determining how safe a medication is for a mother to take while breast-feeding.
- If the RID is less than 10%, most medications are safe to use (depending on the potential toxicity or harm of the individual medication).

FURTHER READING

Buhimschi CS, Weiner CP. Medications in pregnancy and lactation: Part 1. Teratology. *Obstet Gynecol*. 2009;113:166–188.

Hale TW, Baker T. Prescribing during lactation. In: Powrie R, Greene M, Camann W (Eds.), *de Swiet's Medical Disorders in Obstetric Practice*. 5th ed. Oxford: Wiley–Blackwell; 2010.

Matheson I, Kristensen K, Lunde PK. Drug utilization in breast-feeding women: A survey in Oslo. *Eur J Clin Pharmacol*. 1990;38:453–459.

22.

HEADACHE

Kurt F. Dittrich

INTRODUCTION

The pain medicine provider is often asked to wear many hats. The scope of knowledge required to treat pain conditions is expansive. Among the more common conditions a pain provider is likely to encounter is chronic headache. Often, patients will have been seen and treated for headaches by a neurologist or perhaps even by a headache specialist prior to presenting to the provider's clinic. However, patients may also present to a pain management expert with new-onset headaches having never seen another provider for this condition. The provider may be asked to assist in managing headache medications or to provide insight into other etiologies for a patient's headache that may be treatable through interventional procedures. Regardless of the complex or simple nature of the patient's headache history, having a solid grasp of headaches is essential for the pain provider. This required knowledge should include understanding the anatomy and physiology of headaches; knowing how to classify headaches using the second edition of the *International Classification of Headache Disorders* (ICHD-2); recognizing the physical, psychological, and social factors that may contribute to headaches; and understanding the role of counseling and nonpharmacological treatment options. It is essential to understand the pharmacological aspects of headache management as well as some of the nuances of the specific medications most often used. A pain provider should be able to recognize when signs and symptoms of a headache warrant further investigation as well as when to offer alternative treatment options to patients. The questions in this chapter are designed to assist in gathering this knowledge base and assist the pain provider in analyzing the headache condition.

QUESTIONS

1. An 82-year-old female with a history of migraine headaches from the age of 22 years until she was 49 years old has been free of chronic headaches for more than 30 years. She presents to your clinic with onset of a throbbing headache on the right side of her head that has been persistent for the past 8 days. She denies any recent falls, is not on any anticoagulants, and when asked, she states her visual analogue pain score (VAS) to be 7/10. Which of the following is the correct course of management?

A. Perform a greater occipital nerve block.
B. Prescribe a short course of opioids and see her in 2 weeks for follow-up.
C. Ask about any unusual changes in vision, appetite, or general well-being before sending her for blood work to include erythrocyte sedimentation rate (ESR) and/or C-reactive protein (CRP) and prescribing a corticosteroid dose pack.
D. Send her to the emergency department immediately for stat head computed tomography (CT).

2. A 32-year-old female presents to your clinic with complaint of unilateral headaches occurring "in waves" throughout the day. She rates them as a 7–8/10 on the VAS scale and states that when they occur, she has the pain behind her left eye and left temple and that her left eye tears. She also has ptosis of that eyelid. When you ask about the "waves" of pain, she states that these occur up to 20 times per day, each lasting between 5 and 30 minutes. Upon further questioning, she denies any other neurologic changes, and she states that this headache condition has little variation throughout the year. She saw a neurologist 2 years ago for these and had a negative brain magnetic resonance imaging (MRI) for any anomalies. Regarding the most likely diagnosis of this type of headache, which of the following statements is true?

A. This patient should be sent to the emergency department via ambulance for further evaluation.
B. Assuming no contraindications, this patient should receive botulinum toxin (Botox A) 25 units for migraine prophylaxis.

C. Assuming no contraindications, this patient should be prescribed indomethacin.
D. Assuming no contraindications, this patient should be prescribed oxygen for home use.
E. The fourth edition of the *International Classification of Headache Disorders* (ICHD-4) lists this headache as a retinal migraine.

3. All of the following regarding medication overuse headache (MOH) are true except:

A. MOH can occur with the use of aspirin, butalbital, narcotics, and triptans.
B. MOH can occur with the use of nonsteroidal anti-inflammatory drugs (NSAIDs), acetaminophen, and aspirin.
C. The mainstay of treatment for MOH is total withdrawal from analgesics for at least several months.
D. The use of migraine prophylactic medications eliminates the possibility of MOH.

4. A 26-year-old female graduate student has been suffering from neck muscle tightness and headaches for the past 4 months while preparing for her dissertation. You have seen her one time before in your office and provided her with trigger point injections in the upper back and neck as well as greater occipital nerve blocks. During her normal headaches, her VAS ranges between 6/10 and 8/10. Her roommate calls your clinic and states that the patient is reporting this headache to be different. She awoke from her sleep and she states that it is the worst headache she has ever had, rating it as a 10/10. She has vomited twice since onset of the headache 3 hours prior. You ask to speak with the patient and upon doing so find her speech to be incomprehensible. Regarding this patient, which of the following is true?

A. You should advise her roommate to give her acetaminophen 2000 mg PO, Phenergan 25 mg PO, a cup of coffee, and place her in a dark room.
B. She needs to be evaluated in the emergency department immediately.
C. Tension-type headaches often present as VAS 10/10, the "worst headache ever."
D. Preparing for her dissertation is stressful; this headache will likely pass once her stress is reduced. As such, there is no need for any additional workup.

5. You are seeing a 67-year-old left-hand-dominant male, known to your clinic for chronic low back pain and a history of occasional bitemporal headaches, treated in the past with acetaminophen. For the past 2 weeks, he has had a persistent left-sided retro-orbital headache with a VAS of 7/10. He had some blurry vision, which he believes has improved; however, the headache has not subsided. In gathering a history from the patient, he states that the onset occurred immediately after returning from his annual hunting trip. On physical exam, you note ptosis of the left eyelid, as well as slight facial droop on the left. He has pain at the ramus of the mandible on the left, and his left pupil is slightly smaller than his right. Strength in his upper extremities is good; however, it is only 4/5 on the right and 5/5 on the left. His wife reports that he has been squinting for the entire 2 weeks, and that during this time, his headache has not changed; it has been unrelenting despite NSAIDs, acetaminophen, sleep, hydration, and use of gabapentin prescribed for his chronic back pain. He was seen briefly by his primary care physician (PCP), who started him on a medrol dose pack, drew a CRP and ESR (both normal), and asked him to follow up with you. Regarding this patient, which of the following is true?

A. Giant cell arteritis/temporal arteritis is a likely culprit and likely responsible for his neurologic signs.
B. "Side-lock" headaches are always benign and eventually resolve on their own without need for further workup or intervention.
C. His hunting trip and use of a high-powered rifle during that trip have no relation to his current headache.
D. He may have a carotid artery dissection and needs additional workup immediately.

6. An 18-year-old male returns home from basic training in the military. He has no past history of any pain complaints nor any significant past medical history. His mother is a headache patient of yours and calls the clinic because her son has had a severe headache for the past 8 hours. He has had fever and chills; she gave him 1000 mg of acetaminophen 2 hours prior and reports his current temperature to be 102.2°F. She is concerned because he does not want to move and he seems slightly confused, periodically responding to her questions with "sir, yes sir" or "sir, no sir" and reciting his Social Security number. He is lying supine on his bed with his knees and hips flexed. She is concerned because every time he attempts to straighten his leg to get up, his neck hurts and headache worsens. He has vomited several times. Regarding this patient, which of the following is not true?

A. Bacterial meningitis is high on the differential diagnosis.
B. Living in close quarters as the patient was doing when in military barracks has an association with *Neisseria meningitides*.

C. This is a serious condition that needs immediate workup in the emergency department.

D. Antibiotics should be delayed until cerebrospinal fluid (CSF) cultures return a specific organism with sensitivities.

7. You are seeing a 58-year-old male with a long history of migraine headaches with aura. His typical aura involves scintillating scotomas that last for 20–25 minutes just prior to the onset of his migraine headaches. For years, he has been effectively treating his migraine headaches with sumatriptan, as abortive agent. He presents to your clinic because his wife is concerned. She states that he has not consumed much water in the past 3 days. He has had a headache for the past 2 weeks, and in addition to his typical visual aura, he is now hemiplegic. Previous migraine attacks have never lasted more than 2 days and have never involved weakness. The patient states that this is just a prolonged migraine attack and wants to go home. Regarding this patient, which of the following is not true?

A. He may be experiencing a "fatal migraine."

B. Cerebral hypoperfusion can occur during the aura phase of a migraine headache with aura.

C. Migraine infarction is more common than previously thought and occurs more frequently in migraine without aura than in migraine headaches with aura.

D. This patient needs further evaluation immediately.

8. Regarding migraine headaches and the pain-generating structures of the head, which of the following statements is not correct?

A. Pain-generating structures involve the basal meninges, venous sinuses, menigeal arteries, large cerebral arteries, skin, muscle, and cranial nerves V, IX, and X.

B. The trigeminovascular system refers to a plexus of largely unmyelinated fibers from cranial nerve V that innervates the cerebral and pial arteries, venous sinuses, and the dura mater.

C. Migraine headache abortive 5-HT receptor agonists include triptans (sumatriptan, etc.) but not ergot alkaloids.

D. Dorsal roots from the upper cervical nerves innervate structures in the posterior fossa.

9. All of the following statements regarding migraine headache are true except:

A. Medication treatment options generally include abortive agents and prophylactic agents.

B. A migraine with aura that involves visual loss, dysarthria, vertigo, ataxia, or tinitus is referred to as a basilar-type migraine.

C. Aura without migraine exists.

D. Migraine with aura is more common than migraine without aura.

10. A 37-year-old male with no family history of migraine headaches presents to your clinic pacing and agitated, stating that he has had a return of headaches occurring in the left temporal, frontal, and periorbital region. He is currently suffering from a headache and, when asked, reports that they usually last between 15 and 90 minutes. He had similar headaches last year during the same month and states that they eventually went away. Although he did not seek medical attention in the past, he is now concerned because they have returned again this year. On physical exam, he has conjunctival injection on the left, as well as lacrimation and nasal stuffiness also on the left side. Regarding the type of headache that this patient is experiencing, which of the following statements is not correct?

A. Alcohol may be a trigger for his headache.

B. Paroxysmal hemicrania has a similar presentation; however, it more often occurs in women, tends to occur more frequently in shorter durations, and nearly always responds well to indomethacin.

C. He could be provided a prescription for home oxygen use.

D. Valproic acid (Depokote) is not beneficial in treating this kind of headache.

11. A 25-year-old female presents to the emergency department after attempting to manage her migraine without aura with a stratified approach including several of her usual doses of sumatriptan. In addition, she has been on prophylactic medications, including a serotonin–norepinephrine reuptake inhibitor (SNRI) as well as topiramate. In the emergency department, she receives intravenous (IV) fluids, IV ketorolac, and prochlorperazine. Thirty minutes later, she reports not "feeling right" and is notably agitated. She is given an additional dose of prochlorperazine; 10 minutes later, she develops tightening of her sternocleidomastoid and her chin is drawn down toward her shoulder. Which of the following statements is true?

A. Treatment for this condition includes the use of diphenhydramine and/or midazolam.

B. A "stratified approach" to migraine management is generally less agreeable to patients than is a "stepwise" approach to management.

C. The term given for the severe muscle contraction of her sternocleidomastoid is akathisia.

D. Her dystonia is likely to take between 5 and 7 days to resolve spontaneously.

12. Which of the following statements best explains how neck pain can be a trigger for an orbital or fronto-temporal parietal headache?

A. The dorsal rami of C4–C8 nerve roots are involved in supplying the posterior fossa, which precipitates dural irritation with a widespread diffuse headache pattern.

B. The trapezius muscle insertion occurs at the temporal region; cervical pain that creates trapezius muscle tension results in temporal insertion site pain.

C. The spinal nucleus of the trigeminal nerve extends caudally to the outer lamina of the upper cervical (C1–C3) spinal nerves. Convergence of trigeminal and cervical afferents in this trigeminocervical nucleus accounts for this cervical–trigeminal pain referral pattern.

D. None of the above.

13. After evaluating a 34-year-old male for neck pain and associated headaches, you decide to schedule him for an atlantoaxial joint injection. Regarding this procedure, which of the following statements is not correct?

A. This procedure carries risk for potential serious complications, including high spinal damage to the C2 dorsal root ganglion and nerve root if local anesthetic is used; needle insertion into the foramen magnum; and vertebral artery dissection.

B. During the procedure, the needle should be directed toward the anterolateral aspect of the joint to avoid injury to the C2 nerve root and the vertebral artery.

C. The lateral atlantoaxial joint may account for up to 16% of patients with occipital headaches.

D. Diagnosis of atlantoaxial joint pain is often difficult to determine by physical exam alone.

14. The following statements regarding the third occipital nerve and third occipital headaches are false except:

A. The third occipital nerve is actually a superficial medial branch of the dorsal ramus of C4.

B. Radiofrequency ablation provides little benefit in targeting this pain.

C. Tenderness of the C3–C4 zygopophyseal joint is diagnostic of third occipital headaches.

D. It is often involved in patients with whiplash injury.

15. You have been seeing a 42-year-old female who was involved in a car accident 5 months prior. She was rear-ended at 40 mph, and her vehicle struck the car ahead of her. She was wearing a seat belt, and her airbag deployed.

She has been complaining of neck pain and headaches that shoot up the posterior aspect of her head. On physical exam, she has tenderness over the region correlating to the C2–C3 zygopophyseal joint as well as tenderness in the suboccipital region. You diagnose her with third occipital neuralgia and schedule her for C2 and C3 medial branch blocks using 2% lidocaine. This procedure provides her with 6 hours of 100% relief followed by a slow gradual return of her pain toward baseline during the next 24 hours. In contemplating performing radiofrequency ablation in targeting her pain, which of the following should be of consideration?

A. The anatomic location of the third occipital nerve is variable, and as a result, the three-needle technique should be used to ensure good results.

B. Patients should be advised of potential associated conditions such as numbness in the cutaneous distribution of the third occipital nerve (area of skin below the occiput), as well as potential for dysesthesia and hypersensitivity.

C. Denervation of the semispinalis capitis muscle may interfere with tonic neck reflexes, with the result being temporary ataxia.

D. All of the above.

16. A patient has been sent to your clinic from the emergency department for consideration of an epidural blood patch under fluoroscopic guidance for presumed postdural puncture headache (PDPH). A lumbar puncture had been performed 5 days prior, and she presented with positional headache for the past 24 hours. Regarding PDPH, all of the following are true except:

A. The patient had a lumbar puncture 5 days ago with positional headache occurring only in the past 24 hours; this could be a PDPH.

B. Symptoms associated with PDPH can include nausea, vomiting, neck stiffness, lower or upper limb pain, auditory changes including tinnitus and hypoacousia, diplopia, scalp paresthesia, and even mental status changes.

C. Lumbar dural punctures result in PDPH less frequently than those that occur in the cervical region.

D. The incidence of PDPH after a lumbar puncture is impacted by size of the needle, the needle orientation, and the type of needle.

17. Regarding postdural puncture headaches, all of the following are true except:

A. There is a higher incidence in men than in women.

B. There is a higher incidence in thin patients.

C. There is a higher incidence during pregnancy.

D. Treating with an epidural blood patch (EBP) earlier than 24 hours after initial dural puncture has an increased risk of treatment failure.

E. All of the above are false.

18. A 33-year-old female was involved in a motor vehicle accident 2 months prior, during which she sustained a whiplash-like injury. She is being sent to your office by a neurology colleague for consideration of an Epidural Blood Patch (EBP). On physical exam, she has postural bilateral occipital headaches, hypoacusia, and tinnitus, all of which improve when she lays recumbent for more than 20 minutes. No lumbar puncture has been performed, and your visiting medical student asks why you would perform an EBP on this patient. Regarding this patient's condition, all of the following are true except:

A. EBP may be effective for spontaneous intracranial hypotension (SIH), although it is possibly less effective than for a PDPH.

B. Her suspected spontaneous intracranial hypotension may be the result of a dural tear from her whiplash injury.

C. A lumbar puncture is contraindicated in SIH.

D. After two EBPs have been performed 4 days apart without any improved long-term benefit, the next options for aiding in the diagnosis of SIH include MRI, radionucleotide cisternography (RC), CT myelography, MR myelography, and radioisotope myelocisternography.

19. Regarding triggers for migraine headaches, which of the following statements is true?

A. Migraine headaches may be triggered by underlying tension-type headaches.

B. Migraine headaches may be triggered by sleep habits, dietary changes, nitrates, tyramine-containing foods, or monosodium glutamate.

C. Migraine headaches may be triggered by oral contraceptives or changes in hormones, including menstruation.

D. Migraine headaches may be triggered by odors or bright sunlight.

E. Migraine headaches may be triggered by stress or depression.

F. All of the above are true.

20. Regarding the relationship between sleep disorders and headaches, which of the following statements is true?

A. Hypnic headache most commonly has an onset after age 50 years, with women being affected more than men.

B. Snoring is not a trigger for headaches.

C. Sleep apnea can result in hypocarbia, resulting in cerebral vasodilation.

D. There is no relationship between sleep disturbance and headaches; therefore, there is no need to include this line of questioning when gathering a patient's history.

E. Hypnic headache most often presents in people younger than age 30 years and occurs with the same frequency in men and women.

21. A 23-year-old otherwise healthy female presents to your headache clinic with an ongoing migraine. The quality and characteristics of this headache are unchanged from past episodes. She has tried abortive agents, including NSAIDS, acetaminophen, and oral phenergan, without improvement in her condition. In your headache clinic, she receives a subcutaneous injection of sumatriptan. This aborts her headache; however, within several minutes, she develops a new chest pain and neck stiffness that last for approximately 12 minutes. Which of the following statements is true?

A. Had this patient been taking a selective serotonin reuptake inhibitor (SSRI) or SNRI for depression, concomitant use of sumatriptan would be contraindicated.

B. Although she has no cardiac risk factors and her exam is otherwise normal, this patient still needs to be taken to the emergency department to rule out acute coronary syndrome (ACS).

C. Chest pain is a well-recognized side effect of sumatriptan administration.

D. "Triptan sensations" include nonserious side effects such as flushing, paresthesias, and transient neck or chest tightness. These occur more often with the oral route of administration than with the parenteral route.

E. Although sumatriptan was effective at aborting her headache, she should avoid the therapy in the future given the associated chest and neck pain.

22. Regarding hemiplegic migraines, which of the following is true?

A. Episodes of hemiplegic migraine often occur daily and therefore require prophylactic medications.

B. There is no genetic link to hemiplegic migraines.

C. Given that hemiplegic migraines are distinctly different from any other form of migraine (with or without aura), diagnosis can be made on history alone.

D. Triptans are not advised in patients with a family history of hemiplegic migraine headaches.

23. Regarding migraine headaches and the patient wanting to become pregnant, which of the following statements is true?

A. Migraine headaches improve during pregnancy for most patients who have migraine with aura but not for patients who suffer from migraine without aura. The improvement in headaches often occurs immediately after conception.
B. Both topiramate and valproate (divalproex sodium) are safe to use for migraine prophylaxis in the pregnant patient.
C. Acetaminophen should be avoided as a first-line treatment agent in aborting a headache in the pregnant patient.
D. NSAIDS are contraindicated during pregnancy.

24. Regarding the use of topiramate in the prophylactic management of migraine headaches, which of the following statements is true?

A. Topiramate is classified by the US Food and Drug Administration (FDA) as a category "C" drug for use in pregnancy.
B. There are no ophthalmologic concerns with the use of topiramate.
C. Chronic topiramate use is associated with development of nephrolithiasis but not with loss of bone density.
D. Female patients taking oral contraceptive medication should be warned that concomitant use of topiramate may decrease the efficacy of the birth control pill.

25. A 23-year-old female presents to your clinic complaining that she has had headaches for the past 4 months. She has never had migraines but reports being quite overwhelmed with a new job and having broken up with her boyfriend. She now is concerned that she might lose her job because of the number of sick days she has had to take as a result of these headaches. In evaluating and treating her headaches, which of the following statements is true?

A. Trigeminal neuralgia quite often presents in the second and third decades of life.
B. Having this patient keep a headache diary is of no benefit in trying to determine a proper headache diagnosis.
C. Psychological counseling can be beneficial in managing some forms of headaches.
D. Asking her about her diet is rude and has no place in evaluating her condition.

26. Which of the following is not a secondary headache?

A. Headache that develops immediately following head and neck trauma after a motor vehicle accident
B. Headache associated with a cerebral arteriovenous malformation
C. A postdural puncture headache
D. Cough headache
E. Medication overuse headache
F. Chronic post-infection headache

ANSWERS

1. ANSWER: C

This patient is most likely suffering from temporal arteritis. ESR and CRP can often be elevated in this condition. If temporal arteritis is suspected, steroids and a temporal artery biopsy are the next course of action. Although there should always be concern about an intracranial bleed with an elderly patient with new headache, given that this patient has a negative neurologic exam, had not fallen, is not taking anticoagulants, and has had this "less than the worst" headache for 8 days without neurologic changes, a stat head CT is probably not necessary. An auriculotemporal nerve block may provide relief for this patient if she was suffering from auriculotemporal neuralgia; however, a greater occipital nerve block is not likely to alleviate her pain.

FURTHER READING

Benzon H, Raja SN, Fishman SM, et al. (Eds.). *Essentials of Pain Medicine*. 3rd ed. Philadelphia, PA: Saunders; 2011:268.
Kaniecki RG. Diagnostic challenges in headache: Migraine as the wolf disguised in sheep's clothing. *Neurology*. 2002;58:S1–S2.
Moskowitz MA. Neurovascular and molecular mechanisms in migraine headache. *Cerebrovasc Brain Metab Rev*. 1993;5:150–177.
Sobri, M., Lamont AC, Alias NA, et al. Red flags in patients presenting with headache: clinical indications for neuroimaging. *Br J Radiol*. 2014;76(2003), 532–535.

2. ANSWER: C

The description of this patient's headache falls under the diagnosis of paroxysmal hemicrania, a condition with similarities to cluster headaches; however, it tends to occur more often in women, as opposed to cluster headaches, which are more common in men. The headache attacks of paroxysmal hemicranias occur more frequently (15–20 per day) with shorter duration (5–45 minutes) than those of cluster headaches, which can occur twice per day and last up to 180 minutes. Oxygen therapy can be beneficial in the treatment of cluster headaches; however, the treatment of choice for paroxysmal hemicrania is indomethacin at a dose of greater than 150 mg PO per day. This patient's headache condition is stable and unchanged during the past 2 years, and she is denying any new neurologic changes during the headaches. Her previous workup included a negative brain MRI. This patient does not require emergency evaluation. The ICHD-2 lists this headache under Section 3: Cluster Headaches and other Trigeminal Autonomic Cephalalgias. There has been a beta version of ICHD-3 since 2013; however, this currently remains in beta. There is not an ICHD-4. Retinal migraine involves repeated attacks of monocular visual disturbance, including scintillations, scotomata, or blindness, associated with migraine headache (ICHD-2). Botox A is considered a migraine prophylaxis treatment. The botulinum A package insert calls for use of 155 units, not 25 units. This treatment involves 31 different injection sites each with 5 units.

FURTHER READING

Bahra A, May A, Goadsby PJ. Cluster headache. *Neurology*. 2002;58:354–361.
Cohen AS, Burns B, Goadsby PJ. High-flow oxygen for treatment of cluster headache. A randomized trial. *JAMA*. 2009;302:2451–2457.
Gabe U, Spiering CLH. Prophylactic treatment of cluster headache with verapamil. *Headache*. 1989;29:167–168.
International Headache Society. The International Classification of Headache Disorders, 2nd edition. *Cephalalgia*. 2004;24(Suppl. 1):1–150.
Jackson JL, Kuriyama A, Hayashino Y. Botulinum toxin A for prophylactic treatment of migraine and tension headaches in adults: A meta-analysis. *JAMA*. 2012;307(16):1736–1745.
Peres MFP, Silberstein SD, Nahmias S, et al. Hemicrania continua is not that rare. *Neurology*. 2001;57:948–951.
Warner JS. Analgesic rebound as a cause of hemicrania continua. *Neurology*. 1997;48:1540–1541.

3. ANSWER: D

MOH can occur when patients begin using analgesics at a frequency of more than 10 days per month. The use of prophylactic medication should be considered if patients are requiring analgesics more than twice per week. Although prophylactic medications can reduce the risk of developing MOH, they do not eliminate the risk, especially if patients continue to use analgesics with regularity. Analgesics preparations that may be associated with MOH include triptans, ergot derivatives, acetaminophen, NSAIDs, butalbital, and narcotics.

FURTHER READING

Benzon H, Raja SN, Fishman SM, et al. (Eds.). *Essentials of Pain Medicine*. 3rd ed. Philadelphia, PA: Saunders; 2011:268.
Katsarava Z, Limmroth V, Finke M, et al. Rates and predicators for relapse in medication overuse headache: A 1-year prospective study. *Neurology*. 2003;60:1682–1683.
Lipton RB, Bigal ME. Chronic daily headache. *Neurology*. 2003; 61:154–155.
Warner JS. Analgesic rebound as a cause of hemicrania continua. *Neurology*. 1997;48:1540–1541.
Zwart JA, Hagen K, Svebak S, et al. Analgesic use: A predicator of chronic pain and medication overuse headache. *Neurology*. 2003;61:163–164.

4. ANSWER: B

In a general sense, a visit to the emergency department is appropriate when there are "red flag" signs or symptoms that suggest a dangerous cause of headache. These include a headache that is unusually severe or sudden in onset, termed a "thunderclap" headache, or headaches associated with fever or confusion. The 26-year-old graduate student is experiencing a new headache, different than she has experienced in the past. This is the "worst headache of her life" with a VAS of 10/10; she is vomiting and experiencing dysarthria. She needs to be evaluated in the emergency department as soon as possible.

FURTHER READING

Bousser MG, Welch KMA. Relation between migraine and stroke. *Lancet Neurol.* 2005;4:533–542.

Kurth T, Chabriat H, Bousser MG. Migraine and stroke: A complex association with clinical implications. *Lancet Neurol.* 2012;11:92–100.

Loder EW, Burch RC, Rizzoli PB. *Common Pitfalls in the Evaluation and Management of Headache: Case-Based Learning.* Cambridge, UK: Cambridge University Press; 2014.

Parwar BL, Fawzi AA, Arnold AC, et al. Horner's syndrome and dissection of the internal carotid artery after chiropractic manipulation of the neck. *Am J Ophthamol.* 2001;131(4):523–524.

Patel RR, Adam R, Maldjian C, et al. Cervical carotid artery dissection: Current review of diagnosis and treatment. *Cardiol Rev.* 2012;20(3):145–152.

Thigpen MC, Whitney CG, Messonnier NE, et al.; Emerging Infections Programs Network. Bacterial meningitis in the United States, 1998–2007. *N Engl J Med.* 2011;364:2016–2025.

5. ANSWER: D

The 67-year-old left-hand-dominant male returned from a hunting trip. His signs and symptoms are concerning for a possible carotid artery dissection with resulting neurologic sequelae, possible resulting from high-powered rifle-associated trauma to his left shoulder/neck. The differential diagnosis of "side-locked" headaches may include benign conditions such as cluster headache, hemicranias continua, and even migraine. However, more dangerous conditions need to be ruled out, including giant cell arteritis carotid dissection or cervical facet issues. His PCP ordered an ESR and CRP, which were both within normal limits, thus reducing the concern for giant cell arteritis. Suspicion is raised with new-onset Horner's syndrome associated with a headache. The sympathetic fibers lie just outside the carotid artery, and dissections of the carotid artery may result in stretching of these fibers sufficient enough to disrupt functioning. His ipsilateral facial droop and contralateral upper extremity weakness are concerning for possible cerebral embolism and/or ischemia. A patient who presents with headache, new-onset Horner's syndrome, and neck pain should be evaluated with additional imaging, including CT angiogram or MR angiogram of the neck or ultrasound. Given his additional neurologic sequelae, brain imaging is called for as well.

FURTHER READING

Bousser MG, Welch KMA. Relation between migraine and stroke. *Lancet Neurol.* 2005;4:533–542.

Kurth T, Chabriat H, Bousser MG. Migraine and stroke: A complex association with clinical implications. *Lancet Neurol.* 2012;11:92–100.

Loder EW, Burch RC, Rizzoli PB. *Common Pitfalls in the Evaluation and Management of Headache: Case-Based Learning.* Cambridge, UK: Cambridge University Press; 2014.

Parwar BL, Fawzi AA, Arnold AC, et al. Horner's syndrome and dissection of the internal carotid artery after chiropractic manipulation of the neck. *Am J Ophthamol.* 2001;131(4):523–524.

Patel RR, Adam R, Maldjian C, et al. Cervical carotid artery dissection: Current review of diagnosis and treatment. *Cardiol Rev.* 2012;20(3):145–152.

Thigpen MC, Whitney CG, Messonnier NE, et al.; Emerging Infections Programs Network. Bacterial meningitis in the United States, 1998–2007. *N Engl J Med.* 2011;364: 2016–2025.

6. ANSWER: D

The 18-year-old male is having new-onset severe headache with nausea, vomiting, fever, and confusion. By report, his desire to lay still with his knees and hips flexed and not try to sit up is concerning for Kernig's sign. These signs and symptoms are concerning for possible bacterial meningitis. The patient should be seen in the emergency department immediately. Workup should include a lumbar puncture with CSF evaluation and cultures, as well as blood cultures. If concern is high for bacterial meningitis, antibiotics should not be delayed for lab results. Meningococcal meningitis may be caused by several pathogens, including *Haemophilus influenzae* type B, *Neisseria meningitides, Streptococcus pneumoniae*, and *Listeria monocytogenes* (during pregnancy). Bacterial meningitis caused by *N. meningitides* can be transmitted in community settings, such as military personnel living in close quarters.

FURTHER READING

Bousser MG, Welch KMA. Relation between migraine and stroke. *Lancet Neurol.* 2005;4:533–542.

Kurth T, Chabriat H, Bousser MG. Migraine and stroke: A complex association with clinical implications. *Lancet Neurol.* 2012;11:92–100.

Parwar BL, Fawzi AA, Arnold AC, et al. Horner's syndrome and dissection of the internal carotid artery after chiropractic manipulation of the neck. *Am J Ophthamol.* 2001;131(4):523–524.

Patel RR, Adam R, Maldjian C, et al. Cervical carotid artery dissection: Current review of diagnosis and treatment. *Cardiol Rev.* 2012;20(3):145–152.

Thigpen MC, Whitney CG, Messonnier NE, et al.; Emerging Infections Programs Network. Bacterial meningitis in the United States, 1998–2007. *N Engl J Med.* 2011;364: 2016–2025.

7. ANSWER: C

This 58-year-old male with a history of migraine with aura may be experiencing a stroke. There is an association between cerebral hypoperfusion and migraine with aura. Although quite rare, these headaches, termed "fatal migraines," occasionally appear in the neurology literature, usually referring to cases in which a migraine with aura persists and culminates in death from stroke. Decreases in cerebral blood flow are known to occur in the setting of aura but typically are not sufficient to produce ischemic symptoms. True migrainous infarction is quite rare; however, in unusual circumstances, such as volume depletion or hypercoagulability, perhaps the hypoperfusion that occurs during aura is amplified and sufficient to produce a stroke. Current diagnostic criteria in the ICHD-3 beta allow for the diagnosis of migrainous infarction only in patients known to have migraine with aura. The stroke must develop during a typical aura, and imaging must reveal a defect in the relevant brain location. It is a diagnosis of exclusion. Regardless, this patient's new hemiplegia in the setting of history of migraine with aura is concerning and should be worked up further.

FURTHER READING

Bousser MG, Welch KMA. Relation between migraine and stroke. *Lancet Neurol.* 2005;4:533–542.

Kurth T, Chabriat H, Bousser MG. Migraine and stroke: A complex association with clinical implications. *Lancet Neurol.* 2012;11:92–100.

Loder EW, Burch RC, Rizzoli PB. *Common Pitfalls in the Evaluation and Management of Headache: Case-Based Learning.* Cambridge, UK: Cambridge University Press; 2014.

Parwar BL, Fawzi AA, Arnold AC, et al. Horner's syndrome and dissection of the internal carotid artery after chiropractic manipulation of the neck. *Am J Ophthamol.* 2001;131(4):523–524.

Patel RR, Adam R, Maldjian C, et al. Cervical carotid artery dissection: Current review of diagnosis and treatment. *Cardiol Rev.* 2012;20(3):145–152.

Thigpen MC, Whitney CG, Messonnier NE, et al.; Emerging Infections Programs Network. Bacterial meningitis in the United States, 1998–2007. *N Engl J Med.* 2011;364:2016–2025.

8. ANSWER: C

Ergot alkaloids are considered 5-HT agonists, which are believed to reduce the sterile neurogenic inflammation by reducing the release of peptide neurotransmitters such as substance P, Calcitonin gene-related peptide, and neurokinin A. The other choices are true statements.

FURTHER READING

Benzon H, Raja SN, Fishman SM, et al. (Eds.). *Essentials of Pain Medicine.* 3rd ed. Philadelphia, PA: Saunders; 2011:261.

Waeber C, Moskowitz MA: Therapeutic implications of central and peripheral neurologic mechanisms in migraine. *Neurology.* 2003;61(Suppl. 4):S9–S20.

Welch KMA. Contemporary concepts of migraine pathogenesis. *Neurology.* 2003;61:S2–S8.

Moskowitz MA: Neurovascular and molecular mechanisms in migraine headache. *Cerebrovasc Brain Metab Rev.* 1993;5:150–177.

9. ANSWER: D

Although referred to as "classic migraine," migraine with aura occurs less frequently than migraine without aura. Migraine with aura (classic migraine) represents 20% of all migraines, whereas migraine without aura represents 80% of migraines. Medication treatments for migraine headaches consist of abortive agents such as triptans, ergotamines, and isometheptene (Midrin); butalbital-containing agents such as Fioricet; opioids; antinauseants; NSAIDs; corticosteroids; and dihydroergotamines. Treatments also include prophylactic agents such as beta blockers (propanolol); anticonvulsants such as topiramate and valproic acid; antidepressants including tricyclic antidepressants, SSRIs, and SNRIs; calcium channel blockers; lithium; and Botox A. A basilar-type migraine is one in which the aura effects the brainstem and therefore can result in symptoms as reported in the answer choices. Basilar-type migraines do not result in any motor deficits.

FURTHER READING

Benzon H, Raja SN, Fishman SM, et al. (Eds.). *Essentials of Pain Medicine.* 3rd ed. Philadelphia, PA: Saunders; 2011:265.

Denier HC, Limmroth V: The management of migraine. *Rev Contemp Pharmacother.* 1994;5:271–284.

Goldstein J, Silberstein SD, Saper JR, et al. Acetaminophen, aspirin, and caffeine in combination versus ibuprofen for acute migraine: Results from a multicenter, double-blind, randomized, parallel-group, single-dose, placebo-controlled study. *Headache.* 2006;46:444–453.

Hering R, Kuritzky AA. Sodium valproate in the prophylactic treatment of migraine. A double blind study versus placebo. *Cephalalgia.* 1992;12:81–84.

Holroyd KA, Penzien DB. Propranolol in the management of recurrent migraine. A meta-analytic review. *Headache.* 1991;31:33–44.

International Headache Society. The International Classification of Headache Disorders, 2nd edition. *Cephalalgia.* 2004;24(Suppl 1):1–150.

10. ANSWER: D

This patient represents a classic presentation of cluster headache, which is more often seen in males between the ages of 20 and 40 years. Valprioc acid, calcium channel blockers, antidepressants, beta blockers, corticosteroids, oxygen therapy, and NSAIDs such as indomethacin may all be used to treat this condition. Cluster headaches can last between 15 and 180 minutes and may occur up to six to eight times per day. The "clusters" may last weeks to months; headaches may be precipitated during this phase by consumption of alcohol, histamines, or nitroglycerin. Paroxysmal hemicrania, like cluster headaches, is considered a trigeminal autonomic cephalalgia. Unlike cluster headaches, paroxysmal hemicrania occurs more frequently in females; may have up to 20 episodes per day, each lasting 5–45 minutes; and pathognomonically responds to indomethacin.

FURTHER READING

Bahra A, May A, Goadsby PJ. Cluster headache. *Neurology*. 2002;58:354–361.

Benzon H, Raja SN, Fishman SM, et al. (Eds.). *Essentials of Pain Medicine*. 3rd ed. Philadelphia, PA: Saunders; 2011:266–267.

Buse DC, Rupnow MFT, Lipton RB. Assessing and managing all aspects of migraine: Migraine attacks, migraine-related functional impairment, common comorbidities, and quality of life. *Mayo Clin Proc*. 2009;84:422–435.

Cohen AS, Burns B, Goadsby PJ: High-flow oxygen for treatment of cluster headache: A randomized trial. *JAMA*. 2009;302:2451–2457.

Gabe U, Spiering CLH. Prophylactic treatment of cluster headache with verapamil. *Headache*. 1989;29:167–168.

International Headache Society. The International Classification of Headache Disorders, 2nd edition. *Cephalalgia*. 2004;24(Suppl. 1):1–150.

Peres MFP, Silberstein SD, Nahmias S, et al. Hemicrania continua is not that rare. *Neurology*. 2001;57:948–951.

Stewart WF, Lipton RB, Ottman R. Familial risk of migraine: A population-based study. *Neurology*. 1997;41:166–172.

11. ANSWER: A

This patient is likely experiencing neuroleptic-induced extrapyramidal dystonia and akathisia from administration of prochlorperazine. The traditional approach to treating this involves discontinuation of the offending drug. In addition, anticholinergic agents such as diphenhydramine or benztropine or benzodiazepines are often administered to aid in the resolution of symptoms. Anticholinergic agents are believed to work because extrapyramidal effects occur as a result of dopamine/acetylcholine imbalance with the use of neuroleptics. The abnormal muscle contractions with spasm or twisting of the head and abnormal movements of the trunk or limbs are neuroleptic-induced dystonia. Akathisia is characterized by severe motor restlessness and agitation. Episodes of dystonia usually last 20–30 minutes and may often produce pain. In the "stepped care" approach to headache management, patients treat headaches first with a nonspecific agent such as an NSAID and then switch to a specific therapy (usually a triptan) only if the NSAID is not effective. In the "stratified care" approach, patients use the nonspecific agents as first-line therapy for less severe

headaches and use specific therapies as first-line therapy for more severe headaches. A randomized trial comparing the two approaches showed that stratified care was more effective and associated with higher patient satisfaction.

FURTHER READING

Burstein R, Collins B, Jakubowski M. Defeating migraine pain with triptans: A race against the development of cutaneous allodynia. *Ann Neurol*. 2004;55:19–26.

Lima AR, Soares-Weiser K, Bacaltchuk J, et al. Benzodiazepines for neuroleptic-induced acute akathisia. *Cochrane Database Syst Rev*. 2002;(1):CD001950.

Loder EW, Burch RC, Rizzoli PB. *Common Pitfalls in the Evaluation and Management of Headache: Case-Based Learning*. Cambridge, UK: Cambridge University Press; 2014.

Parlak I, Erdur B, Parlak M, et al. Midazolam vs. diphenhydramine for the treatment of metoclopramide induced akathisia: A randomized controlled trial. *Acad Emerg Med*. 2007;14(8):715–721.

Whyte C, Tepper SJ, Evans RW. Expert opinion: Rescue me: Rescue medication for migraine. *Headache*. 2010;50(2):307–313.

12. ANSWER: C

The spinal nucleus of the trigeminal nerve extends caudally to the outer lamina of the dorsal horn of the upper three or four cervical spinal segments. This is known as the trigeminocervical nucleus, which receives afferents from the trigeminal nerve as well as the upper three cervical spinal nerves. Convergence between these accounts for the cervical–trigeminal pain referral.

FURTHER READING

Bartsch T, Goadsby PJ: Stimulation of the greater occipital nerve induces increased central excitability of dural afferent input. *Brain*. 2002;125:1496–1509.

Benzon H, Raja SN, Fishman SM, et al. (Eds.). *Essentials of Pain Medicine*. 3rd ed. Philadelphia, PA: Saunders; 2011:278.

13. ANSWER: B

During an atlantoaxial (AA) joint injection, the needle should be directed toward the posterolateral aspect of the joint in order to avoid the vertebral artery laterally and the C2 nerve root medially. The AA injection has the potential for serious complications. The vertebral artery is lateral as it passes through C2–C1 foramina but then passes medially to go through the foramen magnum; in doing so, it crosses the medial aspect of the atlanto-occipital joint. The lateral AA joint may account for up of 16% of patients with occipital headaches. Clinical presentations suggestive of pain originating from the lateral AA joint include occipital and suboccipital pain, focal tenderness over the suboccipital area, restricted painful rotation of C1 on C2, and pain with passive rotation of C1; however, these are not specific findings and cannot make the diagnosis alone. Diagnosis is made by a diagnostic block with an intra-articular local anesthetic.

FURTHER READING

Aprill C, Axinn MJ, Bogduk N. Occipital headaches stemming from the lateral atlanto-axial (C1–2) joint. *Cephalalgia*. 2002;22:15–22.
Benzon H, Raja SN, Fishman SM, et al. (Eds.). *Essentials of Pain Medicine*. 3rd ed. Philadelphia, PA: Saunders; 2011:279.
Bogduk N. The neck and headache. *Neurol Clin*. 2004;22:151–171.
Narouze SN, Casanova J, Mekhail N. The longitudinal effectiveness of lateral atlanto-axial intra-articular steroid injection in the management of cervicogenic headache. *Pain Med*. 2007;8:184–188.

14. ANSWER: D

Pain stemming from the C2–C3 zygopophyseal joint (third occipital headache) is seen in 27% of patients presenting with cervicogenic headache after whiplash injury. The third occipital nerve innervates the C2–C3 zygophyseal joint and is the superficial medial branch of the dorsal rami of C3. Early reports showed ineffectiveness of radiofrequency ablation; however, with better radiofrequency technique, complete pain relief was obtained in 88% of patients with third occipital headache. Tenderness over the C2–C3 zygopophyseal joint is the only suggestive physical exam finding, and a diagnostic third occipital nerve block is mandatory to confirm the diagnosis of third occipital headache.

FURTHER READING

Benzon H, Raja SN, Fishman SM, et al. (Eds.). *Essentials of Pain Medicine*. 3rd ed. Philadelphia, PA: Saunders; 2011:280.
Bogduk N. The clinical anatomy of cervical dorsal rami. *Spine*. 1982;7:319–330.
Govind J, King W, Baily B, et al. Radiofrequency neurotomy for the treatment of third occipital headache. *J Neurol Neurosurg Psychiatry*. 2003;74:88–93.
Lord SM, Barnsley L, Bogduk N. Percutaneous radiofrequency neurotomy in the treatment of cervical zygapophyseal joint pain: A caution. *Neurosurgery*. 1995;36:732–739.
Lord S, Barnsley L, Wallis B, et al. Third occipital headache: A prevalence study. *J Neurol Neurosurg Psychiatry*. 1994;57:1187–1190.

15. ANSWER: D

The third occipital nerve is the superficial medial branch of the C3 dorsal ramus. It supplies the C2–C3 joint while passing across it laterally. The exact location of the nerve is variable, and the use of the three-needle technique increases the likelihood of capturing the nerve at the lateral C2–C3 joint line, just above or just below. The third occipital nerve supplies part of the semispinalis capitis muscle, and its cutaneous branch supplies a small area of skin below the occiput. Numbness in the cutaneous distribution of the nerve is very common after radiofrequency ablation (RFA), whereas dysesthesia and hyperexcitability occur in up to 50% of cases. Numbness is usually temporary, lasting a few days to weeks. Temporary ataxia has been reported in some patients as third occipital neurotomy partially denervates the semispinalis capitis muscles with resultant interference of tonic neck reflexes.

FURTHER READING

Benzon H, Raja SN, Fishman SM, et al. (Eds.). *Essentials of Pain Medicine*. 3rd ed. Philadelphia, PA: Saunders; 2011:280.
Govind J, King W, Baily B, et al. Radiofrequency neurotomy for the treatment of third occipital headache. *J Neurol Neurosurg Psychiatry*. 2003;74:88–93.
Lord SM, Barnsley L, Bogduk N. Percutaneous radiofrequency neurotomy in the treatment of cervical zygapophyseal joint pain: A caution. *Neurosurgery*. 1995;36:732–739.
Lord S, Barnsley L, Wallis B, et al. Third occipital headache: A prevalence study. *J Neurol Neurosurg Psychiatry*. 1994;57:1187–1190.

16. ANSWER: C

PDPH commonly present within the first 24–48 hours following a dural puncture; however, there are many reports of headaches presenting as much as 7 days later. The higher the lumbar puncture, the less the hydrostatic pressure at the dural puncture site, which may explain why PDPHs are not commonly associated with cervical punctures. The incidence of PDPH ranges from 1% to 63%; determinants of this difference include the needle size, design of the needle tip, and the orientation of the needle bevel during meningeal puncture. Postdural puncture headache is characteristically occipital and/or frontal, and it is always bilateral. Symptoms associated with PDPH include nausea, vomiting, neck stiffness, lower or upper limb pain, auditory changes including tinnitus and hypoacousia, diplopia, scalp paresthesia, and even mental status changes.

FURTHER READING

Benzon H, Raja SN, Fishman SM, et al. (Eds.). *Essentials of Pain Medicine*. 3rd ed. Philadelphia, PA: Saunders; 2011:272–273.
Bussone G, Tullo V, d'Onofrio F, et al. Frovatriptan for the prevention of postdural puncture headache. *Cephalalgia*. 2007;27:809–813.
Gaiser R. Postdural puncture headache. *Curr Opin Anaesthesiol*. 2006;19:249–253.

Hatfield MK, Handrich SJ, Willis JA, et al. Blood patch rates after lumbar puncture with Whitacre versus Quincke 22- and 20-gauge spinal needles. *AJR Am J Roentgenol*. 2008;190:1686–1689.
Reamy BV. Post-epidural headache: How late can it occur? *J Am Board Fam Med*. 2009;22:202–205.
Richman JM, Joe EM, Cohen SR, et al. Bevel direction and postdural puncture headache: A meta-analysis. *Neurologist*. 2006;12:224–228.
Zeidan A, Hamdan F. Occipital blockade for postdural puncture headache: Do we harm? *Pain Pract*. 2009;9:323.

17. ANSWER: A

Independent risk factors of PDPH include a higher incidence in women versus men, pregnancy, a higher incidence in the 20- to 50-year-old age group, and a higher incidence in patients with lower BMI. Risk factors for EBP failure include placement sooner than 24 hours after dural puncture, using inadequate volumes of autologous blood, and performance of the procedure with residual lidocaine in the epidural space.

FURTHER READING

Benzon H, Raja SN, Fishman SM, et al. (Eds.). *Essentials of Pain Medicine*. 3rd ed. Philadelphia, PA: Saunders; 2011:274–275.
Munnur U, Suresh MS. Backache, headache, and neurologic deficit after regional anesthesia. *Anesthesiol Clin North Am*. 2003;21:71–86.
Ong BY, Graham CR, Ringaert KR, et al. Impaired epidural analgesia after dural puncture with and without subsequent blood patch. *Anesth Analg*. 1990;70:76–79.

18. ANSWER: C

The triad of postural headache, low CSF pressure on diagnostic lumbar puncture, and meningeal enhancement on MRI in a patient without any history of dural puncture leads one to suspect the presence of SIH. Diagnostic lumbar puncture usually shows a low CSF pressure, occasionally without spontaneous flow and need for aspiration of CSF during lumbar puncture. MRI of the cranium shows meningeal enhancement, subdural fluid collection, and caudal displacement of the cerebellar tonsils. Radionucleotide cisternography RC is presumed to be the standard confirmatory test in the diagnosis. Some investigators recommend CT myelography, MR myelography, and radioisotope myelocisternography to demonstrate the site of the leak.

FURTHER READING

Benzon H, Raja SN, Fishman SM, et al. (Eds.). *Essentials of Pain Medicine*. 3rd ed. Philadelphia, PA: Saunders; 2011:276.

Diaz JH. Epidemiology and outcome of postural headache management in spontaneous intracranial hypotension. *Reg Anesth Pain Med*. 2001;26:582–587.
Spelle L, Boulin A, Tainturier C, et al. Neuroimaging features of spontaneous intracranial hypotension. *Neuroradiology*. 2001;43:622–627.

19. ANSWER: F

Migraine headaches may be triggered by changes in diet, motion, alcohol, monosodium glutamate, nitrates, tyramine-containing foods, fatigue, stress, menstruation, underlying tension-type headache, strong odors, bright sunlight, or depression.

FURTHER READING

Lewis DW. Headaches in children and adolescents. *Curr Probl Pediatr Adolesc Health Care*. 2007;37:207–246.
Waldman SD. *Pain Review*. Philadelphia, PA: Saunders; 2009:663.

20. ANSWER: A

Hypnic headache represents another syndrome of recurring head pain that awakens patients from rapid eye movement sleep. It most commonly has an onset after age 50 years and is approximately twice as frequent in women as in men. This type of headache responds to indomethacin or lithium. Snoring with or without apnea can be a cause of chronic daily headaches. Sleep apnea can result in hypoxia and hypercarbia, resulting in cerebral vasodilation.

FURTHER READING

Benzon H, Raja SN, Fishman SM, et al. (Eds.). *Essentials of Pain Medicine*. 3rd ed. Philadelphia, PA: Saunders; 2011:270.
Evers S, Goadsby PJ. Hypnic headache. *Neurology*. 2003;60:905–909.
Scher AI, Lipton RB, Stewart WF. Habitual snoring as a risk factor for chronic daily headache. *Neurology*. 2003;60:1366–1368.

21. ANSWER: C

This otherwise healthy 23-year-old female who takes no medications but develops chest pain within minutes of taking sumatriptan is experiencing "triptan sensations." The sensations associated with triptans can include flushing, paresthesias, and transient neck and chest tightness. Given that she is at low risk for cardiovascular disease, has an otherwise normal exam, and has transient chest pain in close temporal relationship to the administration of a triptan, evaluation in the emergency department to rule out ACS is probably not warranted. Triptan sensations have been reported to occur in up to 50% of patients who receive it parenterally and 25% of patients who receive it orally. If this therapy is effective at aborting her headaches, it should not be taken out of her treatment algorithm. Triptan sensations occur with such regularity that patients should be advised of the potential for these before the first use. In 2006, the FDA advised about the potential for serotonin syndrome when triptans are used in patients taking an SSRI/SNRI. In 2010, the American Headache Society position paper stated, "The currently available evidence does not support limiting the use of triptans with SSRIs/SNRIs or the use of triptan monotherapy, due to the concerns for serotonin syndrome." One study suggested that as many as 65 million patients in a 1-year period in the United States were using an SSRI along with a triptan with no documented cases of serotonin syndrome identified among them. Nonetheless, patients should be advised of the theoretical potential for this.

FURTHER READING

Evans RW, Tepper SJ, Shapiro RE, et al. The FDA alert on serotonin syndrome with use of triptans combined with selective serotonin reuptake inhibitors or selective serotonin–norepinephrine reuptake inhibitors: American Headache Society position paper. *Headache.* 2010;50(6):1089–1099.

Loder EW, Burch RC, Rizzoli PB. *Common Pitfalls in the Evaluation and Management of Headache: Case-Based Learning.* Cambridge, UK: Cambridge University Press; 2014:102–105.

Papademetriou V. Cardiovascular risk assessment and triptans. *Headache.* 2004;44(Suppl. 1):S31–S39.

Visser WH, Jaspers NM, de Vriend RH, et al. Chest symptoms after sumatriptan: A two-year clinical practice review in 735 consecutive migraine patients. *Cephalalgia.* 1996;16(8):554–559.

22. ANSWER: D

Vasoconstrictive medications such as triptans that are routinely used for the treatment of patients with migraine with and without aura are contraindicated in patients who have familial hemiplegic migraines. This contraindication is based on the concern that triptans or ergots might be more likely to cause vasoactive complications in patients who have complex forms of aura, such as hemiplegic migraine. Most patients with hemiplegic migraine have relatively infrequent attacks and therefore do not require prophylactic treatment. Patients can often misinterpret sensory and motor deficits so that it is difficult to make the diagnosis of hemiplegic migraine based on reported history alone. Patients suffering from migraine with aura can have sensory deficits such as numbness that can be reported to their provider as a motor deficit. For this reason, it is essential that the patient present for examination during an episode

so that an accurate neurologic exam can be conducted. Patients who experience true motor weakness in association with a migraine are classified separately as having hemiplegic migraine. Hemiplegic migraine is usually an inherited autosomal dominant disorder, and a number of single gene mutations have been identified that are associated with it.

FURTHER READING

Lafreniere RG, Rouleau GA. Identification of novel genes involved in migraine. *Headache.* 2012;52:107–110.

Loder EW, Burch RC, Rizzoli PB. *Common Pitfalls in the Evaluation and Management of Headache: Case-Based Learning.* Cambridge, UK: Cambridge University Press; 2014:97.

Russell MB, Ducros A. Sporadic and familial hemiplegic migraine: Pathophysiological mechanisms, clinical characteristics, diagnosis, and management. *Lancet Neurol.* 2011;10(5):457–470.

23. ANSWER: D

NSAIDs are typically avoided during the first trimester due to increased risk of spontaneous abortion, and they are avoided in the third trimester due to risk of premature closure of the ductus arteriosus and renal abnormalities. Studies consistently show that approximately 70% of women with migraine experience some degree of improvement during pregnancy. This is most noticeable during the second and third trimesters and is most likely to occur in patients who suffer from migraine without aura. Some women who have migraine headaches with aura find that the aura frequency and complexity may increase. For both topiramate and divalproex sodium, there is evidence for potential fetal risk, including orofacial clefts with topiramate and neural tube defects and cognitive deficits with divalproex sodium. Topiramate carries an FDA category "D" rating for use in pregnancy; divalproex sodium carries an "X" rating. Nonpharmacologic treatment options for headache management include biofeedback, proper sleep, adequate hydration, and stress management. When pharmacologic treatment is necessary, acetaminophen is considered first-line symptomatic therapy. It carries an FDA category "B" rating for use in pregnancy.

FURTHER READING

Harirforoosh S, Jamali F. Renal adverse effects of nonsteroidal anti-inflammatory drugs. *Expert Opin Drug Saf.* 2009;8(6):669–681.

Kelley NE, Tepper DE. Rescue therapy for acute migraine: Part 3. Opioids, NSAIDS, steroids and post-discharge medications. *Headache.* 2012;52(3):467–482.

Loder EW, Burch RC, Rizzoli PB. *Common Pitfalls in the Evaluation and Management of Headache: Case-Based Learning.* Cambridge, UK: Cambridge University Press; 2014:128–129.

Lucas S. Medication use in the treatment of migraine during pregnancy and lactation. *Curr Pain Headache Rep.* 2009;13(5):392–398.

24. ANSWER: D

Topiramate decreases serum concentrations of ethinyl estradiol, the active estrogen component in many combined hormonal contraceptives. Studies show that the blood concentration of ethinyl estradiol is reduced by an average of 18% in women taking topirimate 200 mg daily, 21% with 400-mg daily use, and up to 30% with a dose of 800 mg/day. Topiramate is the migraine preventative most commonly associated with increased intraocular pressure. Topiramate may precipitate secondary acute angle-closure glaucoma due to ciliochoroidal effusion, which displaces the lens and the ciliary body. In clinical trials, the incidence of nephrolisthiasis in patients taking topiramate is approximately 1% per year, with cumulative risk increasing with duration of therapy. Bone loss is painless and insidious, and the pharmacologic profile of topiramate suggests that this may be an irreversible complication of long-term topiramate treatment. Several lines of evidence suggest that topiramate may produce bone loss. Topiramate use during pregnancy is associated with orofacial clefts; it has an FDA use-in-pregnancy rating of "D."

FURTHER READING

Ali II, Herial NA, Orris M, et al. Migraine prophylaxis with topiramate and bone health in women. *Headache*. 2011;51:613–616.

Loder EW, Burch RC, Rizzoli PB. *Common Pitfalls in the Evaluation and Management of Headache: Case-Based Learning.* Cambridge, UK: Cambridge University Press; 2014:129, 135–137.

Reddy DS. Clinical pharmacokinetic interactions between antiepileptic drugs and hormonal contraceptives. *Expert Rev Clin Pharmacol*. 2010;3(2):183–192.

25. ANSWER: C

A headache diary kept by the patient for 2 or 3 months may be a useful tool in trying to determine precipitating factors of a migraine headache. Migraines can be triggered by a change in diet, sleep habits, alcohol, hormone fluctuations as occur during menses and oral birth control use, fatigue, stress, bright sunlight, strong odors, environmental or physiological stress, depression, and fatigue. This 23-year-old patient has some psychosocial factors that may be contributing to her headaches. Treatment consideration should include psychological counseling, which may prove beneficial in nonpharmacologically management of her headaches. Trigeminal neuralgia is rarely seen before the third decade unless in association with multiple sclerosis.

FURTHER READING

Lewis DW. Headaches in children and adolescents. *Curr Probl Pediatr Adolesc Health Care*. 2007;37:207–246.

Waldman SD. *Pain Review*. Philadelphia, PA: Saunders; 2009:661–663.

26. ANSWER: D

The ICHD-2 defines primary headaches as follows:

1. Migraine—to include with and without aura, retinal migraine, and childhood periodic syndromes commonly precursors to migraines (cyclical vomiting, abdominal migraines, benign paroxysmal vertigo of childhood)
2. Tension-type headaches
3. Cluster headaches and other trigeminal autonomic cephalalgias, such as paroxysmal hemicranias and short-lasting unilateral neuralgiform headache attacks with conjunctival injection and tearing (SUNCT)
4. "Other primary headaches," which include primary stabbing headache, primary cough headache, primary exertional headache, primary headache associated with sexual activity, primary thunderclap headache, hypnic headache, hemicrania continua, and new daily persistent headaches.

If a new headache occurs for the first time in close temporal relation to another disorder that is a known cause of headache, this headache is coded according to the causative disorder as a secondary headache. This remains true even when the headache has the characteristics of migraine, tension-type headache, cluster headache, or one of the other trigeminal autonomic cephalalgias.

The ICHD lists the following as secondary headaches: headache attributed to head and/or neck trauma; headache attributed to cranial or cervical vascular disorders; headache attributed to nonvascular intracranial disorders (high or low CSF pressure non-infectious inflammatory, intracranial neoplasm, intrathecal injection, and Chiari malformation type 1); headache attributed to substance or its withdrawal (e.g., medication overuse headache); headache attributed to infection (HIV/AIDS, systemic infection, intracranial infection, and post-infection headache); headache attributed to disorders in homeostasis (hypothyroid, hypertension, hypoxia, hypercapnia, dialysis, fasting, and cardiac cephalagia); headache attributed to psychiatric disorders (psychotic or somatiform disorders); and headache or facial pain attributed to disorder of cranium, neck, eyes, ears, nose, sinuses, teeth, mouth, or other facial or cranial structures.

Cough headache is headache precipitated by coughing or straining in the absence of any intracranial disorder; often has a sudden onset, lasting from 1 second to 30 minutes; is brought on by and occurring only in association with coughing, straining, and/or Valsalva maneuver; and is not attributed to another disorder. Cough headache is symptomatic in approximately 40% of cases, and the large majority of these present Arnold–Chiari malformation type I. Other reported causes of symptomatic cough headache include carotid or vertebrobasilar diseases and cerebral aneurysms. Diagnostic neuroimaging plays an important role in differentiating secondary cough headache from a primary cough headache. Primary cough headache is usually bilateral and predominantly affects patients older than age 40 years. Whereas indomethacin is usually effective in the treatment of primary cough headache, a positive response to this medication has also been reported in some symptomatic cases.

FURTHER READING

Headache Classification Subcommittee of the International Headache Society. The International Classification of Headache Disorders. *Cephalalgia* 2004;24:9.

23.

OROFACIAL PAIN

Christopher Sobey

INTRODUCTION

Management of orofacial pain in the general population can be a challenging and demanding undertaking due to the complex neurological anatomy and close proximity to vital structures. Differentiating various syndromes and origins of pain can prove difficult; thus, specific emphasis on establishing the correct diagnosis is of the utmost importance in formatting a successful treatment plan. The questions presented in this chapter delve into the presentations, physical exam findings, diagnostic testing, psychological effects, and evidence-based medical and interventional treatment algorithms of both common and less common craniofacial pain disorders. This chapter covers pathophysiology of the neurological, biomechanical, and central causes of facial pain.

QUESTIONS

1. A patient presents with brief painful episodes of intense, sharp, and stabbing facial pain. What is the most common distribution of pain in idiopathic trigeminal neuralgia?

    A. Bilateral V_2 only
    B. Right-sided V_2 and V_3
    C. Left-sided V_1, V_2, and V_3
    D. Left-sided V_3 only
    E. Right-sided V_1 only

2. A 58-year-old female presents with unilateral sharp, severe stabbing pain precipitated by wiping her nose. She has been trialed on multiple medication regimens, including dual-medication thearpy without significant improvement. Magnetic resonance imaging (MRI) demonstrates compression of the trigeminal root in Meckel's cavity. What is the best treatment option?

    A. Percutaneous radiofrequency thermocoagulation
    B. Pulsed radiofrequency ablation

    C. Gamma knife
    D. Microvascular decompression
    E. Continued trials of medications

3. A 61-year-old male complains of left-sided transient severe, sharp, stabbing pain in the ear, base of tongue, and the tonsillar fossa with swallowing and chewing. What distributions of nerves are transmitting this pain?

    A. Auricular and pharyngeal branches of the glossopharyngeal nerve
    B. Lingual and auriculotemporal branches of the mandibular nerve
    C. Greater and lesser palatine nerves
    D. Chorda tympani branch of facial nerve
    E. Inferior alveolar and myohyoid branches of the mandibular nerve

4. An elderly female presents to clinic for evaluation of pain and drooping on the right side of her face. Symptoms first started 3 days prior with pruritus in her right ear. She was diagnosed with Ramsay–Hunt syndrome (nervus intermedius neuralgia). What is the most likely other physical exam finding present?

    A. Left-sided conductive hearing loss
    B. Deviation of tongue to left
    C. Pain with palpation of the right nasolabial fold
    D. Blanching of right V_2 and V_3 distribution
    E. Herpetiform rash overlying concha and helix of right ear

5. Superior laryngeal neuralgia can result in which of the following signs/symptoms?

    A. Sharp pain in jaw with chewing
    B. Unilateral vocal cord paralysis
    C. Uncontrollable painful coughing

D. Airway obstruction

E. Headache with conjunctival injection and tearing

6. Which trigeminal branch neuralgia is precipitated by touching the ipsilateral nostril and abolished by local anesthetic blockade?

A. Supraorbital neuralgia

B. Nasociliary neuralgia

C. Lacrimal neuralgia

D. Infraorbital neuralgia

E. Supratrochlear neuralgia

7. A 25-year-old female presents with a 1-week history of blurred vision and pain developing behind her right eye with vision impairment. She reports a paracentral "blind spot" in the visual field of her right eye. She has also noted occasional tremor when doing desk work and muscular fatigue. What is the most likely diagnosis?

A. Diabetic neuropathy

B. Encephalomyelitis

C. Lyme disease

D. Multiple sclerosis

E. Vitamin B_{12} deficiency

8. A 59-year-old male with a history of HIV presents with pain involving the right orbital region, forehead, and auriculotemporal area that has persisted for 4 months following eruption of vesicles in the same distribution. Which of the following treatments is considered first-line therapy?

A. Amitriptyline

B. Oxycodone

C. Topical capsaicin

D. Duloxetine

E. Botulinum toxin

9. A 28-year-old female who sustained head trauma in an automobile accident 3 months ago as an unrestrained front seat passenger in which her head shattered the windshield presents complaining of persistent, worsening unilateral pain in the right forehead region. What is the likely cause of her continued pain?

A. Frontal sinusitis

B. Cluster headache

C. Supraorbital neuralgia

D. Whiplash injury

E. Chronic migraine without aura

10. Which of the following procedures would block innervation to the most superior cervical sympathetic ganglion?

A. Trigeminal ganglion block

B. Retrobulbar block

C. Sphenopalatine ganglion block

D. Gasserian ganglion block

E. Stellate ganglion block

11. A 38-year-old female with a history of diabetes, depression, and chronic pain was recently admitted for facial droop, arm weakness, and slurred speech. She now reports unilateral left facial pain with features such as allodynia, pins and needles sensation, and electrical shocks. What would be the next step to confirm the suspected diagnosis?

A. Positron emission tomography scan

B. Lumbar puncture

C. Evoked potential testing

D. Quantitative sensory testing

E. Head computed tomography (CT) scan

12. When performing a fluoroscopically guided sphenopalatine ganglion radiofrequency ablation, confirmation of location using stimulation at 0.5 V at 50 Hz elicits paresthesias in the patient's upper left teeth. Where should the needle be redirected to ensure adequate placement?

A. Anteriorly

B. Laterally

C. Posterior and medially

D. Caudally

E. Current placement is ideal

13. When performing a blockade of the maxillary and mandibular branches of the trigeminal nerve from the lateral approach, a needle will need to be advanced through which of the following structures?

A. Foramen magnum

B. Coronoid notch

C. Foramen spinosum

D. Mandibular foramen

E. Superior orbital fissure

14. A 74-year-old female presents for pain management after a visit to her dentist in which she was diagnosed with severe periodontal disease. Which of the following physical exam findings is likely to be present?

A. Erythema and bleeding of gingival tissue

B. Fractures molars

C. Exposed dentin

D. Lancinating pain throughout the mandible

E. Numbness of the left side of her chin

15. A middle-aged female presents to clinic complaining of generalized burning sensation of the lips and

tongue. On examination, there is no evidence of dry mouth, inflammation, or edema. Extensive laboratory workup includes HbA1C, vitamin levels, erythrocyte sedimentation rate, and C-reactive protein, which are within normal ranges. What is the likely diagnosis?

A. Diabetic neuropathy
B. Folate deficiency
C. Sjögren's syndrome
D. Burning mouth syndrome
E. Mucositis

16. A professional boxer complains of worsening pain in the left jaw, ear, and neck with talking and eating. He reports a clicking sound with mouth opening and closing. What is the expected finding on imaging?

A. Left-sided retropharyngeal abscess on CT
B. MRI demonstrating anteriorly displaced articular disk of the left temporomandibular joint
C. Fracture of the left mandible on plain films
D. Microaneurysm in left temporal artery on angiography
E. Extension of otitis media with effusion into bone on CT

17. A middle-aged stockbroker status post radiation treatment for salivary gland carcinoma complains of a "frozen jaw" and progressively worsening pain with chewing and talking. On examination, he demonstrates minimal jaw oral opening restricted by pain and anxiety. Electromyography (EMG) demonstrates decreased activity with contraction, and MRI shows an intact temporomandibular joint. What is the likely diagnosis and cause of this problem?

A. Oral parafunction from bruxism and clenching
B. Postural hypertonicity secondary to chronic forward neck position at his computer
C. Myofibrotic contracture due to restricted movement after radiation therapy
D. Masticatory muscle injury from distant motor vehicle accident
E. Myositis from direct blow to muscle

18. A college-aged male presents 3 months after parotid gland surgery with unilateral hyperhidrosis and flushing of the right malar region and pinna of the ear when eating or drinking. What interventional treatment option is the treatment of choice for this diagnosis?

A. Auriculotemporal nerve block
B. Buccal fold injection
C. Temporomandibular joint injection
D. Stylohyoid ligament injection
E. Trochlear nerve block

19. A 48-year-old female with poor dentition and newly diagnosed intraoral mass presents with pain at rest with significant aggravation with chewing. You believe an inferior alveolar nerve block is warranted for diagnosis and treatment of the pain source. What is the location of the patient's pain?

A. Left upper canine
B. Hard palate
C. Left upper incisors
D. Right lower molars
E. Left posterior third of the tongue

20. A 32-year-old female presents for evaluation with chronic facial pain lasting greater than 6 months with depressed mood. What symptom is LEAST likely to be present in this patient?

A. Fatigue
B. Anorexia
C. Anhedonia
D. Depressed mood
E. Hyperphagia

21. When examining a 53-year-old male referred for pain in the jaw, teeth periorbital region, and headaches, he complains of a palpable "knot" in his jaw. The pain improves with range-of-motion exercises. He describes weakness when chewing but does not endorse any sensory deficits. Which of the following characteristics would be expected on physical exam?

A. Shooting, paroxysmal pain with light touch
B. Eliciting a grimace when applying pressure to the masseter
C. Purulent discharge from ipsilateral tonsillar fossa
D. Audible painful click with opening of the mandible
E. Bulging ipsilateral tympanic membrane

22. Which of the following statements regarding glossopharyngeal neuralgia is true?

A. It is commonly secondary to vascular compression of the geniculate ganglion.
B. Sensation from the glossopharyngeal nerve receives input from the anterior third of the tongue.
C. Bilateral presentation is six times more likely than in trigeminal neuralgia.
D. Treatment often involves a stylectomy.
E. First-line treatment for mild cases is rhizotomy.

23. A patient presents with unilateral sharp, paroxysmal pain in the right maxillary and mandibular region provoked by touch, such as putting a shirt on over his head. Physical examination of the face demonstrates

no sensory deficits throughout. Which of the following is considered adequate first-line treatment of his condition?

A. Tramadol
B. Gamma knife radiotherapy
C. Diclofenac
D. Carbamazepine
E. Fentanyl

24. Following extraction of the right second molar, a patient develops painful numbness in the right chin and right lower lip, with treatment refractory to antiepileptic medications, nonsteroidal anti-inflammatory drugs (NSAIDs), and short-acting opioids. CT scan of the head, basal skull, mandible, and neck was unremarkable. Which of the following procedures is indicated at this time?

A. Posterior superior alveolar nerve block
B. Auriculotemporal radiofrequency ablation
C. Local infiltration at the mental foramen
D. Injection of the marginal mandibular branch
E. Ketamine infusion

25. Which of the following scales on the Minnesota Multiphasic Personality Inventory (MMPI) is associated with the patient population with postherpetic neuralgia compared to that with trigeminal neuralgia?

A. Depression
B. Psychopathic deviate
C. Schizophrenia
D. Hypomania
E. Paranoia

ANSWERS

1. ANSWER: B

Trigeminal neuralgia is a neuropathic disorder typified by brief episodes of intense facial pain. Diagnosis involves the presence of paroxysmal pain confined to the trigeminal distribution that is generally unilateral in nature, with normal sensory examination on sensory exam and reproduction of pain at areas considered trigger zones by light touch. The distribution can involve all major branches of the trigeminal nerve (CN V), including the ophthalmic (V_1), maxillary (V_2), and mandibular (V_3). Although pain is generally unilateral, bilateral cases do occur. Literature review of trigeminal neuralgia pain demonstrates that right-sided attacks (61%) are more common than left-sided attacks (36%) or bilateral cases (4%). The distribution of pain is most common in $V_2 + V_3$ (36%), followed by $V_1 + V_2 + V_3$ (17%), V_2 alone (17%), V_3 alone (15%), $V_1 + V_2$ (14%), and V_1 alone (4%).

FURTHER READING

Rozen TD. Trigeminal neuralgia and glossopharyngeal neuralgia. *Neurol Clin.* 2004;22:185–206.

2. ANSWER: D

Initial treatment of trigeminal neuralgia typically involves trials of single or multiple antiepileptic drug treatment. In patients who demonstrate symptoms refractory to multiple trials of medication management, or in patients with severe pain, interventional options are generally trialed. When considering the treatment options and the decision process comparing medical and surgical treatments for trigeminal neuralgia, microvascular decompression, percutaneous balloon microcompression, and percutaneous glycerol rhizolysis provide the highest quality of life, or maximum expected utility. Gamma knife or radiofrequency thermoablation may be considered for elderly patients or those with no evidence of vascular compression. Pulsed radiofrequency ablation is a safer alternative than thermal radiofrequency ablation; however, its efficacy is questioned in randomized controlled trials. Patients who are refractory to first- and second-line medication therapies likely will not benefit from further trials.

FURTHER READING

Spatz AL, Zakrzewska JM, Kay EJ. Decision analysis of medical and surgical treatments in trigeminal neuralgia. *Pain.* 2007;131:302–310.

3. ANSWER: A

Glossopharyngeal neuralgia is a fairly uncommon pain syndrome that affects the glossopharyngeal nerve (CN IX) and is characterized by severe, sharp stabbing pain experienced in the ear, base of tongue, tonsillar fossa, or beneath the angle of the jaw. Generally, it is unilateral in nature and lasts for a few seconds up to 2 minutes. The pain is transmitted via the auricular and pharyngeal branches of the glossopharyngeal nerve, along with the auricular and pharyngeal branches of the vagus nerve (CN X). Occasionally, parasympathetic functions of the vagus nerve can be involved with this syndrome, resulting in bradycardia, asystole, syncopal episodes, and convulsions. It is frequently misdiagnosed as trigeminal neuralgia and similarly can be confused with nervus intermedius neuralgia or superior laryngeal neuralgia. Compared to trigeminal neuralgia, it is uncommon, affecting an estimated 0.2–0.7 per 100,000 patients.

FURTHER READING

Pope JE, Narouze S. Orofacial pain. In: Benzon H, Raja S, Fishman S, et al. (Eds.), *Essentials of Pain Medicine.* 3rd ed. Philadelphia, PA: Saunders; 2011:283–293.

4. ANSWER: E

Ramsay–Hunt syndrome (RHS; also known as geniculate neuralgia or nervus intermedius neuralgia) is defined as peripheral facial nerve palsy accompanied by an erythematous vesicular rash on the ear (zoster oticus) or in the mouth. It is often difficult to distinguish from Bell's palsy (facial paralysis without rash); however, RHS patients often have more severe paralysis at onset and are less likely to recover completely. Varicella zoster virus infection of the seventh cranial nerve produces the underlying pathophysiology of RHS. Primary infection (varicella or chicken pox) commonly occurs as a pediatric generalized vesicular rash. Varicella zoster virus remains latent in the neurons of the cranial nerve and the dorsal root ganglion, and it can become reactivated, resulting in localized vesicular rash (herpes zoster). This reactivation in the CN VII distribution can present as RHS. Other frequent symptoms are tinnitus, hearing loss, nausea, vertigo, and nystagmus.

FURTHER READING

Sweeney CL, Gilden DH. Ramsay Hunt syndrome. *J Neurol Neurosurg Psychiatry.* 2001;71:149–154.

5. ANSWER: C

Superior laryngeal neuralgia is a rare disorder characterized by paroxysmal pain, generally unilateral, in the lateral aspect of the throat, submandibular region, and around the ear. The superior laryngeal nerve is a branch of the vagus nerve that arises from the ganglion nodosum and descends lateral to the pharynx behind the internal carotid artery. It receives a branch of sympathetic fibers from the superior cervical ganglion. The nerve splits into the external and internal laryngeal nerves, which innervate the cricothyroid and provide sensory innervation above the vocal cords, respectively. Superior laryngeal neuralgia can occur from trauma, postoperative complication, laryngitis, and compression from hematoma or tumor. Triggers include compression of the hyoid bone, chewing, and head extension or rotation. It can be associated with uncontrollable coughing. Sharp pain in the jaw with chewing is typical of trigeminal neuralgia in the V_3 distribution. Unilateral vocal cord paralysis and airway obstruction occur with damage to the recurrent laryngeal nerve(s), unilaterally and bilaterally, respectively. Short-lasting unilateral neuralgiform headache with conjunctival injection and tearing is the definition of SUNCT syndrome.

FURTHER READING

De Simone R, Ranieri A, Bilo L, et al. Cranial neuralgias: From physiopathology to pharmacological treatment. *Neurol Sci.* 2008;29:S69–S78.

6. ANSWER: B

The nasociliary nerve is a branch of the ophthalmic nerve (V_1) that enters the orbit in close proximity to the oculomotor nerve (CN III) and optic nerve (CN II). It passes through the anterior ethmoidal opening, where it becomes the anterior ethmoidal nerve. It supplies branches to the mucous membrane of the nasal cavity and external nares. When pathologic processes exist, nasociliary neuralgia can produce transient lancinating pain in the ipsilateral nostril. The supraorbital nerve produces pain in the forehead. The supratrochlear region is just superior to the superior orbital ridge, including the eyebrows. The lacrimal nerve is present on the lateral aspect of the orbits. The infraorbital nerve is a branch of V_2 and is lateral and inferior to the nostril. Essentially all trigeminal branch neuralgias can be abolished, at least temporarily, by blockade from local anesthetic.

FURTHER READING

Pope JE, Narouze S. Orofacial pain. In: Benzon H, Raja S, Fishman S, et al. (Eds.), *Essentials of Pain Medicine.* 3rd ed. Philadelphia, PA: Saunders; 2011:283–293.

7. ANSWER: D

Optic neuritis (pain in CN II) is a clinical diagnosis described as pain behind one or both eyes that coexists with central vision impairment from a scotoma. It is secondary to optic nerve inflammation. Acute demyelinating optic neuritis is often the first clinical presenting manifestation of multiple sclerosis, which also has features of blurred/double vision, muscle weakness, tremor, loss of balance, numbness, and tingling. During a 10-year follow-up, multiple sclerosis was diagnosed in 38% of patients with a first episode of optic neuritis. Gadolinium-enhanced MRI of the brain should be performed, with the orbits often showing enlargement of the optic nerves. However, more importantly, imaging can demonstrate the presence of demyelinating lesions, indicating multiple sclerosis.

Diabetic neuropathy can produce progressive vision loss. Encephalomyelitis is inflammation of both the brain and the spinal cord that often presents with meningeal signs (neck stiffness, headache, and fever). Lyme disease is a tick-borne illness with systemic signs such as rash and flu-like symptoms. Vitamin B_{12} deficiency can cause neuropathy involving the central and peripheral nervous system, which can rarely affect the optic nerves (0.5%). However, generally these symptoms appear with paresthesias in the extremities, weakness, and sore tongue.

FURTHER READING

Balcer LJ. Optic neuritis. *N Engl J Med.* 2006;354:1273–1280.

8. ANSWER: A

Facial postherpetic neuralgia (PHN) is defined as pain in the distribution of the affected nerve of a herpes zoster (shingles) outbreak persisting for 3 months following the skin manifestations. Zoster entails the reactivation in the dorsal root ganglion of varicella zoster virus. It is often seen in the elderly and immunocompromised patients. Pain can be severe and debilitating in nature. Multiple agents have been trialed as treatment options for this disease. Recent guidelines by the International Association for the Study of Pain and the American Academy of Neurology recommend the following medications in the treatment based on evidence-based algorithms. First-line agents include tricyclic antidepressants and gabapentinoids. Second-line agents include lidocaine patches (5%), capsaicin patches (8%), and tramadol. Third-line agents include stronger opioids (oxycodone, hydrocodone, methadone, etc.) and botulinum toxin. Serotonin and norepinephrine reuptake inhibitors have not been effectively studied for treatment of PHN. There is inconclusive evidence on the efficacy of antiepileptics, capsaicin cream, topical clonidine, selective serotonin reuptake inhibitors, and NMDA antagonists.

FURTHER READING

Haanpaa M, Rice ASC, Rowbotham MD. Treating herpes zoster and postherpetic neuralgia. *Pain Clin Update*. 2015;23(4).

9. ANSWER: C

The supraorbital nerve is the terminal branch of the frontal nerve (the largest branch of the ophthalmic nerve, V_1). It passes through the supraorbital foramen and supplies sensation to the upper eyelid, the conjunctiva of the eye, the frontal sinus, and the skin from the forehead to the middle of the scalp. It can be impacted after blunt trauma (e.g., deceleration trauma against a car windshield) at the area of the supraorbital notch. Scar formation can occur around the nerve, causing worsening pain as the scar enlarges. Diagnosis can be made with local injection of the supraorbital nerve at the supraorbital notch, which can be following by cryoablation if conservative treatment fails to provide long-lasting relief. This can frequently be confused with migraines or frontal sinusitis often co-occurring with blurred vision, nausea, and photophobia, but supraorbital neuralgia is generally diagnosed by history and response to diagnostic nerve blocks. Although typically unilateral, cluster headaches have a cyclical time course and are not related to trauma. Whiplash injury is typically muscular in nature, involving the posterior cervical paraspinous musculature.

FURTHER READING

Klein DS, Schmidt RE. Chronic headache resulting from postoperative supraorbital neuralgia. *Anesth Analg*. 1991;73:490.

10. ANSWER: C

The superior cervical ganglia are a part of the sympathetic nervous system. The sphenopalatine ganglion (also called the pterygopalatine ganglion) is the superior most constellation of this system and is located in the pterygopalatine fossa inferior to the maxillary nerve on the posterior wall of the nasopharynx. The sympathetic fibers originate in the superior cervical plexus and ascend through the carotid plexus. The deep petrosal nerve enters the sphenopalatine ganglion to provide vasoconstrictive functionality. The ganglion also receives parasympathetic and sensory input. Trigeminal ganglion block and gasserian ganglion block are synonymous, with the trigeminal

ganglion providing no sympathetic contribution. A retrobulbar block would block cranial nerves II, III, IV, and VI, providing akinesia and anesthesia for eye surgery. A stellate ganglion injection does block innervation of the cervical sympathetic chain; however, it is inferior to the sphenopalatine ganglion.

FURTHER READING

Day M. Sympathetic blocks: The evidence. *Pain Pract*. 2008;4(2): 98–109.

11. ANSWER: E

This patient demonstrates a history and symptoms suggestive of central post-stroke pain. Pain is a direct result from the cerebrovascular lesion in the somatosensory nervous system. The criteria were clarified in 2009 in an attempt to exclude other causes of pain in patients suspected of having a cerebrovascular accident. These criteria include both mandatory and supportive conditions. The mandatory conditions are (1) pain within an area of the body corresponding to a central nervous system (CNS) lesion, (2) a history suggestive of stroke and onset of pain at or after stroke onset, (3) confirmation of a CNS lesion by imaging and/ or negative or positive sensory signs confined to the area of the body corresponding to the CNS lesion, and (4) exclusion of other possible causes. The supportive criteria are (1) no primary association with movement, inflammation, or other local tissue damage; (2) certain descriptions such as burning, painful cold, electric shocks, aching, pressing, stinging, and pins and needles; and (3) allodynia or dysesthesia to touch.

FURTHER READING

Kilt HM, Finnerup NB, Jensen TS. Diagnosis, prevalence, characteristics and treatment of central poststoke pain. *Pain Clin Update*. 2015;23(3).

12. ANSWER: D

Sphenopalatine ganglion blockade can be performed with several different approaches. The most common is the anterior transnasal approach, which involves utilizing pledgets or cotton tip swabs soaked in local anesthetic that are placed through the nares to the mucosa of the posterior nasopharynx, allowing diffusion of local anesthetic to the sphenopalatine ganglion. The intraoral approach accesses the ganglion via the greater palatine foramen, identified by a dimple on the medial aspect of the posterior hard palate. Using fluoroscopy in the lateral view, aligning the two pterygopalatine plates within the pterygopalatine fossa provides a targeted approach, thus allowing the utilization of radiofrequency ablation for longer duration blockade if diagnostic blocks have produced significant temporary relief. The needle is placed under the zygoma in the coronoid notch and advanced into the lateral aspect of the wall of the pterygopalatine fossa but medial to the maxillary sinus. To confirm adequate positioning with nerve stimulation, when positioned correctly, the patient will describe paresthesia at the root of the nose. If the needle is too close to the maxillary nerve, sensation will be felt in the upper teeth, and it should be repositioned more caudally. If stimulation produces paresthesias in the hard palate, this indicates that the location is too lateral and anterior, at the greater and lesser palatine nerves. The needle should be redirected posteriorly and medially.

FURTHER READING

Leong MS, Glolaj MP, Gaeta RR. Sphenopalatine ganglion block. In: Deer TR, Leong MS, Buvanendran A, et al. (Eds.), *Comprehensive Treatment of Chronic Pain by Medical, Interventional and Integrative Approaches*. New York, NY: Springer; 2013:303–307.

13. ANSWER: B

Blockade of the maxillary and mandibular branches of the trigeminal nerve is usually done in the lateral approach under fluoroscopic guidance passing through the mandibular notch, also known as the coronoid notch. The patient opens and closes his or her mouth multiple times to identify the mandibular notch. The needle is advanced through the notch and through the infratemporal fossa, with the end point at the lateral pterygoid plate. End positioning is slightly superior and posterior for the maxillary nerve, whereas the mandibular nerve requires slight caudad and anterior angulation. The foramen magnum and spinosum are foramina in the base of the skull posterior to the mandibular and maxillary branches that would not be accessed in this block. The superior orbital fissure contains CN II, IV, V_1, and VI, as well as the superior ophthalmic vein. The mandibular foramen houses the mandibular nerve on the medial aspect of the angle of the jaw, which would not be traversed in this block.

FURTHER READING

Mchaourab A, Kabbara AI. Neural blockade for trigeminal neuralgia. In: Deer TR, Leong MS, Buvanendran A, et al. (Eds.), *Comprehensive Treatment of Chronic Pain by Medical, Interventional and Integrative Approaches*. New York, NY: Springer; 2013:319–328.

14. ANSWER: A

Periodontal disease is classified as an immune-mediated inflammatory process that can result in focal or generalized areas of destruction of the gingiva, periodontal ligament, cementum, and alveolar bone. Patients typically experience tenderness or gingival enlargement, with inflammation and bleeding with probing or brushing. The roots of the teeth can become exposed with loss of bone support, resulting in tooth sensitivity, tenderness, and mobility. Tooth percussion over compromised periodontium can provoke pain, and inflammation or abscess can be present on exam. Treatment is generally with NSAIDs, non-opiate analgesics, antibiotics, mouthwashes, or drainage/debridement of tissues.

A cracked or fractured tooth should be detectable on examination or X-ray. Dentinal pain is brief, sharp pain evoked by various stimuli to the dentin, such as hot or cold drinks. Lancinating pain is characteristic of trigeminal neuralgia, and numbness of the chin is suggestive of mental neuropathy.

FURTHER READING

Mehta NR, Scrivani SJ, Spierings ELH. Dental and facial pain. In: Benzon H, Rathmell JP, Wu CL, et al. (Eds.), *Practical Management of Pain*. 5rd ed. Philadelphia, PA: Mosby; 2013: 424–440.

15. ANSWER: D

The diagnosis of burning mouth syndrome is one of exclusion after no underlying dental or medical causes are identified and no oral signs are found in a patient experiencing focal or generalized burning sensation. This disorder is most common in postmenopausal females. It is thought to be a disorder of neuropathic pain of either central or peripheral origin. Unfortunately, although multiple interventions have been trialed in treatment of this disorder, little evidence indicates that any specific medication or cognitive-based treatment is effective.

Lack of objective findings on exam or laboratory values excludes the other options as correct answers.

FURTHER READING

Lauria G, Majorana A, Borgna M, et al. Trigeminal small-fiber sensory neuropathy causes burning mouth syndrome. *Pain*. 2005; 115:332–337.

16. ANSWER: B

Temporomandibular joint (TMJ) disk displacement is frequently the underlying pathology when clicking sounds are audible with mouth opening and closing. The term *reduction* is used when the disc moves back into alignment between the condyl and fossa during opening, with displacement with closing of the jaw. TMJ commonly involves pain of the joint itself with radiation to the ipsilateral ear, as well as pain and neck stiffness. TMJ disorder is often secondary to trauma (e.g., blunt trauma to the head/jaw) or bruxism. MRI and CT are often utilized to rule out tumors or determine the extent of advanced degenerative stages, if suspected. Internal derangement of the TMJ disc on imaging identifies articular causes compared to muscular or myofascial origins of TMD.

FURTHER READING

Mehta NR, Scrivani SJ, Spierings ELH. Dental and facial pain. In: Benzon H, Rathmell JP, Wu CL, et al. (Eds.), *Practical Management of Pain*. 5rd ed. Philadelphia, PA: Mosby; 2013: 424–440.

17. ANSWER: C

The muscles of mastication can demonstrate multiple types of pathology that affect the ability to open the jaw adequately and elicit pain. They are often difficult to distinguish because frequently there are overlapping symptoms. The patient in question works as a stockbroker and could demonstrate TMJ disorder from bruxism/clenching from a high-stress occupation, postural tonicity from exaggerated forward positioning sitting at a desk, and muscle injury from a trauma. However, due to the progressively worsening nature following radiation treatment near the area in question, decreased EMG activity, and no pathology at the joint, the likely diagnosis is myofibrotic contracture. This occurs in muscles that are not allowed to function within their full range of motion and, as a result a gradual shortening of the muscle takes place. There occurs fibrotic healing of damaged tissues, as would occur following radiation, which results in limited interincisal opening.

FURTHER READING

Mehta NR, Scrivani SJ, Spierings ELH. Dental and facial pain. In: Benzon H, Rathmell JP, Wu CL, et al. (Eds.), *Practical Management of Pain*. 5rd ed. Philadelphia, PA: Mosby; 2013: 424–440.

18. ANSWER: A

Frey syndrome (also known as auriculotemporal syndrome, Baillarger syndrome, gustatory sweating syndrome, Dupuy syndrome, or salivosudoriparous syndrome) is a constellation of unilateral symptoms that occur in the malar area anterior to the ear in the auriculotemporal distribution. It can occur 2–14 months after surgery, open trauma, or infection of the parotid gland. It is thought to be secondary to improper regeneration of the sympathetic and parasympathetic nerves following an injury. Medical management can consist of topical antiperspirants or scopolamine cream; however, in severe cases, blockade of the auriculotemporal nerve is the treatment of choice. This can be combined this intradermal injection of botulism toxin.

The technique of blockade of the auriculotemporal nerve involves identifying the ipsilateral temporal artery above the origin of the zygoma. A 25-gauge, 1.5-in. needle is inserted in a perpendicular manner anterior to the auricle toward the periosteum. A paresthesia can be elicited. After negative aspiration, 3 ml of local plus steroid is administered. An additional 2 ml of solution can be injected cephalad to this point in a fan-like manner for field block in the auriculotemporal distribution.

FURTHER READING

Waldman SD. Auriculotemporal nerve block. In: Waldman SD (Ed.), *Atlas of Pain Management Injection Techniques*. 3rd ed. Philadelphia, PA: Saunders; 2012:40–41.

19. ANSWER: D

The inferior alveolar nerve block can provide emergency pain relief for lower molar dental pain while waiting for definitive treatment of dental pain. It is a branch of the mandibular nerve, which dives into the mandible through the mandibular foramen. The lingual nerve also innervates the lingual gingiva of the lower molars and thus should be concomitantly blocked for satisfactory anesthesia. Both can be blocked with one injection site through the oral mucosa on the medial aspect of the mandibular ramus at the lateral margin of the pterygoid muscle.

Innervation of the hard palate is by the maxillary branch of the trigeminal nerve. The superior alveolar nerve innervates the upper canines and incisions. The sensory innervation of the tongue is split between the mandibular nerve covering the anterior two-thirds, the glossopharyngeal nerve covering the posterior third, and the vagus contributing to the posterior root of the tongue.

FURTHER READING

Waldman SD. Auriculotemporal nerve block. In: Waldman SD (Ed.), *Atlas of Pain Management Injection Techniques*. 3rd ed. Philadelphia, PA: Saunders; 2012:40–41.

20. ANSWER: E

There appears to be a significant connection between chronic pain and psychiatric comorbidities such as depression, and facial pain is not exempt from this. In a study by Korszun et al., 53% of patients presenting for tertiary referral for chronic facial pain met criteria for major or minor depression, with an additional 22% demonstrating some depressive symptoms. This compares to approximately 20% of the general population. However, the distribution of depression did not differ between patients with or without objective physical or imaging findings to account for their pain symptoms. This suggests that the experience of the pain itself, and not the pathology, drives the association. Given this high association, screening for symptoms of depression and subsequent treatment should be considered an integral part of the evaluation. Of the patients exhibiting chronic facial pain, the symptoms that had the largest discrepancies in those diagnosed with or without depression were depressed mood, anhedonia, and anorexia. Symptoms of fatigue, insomnia, and a precipitating life event were higher in the depressed group but not to the same extent of significance. Hyperphagia was uncommon in both groups, but it occurred slightly more commonly in those without depression.

FURTHER READING

Korszun A, Hinderstein B, Wong M. Comorbidity of depression with chronic facial pain and temporomandibular disorders. *Oral Surg Oral Med Oral Pathol Oral Radiol Endod*. 1996;82:496–500.

21. ANSWER: B

This patient presents with symptoms suggestive of myofascial pain disorder with muscle trigger points. The features of trigger points include (1) local tenderness over a discrete area in muscle; (2) referred pain, tenderness, and autonomic phenomena; (3) palpable taut band associated with trigger point; (4) a local twitch response usually present in a taut band; (5) therapeutic effect with stretching of the trigger point; (6) perpetuation of the trigger point; and (7) weakness/fatigability of muscles afflicted by the trigger point. Pain is generally dull or aching in nature rather than sharp or shooting. There can be restricted movement with active or passive range of motion. Applying pressure on the trigger point can elicit a "jump sign," which is a grimace or involuntary sound from the patient. Treatment can involve stretching; hot compress; range-of-motion exercises; injection with local anesthetic or botulinum toxin; acupuncture; or pharmacological treatment with NSAIDs, muscle relaxants, antidepressants, or other analgesics. These pain mediators can be compounded by stress, nutrition, and hormonal factors, which should also be considered in the treatment plan.

Shooting pain with light touch in this location is generally indicative of trigeminal neuralgia. Purulent discharge from the tonsillar fossa is suggestive of an abscess formation. Clicking sounds from the mandible suggest disorders of the articular component of the TMJ, which would not improve with stretching or demonstrate a taut band of muscle. Otitis media with effusion presents with a bulging tympanic membrane.

FURTHER READING

Travell JG, Simons DG. *Myofascial Pain and Dysfunction: The Trigger Point Manual*. Baltimore, MD: Williams & Wilkins, 1983.

22. ANSWER: C

Glossopharyngeal neuralgia (GN) is a syndrome that manifests as repeated episodes of sharp, stabbing paroxysmal pain in the throat, tongue, ear, and/or tonsils. Causes are generally attributed to compression of the glossopharyngeal nerve by blood vessels, tumors, or abscesses during its course. Pain is generally short-lasting, between 1 or 2 seconds and 2 minutes; can range from mild to severe; and can be triggered by actions such as chewing, coughing, laughing, speaking, or swallowing. Diagnostic tests generally include MRI/MR angiography, head CT, or angiography. It is a rare condition that occurs in approximately 0.2–0.7 per 100,000 patients; however, almost one-fourth of these patients demonstrate bilateral symptoms compared to 4% of patients with trigeminal neuralgia.

Vascular compression of the geniculate ganglion occurs in nervus intermedius neuralgia, a branch of the facial nerve. Sensation from the glossopharyngeal nerve includes the skin of the external ear, internal surface of the tympanic membrane, walls of the upper pharyx, and posterior one-third of the tongue. The trigeminal nerve provides sensation to the anterior two-thirds of the tongue. A rare cause of GN is compression due to the styloid bone, which occasionally will require its surgical removal. First-line treatment for GN is medical management, including carbamazepine, oxcarbazepine, gabapentin, pregabalin, and phenytoin. In severe cases, surgical options such as microvascular decompression and rhizotomy have been shown to be effective as well.

FURTHER READING

Reddy GD, Viswanathan A. Trigeminal and glossopharyngeal neuralgia. *Neurologic Clin*. 2014;32(2):539–552.

23. ANSWER: D

The diagnosis of trigeminal neuralgia is based on the presence of specific criteria, including (1) paroxysmal pain, (2) confined to the trigeminal distribution, (3) generally unilateral in nature, (4) normal sensory examination on sensory exam, and (5) production of pain at areas considered trigger zones by light touch. Treatment of trigeminal neuralgia generally starts with medical options, with surgical treatments available for severe or refractory pain. Multiple trials of antiepileptic drugs (AEDs) have been performed, with evidence showing that carbamazepine, oxcarbazepine, lamotrigine, gabapentin, topiramate, and baclofen are effective in the treatment of this disorder. If a patient does not respond to a single medication, often adding a second AED may increase the probability of a therapeutic response; this produces a satisfactory pain response in 70% of patients. Those whose pain is refractory to multiple combinations of the various AED options can be considered for peripheral local anesthetic blockade or surgical treatment, including percutaneous retrogasserian, radiofrequency lesioning, posterior fossa microvascular decompression, or gamma knife radiotherapy.

FURTHER READING

Mehta NR, Scrivani SJ, Spierings ELH. Dental and facial pain. In: Benzon H, Rathmell JP, Wu CL, et al. (Eds.), *Practical Management of Pain*. 5rd ed. Philadelphia, PA: Mosby; 2013:424–440.

24. ANSWER: C

The trigeminal nerve has three primary branches—the ophthalmic, maxillary, and mandibular—that exit the skull through three separate foramina (the superior orbital fissure, the foramen rotundum, and the foramen ovale, respectively). The mandibular nerve (V_3) has nine branches—recurrent meningeal, medial pterygoid, masseteric, deep temporal, lateral pterygoid, buccal, auriculotemporal, lingual, and inferior alveolar—that combine to provide sensory information from the lower lip, lower teeth, gums, chin, and jaw. The angle of the mandible is supplied by C2–C3 and is not supplied by V_3. The inferior alveolar nerve accompanies the inferior alveolar artery as it travels through the mandibular foramen and canal, where it exits at the mental foramen as the mental nerve. Mental nerve neuropathy, also called numb chin syndrome, can manifest as a painful numbness overlying unilateral lower limb and chin. Its presence is often linked to the presence of metastatic cancer compressing the coursing inferior alveolar or exiting mental nerves; however, it can be caused by dental disease/extractions, trauma, cysts, mandibular atrophy, temporomandibular disorders, and others causes. Diagnosis and treatment can be confirmed following successful local infiltration at the mental foramen, with reports of subsequent radiofrequency ablation providing longer term results.

The posterior superior alveolar nerve is a branch of the maxillary nerve that innervates the second and third maxillary molars and two of the three roots of the first molar. The auriculotemporal nerve is one of the proximal branches of the mandibular nerve (V_3) that is somatosensory in nature, supplying the auricle, external acoustic meatus, outer side of the tympanic membrane and skin in the temporal region, in addition to some of the TMJ. The marginal mandibular branch of the facial nerve passes beneath the platysma and depressor anguli oris, providing motor innervation of the muscles and the lower lip and chin, including the depressor labii inferioris, the depressor anguli oris, and mentalis. It communicates with the mental branch of the inferior alveolar nerve, but it is not involved in sensation. Intravenous ketamine infusion has not been described in the literature as a treatment for mental nerve neuropathy.

FURTHER READING

Divya KS, Moran NA, Atkin PA. Numb chin syndrome: A case series and discussion. *Br Dental J.* 2010;208:157–160.

25. ANSWER: A

Patients experiencing chronic pain have been shown to report more frequent psychosocial problems compared to patients with other chronic illnesses. It is believed that the experience of pain itself is a strong contributor to the manifestation of these psychological comorbidities. In comparing the patient populations with postherpetic neuralgia and those with trigeminal neuralgia, those with postherpetic neuralgia demonstrate significantly greater psychological dysfunction and disability. The MMPI is the most widely used and researched standardized psychometric test of adult personality and psychopathology. Examining the characteristics on the MMPI psychometric test, patients with PHN demonstrated elevations in the H (hypochondriasis), D (depression), and Hy (hysteria) scales compared to the trigeminal neuralgia group. This profile mimics that of other chronic pain conditions, suggesting that the temporal distribution of pain significantly affects the amount of disturbance. It is hypothesized that the continuous unrelenting pain of conditions such as postherpetic neuralgia that are without substantial periods of relief account for the difference; compared to TN, which produces sharp intermittent pain, these conditions produce a significantly greater amount of psycho-social dysfunction.

The MMPI scales measuring psychopathic deviate, schizophrenia, hypomania, and paranoia showed no significant difference between the postherpetic neuralgia group and the trigeminal neuralgia group.

FURTHER READING

Graff-Raford SB, Kames LD, Naliboff BD. Measures of psychological adjustment and perception of pain in postherpetic neuralgia and trigeminal neuralgia. *Clin J. Pain*. 1986;2(1):55–58.

24.

NEUROPATHIC PAIN

Ian M. Fowler, Robert J. Hackworth, and Erik P. Voogd

INTRODUCTION

Neuropathic pain encompasses a vast number of clinical conditions that share the common characteristic of pain resulting from nerve injury or damage. Upon injury, pathophysiologic changes in the peripheral nervous system occur, including hyperexcitability and the spontaneous generation of impulses (ectopia). As a result of these peripheral changes, alterations in signal processing and intrinsic changes within the central nervous system occur. All of these changes contribute to the generation of neuropathic pain. This chapter attempts to capture the essence of the objectives and goals set forth by the International Association for the Study of Pain's Core Curriculum for Professional Education in Pain for the topic of neuropathic pain. The questions cover topics including definitions, common clinical conditions, uncommon clinical conditions, therapeutic interventions, pathophysiological mechanisms, and current investigations.

QUESTIONS

1. Neuropathic pain describes painS arising as a direct consequence of a lesion or disease affecting which of the following systems?

A. Motor system
B. Parasympathetic system
C. Somatosensory system
D. Limbic system
E. Sympathetic system

2. A 56-year-old male patient with long-standing, poorly controlled diabetes presents to your clinic complaining of a burning and stinging sensation to his bilateral lower extremities from the mid-calf region distally to the toes. Examination reveals diminished sensation to both tuning fork and coarse monofilament from the mid-calf region distally to the toes in a nondermatomal pattern. Which of the following is a proposed mechanism for the etiology of this condition?

A. Thickening of capillary basement membranes
B. Deposition of glycosylation end products around peripheral nerves
C. Dysregulation of inhibitory interneurons in the spinal cord
D. A and B
E. All of the above

3. A 35-year-old male patient with HIV presents to your clinic complaining of burning and tingling sensations in the bilateral feet. Recent laboratory testing revealed an undetectable viral load. Examination reveals diminished sensation to coarse monofilament across the feet in a nondermatomal pattern. Current medications include didanosine (ddI), lamivudine, rilpivirine, tipranavir, and gabapentin. Which of the following would be your next step in the management of this patient?

A. Discontinuation of ddI in consultation with an HIV specialist
B. Discontinuation of lamivudine in consultation with an HIV specialist
C. Discontinuation of rilpivirine in consultation with an HIV specialist
D. Discontinuation of tipranavir in consultation with an HIV specialist
E. Trial of methadone

4. A 65-year-old male patient is being treated with isoniazid, rifampicin, pyrazinamide, and ethambutol for tuberculosis. The patient develops a deep aching pain in the bilateral calf muscles along with burning sensations in the bilateral upper and lower extremities that he states developed several months after starting these

medications. What medication would best treat this condition?

A. Gabapentin
B. Nortriptyline
C. Vitamin B_{12}
D. Vitamin B_6
E. Vitamin E

5. A 43-year-old male patient with HIV and diabetes mellitus type 2 presents to your clinic with a diagnosis of peripheral neuropathy and complains of severe burning pain to his bilateral distal lower extremities in addition to insomnia secondary to pain. He is currently receiving only non-nucleoside reverse transcriptase inhibitors and protease inhibitors for his HIV treatment, and he has an undetectable viral load. A hemoglobin A1C level from 1 month prior is 4.9. He is currently taking oral meloxicam and acetaminophen for pain control. What would be the next step in management of this patient?

A. Trial of spinal cord stimulation
B. Trial of oxymorphone
C. Trial of valproic acid
D. Trial of oral tramadol
E. Trial of nortriptyline

6. After an axon is injured, the portion of the axon distal to the injury begins to degenerate. This is an example of:

A. Dying back
B. Sprouting
C. Wallerian degeneration
D. Collateral sprouting
E. Neuroma formation

7. Following peripheral nerve injury in animal models, which of the following neuropeptides is associated with upregulation and increased expression in the dorsal root ganglia of the injured nerves?

A. Vasoactive inhibitory peptide (VIP)
B. Calcitonin gene-related peptide (CGRP)
C. Galanin
D. Substance P
E. A and C only

8. Following injury of a peripheral nerve, which of the following occurs within the central nervous system?

A. Gliosis of microglia and astrocytes within the spinal cord
B. Reduced γ-aminobutyric acid (GABA)-mediated spinal cord inhibitory mechanisms
C. Increased spontaneous activity in the thalamus

D. A and B only
E. All of the above

9. Local anesthetic blockade of the nerve identified by white arrows in Figure 24.1 will provide temporary relief of which of the following conditions?

A. Ilioinguinal neuralgia
B. Postoperative medial ankle pain
C. Meralgia paresthetica
D. Orchialgia
E. Plantar fasciitis

10. An 85-year-old female patient presents with a rash on the right side of her mid-back that radiates around the flank to the nipple in a dermatomal pattern that started 2 days ago. She also complains of burning, itching, and severe pain in the vicinity of the rash in addition to a headache and malaise. Which of the following treatments would be appropriate for this patient?

A. Valacyclovir
B. Epidural injection of methylprednisolone
C. Topical capsaicin
D. A and C only
E. All of the above

11. The most common facial site for acute herpes zoster infection and postherpetic neuralgia is the:

A. Facial nerve (CN VII)
B. Trigeminal nerve ophthalmic branch (CN V1)
C. Trigeminal nerve maxillary branch (CN V2)
D. Trigeminal nerve mandibular branch (CN V3)
E. Optic nerve (CN II)

12. A 29-year-old male patient presents with a recent history of a gastrointestinal illness followed by the onset of bilateral lower extremity weakness 1 week following the illness. Examination reveals arreflexia of the knee and ankle jerk reflexes. What percentage of patients with this condition will require ventilatory support?

A. 1%
B. 10%
C. 25%
D. 50%
E. 90%

13. All of the following pharmacologic agents have been shown to be effective in the treatment of postherpetic neuralgia except:

A. Pregabalin
B. Mexiletine

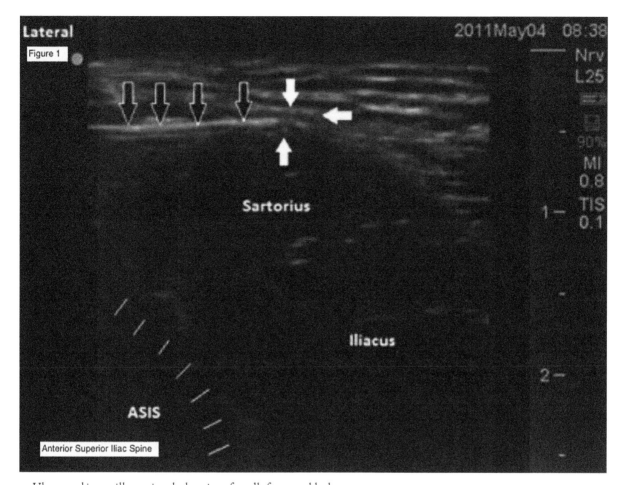

Figure 24.1 Ultrasound image illustrating the location of needle for nerve block.

SOURCE: Reprinted with permission from Fowler IM, Tucker AA, Mendez RJ. Treatment of meralgia paresthetica with ultrasound-guided pulsed radiofrequency ablation of the lateral femoral cutaneous nerve. *Pain Practice*, Volume 12, Issue 5, 2012 394–398.

C. Desipramine
D. Topical TRPV1 agonists
E. Tramadol

C. C7
D. C8
E. T1

14. A delayed F-wave on a nerve conduction study is most useful in diagnosing which of the following neuropathic pain conditions?

A. Cervical radiculopathy
B. Early onset Guillain–Barré syndrome
C. Carpal tunnel syndrome
D. Cubital tunnel syndrome
E. Diabetic peripheral neuropathy

15. You are examining a patient with chronic neck pain with tingling, numbness, radiating pain, and weakness in the left arm. You note decreased sensation to pinprick over the lateral forearm, thumb, and index fingers; diminished brachioradialis reflex; and 4/5 motor strength to biceps flexion and wrist extension. Which spinal nerve root is most likely compromised in this patient?

A. C5
B. C6

16. Which of the following pain quality assessment questionnaires used to help differentiate between nociceptive and neuropathic pain must be administered by a clinician?

A. Neuropathic Pain Questionnaire
B. Leeds Assessment of Neuropathic Symptoms and Signs (LANSS)
C. Neuropathic Pain Diagnostic Questionnaire
D. B and C
E. All of the above

17. All of the following drugs have demonstrated clinical efficacy in randomized trials for the treatment of painful diabetic neuropathy except:

A. Duloxetine
B. Divalproex
C. Pregabalin
D. Fluoxetine
E. B and D

18. A 72-year-old male with diabetic peripheral neuropathy, chronic obstructive pulmonary disease, and renal failure presents to your clinic. The patient complains of moderate to severe burning pain to his feet and ankles. He is currently taking acetaminophen for his pain. Which of the following medications would be the best first choice for treatment of this neuropathic pain?

A. Amitriptyline
B. Morphine
C. Gabapentin
D. Naproxen
E. Clonidine

19. A patient is started on a medication for treatment of a neuropathic pain condition. Several days after starting the medication, the patient complains of sore throat, fever, fatigue, and pain of the tongue and mouth. On examination, ulcerative lesions on the mouth and lips are seen consistent with Stevens–Johnson syndrome. Which of the following medications is the most likely the cause?

A. Pregabalin
B. Lamotrigine
C. Gabapentin
D. Phenobarbital
E. Valproic acid

20. A 55-year-old male undergoes amputation of the right lower extremity. Which of the following factors is a predictor of an increased risk for the development of phantom limb pain?

A. The presence of pre-amputation pain
B. Telescoping
C. Phantom sensations
D. Side of amputation
E. All of the above

21. A 56-year-old male patient who works as a painter at a car body shop presents with complaints of a dull ache in his right upper arm, forearm, and hand. He presents to the clinic with a cervical magnetic resonance imaging (MRI) report that was normal. Upon questioning, he reports decreased strength when gripping objects. His pain is worse at night and while driving. Shaking the hand can temporarily relieve the pain. Neurological exam of the hand is normal to light touch sensation, and motor strength is 5/5 across all muscle groups of the hand and forearm. The provocative test that would most likely elicit painful symptoms or help with the diagnosis would be:

A. Spurling's (neck extension, lateral bending, and rotation with axial compression)
B. Yergason's (forced supination and flexion at the elbow)
C. Phalen's (acute wrist flexion held for 30–60 seconds)
D. Hawkin's (arm fully pronated and forcibly fully flexed)

22. A 47-year-old female violinist presents with forearm and hand pain on the right side for 2 months. She has noticed a decrease in ability to grasp items with her right hand. She denies neck or shoulder pain. Her physical exam is positive for decreased sensation in a median nerve distribution sparing the thenar eminence and a positive Tinel's sign over the carpal tunnel. Phalen's test is positive at 60 seconds. You suspect she has carpal tunnel syndrome. The next most appropriate step would be:

A. Order an electromyogram (EMG) and nerve conduction study (NCS)
B. Consult a hand surgeon
C. Order a cervical spine MRI to rule out radiculopathy
D. Prescribe a hand splint and perform a glucocorticoid injection into the carpal tunnel

23. A 23-year-old male patient underwent a right-sided open inguinal hernia repair 3 months prior. He reports that he received some type of "nerve block" during the perioperative period for pain. He now complains of ongoing lancinating pain and burning paresthesias into his right hemiscrotum, groin, and inner thigh that began soon after the surgery. What is the most likely etiology for his presentation?

A. Herpes zoster recrudescence
B. Surgical trauma to the ilioinguinal and iliohypogastric nerves
C. Ilioinguinal and iliohypogastric nerve injury from a perioperative transversus abdominis plane (TAP) block
D. Surgical trauma to the genitofemoral nerve
E. Ilioinguinal and iliohypogastric nerve injury due to patient positioning

24. An 82-year-old male patient presents with constant burning dysesthesias and allodynia in a band-like distribution encompassing his chest, axilla, and back from approximately T3 to T6, resulting in severe insomnia. He states that he had an open thoracotomy to perform a right upper lobectomy to resect bronchogenic carcinoma 18 months ago and has received radiation treatments to his right upper chest and chemotherapy treatment since then. Careful questioning also elicits the history of a very painful rash in roughly the same

area 12 months ago composed of erythematous vesicular lesions that crusted over after 1 week and finally resolved after 3 weeks. Which of the following etiologies is most likely to explain this patient's current pain complaint?

A. Post-thoracotomy neuropathic pain
B. Radiation-induced neuropathy
C. Chemotherapy-induced neuropathy
D. Postherpetic neuralgia
E. Intraoperative patient positioning

25. A 32-year-old right-hand-dominant woman presents with an insidious onset of pain and numbness in the palm and in her first three digits bilaterally, right worse than left. She states that the numbness and pain are usually worse at night and upon waking, with minimal improvement throughout the day. She is concerned that she may lose her job because she has started dropping expensive electronic components frequently during her work on the assembly line. You are concerned that she may be developing worsening carpal tunnel syndrome. Which of the following tests and examinations would be useful in confirming the diagnosis?

A. Tinel's sign with light percussion over the median nerve at the wrist
B. EMG and NCS
C. MRI of the wrist
D. Phalen's sign
E. All of the above

26. A 34-year-old male patient presents to your clinic in a motorized wheelchair with a 2-year history of worsening burning pain and allodynia in a sock-like distribution on the right lower extremity from his toes to mid-calf that began after a pronation injury to his ankle. In the past year, he noted the onset of hair loss, mottling, increased sweating, and significant decreases in skin temperature in the right lower extremity compared to his left lower extremity. His primary care provider has been treating his pain since the original injury with high-dose opioids but is concerned about rapid dose escalations during the past few months. His pain at rest is rated as 8/10 (numeric rating scale) and escalates to 10/10 when the limb is touched or upon ambulation. His medications include sustained-release oxycodone 80 mg PO BID, immediate-release oxycodone 15 mg PO Q4 hours as needed (averaging five or six tabs per day), and gabapentin 300 mg PO TID. The patient also reports a transcutaneous electrical nerve stimulator makes the pain worse. Which of the following

treatment recommendations would likely be advisable for this patient?

A. Increase his sustained-release oxycodone to 110 mg PO BID with the same immediate-release oxycodone dose.
B. Order a three-phase bone scintigraphy and consider a series of lumbar sympathetic blocks for diagnosis and treatment.
C. Titrate his gabapentin upward to a goal of 2700 mg PO TID as tolerated while decreasing his oral opioid dose and enroll the patient in a physical therapy program.
D. If the patient meets the Budapest clinical criteria for the diagnosis of complex regional pain syndrome, consider a dorsal column spinal cord stimulator trial at the T12–L1 level.
E. B, C, and D.

27. Which of the following symptoms are parts of the Budapest criteria for diagnosing complex regional pain syndrome (CRPS)?

A. Evidence of hyperalgesia (to pinprick) and/or allodynia (to light touch and/or deep somatic pressure and/or joint movement)
B. Evidence of edema and/or sweating changes and/or sweating asymmetry
C. Evidence of temperature asymmetry and/or skin color changes and/or asymmetry
D. Evidence of decreased range of motion and/or motor dysfunction (weakness, tremor, and dystonia) and/or trophic changes (hair, nail, and skin)
E. All the above

28. A 37-year-old male with a 10-year history of severe brachial plexus neuralgia pain after a work-related injury is referred to you by his primary care physician. Psychological assessments completed by the patient indicate he has depression and anxiety. Which of the following medications would most likely be beneficial in this patient to improve his psychiatric symptoms as well as his pain?

A. Milnacipran
B. Citalopram
C. Venlafaxine
D. Duloxetine
E. A, C, and D

29. A 26-year-old female patient complains of a 6-month history of sharp, lancinating pain and burning sensation in a T6 dermatomal pattern along her anterior chest wall. She denies any history of surgery, trauma, or infection

prior to the onset of symptoms. An ultrasound-guided intercostal nerve block provides nearly 100% relief of her pain. You diagnose her as having idiopathic intercostal neuralgia. Which of the following medications would likely be most beneficial for reducing this patient's pain with the least dangerous side effects?

A. Hydrocodone
B. Gabapentin
C. Carisoprodol
D. Naproxen
E. A and C

30. Several limbic structures in the brain are involved in processing pain signals as is demonstrated on functional magnetic resonance imaging (fMRI) and positron emission tomography–computed tomography (PET-CT) imaging when patients experience acute and/or chronic pain. The structure outlined in black in the sagittal depiction of the human brain (Figure 24.2) is which of the following?

A. Amygdala
B. Hippocampus
C. Anterior cingulate cortex
D. Thalamus
E. All of the above

31. The structure outlined in the sagittal depiction of the human brain (Figure 24.2) is involved in which of the following with regard to noxious stimuli?

A. Avoidance behaviors
B. The emotional experience of pain

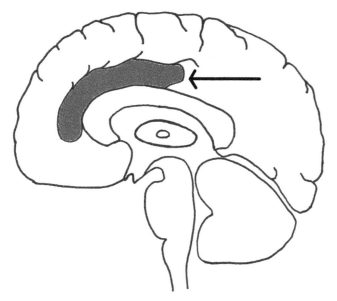

Figure 24.2 Sagittal depiction of human brain.

C. Precise localization of the area where pain is being generated
D. A and B
E. A and C
F. None of the above

32. Which of the following drugs has NMDA receptor antagonist activity and thus can be useful in the treatment of neuropathic pain states?

A. Methadone
B. Ketamine
C. Dextromethorphan
D. Memantine
E. A and C
F. A, B, and C
G. All of the above

33. A patient presents with allodynia that has continued for several years following a peripheral nerve injury. This abnormal and prolonged response is most likely caused in part by which of the following?

A. Increased substance P in the nerve terminals
B. Increased activity in the cingulate gyrus
C. Continued tissue destruction and abnormalities at the site of the injury
D. Increased activity in the peripheral nociceptors

34. A 23-year-old male patient sustained a gunshot injury to the left lower quadrant causing a lumbar plexus injury. He complains of a burning pain in his left foot. On exam, he tolerates light touch, but he winces and moves his foot away with very light pressure. This type of response is described by which of the following terms?

A. Hyperdysthesia
B. Allodynia
C. Hyperalgesia
D. Paresthesia

35. A 68-year-old diabetic female patient with severe bilateral lower extremity neuropathy was treated with 8% topical capsaicin. She reported an 80% reduction from her usual pain symptoms. The result of this pain relief likely occurs through which of the following mechanisms?

A. TRPV1 agonism
B. TRPV1 antagonism
C. TRPV2 agonism
D. TRPV2 antagonism
E. Sodium channel blockade

36. A 75-year-old male with preexisting urinary retention presents with painful postherpetic neuralgia. He has not been able to tolerate gabapentin or pregabalin. You would like to start him on a low-dose tricyclic antidepressant (TCA). The best first-choice TCA would be which of the following?

A. Amitriptyline
B. Selegiline
C. Nortriptyline
D. Desipramine
E. Duloxetine

37. Dorsal root entry zone lesioning would most likely be effective in a patient who has which of the following symptoms and signs?

A. Severe dysesthesia and continued allodynia and constant burning pain in the upper extremities following a thalamic stroke
B. Severe constant pain down the posterior aspect of the left arm with grip strength weakness and a positive Spurling's exam on the left side
C. Constant pain of the an entire arm that is burning with a sensation of a deep ache; the arm is nonfunctional after an injury several years prior
D. Burning and tingling in all extremities with severe pain and burning in the left hand only

38. A 63-year-old male smoker presents to your clinic with pain around her horizontal surgical scar on the right chest wall after removal of a right lung mass. She describes a burning, constant pain around the area of the scar, but she also complains of intermittent and sudden increases in sharp and debilitating pain. On exam, she has noticeable allodynia to light touch and pressure two or three dermatomal levels above and below the scar, with hyperesthesia extending beyond the allodynic area. Which explanation best describes the most likely reason for this pain pattern?

A. The scalpel and surgical instruments during the surgery likely cut or injured several nerves underneath the scar, resulting in pain beyond the boundaries of the incision.
B. Surgical trespass causes a large inflammatory response, thus creating a milieu of inflammatory mediators that are damaging to surrounding nerves. This inflammatory response spreads and likely causes lasting damage to a large tissue area.
C. Transection of a nerve results in a regenerative process that can cause sprouting. This sprouting is widespread, and new neural structures can grow in many directions, resulting in pain to a large area.
D. Class switching of non-nociceptive neurons and increased efficacy of the dorsal horn results in

receptor field expansion; this causes a large area around the original site of injury to activate the spinal cord and cause pain.

39. A 65-year-old male presents with severe, paroxysmal right-sided facial pain described as electrical shocks to the corner of the mouth and angle of the jaw. The pain is elicited by chewing and drinking cold water. No neurologic deficits are reported by the patient nor identified on physical examination. MRI/MR angiography of the brain reveal no space-occupying lesions. If the patient fails conservative therapy, which of the following treatments is least likely to result in a recurrence of symptoms?

A. Glycerol rhizotomy of the trigeminal ganglion
B. Radiofrequency rhizotomy of the trigeminal ganglion
C. Balloon compression of the trigeminal ganglion
D. Microvascular decompression of the trigeminal nerve
E. Focused radiation therapy to the trigeminal nerve

40. A patient undergoes a unilateral radiosurgical thalamotomy procedure for treatment of refractory pain associated with metastatic cancer. Which of the following is true regarding this specific treatment for pain?

A. Neuropathic pain symptoms respond more favorably than nociceptive pain symptoms.
B. Recurrence of pain in long-term follow-up is common.
C. The occurrence of neurological deficits is a common complication.
D. Radiosurgical ablative techniques result in immediate onset of pain relief, whereas surgical ablative techniques result in delayed onset of pain relief.
E. All of the above are true.

41. A 72-year-old male patient has multiple metastatic lesions throughout the spine and brain from advanced prostate cancer and has a prognosis of only a few months to live. He suffers from severe bilateral upper and lower extremity burning pain thought to be due to compressive lesions throughout the cervical, thoracic, and lumbar spine and has a severe emotional component to his pain, including crying spells, depressed mood, and anxiety. Current treatments include high-dose opioids delivered systemically and adjuvant medications including gabapentin, amitriptyline, and naproxen; however, his pain is still uncontrolled. He is not a candidate for intrathecal opioid delivery or spinal cord stimulation due to the compressive lesions in the spine. Which of the following procedures would represent the best option for surgical management of his pain?

A. Stereotactic cingulotomy
B. Anterolateral cordotomy
C. Brainstem caudalis dorsal root entry zone (DREZ) procedure
D. Extralemniscal myelotomy
E. All of the listed procedures are reasonable options for this patient.

42. Which of the following agents has been used in animals to induce a neuropathic pain condition similar to postherpetic neuralgia?

A. Pyridoxine
B. Streptozotocin
C. Paclitaxel
D. Acrylamide
E. Resiniferotoxin

43. Which of the following statements is true regarding CRPS in pediatric patients?

A. The International Association for the Study of Pain (IASP) criteria for diagnosis of CRPS in adults is also applicable to the pediatric population.
B. CRPS occurs more frequently in male patients compared to female patients.
C. Treatment with physical therapy is used to a lesser degree in pediatric patients than in adult patients.
D. A and B are true.
E. All of the above are true.

44. Which of the following are associated with hereditary sensory and autonomic neuropathy type 4?

A. Anhidrosis
B. Multiple accidental injuries, fractures, and burns
C. Autosomal recessive pattern of inheritance

D. A and B
E. All of the above

45. Which term describes nerve injury that involves disruption of the myelin sheath and axon?

A. Neuropathy
B. Axonotomesis
C. Neuropraxia
D. Neurotmesis
E. Wallerian degeneration

46. Which of the following statements is true regarding neuropathic pain conditions?

A. In idiopathic polyneuropathy, motor dysfunction, loss of balance, autonomic dysfunction, and sensory loss are much more common than painful symptoms.
B. Pain as a consequence after stroke, spinal cord injury, multiple sclerosis, and synringomyelia is difficult to treat; however, the occurrence is rare. On the other hand, pain that often occurs from central nervous system (CNS) tumors and CNS infections responds well to typical neuropathic pain treatment.
C. One in three patients with Guillain-Barré syndrome suffer from neuropathic pain.
D. Neuropathic pain after mastectomy is rare.

47. A patient presents with painful peripheral neuropathy. Small fiber neuropathy is suspected. Which of the following statements is true regarding this diagnosis?

A. EMG studies will confirm the diagnosis.
B. Diagnosis is made with a skin biopsy.
C. A detailed neurological examination will usually reveal certain abnormalities that make the diagnosis more likely, such as loss of deep tendon reflexes.
D. Unlike most peripheral neuropathies, symptoms start in the short nerves and progress to the longer nerves.

ANSWERS

1. ANSWER: C

The 2007 revised research and clinical definition of neuropathic pain is described as "pain arising as a direct consequence of a lesion or disease affecting the somatosensory system." The older 1994 IASP definition describes neuropathic pain as "pain initiated or caused by a primary lesion or dysfunction in the nervous system." The newer 2007 definition is much more specific, whereas the older 1994 definition is much more sensitive.

FURTHER READING

Hurley RW, Henriquez OH, Wu CL. Neuropathic pain syndromes. In: Benzon HT, Rathmell JP, Wu CL, et al. (Eds.), *Practical Management of Pain*. 5th ed. Philadelphia, PA: Mosby; 2014:347–360.

2. ANSWER: E

The proposed mechanisms behind the pathophysiology of diabetic peripheral neuropathy (DPN) include the following: (1) polyol pathway—high fructose and sorbitol levels result in oxidative injury and chronic ischemia to neurons; (2) microvascular damage—capillary membranes thicken and endothelial cells become hyperplastic, resulting in ischemic conditions to neurons; and (3) deposition of end products of glycosylation around nerves leading to direct damage. In addition, experimental models have been used to study the etiology of DPN, and these models have shown the pain caused by DPN may result from dysfunction at multiple sites throughout both the peripheral and the central nervous system, including alterations in the expression of sodium channels in primary afferent neurons, release of COX-2 from oligodendrocytes in the CNS, abnormalities in inhibitory interneurons within the spinal cord, and dysfunction of the descending inhibitory pathways.

FURTHER READING

Hurley RW, Henriquez OH, Wu CL. Neuropathic pain syndromes. In: Benzon HT, Rathmell JP, Wu CL, et al. (Eds.), *Practical Management of Pain*. 5th ed. Philadelphia, PA: Mosby; 2014:347–360.
Walk D, Backonja MM. Painful neuropathies. In: Fishman SM, Ballantyne JC, Rathmell JP (Eds.), *Bonica's Management of Pain*. 4th ed. Philadelphia, PA: Lippincott Williams & Wilkins; 2010:303–313.

3. ANSWER: A

HIV infection itself or the use of antiretroviral therapies for HIV (HAART) can cause a distal symmetrical polyneuropathy, and often the ability to distinguish whether HIV infection or HAART is the etiology is difficult. Factors associated with neuropathy in HIV patients include high viral load; age older than 50 years; alcohol, amphetamine, or cocaine use; or coexisting diabetes, vitamin B_{12}, or vitamin E deficiencies. HAART medications most often associated with HIV neuropathies are the dideoxynucleoside analogues (or "d" drugs), including stavudine (D4T), zalcitabine (ddC), and didanosine (ddI). Other nucleoside analogues (zidovudine, lamivudine, and abacavir), protease inhibitors (tipranavir and ritonavir), and non-nucleoside reverse transcriptase inhibitors (rilpivirine and etravirine) are rarely associated with neuropathies.

FURTHER READING

Walk D, Backonja MM. Painful neuropathies. In: Fishman SM, Ballantyne JC, Rathmell JP (Eds.), *Bonica's Management of Pain*. 4th ed. Philadelphia, PA: Lippincott Williams & Wilkins; 2010:303–313.

4. ANSWER: D

Patients being treated with isoniazid in doses greater than 5 mg/kg/day are at risk of developing a nutritional neuropathy. Isoniazid interferes with the functions of pyridoxine (or vitamin B_6) and results in axonal damage to both small and larger fibers. Patients may have sensory and motor deficits in addition to pain. The treatment for isoniazid-induced peripheral neuropathy is supplementation with vitamin B_6 (pyridoxine) at doses of 30–100 mg/day.

FURTHER READING

Walk D, Backonja MM. Painful neuropathies. In: Fishman SM, Ballantyne JC, Rathmell JP (Eds.), *Bonica's Management of Pain*. 4th ed. Philadelphia, PA: Lippincott Williams & Wilkins; 2010:303–313.

5. ANSWER: E

One of the cornerstones for treatment of painful peripheral neuropathies in both diabetes and HIV is ensuring both diseases are well-controlled (i.e., HbA1C levels in the range of 4–6 in diabetes and viral load suppression in

HIV) and patients are not taking medications that could possibly induce the painful neuropathy (i.e., dideoxynucleoside analogues). In this particular patient, all disease states are well-controlled. Treatment with first-line agents for painful DPN includes gabapentin/pregabalin, TCAs (i.e., nortriptyline and amitriptyline), or serotonin–norepinephrine reuptake inhibitors (i.e., duloxetine and venlafaxine), whereas opioids would be a second-line agent. Invasive procedures such as spinal cord stimulation should not be considered until medication therapy has been maximized. In this patient, the best option is the TCA nortriptyline because it is a first-line agent and has the most favorable number needed to treat (NNT) (Table 24.1). Moreover, it also has the added side effect of sedation, which may help this patient with insomnia.

Table 24.1 **NNT FOR PAIN REDUCTION IN PAINFUL DPN**

AGENT	NNT
Gabapentin	3
Pregabalin	4
TCAs	1.3
Duloxetine	4.5
Tramadol	4.3
Capsaicin Cream	6.6

NNT, number needed to treat; TCAs, tricyclic antidepressants.

FURTHER READING

Hurley RW, Henriquez OH, Wu CL. Neuropathic pain syndromes. In: Benzon HT, Rathmell JP, Wu CL, et al. (Eds.), *Practical Management of Pain*. 5th ed. Philadelphia, PA: Mosby; 2014:347–360.

6. ANSWER: C

When nerve injury occurs, several processes occur both proximal and distal to the site of injury. The portion of the axon proximal to the nerve injury may "die back" a few millimeters (*retrograde degeneration*). The stump of the axon proximal to the injury that is still connected to the cell body forms an "end bulb," and several processes begin to grow outward from this end bulb know as *sprouts*. These sprouts will reconnect with the axon that is distal to the injury in ideal conditions and re-form the neural connections. However, if the sprouts are unable to reconnect with the distal axon (as in amputations), the sprouts form a web of sprouts known as a *neuroma*. Likely due to high concentrations of nerve growth factor in the vicinity, normal or uninjured axons in the vicinity may begin producing sprouts, and this is known as *collateral sprouting*. The portion of the axon distal to the injury will also degenerate, and this is known as *Wallerian degeneration* or *anterograde degeneration*.

FURTHER READING

Devor M. Neuropathic pain: Pathophysiological response of nerves to injury. In: McMahon S, Koltzenburg M, Tracey I, et al. (Eds.), *Wall and Melzack's Textbook of Pain*. 6th ed. Philadelphia, PA: Saunders; 2013:861–888.

7. ANSWER: D

Injury to peripheral nerves leads to changes in the expression or the new expression of molecules, including neuropeptides, receptors, ion channels, and enzymes. Specific neuropeptides that are upregulated include VIP, galanin, and neuropeptide Y. Specific neuropeptides that are downregulated include CGRP and substance P.

FURTHER READING

Hökfelt TGM, Zhang X, Villar M, et al. Central consequences of peripheral nerve damage. In: McMahon S, Koltzenburg M, Tracey I, et al. (Eds.), *Wall and Melzack's Textbook of Pain*. 6th ed. Philadelphia, PA: Saunders; 2013:902–914.

8. ANSWER: D

Following peripheral nerve injury, several processes occur centrally within the spinal cord and brain. These activities include central sensitization; ectopic activity within the dorsal horn; receptor field expansion within the dorsal horn; sensitization in regions including the rostroventral medulla, amygdala, anterior cingulate gyrus, and brainstem; and increased activity in the thalamus. Gliosis (or proliferation and hypertrophy) of spinal microglia and astrocytes occurs as well as loss of GABA and cannabinoid-mediated inhibition in the spinal cord.

9. ANSWER: C

The ultrasound image shown in Figure 24.1 represents the sonographic view of the lateral femoral cutaneous nerve (LFCN) that lies medial to the anterior superior iliac spine and superficial to the iliacus and sartorius muscles. It lies between the fascial lata and fascia iliaca layers, which are not visualized in Figure 24.1. The black arrows point to a needle inserted from lateral to medial within the vicinity of the LFCN. Blockade of the LFCN will treat the condition meralgia paresthetica, which is a peripheral sensory mononeuropathy characterized by pain, numbness, and paresthesias to the anterolateral thigh often secondary to compression.

FURTHER READING

Fowler IM, Tucker AA, Mendez RJ. Treatment of meralgia paresthetica with ultrasound-guided pulsed radiofrequency ablation of the lateral femoral cutaneous nerve. *Pain Pract*. 2012;12(5):394–398.

10. ANSWER: E

Pain, burning, and itching with a maculopapular vesicular rash in a dermatomal pattern with prodromal symptoms including headache, malaise, fever, and photophobia are characteristic of acute herpes zoster (HZ) infection. Treatment of acute HZ that reduces the duration of the disease is with antiviral medications including acyclovir, valacyclovir, and famciclovir when administered with the first 72 hours of onset. Data showing whether antiviral medications help reduce the incidence of postherpetic neuralgia (PHN) are lacking. Medications that may be used for pain control include acetaminophen, NSAIDs, opioids, and topical agents. Membrane stabilizers, TCAs, and selective norepinephrine reuptake inhibitors (SNRIs) may be used as adjuvant agents in refractory severe pain. Corticosteroids (administered via the oral or epidural route) are effective in decreasing the intensity of pain; however, they are not effective in preventing the development of PHN. Topical high-strength capsaicin cream helps relieve pain in patients with PHN, but it has not been used for acute HZ infection; therefore, it is not an appropriate treatment for this patient.

FURTHER READING

Hurley RW, Henriquez OH, Wu CL. Neuropathic pain syndromes. In: Benzon HT, Rathmell JP, Wu CL, et al. (Eds.), *Practical Management of Pain*. 5th ed. Philadelphia, PA: Mosby; 2014:347–360.

11. ANSWER: B

The most common sites for both acute HZ infection and PHN are the mid-thoracic dermatomes (trunk) and trigeminal nerve. The ophthalmic branch of the trigeminal nerve (CN V1) is the most common site.

FURTHER READING

Scadding JW, Koltzenburg M. Painful peripheral neuropathies. In: McMahon S, Koltzenburg M, Tracey I, et al. (Eds.), *Wall and Melzack's Textbook of Pain*. 6th ed. Philadelphia, PA: Saunders; 2013:926–951.

12. ANSWER: B

Guillian–Barré syndrome (GBS) is an inflammatory polyneuropathy that presents as a rapid-onset weakness of the limbs and facial muscles. Generally, the onset occurs from descending (lower limbs) to ascending (upper limbs and face). After the maximum point of weakness, which is 4 weeks, patients often have a spontaneous recovery. Approximately 10% of those with GBS will require ventilatory support. Other presenting symptoms of GBS include back and leg pain, myalgias, dysesthesias, and paresthesias. GBS usually occurs after infection with upper respiratory viruses or gastrointestinal illnesses (*Campylobacter jejuni*). The pathophysiology of GBS is demyelination of nerve roots and peripheral nerves.

FURTHER READING

Walk D, Backonja MM. Painful neuropathies. In: Fishman SM, Ballantyne JC, Rathmell JP (Eds.), *Bonica's Management of Pain*. 4th ed. Philadelphia, PA: Lippincott Williams & Wilkins; 2010:303–313.

13. ANSWER: B

The available pharmacologic agents for which there is evidence of efficacy for treatment of PHN are shown in Table 24.2. Although other agents may have efficacy for

Table 24.2 **PHARMACOLOGIC TREATMENTS FOR PHN**

TCAs
    Nortriptyline
    Desipramine
    Amitriptyline

Calcium channel receptor antagonists
    Pregabalin
    Gabapentin

Topical agents
    Lidocaine
    Capsaicin (TRPV1 antagonist)

Opioids
    Tramadol
    Oxycodone
    Morphine
    Methadone

PHN, postherpetic neuralgia; TCA, tricyclic antidepressant.

the treatment of other types of neuropathic pain, only those listed in Table 24.2 have available evidence for their use in PHN. Agents such as SNRIs (e.g., duloxetine and venlafaxine) and NMDA receptor antagonists (e.g., ketamine and dextromethorphan) have not been studied in the treatment of PHN. Mexiletine, a sodium channel receptor antagonist, has not been shown to be effective in the treatment of PHN.

FURTHER READING

Kent JL, Dworkin RH. Herpes zoster and postherpetic neuralgia. In: Fishman SM, Ballantyne JC, Rathmell JP (Eds.), *Bonica's Management of Pain*. 4th ed. Philadelphia, PA: Lippincott Williams & Wilkins; 2010:338–357.

14. ANSWER: B

The F-wave on an NCS represents a delayed response from axons of motor neurons in both the spinal cord and the peripheral nerves. When the F-wave is delayed or absent, in the presence of normal distal motor conduction velocities, it often suggests a lesion proximal to the region of the nerve being stimulated. The most accepted use of the F-wave in NCS is for the early detection of GBS due to proximal neural inflammation and myelin erosion. Although the F-wave could theoretically be used to detect other proximal lesions such as spinal nerve root compression from herniated discs or nerve entrapment syndromes, use of the F-wave is controversial and not recommended in the diagnosis of these conditions.

FURTHER READING

Chang DG, Date ES. Electrodiagnostic evaluation of acute and chronic pain syndromes. In: Fishman SM, Ballantyne JC, Rathmell JP (Eds.), *Bonica's Management of Pain*. 4th ed. Philadelphia, PA: Lippincott Williams & Wilkins; 2010:223–234.

15. ANSWER: B

This patient demonstrates a likely radiculopathy to the C6 nerve root based on sensory, motor, and reflex exams. See Table 24.3 for a comprehensive review of motor, sensory, and reflex patterns for each nerve root that contributes to the brachial plexus and hence innervation of the upper extremities.

FURTHER READING

Dubin A, Lalani I, Argoff CE. History and physical examination of the pain patient. In: Benzon HT, Rathmell JP, Wu CL, et al. (Eds.),

Table 24.3 **MOTOR, SENSORY, AND REFLEX PATTERNS FOR EACH NERVE ROOT OF THE BRACHIAL PLEXUS**

NERVE ROOT	MOTOR	SENSATION	REFLEX
C5	Biceps flexion (C5–C6 musculocutaneous nerve)	Lateral arm	Biceps
	Deltoid (C5–C6 axillary nerve)	•	•
C6	Biceps flexion (C5–C6 musculocutaneous nerve)	Lateral forearm	Brachioradialis
	Wrist extension (C6–C7 radial nerve)	Thumb	•
		Index finger	•
		Half of middle finger	•
C7	Triceps (C6–C8 radial nerve)	Middle finger	Triceps
	Finger extension (C7 radial nerve)	•	•
	Wrist flexion (C7 median and ulnar nerves)	•	•
	Pronator teres (C6–C7 median nerve)	•	•
C8	Finger flexion	Medial forearm	None
	Finger abduction (C8, T1)	Ring finger	•
	Finger adduction (C8, T1)	Fifth digit ("pinky")	•
T1	Finger abduction (C8, T1)	Medial arm	None
	Finger adduction (C8, T1)	•	

Practical Management of Pain. 5th ed. Philadelphia, PA: Mosby; 2014:151–161.

16. ANSWER: D

Several measurement tools have been developed to aid clinicians in distinguishing between neuropathic and nociceptive pain. Table 24.4 explains their uses and whether a clinician is required for their completion.

FURTHER READING

Jensen MP. Measurement of pain. In: Fishman SM, Ballantyne JC, Rathmell JP (Eds.), *Bonica's Management of Pain*. 4th ed. Philadelphia, PA: Lippincott Williams & Wilkins; 2010:251–270.

Table 24.4 MEASUREMENT TOOLS FOR DISTINGUISHING BETWEEN NEUROPATHIC AND NOCICEPTIVE PAIN

TOOL NAME	DESCRIPTION	CLINICIAN NEEDED	ACCURACY (%)
Leeds Assessment of Neuropathic Symptoms and Signs (LANSS)	Two components Questionnaire (by patient) Sensory Testing (by clinician)	Yes	82
Self-report LANSS	Includes same questionnaire as LANSS Patient does self-sensory examination	No	75
Neuropathic Pain Questionnaire (NPQ)	Questionnaire only that assesses both pain effect and descriptors	No	75
NPQ Short Form	Shortened NPQ that asks about numbness, tingling, and increased pain with light touch	No	73
Neuropathic Pain Diagnostic Questionnaire	History and physical exam Fully administered by clinician	Yes	86

17. ANSWER: D

Pharmacologic agents that have shown efficacy in the treatment of painful diabetic neuropathy with positive results in randomized trials include gabapentin, pregabalin, divalproex, duloxetine, TCAs (amitriptyline and nortriptyline), and some opioids (tramadol and oxycodone). At no time have any serotonin reuptake inhibitors (e.g., fluoxetine and escitalopram) been shown to be effective in the treatment of pain for any neuropathic pain condition.

FURTHER READING

Toelle TR, Backonja MM. Pharmacological therapy for neuropathic pain. In: McMahon S, Koltzenburg M, Tracey I, et al. (Eds.), *Wall and Melzack's Textbook of Pain*. 6th ed. Philadelphia, PA: Saunders; 2013:1003–1011.

18. ANSWER: C

In deciding on an initial treatment for PDN, one must also consider the medical comorbidities of the patient being treated and the patient's age. This particular question emphasizes the necessity to choose the best treatment for an elderly patient with coexisting renal dysfunction. Although amitriptyline is a first-line agent and has shown considerable efficacy for the treatment in PDN, it is not the best choice in elderly patients due to cardiac, sedative, and anticholinergic side effects. Morphine is metabolized by the liver to a renally cleared metabolite called morphine-6-glucoronide, which can accumulate in renal failure patients and has a high potential to cause excessive sedation or respiratory depression. The American Geriatrics Society recommends that all NSAIDs be avoided in elderly patients; moreover, NSAIDs can worsen coexisting renal dysfunction. Finally, clonidine has very limited evidence in the treatment of neuropathic pain and also carries a caution with use in the elderly because it can cause excessive sedation. Therefore, the correct answer is the first-line agent gabapentin; the dose of this medication can be reduced in renal failure based on calculated creatinine clearance.

FURTHER READING

Arnstein P, Herr K. Pain in the older person. In: Fishman SM, Ballantyne JC, Rathmell JP (Eds.), *Bonica's Management of Pain*. 4th ed. Philadelphia, PA: Lippincott Williams & Wilkins; 2010:782–790.

19. ANSWER: B

Stevens–Johnson syndrome (SJS) usually develops over a course of 1 day to 2 weeks in response to various triggers, such as medications and infections, or it can be idiopathic. Patients present with fever, sore throat, and fatigue, with the development of oral mucous membrane and oral cutaneous lesions. Although the oropharynx is the most common part of the body to be involved, the esophagus, anus, trachea, vagina, urethra, and eyes can also be involved. A retrospective review of all patients hospitalized with SJS from 1998 to 2001 in a German registry revealed that 90% of SJS occurred within the first 63 days of starting an anticonvulsant drug. Although carbamazepine, phenobarbital, phenytoin, valproic acid, and lamotrigine all carry a risk for the development of SJS, lamotrigine carries the highest risk and incidence. SJS is very rare with gabapentin and pregabalin.

FURTHER READING

Mockenhaupt M, Messenheimer J, Tennis P, et al. Risk of Stevens–Johnson syndrome and toxic epidermal necrolysis in new users of antiepileptics. *Neurology*. 2005;64(7):1134–1138.

20. ANSWER: A

Phantom limb pain (PLP) refers to the sensation of pain referred to the missing limb, whereas phantom sensation refers to the sensation of the missing limb without the presence of pain. Phantom sensations are very common and are reported to occur in 54–100% of patient undergoing amputations, whereas PLP occurs in 2–80% of these patients. The presence of phantom sensations does not predict the occurrence of PLP. Telescoping, which refers to the sensation that the distal phantom (i.e., hand or foot) approaches and then is attached to stump, is a sensation and not a predictor of PLP. Predictors for the development of PLP include pre-amputation pain. Genetic factors have been shown to contribute to the development of neuropathic pain conditions, but conflicting evidence has shown that genetic components do not always play a role in the development of PLP. Psychological conditions such as depression and anxiety can predict the intensity of PLP. Although age, gender, and side and cause of amputation are likely not predictors of the development of PLP, recent prospective studies have shown that female gender and upper limb amputations are associated with higher risk for PLP.

FURTHER READING

Nikolajsen L. Phantom limb. In: McMahon S, Koltzenburg M, Tracey I, et al. (Eds.), *Wall and Melzack's Textbook of Pain*. 6th ed. Philadelphia, PA: Saunders; 2013:915–925.

21. ANSWER: C

This patient has the likely diagnosis of carpel tunnel syndrome (CTS). With a normal MRI, radiculopathy is unlikely. CTS is often associated with occupational tasks such as repetitive hand motions, strong gripping (e.g., holding a spray paint gun), vibration, or awkward positioning. Although the sensory symptoms of CTS are usually limited to the median-innervated fingers, there is a wide range of variability. Pain is often worse at night, and not infrequently the patient will complain of whole arm pain. Pain can be relieved with shaking the hand. Weakness of the hand can also occur, causing difficulty with pinch and grasp. Sensory changes in the palm and hand can occur, but these are usually a later finding. Sensory testing spares the area of skin over the thenar eminence because this branch of the nerve branches early and passes over the carpal canal. In addition, with severe cases, there may be the-nar eminence atrophy. Spurling's test is usually positive in patients with radiculopathy. Yergason's maneuver is a test for bicep tendinopathy. Hawkin's sign tests for impingement of the rotator cuff.

FURTHER READING

Middleton SD, Anakwe RE. Carpal tunnel syndrome. *Br Med J.* 2014;349:g6437–g6437.

22. ANSWER: D

CTS is often associated with occupational tasks such as repetitive hand motions, strong gripping, vibration, or awkward positioning (e.g., playing a violin). The treatment of CTS depends on the severity of nerve dysfunction. For patients with mild to moderate symptoms that have not been in place for a long time, conservative treatment (splinting, glucocorticoid orally or locally, exercise, or therapy) is likely the best approach. EMG and NCS are certainly useful in confirming the diagnosis. However, EMG/NCS are probably most useful in ruling out other pathologies or determining if surgical decompression is an option. Surgery can be useful in CTS. However, this should not be the first treatment option. A cervical spine MRI is not needed in this patient as the initial next step in management because she denies neck or shoulder pain. If the patient does not respond to treatment, further workup (e.g., an MRI) may be necessary.

FURTHER READING

Middleton SD, Anakwe RE. Carpal tunnel syndrome. *Br Med J.* 2014;349:g6437–g6437.

23. ANSWER: B

Post-inguinal herniorrhaphy has a high rate of postoperative neuropathic pain primarily due to the surgical approach to the hernia sac and the anatomic locations where the ilioinguinal and iliohypogastric nerves traverse. It is common for 30–40% of patients to have significant pain (up to 10% severe). There has been no statistically significant difference in postoperative pain rates between open or laparoscopic techniques. Injury of these nerves from positioning or TAP blocks is very rare.

FURTHER READING

Haroutiunian S, Nikolajsen L, Finnerup NB, et al. The neuropathic component in persistent postsurgical pain: A systematic literature review. *Pain.* 2013;154(1):95–102.
Neumayer L, Giobbie-Harder A, Jonasson O, et al. Open mesh versus laparoscopic mesh repair of inguinal hernia. *N Engl J Med.* 2004;350(18):1819–1827.

24. ANSWER: D

Any one of these can cause various forms of neuropathic pain, and his history is consistent with exposure to all of the listed potential insults and all of them can cause significant neuropathic pain. However,

1. Patient positioning during open (or video-assisted) thoracotomy or thoracoscopy is more likely to cause a brachial plexus injury, with arm pain being the primary complaint.
2. Although chemotherapy in an 82-year-old male patient may have severely compromised his immune system and led to herpes zoster infection, chemotherapy-induced neuropathy itself most commonly presents peripherally (not on the trunk) and is usually manifested in the hands and feet in a "stocking and glove" pattern.
3. Radiation therapy as described in this case would be unlikely (although not impossible) as a cause of bilateral thorax pain.
4. Post-thoracotomy neuropathic pain is relatively common; however, it usually affects only the surgical side and only rarely does it spread to multiple dermatomes caudally or cephalad.
5. Patients in their seventh decade of life with herpes zoster have a 50% chance of developing PHN, whereas patients younger than age 40 years rarely develop this condition. The following are risk factors for the development of PHN: advanced age, greater severity of the rash during the acute phase, female gender, and greater acute pain severity. The sites most commonly observed to have been affected are ophthalmic in 32%, thoracic in 16.5%, and facial in 16%.

FURTHER READING

Hurley RW, Henriquez OH, Wu CL. Neuropathic pain syndromes. In: Benzon HT, Rathmell JP, Wu CL, et al. (Eds.), *Practical Management of Pain*. 5th ed. Philadelphia, PA: Mosby; 2014:347–360.
Kent JL, Dworkin RH. Herpes zoster and postherpetic neuralgia. In: Fishman SM, Ballantyne JC, Rathmell JP (Eds.), *Bonica's Management of Pain*. 4th ed. Philadelphia, PA: Lippincott Williams & Wilkins; 2010:338–357.

25. ANSWER: E

CTS is a neuropathy of the median nerve caused by compression as it passes through the carpal tunnel, and it is considered the most frequent compression neuropathy. Based on clinical symptoms and nerve conduction studies, the prevalence is 3.0–5.8% among women and 0.6–2.1% among men in the general population. Exposure to hand–arm vibrations and exposure to a combination of repetitive hand use and the use of hand force are the usual causal agents (i.e., repetitive tasks). Physical exam findings include Tinel's sign (a tingling sensation radiating out into the hand on the palmar aspect of the first three digits proximally to the thenar eminence elicited by light percussion over the median nerve at the wrist) and Phalen's maneuver (elicitation of a paresthesia when the hands are held in forced flexion for 30–60 seconds). After appropriate screening with a consistent history and physical examination, the "gold standard" test is an electrophysiologic study of the nerves at the wrist. Last, MRI can be useful in elucidating anatomic abnormalities that may lead to inconsistent physical exam and electrophysiologic study findings.

FURTHER READING

Palmer KT, Harris EC, Coggon D. Carpal tunnel syndrome and its relation to occupation: A systematic literature review. *Occup Med*. 2007;57(1):57–66.

26. ANSWER: E

Every listed answer except for increasing the opioid dose would be a reasonable option, and, indeed, all could be pursued simultaneously. This patient has noncancer pain that will likely continue for many years, and he is currently taking high doses of opioids with minimal efficacy for his pain and no improvement in his activity or quality of life. Increasing this patient's opioid dose for noncancer pain (with no prior evidence of improvement from opioids) to higher levels would place the patient at significant risk of death or disability due to respiratory depression and is contraindicated.

FURTHER READING

Hurley RW, Henriquez OH, Wu CL. Neuropathic pain syndromes. In: Benzon HT, Rathmell JP, Wu CL, et al. (Eds.), *Practical Management of Pain*. 5th ed. Philadelphia, PA: Mosby; 2014:347–360.

27. ANSWER: E

All of the listed symptoms are part of the Budapest criteria for diagnosing CRPS. The Budapest criteria are as follows:

1. Continuing pain, which is disproportionate to any inciting event

2. Must report at least one symptom in three of the four following categories
    a. Sensory: Reports of hyperesthesia and/or allodynia
    b. Vasomotor: Reports of temperature asymmetry and/or skin color changes and/or skin color asymmetry
    c. Sudomotor/edema: Reports of edema and/or sweating changes and/or sweating asymmetry
    d. Motor/trophic: Reports of decreased range of motion and/or motor dysfunction (weakness, tremor, and dystonia) and/or trophic changes (hair, nail, and skin)
3. Must display at least one sign at time of evaluation in two or more of the following categories
    a. Sensory: Evidence of hyperalgesia (to pinprick) and/or allodynia (to light touch and/or deep somatic pressure and/or joint movement)
    b. Vasomotor: Evidence of temperature asymmetry and/or skin color changes and/or asymmetry
    c. Sudomotor/edema: Evidence of edema and/or sweating changes and/or sweating asymmetry
    d. Motor/trophic: Evidence of decreased range of motion and/or motor dysfunction (weakness, tremor, and dystonia) and/or trophic changes (hair, nail, and skin)
4. There is no other diagnosis that better explains the signs and symptoms

FURTHER READING

Harden NR, Bruehl SP. Complex regional pain syndrome. In: Fishman SM, Ballantyne JC, Rathmell JP (Eds.), *Bonica's Management of Pain*. 4th ed. Philadelphia, PA: Lippincott Williams & Wilkins; 2010:314–331.

28. ANSWER: E

Depression and anxiety are commonly associated with neuropathic pain and need to be medically and psychologically managed. The selected antidepressants, often referred to as selective norepinephrine reuptake inhibitors (SNRIs), all have a relatively high norepinephrine to serotonin selectivity relative to most selective serotonin reuptake inhibitors (SSRIs) and as such can also be very useful in treating chronic pain symptoms in addition to depression and anxiety (Table 24.5).

FURTHER READING

Montgomery SA. Tolerability of serotonin norepinephrine reuptake inhibitor antidepressants. *CNS Spectr.* 2008;13:27–33.

Table 24.5 **SSRI AND SNRI AFFINITY OF SELECTED ANTIDEPRESSANTS**

DRUG	SSRI AFFINITY	SNRI AFFINITY
Venlafaxine	30	1
Duloxetine	10	1
Milnacipran	1	1

SNRI, selective norepinephrine reuptake inhibitor; SSRI, selective serotonin reuptake inibitor.

29. ANSWER: B

Intercostal neuralgia and idiopathic polyneuropathy symptoms can present without any identifiable cause. They are typically poorly responsive to NSAIDs and opioids but often respond well to antiepileptic drugs such as gabapentin, pregabalin, carbamazepine, topiramate, oxcarbazepine, levetiracetam, and lamotrigine.

FURTHER READING

Toelle TR, Backonja MM. Pharmacological therapy for neuropathic pain. In: McMahon S, Koltzenburg M, Tracey I, et al. (Eds.), *Wall and Melzack's Textbook of Pain*. 6th ed. Philadelphia, PA: Saunders; 2013:1003–1011.

30. ANSWER: C

The structure identified in this depiction is the anterior cingulate cortex (ACC), which is an important part of the limbic system and its involvement in the processing and interpretation of noxious stimuli.

FURTHER READING

Vogt BA. Pain and emotion interactions in subregions of the cingulate gyrus. *Nat Rev Neurosci.* 2005;6(7):533–544.

31. ANSWER: D

The ACC has been identified with function imaging studies to be the area of the brain that provides the "experience of suffering" associated with pain (particularly chronic pain). It also appears to be the area most involved with the development of "avoidance" as it relates to pain and behaviors previously associated with a painful experience. Interestingly, the ACC also appears to be the area of the brain affected by mindfulness, with its resulting positive impact on pain and anxiety experienced by its practitioners.

Price DD. Psychological and neural mechanisms of the affective dimension of pain. *Science*. 2000;288(5472):1769–1772.

Vogt BA. Pain and emotion interactions in subregions of the cingulate gyrus. *Nat Rev Neurosci*. 2005;6(7):533–544.

Zeidan F, Grant JA, Brown CA, et al. Mindfulness meditation-related pain relief: Evidence for unique brain mechanisms in the regulation of pain. *Neurosci Lett*. 2012;520(2):165–173.

32. ANSWER: G

Ketamine, dextromethorphan, methadone, and memantine are four of the most well-known and clinically relevant NMDA receptor antagonists commercially available, and all have some evidence of efficacy in the treatment of neuropathic pain as described in the peer-reviewed literature.

Correll GE, Maleki J, Gracely EJ, et al. Subanesthetic ketamine infusion therapy: A retrospective analysis of a novel therapeutic approach to complex regional pain syndrome. *Pain Med*. 2004;5(3):263–275.

Morel V, le Pickering G, Etienne M, et al. Low doses of dextromethorphan have a beneficial effect in the treatment of neuropathic pain. *Fundam Clin Pharmacol*. 2014;28(6):671–680.

Sinis N, Birbaumer N, Schwarz A, et al. Memantine and complex regional pain syndrome (CRPS): Effects of treatment and cortical reorganisation. *Handchir Mikrochir Plast Chir*. 2006;38(3):164–171.

33. ANSWER: D

Allodynia is a consequence of central sensitization. Central sensitization is a complex neuropathic state that can occur regardless of continued nociceptive input. The pain can persist long after tissue is healed and returned to a non-injured or non-inflamed state. Although inflammatory mediators are involved in the development of central sensitization, this is usually not ongoing at the periphery but likely is ongoing centrally. Theories of mechanisms for central pain are abundant, and the science is changing, with many areas being implicated. However, cingulate gyrus is not considered to be involved with this phenomenon. Central sensitization occurs long after the tissue has healed and often even repaired. Nonetheless, even with this, the peripheral nerves show continued activity with lower thresholds for activation. This continued activity promotes an increase in synaptic efficacy in the dorsal horn and even increases responsiveness of dorsal horn neurons. In addition, the continued activity results in expansion of their receptive fields and explains why pain and allodynia continue temporally and geographically well beyond the boundaries of the original injury.

Jensen TS, Finnerup NB. Central pain. In: McMahon S, Koltzenburg M, Tracey I, et al. (Eds.), *Wall and Melzack's Textbook of Pain*. 6th ed. Philadelphia, PA: Saunders; 2013:990–1002.

Ji RR, Kohno T, Moore KA, et al. Central sensitization and LTP: Do pain and memory share similar mechanisms? *Trends Neurosci*. 2003;26(12):696–705.

34. ANSWER: B

Allodynia is the perception of pain from a nonpainful stimulus. Allodynia can be mechanical from light touch (dynamic) or light pressure (static), thermal (pain from mild temperature changes or exposures), or movement (pain triggered by normal movement of joint or muscle). In this case, the patient suffers from mechanical static allodynia. Hyperdysthesia is not a pain descriptor. Hyperalgesia describes increased pain from a normally painful stimulus. Paresthesia is an abnormal sensation, whether spontaneous or evoked.

Devor M. Neuropathic pain: Pathophysiological response of nerves to injury. In: McMahon S, Koltzenburg M, Tracey I, et al. (Eds.), *Wall and Melzack's Textbook of Pain*. 6th ed. Philadelphia, PA: Saunders;2013:861–888.

Merskey H. The taxonomy of pain. *Med Clin North Am*. 2007; 91(1):13–20.

35. ANSWER: A

Capsaicin is a very potent TRPV1 agonist. The TRPV1 receptor is a nonspecific cation channel. Activation with capsaicin causes a prolonged and sustained ion channel opening that causes depolarization and subsequently nerve dysfunction. TRPV1 is heat sensitive. Because capsaicin acts on this channel originally causing nerve activation, it generates a sensation of burning and heat. TRPV2 is a close homolog of TRPV1 and can be activated by plant cannabinoid, probenecid, or high temperatures; it can be blocked by ruthenium red. Lidocaine transdermal patches work by blocking sodium (Na) channels.

Derry S, Sven-Rice A, Cole P, et al. Topical capsaicin (high concentration) for chronic neuropathic pain in adults. *Cochrane Database Syst Rev*. 2013;2:CD007393.

Martini C, Yassen A, Olofsen E, et al. Pharmacodynamic analysis of the analgesic effect of capsaicin 8% patch (Qutenza) in diabetic neuropathic pain patients: Detection of distinct response groups. *J Pain Res*. 2012;5:51–59.

36. ANSWER: D

TCAs have fairly robust evidence for treatment in painful neuropathies. They should always be considered when treating neuropathic pain. Their mechanism of action for this condition is not entirely clear, but they may work by indirectly modulating the opioid system centrally via the serotonergic and noradrenergic neuropathways. They also are potent sodium channel blockers and NMDA receptor antagonists. However, they can have significant anticholinergic side effects. Desipramine has the lowest anticholinergic effect and would be the best choice in this patient. Amitriptyline has one of the higher anticholinergic profiles. Selegiline is not a TCA but, rather, a monoamine oxidase inhibitor. Nortriptyline has anticholinergic side effects similar to amitriptyline, it has slightly fewer. Although duloxetine also blocks both serotonin and norepinephrine, it is not classified as a TCA.

FURTHER READING

McQuay HJ, Tramèr M, Nye BA, et al. A systematic review of antidepressants in neuropathic pain. *Pain*. 1996;68(2–3):217–227.

37. ANSWER: C

DREZ lesioning can be an effective treatment for certain spinal cord injuries or avulsion injuries such as a brachial plexus stretch injury. These injuries can be extremely difficult to manage, and usually the severe pain is not responsive to traditional neuropathic pain treatments. Using this treatment for other types of pain syndromes (e.g., radicular pain or central stroke pain) may lead to worsening symptoms. DREZ lesioning is not effective for central stroke pain. The signs and symptoms in choice B are suggestive of a radiculopathy and are not appropriate for DREZ lesioning. Polyneuropathies, as described in option D, often have an extremity that is the most bothersome. Over time, this can migrate. It would not be appropriate to treat these with DREZ lesioning.

FURTHER READING

Prestor B. Microsurgical junctional DREZ coagulation for treatment of deafferentation pain syndromes. *Surg Neurol*. 2001;56(4):259–265.

Sindou M, Mertens P, Wael M. Microsurgical DREZotomy for pain due to spinal cord and/or cauda equina injuries: Long-term results in a series of 44 patients. *Pain*. 2001;92(1–2):159–171.

38. ANSWER: D

After injury, tactile fibers have been shown to converge onto dorsal horn cells that already receive inputs from nociceptive primary afferents. Presumably, the inputs from the nociceptors in the injury zone are sensitized wide-dynamic range neurons, which enhance the synaptic efficacy of the tactile fibers. Nociceptive-specific neurons (dorsal horn neurons in lamina I) may be sensitized in a similar manner. Both animal and human volunteer studies have shown that the tactile pain can arise from central sensitization to the inputs of A and β fibers. Choice A is an unlikely scenario in a horizontal incision along a dermatome. For choice B, although it is true that trauma induces a large inflammatory response and these mediators sensitize nerve endings, it would be unlikely to produce long-lasting damage. Inflammation is a natural and necessary response to injury or trauma that starts the repair cycle. In choice C, sprouting certainly does occur and can be a source of difficult-to-treat pain, such as when a large neuroma forms after nerve injury. However, this phenomenon would be unlikely to explain the clinical scenario presented.

FURTHER READING

Nickel FT, Seifert F, Lanz S, et al. Mechanisms of neuropathic pain. *Eur Neuropsychopharmacol*. 2012;22(2):81–91.

39. ANSWER: D

All of the choices are potential treatments for the neuropathic pain condition of trigeminal neuralgia. Microvascular decompression is a surgical procedure in which a compressing vessel and trigeminal nerve are physically separated. The recurrence of symptoms with this procedure is approximately 15%. Glycerol rhizotomy involves injecting the chemical neurolytic medication glycerol into the cistern posterior to the trigeminal ganglion. Recurrence of symptoms is approximately 54%. Radiofrequency rhizotomy involves percutaneous neuroablation of the trigeminal ganglion, and recurrence of symptoms is approximately 23%. Use of percutaneous balloon compression devices introduced into Meckel's cave results in mechanical compression of the trigeminal ganglion to produce a functional lesion and blockade of nerve signals; this is associated with a 21% rate of recurrence. Finally, the delivery of a focused dose of radiation to the trigeminal ganglion (e.g., gamma knife) results in delayed-onset pain relief, but it has a recurrence rate of 40–84%.

FURTHER READING

Asaad WF, Eskandar EN. The surgical management of trigeminal neuralgia. In: Fishman SM, Ballantyne JC, Rathmell JP (Eds.), *Bonica's Management of Pain*. 4th ed. Philadelphia, PA: Lippincott Williams & Wilkins; 2010:1507–1514.

40. ANSWER: B

The thalamotomy procedure involves the destruction of several medial thalamic structures that are involved in the processing of painful stimuli. This procedure has better results in reducing nociceptive pain symptoms compared to neuropathic pain symptoms. Recurrence of pain in long-term follow-up studies is very common, and the occurrence of neurologic deficits after this procedure is rare. The procedure can be performed surgically via craniotomy or radiosurgically by using focused beams of radiation. Although the outcomes between the surgical and radiosurgical thalamotomy procedures are similar, radiosurgical procedures have a 2- or 3-month delay in the onset of pain relief.

FURTHER READING

Shields DC, Eskandar EN. Ablative neurosurgical procedures for chronic pain. In: Fishman SM, Ballantyne JC, Rathmell JP (Eds.), *Bonica's Management of Pain*. 4th ed. Philadelphia, PA: Lippincott Williams & Wilkins; 2010:1515–1522.

41. ANSWER: A

Stereotactic cingulotomy targets the anterior cingulate gyrus and also interrupts the Papez circuits, which are responsible for the emotional reactions to painful stimuli. This procedure is appropriate for patients who are terminally ill and have widespread metastatic disease and intrathecal or intraventricular delivery of opioids is difficult. In addition, patients with a substantial emotional component to their pain may also benefit from this procedure. The anterolateral cordotomy procedure targets the lateral spinothalamic tract and results in a contralateral deficit in both pain and temperature sensation two to five levels below the cordotomy. Patients who have unilateral cancer pain that is nociceptive somatic and located distal to the upper thoracic cord are good candidates for this procedure. Brainstem caudalis DREZ procedures target the spinal trigeminal nucleus located in the brainstem, and

appropriate patients for this procedure include those with PHN involving the ophthalmic branch of the trigeminal nerve or other types of neuropathic facial pain. The extralemniscal myelotomy procedure targets the medulla and interrupts the fibers of the spinothalamic tract at the point where they decussate. Patients with pelvic and lower extremity pain that is nociceptive visceral are good candidates for this procedure.

FURTHER READING

Raslan AM, Burchiel KJ. Neurosurgical approaches to pain management. In: Benzon HT, Rathmell JP, Wu CL, et al. (Eds.), *Practical Management of Pain*. 5th ed. Philadelphia, PA: Mosby; 2014:328–334.

42. ANSWER: E

Resiniferotoxin (RTX) is a TRPV1 agonist that produces mechanical and thermal sensitivity in rats, and this sensitivity is similar to that of PHN. The mechanism of action is thought to be due to the depletion of nerve endings that are sensitive to capsaicin; moreover, behavioral changes in RTX-treated rats mimic those of rats with PHN. Pyridoxine (vitamin B_6) is a coenzyme that is vital for many reactions within humans and animals, and intoxication with this substance results in sensory neuropathies. Streptozotocin is a toxin that destroys pancreatic beta cells and can induce a diabetic neuropathy in rats. Paclitaxel is an antineoplastic medication that can induce peripheral sensory polyneuropathies in a "stocking and glove" pattern. Acrylamide is used in polymer production and can induce central and peripheral nervous system damage.

FURTHER READING

Jaggi AS, Jain V, Singh N. Animal models of neuropathic pain. *Fundam Clin Pharmacol*. 2011;25:1–28.

43. ANSWER: A

The IASP criteria are applicable to both children and adults in the diagnosis of CRPS. Management of CRPS in children has been extrapolated from the treatment in adults. Physical therapies are a major component in the treatment of CRPS and neuropathic pain in both populations, but especially in children. Pharmacologic and interventional treatments for CRPS in children have little to no evidence. CRPS is most often seen in girls aged 11–13 years.

FURTHER READING

Suresh S, Shah R. Pediatric chronic pain management. In: Hurley RW, Henriquez OH, Wu CL. Neuropathic pain syndromes. In: Benzon HT, Rathmell JP, Wu CL, et al. (Eds.), *Practical Management of Pain*. 5th ed. Philadelphia, PA: Mosby; 2014: 449–466.

44. ANSWER: E

Hereditary sensory and autonomic neuropathy type 4 is also known as congenital insensitivity to pain with anhidrosis. It is a very rare inherited disease with an autosomal recessive pattern of inheritance. There are 56 cases reported in the literature, and many of these cases show a mutation in the tropomyosin receptor kinase A (TrkA) gene, which is important in determining sensory neuron subtypes. Patients usually present with symptoms early on in life; these include fever of unknown origin, multiple fractures and burns, self-mutilation, mental retardation, and anhidrosis. Most patients succumb to death within the first few years of life.

FURTHER READING

Shorer Z, Moses SW, Hershkovitz E, et al. Neurophysiologic studies in congenital insensitivity to pain with anhidrosis. *Pediatr Neurol*. 2001;25(5):397–400.

45. ANSWER: D

Peripheral nerve injury can be classified into three categories:

1. Neuropraxia: This is the least severe of nerve injuries. Although it does not result in disruption of the myelin sheath, interruption of nerve conduction occurs. Neuropraxia generally occurs from ischemic conditions or temporary nerve compression and resolves in days to months following the injury. Wallerian degeneration does not occur with neuropraxia.
2. Axonotmesis: This type of nerve injury is more severe than neuropraxia and involves complete disruption of the myelin sheath with sparing of the epineurium and may lead to paralysis. Axonotmesis often occurs from crush injuries, and Wallerian degeneration does occur, with regeneration taking months to years.

3. Neurotmesis: This is the most severe of nerve injuries and involves damage to the axon itself as well as the epineurium and is often due to stretch or laceration injuries. Wallerian degeneration does occur, and recovery is rare. Neuropathy refers to a clinical condition of autonomic, sensory, and/or motor dysfunction resulting from damage to nerve(s).

FURTHER READING

Lee SK, Wolfe SW. Peripheral nerve injury and repair. *J Am Acad Orthop Surg*. 1999;8(4):243–252.

46. ANSWER: C

Regarding choice A, neuropathic pain occurs in four out of five patients with idiopathic polyneuropathy, along with the other symptoms mentioned. Regarding choice B, pain after CNS injury is very common except in the cases of tumor and infection, in which neuropathic pain is much less common. Regarding choice D, many surgical procedures have a very high incidence of neuropathic pain, including mastectomy, thoracotomy, and herniorrhaphy. In addition, many chemotherapeutic agents can cause neuropathic pain post treatment.

FURTHER READING

Hökfelt TGM, Zhang X, Villar M, et al. Central consequences of peripheral nerve damage. In: McMahon S, Koltzenburg M, Tracey I, et al. (Eds.) *Wall and Melzack's Textbook of Pain*. 6th ed. Philadelphia, PA: Saunders; 2013:902–914.

47. ANSWER: B

Small fiber neuropathy is a type of peripheral neuropathy that occurs from damage to C fibers found in skin, peripheral nerves, and organs. Damage to these nerves can cause autonomic dysfunction, which plays a major role in symptomatology. Symptoms of the disease are highly variable. Regarding choice A, EMG studies are normal in small fiber neuropathies. Regarding choice C, on neurological exam, the abnormities found are usually with qualitative sensory testing and skin sensory testing, not with large nerve testing such as deep tendon reflexes. Regarding choice D, most peripheral neuropathies affect the longer nerves first, thus causing pain in the feet before the hands. This disease is no exception.

FURTHER READING

Scadding JW, Koltzenburg M. Painful peripheral neuropathies. In: McMahon S, Koltzenburg M, Tracey I, et al. (Eds.), *Wall and Melzack's Textbook of Pain*. 6th ed. Philadelphia, PA: Saunders; 2013:926–951.

Walk D, Backonja MM. Painful neuropathies. In: Fishman SM, Ballantyne JC, Rathmell JP (Eds.), *Bonica's Management of Pain*. 4th ed. Philadelphia, PA: Lippincott Williams & Wilkins; 2010:303–313.

25.

COMPLEX REGIONAL PAIN SYNDROME

Jenna L. Walters

INTRODUCTION

Complex regional pain syndrome (CRPS) is a neuropathic pain condition originally recognized during the Civil War. Silas Weir Mitchell documented that some of the soldiers suffering traumatic injuries developed severe pain and motor dysfunction. In 1993, the International Association for the Study of Pain (IASP) developed the first CRPS clinical diagnostic criteria. CRPS is currently classified as type 1 and type 2, which were previously referred to as reflex sympathetic dystrophy and causalgia, respectively. The two classifications are distinguished by the presence of documented nerve injury in CRPS type 2. The initial criteria by the IASP led to an overdiagnosis of the painful syndrome and were eventually replaced with the Budapest criteria in 2003.

CRPS type 1 and type 2 are believed to originate from peripheral nociceptive dysfunction causing unregulated central input and central sensitization. The release of neuropeptides activates NMDA receptors and leads to hyperesthesia. Altered central input also causes reorganization of the sensory cortex, as evidenced by neuroimaging studies in patients diagnosed with CRPS. The characteristic symptoms of CRPS, including cold, blue, and painful extremities, are believed to occur from vasoconstriction caused by sympathetic dysfunction. Coupling between sympathetic postganglionic and afferent neurons also creates dysregulation of peripheral nociceptors in sympathetically mediated CRPS.

Treatment in CRPS focuses on targeting neuropathic and sympathetically maintained pain. Traditional antineuropathic pain medications include membrane stabilizers and serotonin and norepinephrine reuptake inhibitors. Corticosteroids and nonsteroidals target the inflammatory process present in the initial stages of CRPS. Bone resorption, which is primarily seen in the first year of diagnosis, has been treated with calcium-modulating drugs such as calcitonin and bisphosphonates. Interventional therapies include sympathetic blockade of the affected extremity,

spinal cord stimulation, and intrathecal drug delivery. All of these therapies have been implemented in an effort to facilitate functional restoration of the affected limb. Physical and occupational therapies, such as desensitization and mirror box treatments, have demonstrated some of the most significant improvements in pain, mobility, and function.

QUESTIONS

1. A 45-year-old female is referred to your clinic with complaints of severe hand pain 6 months after falling on the extremity. There was no documented fracture on initial imaging. She is unable to wear long sleeves over the arm due to associated pain. On examination, the arm is swollen and has a blue discoloration. She has decreased flexion and extension at the wrist. What is the most likely diagnosis?

A. Cellulitis
B. CRPS type 1
C. Radial neuropathy
D. CRPS type 2

2. A 32-year-old male underwent an internal fixation of his right ankle after a distal tibia fracture with documented nerve injury and associated sensory deficit. He presents to your office with continued pain in his right leg 3 months after his surgery. You are unable to perform a full physical exam because even lightly touching the extremity elicits extreme pain. The right leg is cold and has decreased hair growth compared to the left. According to the Budapest criteria, what is the patient's diagnosis?

A. CRPS type 2
B. Peripheral neuropathy
C. Failed back surgery syndrome
D. CRPS type 1

3. Which of the following statements is true regarding CRPS type 2?

A. Abnormal sweating is not part of the diagnostic criteria.
B. Documented nerve injury is required for diagnosis.
C. Allodynia must be present for the diagnosis.
D. It is typically not associated with surgery or trauma.

4. Which of the following statements regarding CRPS type 1 is false?

A. Documented nerve injury is not required for diagnosis.
B. Dystonia and tremor are not considered signs of motor dysfunction.
C. Pain is out of proportion to the inciting event.
D. Sudomotor changes include hyper- or hypohidrosis.

5. Which medication is not considered appropriate for the pain associated with CRPS?

A. Methadone
B. Nonsteroidal anti-inflammatory drugs (NSAIDs)
C. Amitriptyline
D. All of the above

6. A patient is referred to your clinic with a diagnosis of CRPS type 1 of the right leg following an operative fixation of the left ankle related to a work injury. He has trialed multiple medications without improvement. What interventional procedure is indicated for CRPS of the lower extremity?

A. Lumbar epidural steroid injection
B. Femoral nerve block
C. Lumbar sympathetic block
D. All of the above

7. The activation of which types of receptors is believed to be responsible for the hyperalgesia and allodynia associated with CRPS?

A. Serotonin
B. GABA
C. NMDA
D. Norepinephrine

8. Which of the following medications may be beneficial in the treatment of CRPS-related hyperalgesia due to its action as an NMDA antagonist?

A. Methadone
B. Ketamine
C. Dextromethorphan
D. All of the above

9. Which statement is not a component of the Budapest criteria for CRPS?

A. Two of four symptoms must be present for the diagnosis.
B. It has less false positives than the original IASP criteria.
C. For a clinical diagnosis of CRPS, the criteria are more specific than the original IASP criteria.
D. Vasomotor changes are the most commonly reported symptom.

10. Which pro-inflammatory cytokine is not believed to be involved in the peripheral sensitization associated with CRPS?

A. Tumor necrosis factor-α (TNF-α)
B. Dynorphin
C. Interleukin-1 (IL-1)
D. Substance P

11. Which of the following is not a risk factor for the development of CRPS?

A. Male gender
B. Work-related injury
C. Fracture as the initiating injury
D. Electromyography (EMG) documenting motor nerve damage

12. Which diagnostic test evaluates the sudomotor signs and symptoms characteristic of CRPS?

A. EMG
B. Three-phase bone scintigraphy
C. Magnetic resonance imaging (MRI)
D. Quantitative sudomotor axon reflex test (QSART)

13. You performed a stellate ganglion block on a patient for CRPS of the left arm. Which of the following indicates that the procedure successfully blocked sympathetic outflow to the left upper extremity?

A. Horner's syndrome on the left side of the face
B. Temperature increase in the left arm
C. Edema in the left arm
D. Hoarseness

14. Which of the following diagnostic tests has a high specificity for the diagnosis of CRPS if performed within the first year of presentation?

A. Three-phase bone scintigraphy
B. Computed tomography of the extremity
C. EMG of the extremity
D. All of the above

15. Functional restoration is the primary treatment modality for CRPS. Which of the following statements regarding its application is incorrect?

A. Immobilization therapy is a critical component of functional restoration in the early stages of CRPS to limit further trauma.
B. Modalities include isometric strengthening, active range of motion, and myofascial release.
C. Physical therapy can include aquatherapy and desensitization therapy.
D. Regular use of the limb is promoted during therapy sessions.

16. Which of the following medications is indicated for the pharmacologic management of CRPS?

A. Gabapentin
B. Duloxetine
C. Steroids
D. Bisphosphonates
E. All of the above

17. Which statement is true regarding the use of calcium-modulating drugs in the treatment of CRPS?

A. Bisphosphonates are believed to improve range of motion but not pain.
B. Bisphosphonates primarily target osteoblastic activity.
C. Intranasal calcitonin has been proven to be more effective in pain relief than bisphosphonates.
D. Bone resorption is believed to contribute to the pain of CRPS.

18. Which interventional procedure is not considered a commonly accepted interventional treatment strategy for CRPS?

A. Spinal cord stimulation
B. Intrathecal ziconotide
C. Trigger point injections
D. Lumbar sympathetic block

19. Multiple studies have suggested a central component in the development and progression of CRPS. Which of the following is true regarding the association of central sensitization and CRPS?

A. Neuropeptides are indicated in the development of central sensitization.
B. Neuroimaging studies support increased brain responsiveness, supporting a theory of central sensitization.

C. Central sensitization may be reversible if afferent nerve activity is regulated.
D. All of the above are true.

20. Which of the following statements is not true regarding sympathetically maintained pain in CRPS?

A. Coupling of sympathetic neurons and nociceptive afferents leads to the sympathetically maintained pain of CRPS.
B. Pain relieved by sympathetic blockade is required for the diagnosis of CRPS.
C. Many of the motor changes associated with CRPS are attributed to sympathetic dysfunction.
D. Vasoconstriction mediated by the sympathetic nervous system is believed to create the mottled, cold, and glossy extremity representative of CRPS.

21. Based on current data regarding pharmacologic management of CRPS, which of the following statements is false?

A. The combination of gabapentin and nortriptyline is more effective than either alone.
B. Subanesthetic doses and anesthetic doses of ketamine were shown to improve the hyperalgesia and allodynia associated with CRPS.
C. NSAIDs are not typically effective due to the extreme pain involved in CRPS.
D. Membrane stabilizers are considered first-line therapy for CRPS.

22. Which of the following symptoms and signs is related to the sympathetic dysfunction associated with CRPS?

A. Blue discoloration
B. Cold extremity
C. Decreased or increased sweat production
D. All of the above

23. Which of the following motor symptoms is not consistent with a diagnosis of CRPS?

A. Dystonia
B. Tremor
C. Weakness
D. All of the above are consistent with CRPS.

24. Which of the following statements is true regarding the somatosensory abnormalities found in patients with a diagnosis of CRPS?

A. Patients exhibit somatotopic reorganization leading to hyperalgesia.

B. Changes in the somatosensory cortex are not reversible, even if pain improves.
C. There is a higher density of Aδ and C fibers in the affected limb compared to the unaffected limb.
D. Mirror box therapy has been shown to improve pain but not tactile acuity.

25. You have been treating a patient for lower extremity CRPS for 6 months. Despite aggressive pharmacologic and interventional therapy, the patient still reports uncontrolled pain during his home physical therapy. He also reports depression related to his pain. What modality would provide the most significant benefit for continued physical therapy?

A. Medication weaning
B. Discontinuation of physical therapy
C. Cognitive–behavioral therapy
D. Weekly office visits for further medication changes

26. Which of the following statements regarding spinal cord stimulation as a treatment modality for CRPS is true?

A. Spinal cord stimulation has been proven to provide significant improvements in pain for decades after implantation.
B. The mechanism of action of spinal cord stimulation in relieving the pain associated with CRPS is poorly understood.
C. Spinal cord stimulation should be not be combined with physical therapy due to the risk of lead migration.
D. Spinal cord stimulation is considered first-line therapy for CRPS.

27. You are performing your first of three scheduled stellate ganglion blocks on a patient with a diagnosis of CRPS type 1 in the right hand. Which of the following should be included in the consent process as a side effect or complication?

A. Pneumothorax
B. Hoarseness

C. Horner's syndrome
D. All of the above

28. A colleague is treating a patient with newly diagnosed CRPS of the upper extremity. He asks you about possible pharmacologic interventions. Which of the following statements is correct?

A. Gabapentin and pregabalin, which block sodium channels, are indicated for the treatment of neuropathic pain.
B. Nortriptyline decreases norepinephrine and serotonin and augments the inhibitory pain pathway.
C. Bisphosphonates decrease osteoclast overactivity and have been shown to improve pain and mobility.
D. Oral steroids have no indication in the treatment of CRPS because there is no inflammatory component.

29. Which of the following symptoms is not included in the Budapest criteria for the diagnosis of CRPS?

A. Documented nerve injury
B. Motor dysfunction
C. Edema
D. Pain out of proportion to the inciting event

30. A 28-year-old male presents as a referral for evaluation of suspected CRPS. He reports burning pain in his right foot after a fall at work 4 weeks ago. He denies any color changes but does report swelling at night. On physical exam, he has decreased range of motion due to pain, but otherwise his extremity appears normal. Which of the following is true?

A. The patient meets diagnostic criteria for CRPS type 2.
B. Physical therapy is not indicated given his extreme pain complaints.
C. The patient meets diagnostic criteria for CRPS type 1.
D. None of the above are true.

ANSWERS

1. ANSWER: B

CRPS is a clinical diagnosis based on signs and symptoms. The low specificity of the previous IASP criteria led to a potential overdiagnosis of CRPS. In 2003, the Budapest criteria were developed in Budapest, Hungary, in an effort to improve the diagnostic accuracy of CRPS. The Budapest criteria include the following:

1. Continued pain disproportionate to the inciting event
2. At least one symptom in three of the four following categories
   a. Sensory—Hyperesthesia and/or allodynia
   b. Vasomotor—Temperature asymmetry, skin color changes, hyper- or hypohidrosis
   c. Sudomotor/edema—Edema and/or sweating asymmetry
   d. Motor/trophic—Decreased range of motion, motor dysfunction (weakness, tremor, dystonia) and/or trophic changes (skin, hair, nail)
3. At least one sign in two of the four following categories
   a. Sensory—Hyperalgesia and/or allodynia on exam
   b. Vasomotor—Temperature asymmetry, skin color changes, hyper- or hypohidrosis
   c. Sudomotor/edema—Edema and/or sweating asymmetry
   d. Motor/trophic—Decreased range of motion, motor dysfunction (weakness, tremor, dystonia) and/or trophic changes (skin, hair, nail)
4. There is no other diagnosis that explains the signs and symptoms

CRPS type 1 and type 2 differ in that CRPS type 2 patients have evidence of nerve damage.

2. ANSWER: A

This patient has CRPS based on his symptoms of hyperalgesia, allodynia, sudomotor and trophic changes, along with associated findings on physical exam. Due to the documented nerve injury with sensory deficit, his diagnosis can be further classified as CRPS type 2 based on the Budapest criteria (see answer to Question 1). In contrast, CRPS type 1 has similar signs and symptoms but no documentation of nerve injury. Peripheral neuropathy involves damage to peripheral nerves and can have many etiologies, including toxins, trauma, systemic disease, or vitamin deficiencies. Failed back surgery syndrome is a term used to describe patients who have undergone an unsuccessful spine surgery or have continued pain despite successful spine surgery.

3. ANSWER: B

CRPS type 2 requires a documented nerve injury for diagnosis. Compared to CRPS type 1, it is more commonly associated with a traumatic event. Sweating asymmetry is one of the diagnostic signs and symptoms included in the Budapest criteria. Allodynia is also one of the diagnostic criteria, but it is not required to make the diagnosis.

4. ANSWER: B

Documented nerve damage is required for the diagnosis of CRPS type 2 but not for CRPS type 1. As part of the Budapest criteria, motor dysfunction is defined as tremor, dystonia, or weakness. Sudomotor changes are defined as hyper- or hypohidrosis, temperature asymmetry, or skin color change. Pain out of proportion to the inciting event is required to make the diagnosis of CRPS.

5. ANSWER: D

Pharmacologic therapy for CRPS focuses on a multimodal approach targeting inflammatory, neuropathic, sympathetic, and centrally mediated pain. Medication regimens can include NSAIDs and corticosteroids to decrease inflammation. Opioid therapy treats both somatic and neuropathic pain, whereas NMDA antagonists improve hyperalgesia and allodynia associated with CRPS. Anticonvulsants and tricyclic antidepressants primarily target neuropathic pain. Calcium modulators include bisphosphonates and calcitonin, which have been shown to improve pain and bone resorption. Sympathetic and central pain pharmacotherapy includes α_2 agonists such as clonidine.

6. ANSWER: C

Excessive sympathetic outflow is believed to be responsible for many of the signs and symptoms, including the pain, associated with CRPS. The lumbar sympathetic chain is located anterior to the L2–L4 vertebral bodies. Lumbar sympathetic blocks are frequently performed to block the sympathetic outflow to the lower extremities and diagnose sympathetically mediated CRPS. Due to the relatively short duration of pain relief typically associated with sympathetic blockade, these therapies should be performed in conjunction with occupational and/or physical therapy.

7. ANSWER: C

NMDA receptors are likely responsible for the hyperalgesia and allodynia associated with CRPS. The release of neuropeptides in response to painful stimuli leads to activation of NMDA receptors located in the peripheral and central nervous system, including the dorsal root ganglia. NMDA receptor hyperactivity and coupling to somatic and nociceptive receptors results in pain with light touch and increased intensity of painful stimuli. NMDA receptor antagonists, such as ketamine and methadone, may be beneficial in patients who experience these symptoms.

8. ANSWER: D

NMDA receptors are believed to be responsible for the hyperesthesia and allodynia associated with CRPS. NMDA antagonists, including ketamine, methadone, and dextromethorphan, block further excitability of nociceptive neurons located in the dorsal horn. Serotonin and norepinephrine modulate the descending inhibitory pathways. Medications that increase these neurotransmitters, such as tricyclic antidepressants and selective norepinephrine reuptake inhibitors, can be useful in the treatment of neuropathic pain.

9. ANSWER: A

The Budapest criteria were developed in Budapest, Hungary, in 2003 to improve the diagnostic accuracy of CRPS. The criteria include identification of three symptoms and two physical signs to make a positive diagnosis. The Budapest criteria have a higher specificity and lower false-positive rate compared to the IASP criteria. Vasomotor criteria are the most frequently reported symptom of CRPS, with an incidence of 86.9%.

10. ANSWER: B

Inflammatory cytokines, including IL-1, TNF-α, substance P, bradykinin, and prostaglandin E_2, are released after peripheral tissue injury and activate peripheral nociceptors. This can eventually lead to peripheral nociceptor firing at lower thresholds, creating an environment for peripheral sensitization. Dynorphin is an endogenous opioid that binds to κ receptors and is not indicated in the peripheral inflammatory cascade associated with CRPS.

11. ANSWER: A

Risk factors associated with the development of CRPS include female gender, age, workplace-related injury, fracture as the mechanism of injury, and associated motor damage.

12. ANSWER: D

A QSART measures sweat output and can provide evidence of sudomotor dysfunction. A QSART showing abnormal sudomotor activity is indicative of a diagnosis of CRPS. EMG records electrical activity in skeletal muscle, which is indicated for the diagnosis of neuromuscular diseases. MRI is an imaging technique that uses magnetic fields and radio waves to form images of the body. Three-phase bone scintigraphy is a radionucleotide study that demonstrates perfusion to certain areas of bone. Increased radionucleotide uptake in an extremity supports a diagnosis of CRPS but is not evidence of sudomotor dysfunction.

13. ANSWER: B

The stellate ganglion is formed by the fusion of the inferior cervical and first thoracic sympathetic ganglia. It is anatomically located anterior to the C7 transverse process. The stellate ganglion block is typically performed at the transverse process of C6, Chassaignac's tubercle, to avoid puncture of the vertebral artery. Horner's syndrome indicates a successful sympathetic blockade of the face, but it does not necessarily ensure sympathetic blockade of the arm. Hoarseness is a common complication of a stellate ganglion block due to concomitant blockade of the recurrent laryngeal nerve. Edema is a symptom of CRPS but not an indication of a successful stellate ganglion block.

14. ANSWER: A

Three-phase bone scintigraphy is a radionucleotide study that demonstrates perfusion to certain areas of bone. The uptake of radionucleotide tracer can indicate changes in bone metabolism. Increased uptake in the affected limb compared to the normal limb suggests a diagnosis of CRPS. It is most specific if performed within the first year of diagnosis.

15. ANSWER: A

Functional restoration is the foundation for the treatment of CRPS to improve physical rehabilitation. The goal of this therapy includes desensitization, normalization of peripheral and central transmission, and regulation of sympathetic tone in the affected extremity. Functional restoration modalities include isometric strengthening, active range of motion, and myofascial release. Aquatherapy can also be employed as a form of gentle physical therapy. Immobilization of the extremity is now recognized as a possible contributing factor in the development of CRPS and should be avoided to prevent further motor dysfunction and pain.

16. ANSWER: E

Gabapentin is a calcium channel blocker used to treat neuropathic pain. It is considered first-line therapy in the treatment of CRPS. Duloxetine is a serotonin and norepinephrine reuptake inhibitor (SNRI) that is also indicated for the treatment of neuropathic pain, including CRPS. Increases in serotonin and norepinephrine augment the inhibitory pain pathways, which originate in the central nervous system. Some studies indicate that the combination of membrane stabilizer and an SNRI may be more helpful than either one alone. Corticosteroids may be beneficial in the acute inflammatory phase of CRPS. Bisphosphonates regulate osteoclast activity and bone resorption at the site of inflammation. Corticosteroids and bisphosphonates are believed to be most beneficial during the acute stage of CRPS.

17. ANSWER: D

Calcitonin and bisphosphonates have both been used in the treatment of CRPS. Intranasal calcitonin and oral bisphosphonates are used to augment increased osteoclast activity. Hyperactive osteoclasts lead to bone resorption that can be documented in the affected limb by increased radionucleotide uptake on triple-phase bone scintigraphy. Calcium modulators have been shown to improve pain and range of motion. Side effects of calcium modulators include stomach and esophageal erosion and osteonecrosis of the mandible.

18. ANSWER: C

Interventional therapy includes targets for sympathetically mediated and neuropathic pain. Stellate and lumbar sympathetic blocks target sympathetic input to the upper and lower extremities, respectively. A stellate ganglion block is classically performed by injecting local anesthetic at Chassaignac's tubercle near the transverse process of C6. The actual stellate ganglion is typically just inferior at the C7 transverse process. A lumbar sympathetic block is performed anterior to the L3 vertebral body. The procedure blocks the sympathetic ganglion from approximately L2 to L4. Spinal cord stimulation utilizes electrical stimulation of the dorsal column to prevent transmission of neuropathic pain through largely unknown mechanisms. Intrathecal ziconotide is an ω conotoxin from sea snail venom that blocks N-type calcium channels. It is only available via the intrathecal (IT) route and is one of three current US Food and Drug Administration-approved IT medications. It has been shown to improve pain, trophic changes, and edema in CRPS. All interventional therapies are ultimately implemented to allow the patient to regain functionality through physical and occupational therapy.

19. ANSWER: D

Constant firing of peripheral nociceptors due to an increase in local inflammatory markers is the characteristic sign of peripheral sensitization. Repetitive nociceptive input to the spinal cord is believed to result in the central sensitization associated with CRPS. Increased nociceptive firing results in the release of neuropeptides and activation of NMDA receptors in the central nervous system. Neuroimaging studies performed on patients with CRPS show changes in afferent activity causing sensory reorganization along with increased brain responsiveness. Imaging studies also indicate that these changes are reversible if the patient undergoes effective treatment and functional restoration.

20. ANSWER: B

Sympathetic dysfunction seen in CRPS, either inhibition or enhancement, is responsible for many of the characteristic clinical symptoms. Enhanced sympathetic activity leads to vasoconstriction causing the cold, blue, and sweaty appearance of most extremities acutely affected by CRPS. Animal models in which extremities were injected with norepinephrine showed a similar clinical picture to CRPS. Coupling of sympathetic neurons and nociceptive afferents occurs in most patients with CRPS. Increased sympathetic neuron activity then leads to aberrant nociceptive firing. A small group of patients with CRPS do not have sympathetically mediated pain and do not respond to sympathetic blockade despite a similar clinical picture.

21. ANSWER: C

Membrane stabilizers, such as gabapentin and pregabalin, are considered first-line therapy in the treatment of CRPS via the blockade of calcium channels. The combination of a membrane stabilizer with an SNRI has been shown to be more beneficial than either medication alone. NSAIDs are indicated, especially in the early stages of CRPS when the peripheral inflammatory cascade is believed to predominate. Ketamine is an NMDA antagonist that acts in the central nervous system to target the central sensitization associated with CRPS. Subanesthetic and anesthetic doses of ketamine have been shown to provide short-term relief of pain in CRPS.

22. ANSWER: D

Sympathetic enhancement and increases in norepinephrine lead to vasoconstriction in the limb affected by CRPS. This causes a clinical picture of a cold, blue, and sweaty extremity. Animal models injected with norepinephrine exhibit similar symptoms.

23. ANSWER: D

The signs of motor dysfunction associated with CRPS include decreased range of motion, weakness, tremor, dyskinesia, and muscle spasm. Pain primarily contributes to the decreased range of motion that develops over time. Tremor has been documented in up to 70% of patients with CRPS of the upper extremity. Improvement following sympathetic blockade suggests that this symptom may be mediated by the sympathetic nervous system. Continued neglect and disuse of the extremity can worsen motor function and the associated weakness.

24. ANSWER: A

Brain plasticity and somatosensory changes are a relatively recent feature discovered in patients with CRPS. This finding supports the theory that CRPS involves modulation in both the peripheral and the central nervous system. Skin biopsies in patients with CRPS show a lower density of Aδ and C fibers in the affected limbs. This can lead to peripheral sensory deficits and altered central nervous system input. Neuroimaging studies reveal that patients have decreased sensory input to the affected side and associated somatotopic reorganization. This evidence supports the implementation of mirror therapy in an attempt to normalize input in the sensory cortex. Studies involving patients undergoing mirror therapy have shown improved two-point acuity and pain. Successful functional restoration programs have also led to the reversal of sensory cortex reorganization and improvement in pain scores.

25. ANSWER: C

No study has shown a clear association between CRPS and specific psychiatric diagnoses; however, psychological and behavioral therapies are essential to improve function. Over time, these patients can exhibit signs of disuse and fear of pain and emotional stress related to their diagnosis. Cognitive–behavioral therapies such as biofeedback, relaxation techniques, and pain coping skills can provide patients some control over their disease while improving the success of interventional therapies. Referral to a psychiatrist or pain psychologist should be considered in the treatment regimen.

26. ANSWER: B

Spinal cord stimulation involves placing electrical leads in the epidural space, which conduct electrical impulses to the dorsal column of the spinal cord. The mechanism of action of spinal cord stimulation in the treatment of CRPS is still poorly understood. Short-term studies involving spinal cord stimulation show improvements in pain but not necessarily function. Optimally, spinal cord stimulation should be combined with an effective functional restoration program. No studies have proven long-term efficacy of spinal cord stimulation; however, definitive studies are still lacking.

27. ANSWER: D

The stellate ganglion is a fusion of the inferior cervical and upper thoracic sympathetic ganglions. The stellate ganglion provides sympathetic input to the upper extremity. Traditionally, it is blocked at the anterior tubercle of the C6 vertebrae to avoid puncture of the vertebral artery. Successful sympathetic blockade to the affected extremity results in vasodilation and an associated increase in temperature.

Sympathetic blockade to the face causes Horner's syndrome that includes ptosis, miosis, and anhidrosis. The volume of injectate typically results in block of the recurrent laryngeal nerve causing hoarseness and phrenic nerve block leading to shortness of breath. Complications include pneumothorax, hematoma, hypotension, seizure, apnea, loss of consciousness, and cardiorespiratory arrest. These side effects should be considered when determining if a patient is a candidate for interventional therapy.

28. ANSWER: C

First-line pharmacologic therapy for neuropathic pain includes gabapentin and pregabalin, which are both calcium channel blockers. Tricyclic antidepressants, such as nortriptyline and amitriptyline, act by inhibiting the reuptake of serotonin and norepinephrine. These medications are believed to target the descending spinal inhibitory pathways that augment peripheral nociceptive input. Bisphosphonates have shown the most clinical benefit in the first year following the diagnosis of CRPS. These medications decrease osteoclast activity and have been shown to be beneficial with regard to pain and mobility. Corticosteroids may be useful during the acute inflammatory process initially present in CRPS.

29. ANSWER: A

Documented nerve injury is not included in the Budapest criteria for the diagnosis of CRPS. The Budapest criteria include the following:

1. Continued pain disproportionate to the inciting event
2. At least one symptom in three of the four following categories
   a. Sensory—Hyperesthesia and/or allodynia
   b. Vasomotor—Temperature asymmetry, skin color changes, hyper- or hypohidrosis
   c. Sudomotor/edema—Edema and/or sweating asymmetry

   d. Motor/trophic—Decreased range of motion, motor dysfunction (weakness, tremor, dystonia) and/or trophic changes (skin, hair, nail)
3. At least one sign in two of the four following categories
   a. Sensory—Hyperalgesia and/or allodynia on exam
   b. Vasomotor—Temperature asymmetry, skin color changes, hyper- or hypohidrosis
   c. Sudomotor/edema—Edema and/or sweating asymmetry
   d. Motor/trophic—Decreased range of motion, motor dysfunction (weakness, tremor, dystonia) and/or trophic changes (skin, hair, nail)
4. There is no other diagnosis that explains the signs and symptoms

CRPS type 1 and type 2 differ in that CRPS type 2 patients have evidence of nerve damage.

30. ANSWER: D

This patient displays some of the signs and symptoms of CRPS, including decreased range of motion and reported edema and pain. However, according to the Budapest criteria, he does not meet the diagnosis. He does not describe symptoms in three of the four diagnostic categories and does not exhibit physical signs in two of the four diagnostic categories. Pain may limit physical therapy, but it is not an indication to avoid this treatment strategy.

FURTHER READING

Harden NR, Bruehl SP. Complex regional pain syndrome. In: Fishman SM, Ballantyne JC, Rathmell JP (Eds.), *Bonica's Management of Pain*. 4th ed. Philadelphia, PA: Lippincott Williams & Wilkins; 2010:314–331.

Hurley RW, Henriquez OH, Wu CL. Neuropathic pain syndromes. In: Benzon HT, Rathmell JP, Wu CL, et al. (Eds.), *Practical Management of Pain*. 5th ed. Philadelphia, PA: Mosby; 2014:346–360.

Williams K, Guarino A, Raja SN. Complex regional pain syndrome. In: Benzon H, Raja S, Fishman S, et al. (Eds.), *Essentials of Pain Medicine*. 3rd ed. Philadelphia, PA: Saunders; 2011:351–357.

PEDIATRIC PAIN AND DEVELOPMENT OF PAIN SYSTEMS

Ellen W. K. Rosenquist and Natalie Strickland

INTRODUCTION

The diagnosis and treatment of pain in the pediatric population are challenging because there is still much that is not understood about the development of pain systems in the human body. Many common pain syndromes manifest unique characteristics in the pediatric population that vary greatly from those in adults. In addition, pediatric treatments vary greatly from those used for adults and typically rely to a far greater degree on physical therapy or other nonpharmacologic treatments before resorting to pharmacologic or interventional therapies. Furthermore, there are many factors that must be taken into consideration when treating children, such as a child's stage of development, pharmacokinetic and pharmacodynamic variables, caregiver concerns, psychosocial considerations, ethical considerations, and the ability of the child to describe his or her pain. This chapter highlights important topics to be considered when managing pain in pediatrics.

QUESTIONS

1. Which of the following statements is true?

A. Newborns do not feel pain because myelination is incomplete at birth, and therefore it is unnecessary to provide analgesia.
B. Newborns do not feel pain until 12 weeks after birth when myelination is complete, and therefore it is unnecessary to provide analgesia.
C. Newborns feel pain because myelination is complete, and therefore analgesia is required.
D. Newborns feel pain even though myelination is incomplete, and therefore analgesia is required.
E. Newborns only feel certain types of pain because myelination is incomplete, and therefore analgesia is required.

2. What is the mechanism of action of sucrose for the reduction in pain in infants undergoing needle procedures?

A. Taste-induced release of endogenous opioids
B. Calming effect of sucking
C. Distraction
D. Increased activity in the rostral ventral medulla
E. A, B, and C

3. A 15-year-old African American female with an ear infection spent 5 hours yesterday sunbathing in 95° weather. She presents to the emergency department with chest pain and shortness of breath. When examining her medical records on the computer, you notice many hospital admissions that usually last 3–7 days. Which of the following diseases does she most likely have?

A. Costochondritis
B. Asthma
C. Malingering
D. Congenital heart disease
E. Sickle cell

4. A 13-year-old female has been complaining of stomach pain that is so bad that she cannot go to soccer practice. During the past few months, she has had multiple episodes of periumbilical pain described as aching and cramping. There is no relationship to food or her menses. She has seen her primary care physician and is now being referred to a gastroenterologist. The gastroenterologist diagnoses her with functional gastrointestinal disorder (FGID). FGID includes the all of the following diagnoses except:

A. Recurrent abdominal pain
B. Functional abdominal pain

C. Irritable bowel syndrome
D. Abdominal migraine
E. Functional dyspepsia

5. A 9-year-old female presents to her doctor's office with abdominal pain. Her pain is located on the lateral border of the rectus sheath on the left side approximately 2 inches below her umbilicus. On palpation, it is tender, and it is worsened by Carnett's sign. Which of the following diagnoses does she have?

A. Cholecystitis
B. Anterior cutaneous nerve entrapment
C. Interstitial cystitis
D. Diverticulitis
E. Functional abdominal pain

6. Which of the following statements is correct regarding volumes of distribution in neonates and infants compared to those in adults?

A. Neonates and infants have larger distribution volumes for water-soluble drugs and smaller volumes for lipophilic drugs.
B. Neonates and infants have smaller distribution volumes for water-soluble drugs and larger volumes for lipophilic drugs.
C. Neonates and infants have larger distribution volumes for water-soluble drugs and larger volumes for lipophilic drugs.
D. Neonates and infants have smaller distribution volumes for water-soluble drugs and smaller volumes for lipophilic drugs.
E. Neonates and infants have the same distribution for water-soluble and lipophilic drugs.

7. Transdermal, intramuscular, and rectal bioavailability are greatest in which age group?

A. Neonates and infants
B. Small children
C. Adolescents
D. Adults
E. Elderly

8. A 4-week-old, full-term, otherwise healthy male is taken to the operating room for club foot cast exchange. After intravenous (IV) sedation was given, he had extensor spasms and opisthotonos. What medication is associated with this side effect in infants?

A. Etomidate
B. Ketamine
C. Midazolam
D. Propofol
E. Thiopental

9. Which of the following statements is correct regarding epidural-administered local anesthetics?

A. Peak plasma concentrations occur later and are lower in neonates and infants compared to adults.
B. Peak plasma concentrations occur later and are higher in neonates and infants compared to adults.
C. Peak plasma concentrations occur earlier and are lower in neonates and infants compared to adult.
D. Peak plasma concentrations occur earlier and are higher in neonates and infants compared to adults.
E. Peak plasma concentrations occur at the same time and amount in neonates and infants as they do in adults.

10. Blake is an 11-year-old male who sprained his wrist wrestling at school 2 months ago. The orthopedic surgeon has cleared him to resume all activities. Blake continues to use the wrist splint and will not allow anyone to touch his arm. On exam, there is no swelling, atrophy, discoloration, or skin changes. He has very limited range of motion. He will not allow you to perform any strength exam or touch his wrist. Which of the following responses from his parents is most appropriate?

A. "You can't touch his wrist, it hurts him too much."
B. "Only when he is pain free will I ask him to participate in activities."
C. "The doctor said he is fine, I don't understand why he can't just start wrestling again."
D. "Quit being a wimp, and let the doctor do the exam."
E. "I know it is going to be uncomfortable for you, but the doctor needs to examine your wrist. Why don't you listen to music while she does the exam."

11. Maddie is a 2-year-old who was playing in the yard when she fell on the grass while running after her dog. She has a small cut on her knee but has been crying for the past 20 minutes. Which of the following statements is correct?

A. Maddie needs a Band-Aid to make her booboo all better.
B. Maddie needs to be taken to the nearest emergency room to be evaluated.
C. Her parents need to learn some tough love strategies.
D. Maddie deserved to have pain because she was chasing the dog after being told not to do so.
E. Maddie should have ice placed on her knee and not be allowed to stand for the rest of the day.

12. What is the suggested maximum acetaminophen dose for a 5-week-old otherwise healthy male who underwent pyloric stenosis repair?

A. 55 mg/kg/day
B. 60 mg/kg/day

C. 65 mg/kg/day

D. 70 mg/kg/day

E. 75 mg/kg/day

13. Which of the following statements is true in reference to morphine elimination half-life ($t\frac{1}{2}\beta$) in newborns younger than 1 week old?

A. Elimination is one-fourth as long in newborns compared to older children.

B. Elimination is one-half as long in newborns and older children.

C. Elimination is the same in newborns and older children.

D. Elimination is twice as long in newborns and older children.

E. Elimination is four times as long in newborns and older children.

14. A 10-year-old female patient suffered from second-degree burns to 15% of her upper extremity after an accidental burn. She is having severe pain with a neuropathic component. Which of the following opioids would be most appropriate?

A. Morphine

B. Demerol

C. Dilaudid

D. Fentanyl

E. Methadone

15. A 5-year-old male undergoes tonsillectomy and adnoidectomy for recurrent pharyngitis infections. He is otherwise healthy and has no known drug allergies. He is given a prescription for oral pain medications and is discharged home after meeting post-anesthesia care unit requirements. At approximately 2 a.m., his mother places a 911 call that he is unresponsive. Which opioid was he most likely given?

A. Codeine

B. Morphine

C. Hydrocodone

D. Oxycodone

E. Dilaudid

16. A 12-year-old is scheduled for a slipped capital femoral epiphysis repair. Because this surgery is expected to have significant postoperative pain, you talk to his parents about placing an epidural. They refuse to give consent. You talk with the orthopedic intern and suggest that she order an opioid patient-controlled analgesia (PCA). She says she has never ordered one and asks for recommendations. Which of the following is correct?

A. Morphine continuous basal infusion of 100 µg/kg/hr with a demand dose of 100 µg/kg every 8 minutes

B. Morphine continuous basal infusion of 100 µg/kg/hr without a demand dose

C. Morphine without a continuous basal infusion and a demand dose of 100 µg/kg every 8 minutes

D. Morphine continuous basal infusion of 20 µg/kg/hr with a demand dose of 20 µg/kg every 8 minutes

E. Morphine continuous basal infusion of 20 µg/kg/hr without a demand dose

17. A 7-year-old male is scheduled for an umbilical hernia repair. His mother states that after his ear tubes and elbow fracture surgeries, he woke up like a crazy man, hitting, screaming, and he did not know where he was. You recently read an article about an opioid that can decrease emergence delirium. Which opioid was the article about?

A. Morphine

B. Dilaudid

C. Methadone

D. Nalbuphine

E. Buprenorphine

18. Aubrey is a 16-year-old female who had a right ankle sprain 6 months ago. She continues to use crutches and frequently misses school because she is having pain. Her parents state that her ankle frequently has swelling and discoloration and that even wearing a sock is painful. Her parents have been doing their best to help minimize activities that exacerbate Aubrey's pain. She no longer participates in soccer, and her chores have been eliminated. Which of the following treatment options is most appropriate?

A. Lumbar sympathetic block

B. Referral for physical therapy

C. Referral for biofeedback

D. Prescription for Dilaudid

E. Tell her parents to make her play soccer and do her chores

19. Karlie is a 9-year-old female with chronic abdominal pain. She has been seen by many specialists, and all workup for an organic etiology has been ruled out. Which of the following should her parents not do?

A. Encourage Karlie to go to school even when her stomach hurts.

B. Ask Karlie in the mornings if she has a stomachache before getting her out of bed.

C. Ignore Karlie slowly walking around holding her stomach.

D. Praise Karlie for using diaphragmatic breathing techniques.

E. Avoid negative words and reframe Karlie's distress.

20. At what age can a child reliably self-report his or her pain?

A. 5 years
B. 3 years
C. 4 years
D. 7 years
E. 2 years

21. Faces scales are often more suitable for younger children than the visual analogue scale (VAS) or the numerical rating scale (NRS) for the following reason(s):

A. A faces scale requires the ability to count and put things in a specific order.
B. A faces scale only requires matching one of the pictures to the state of the distress the patient is feeling.
C. The ability to estimate the magnitude of pain is not well developed in children younger than age 6 years.
D. A faces scale requires an ability to draw a face.
E. B and C.

22. The most common source of pain in pediatric patients with cancer is:

A. Tumor growth
B. Venipuncture
C. Chemotherapy
D. Radiation
E. Surgeries

23. Sara is a 10-year-old female who complains of constant burning pain in her hands and feet that developed 3 weeks after completing chemotherapy using cisplatin. What are the most commonly used medications to treat neuropathic pain in children?

A. Tricyclic antidepressants (TCAs)
B. Opioids
C. Serotonin–norepinephrine reuptake inhibitors (SNRIs)
D. Calcium channel $\alpha_2\delta$ ligands
E. Lidocaine patches

24. Withholding opioids for pain management in children and adolescents using the reasoning that the risk of becoming addicted to these medications outweighs the benefits of using them in this patient population is an example of which type of ethical justification?

A. Comparative justification
B. Revisionist justification
C. Pragmatic justification
D. Competitive justification
E. None of the above

25. A 12-year-old male with cerebral palsy and scoliosis recently underwent implantation of an intrathecal baclofen pump to treat severe spasticity. His mother reports that he has been more irritable during the past few days as well. He presents to your office 3 weeks after the procedure with fever, tachycardia, and pain in his back. A viral illness has been affecting many children at the patient's school. What is the next step in the management of this patient?

A. Obtain an X-ray of the spine as an outpatient
B. Prescribe a 2-week course of antibiotics
C. Transport the patient to the nearest emergency room
D. Reassure the patient's mother and recommend fluids and rest

26. A 6-year-old female with a history of osteomyelitis of the left lower extremity has been admitted for the past 2 weeks for intravenous antibiotics and pain control. The patient's pain has been well controlled using a morphine PCA. At the time of discharge, the patient reports only mild pain in the left lower extremity. The patient was discharged to home with a prescription for oral acetaminophen and a course of oral antibiotics. Three days after discharge, the patient becomes increasingly anxious, agitated, and has difficulty sleeping. She also developed diarrhea, has been vomiting, and has a fever. What is the most likely cause of this patient's symptoms?

A. Recurrence of infection
B. Allergic reaction to the antibiotics
C. Opioid withdrawal
D. Viral illness

27. What factor(s) increases the risk of a child developing phantom limb pain?

A. Congenital deficient limb
B. Cancer and chemotherapy
C. Major burns due to flame injury
D. No preoperative pain
E. Younger at time of amputation

28. It is often difficult to determine if musculoskeletal symptom and pain complaints are related to an inflammatory process such as juvenile idiopathic arthritis (JIA). However, the prompt diagnosis of this disorder is

important to allow for early treatment and reduce pain. Which of the following is not a common sign or symptom in patients presenting with JIA?

A. Swelling and/or pain on movement with limitation of motion
B. Pain that is worst after prolonged inactivity and better with movement
C. Pain that wakes the patient up at night
D. Tenderness at the joint line
E. Pain described as dull and achy

29. Kaitlyn is a 15-year-old female who presents to the clinic complaining of constant ankle pain and swelling in her left ankle. She twisted her left ankle during softball practice 4 months ago and has complained of severe pain since that time. She describes the pain as burning and as if there are bugs crawling under her skin. Furthermore, she states that her left foot can turn blue and feel ice cold compared to the right foot. Which other symptom(s) would be consistent with a diagnosis of complex regional pain syndrome?

A. Decreased range of motion in the left foot with weakness in the left lower extremity

B. Thickened toenails on the left foot compared to the right
C. Increased hair growth on the left lower extremity compared to the right
D. Inability to wear a sock on the left foot due to severe pain when touching the foot
E. All of the above

30. Meghan is a 12-year-old female who presents to your office complaining of headaches. The patient describes the headache as a pulsating pain in the front of the head on both sides. The headaches initially lasted only for as little as a few hours to a few days. However, she states that she now has the headaches almost every day. The headaches are worse when she is moving around, and she finds the most comfort in a dark and quiet room. What type of headache is the patient most likely experiencing?

A. Migraine headaches without aura
B. Tension-type headaches
C. Cluster headaches
D. Chronic migraines
E. Hemicranias continua

ANSWERS

1. ANSWER: D

By 24 weeks of gestation, most of the nerve pathways are established for the transmission, perception, and modulation of pain. At birth, the pain pathways are present but immature. Myelination is incomplete at birth, and this results in slower transmission. Furthermore, inhibitory mechanisms in the dorsal horn of the spinal cord are also immature, resulting in less inhibition of nociceptive input. Dorsal horn neurons also have a wider receptive field and lower excitatory threshold, which may contribute to more pain transmission.

KEY FACTS: PHYSIOLOGY AND DEVELOPMENT

- Pain pathways are mostly developed by 24 weeks of gestation.
- At birth, pain pathways are established but immature.
- At birth, myelination is incomplete.

FURTHER READING

Davis P, Cladis F, Motoyoma E (Eds.). *Smith's Anesthesia for Infants and Children*. 8th ed. Philadelphia, PA: Mosby; 2011:418–419.

2. ANSWER: E

Utilization of sweet solutions can have analgesic effects in infants up to 12 months old. The mechanism of action is unknown, but it is thought to be due to release of endogenous opioids, a calming effect of sucking, and distraction from the painful procedure. There was no evidence of change in brain activity on functional magnetic resonance imaging following the administration of sweet solutions. The most widely used sweet solution is sucrose, but other artificial sweet compounds can also be used. The onset of action is usually within 2 minutes, and the effects can last up to 10 minutes.

KEY FACTS: PAIN MANAGEMENT IN INFANTS

- Sweet solutions can have analgesic effects in infants up to 12 months of age.
- Sweet solutions offer a safe method of analgesia for needle procedures in infants.

FURTHER READING

McGrath PJ, Stevens BJ, Walker SM, et al. (Eds.). *Oxford Textbook of Paediatric Pain*. Cambridge, UK: Oxford University Press; 2014:187.

3. ANSWER: E

Sickle cell disease results from a point mutation causing the amino acid valine to be replaced with glutamine acid. This replacement leads to sickling of the hemoglobin and vaso-occlusive crisis. The frequent hypoxia causes multiorgan dysfunction and increased risk of infections. Chronic consequences include infections, gallstones, splenic autoinfarction, priapism, stroke, and avascular necrosis. Acute chest syndrome caused by infection or emboli is the leading cause of death.

Sickle cell crisis can be triggered by dehydration, cold, alcohol, stress, and underlying infections, but 50% of cases have no known triggering events. Young children often have crisis that involve an extremity, whereas adolescents and adults have pain in their backs, abdomen, and chest.

Treatment of a crisis often involves hydration and oral medication such as acetaminophen, nonsteroidal anti-inflammatory drugs, and opioids at home. When the pain is not controlled at home, they are admitted to the hospital for IV opioid treatment, hydration, and to rule out underlying infections. Sometimes blood transfusions are needed for severe hemolysis. Hydroxyurea increases the amount of fetal hemoglobin and reduces further sickling; it also decreases hemolysis.

Treating sickle cell patients can be frustrating at times because patients will have pain of 10/10 but objectively are not in any distress. The post-infarctive phase of their crisis includes inflammation and continued severe pain. Inadequate dosing can lead to pseudo-addiction. Sickle cell patients will experience tolerance and physical dependence like all chronic opioid patients. The rate of addiction in the sickle cell patient population is not higher than that of the general population.

KEY FACTS: PAIN IN ADOLESCENTS—SICKLE CELL

- The leading cause of death in a sickle cell crisis is acute chest syndrome from infection or emboli.
- Young children usually have pain in extremities, and older children or adults usually have pain in the back, abdomen, or chest.

FURTHER READING

Davis P, Cladis F, Motoyoma E (Eds.). *Smith's Anesthesia for Infants and Children*. 8th ed. Philadelphia, PA: Mosby; 2011:447–449.

4. ANSWER: A

FGID is a group of four disorders in which children experience at least three episodes of abdominal pain that interfere with activity in a 3-month period. The categories are functional abdominal pain, functional dyspepsia, irritable bowel syndrome, and abdominal migraine. Recurrent abdominal pain describes the symptoms the patient is experiencing, not a disorder. The Rome II criteria shown in Table 26.1 are used to diagnose FGID.

Almost 40% of school-aged children complain of abdominal pain each week, making this a common reason for doctor visits as well as missed school. The cause of FGID is unknown, but causes such as altered pain processing, visceral hyperalgesia, viral infections, and the biopsychosocial model have been used to explain it. Chronic abdominal pain in children is associated with missing school, social isolation, anxiety, depression, and poor quality of life. Children with a history of FGID have increased use of medications as adults, socialization problems, and a higher incidence of psychiatric conditions.

There is little evidence for the treatment of FGID, so a multimodal approach is usually taken. Therapies may include acid suppression, bowel regimens, cyproheptadine, antispasmotic, prokinetics, TCAs, selective serotonin reuptake inhibitors, lactose-free diets, fiber supplements, and psychological treatments to improve pain coping skills.

Alarming signs and symptoms to look for in children who present with frequent abdominal pain include fever, weight loss or decreased growth, hematemesis, hematochezia, significant vomiting, right upper quadrant or right lower quadrant pain, localized fullness on exam, hepatomegaly, splenomegaly, costovertebral angle tenderness, perianal abnormalities, or spine tenderness. Children who present with these symptoms should be further evaluated for an organic cause.

Table 26.1 **ROME II CRITERIA FOR DIAGNOSIS OF FGID**

DISORDER	SYMPTOMS
Childhood functional abdominal pain	• Intermittent or constant pain • Minimal evidence for other FGID disorders • No evidence of inflammatory, anatomic, metabolic, or neoplastic process
Childhood functional abdominal pain syndrome	Includes childhood functional abdominal pain at least 25% of the time and one or both of the following: • **Decreased daily functioning or trouble sleeping** • **Additional somatic symptoms (headache or limb pain)**
Functional dyspepsia	• **Intermittent or constant pain or discomfort in the upper abdomen** • **Pain not improved with defecation or associated with the onset of change in stool frequency or form** • No evidence of inflammatory, anatomic, metabolic, or neoplastic process
Irritable bowel syndrome	Discomfort or pain associated with two or more of the following at least 25% of the time: • **Pain improved with defecation** • **Onset associated with a change in stool frequency or form** • No evidence of inflammatory, anatomic, metabolic, or neoplastic process
Abdominal migraine	Paroxysmal, intense, periumbilical pain lasting more than or equal to 1 hour. Interferes with normal activities Associated with two or more of the following: • Anorexia, nausea, vomiting, headache, photophobia, and pallor • Intervening periods of health • No evidence of inflammatory, anatomic, metabolic, or neoplastic process

KEY FACTS: ABDOMINAL PAIN— FUNCTIONAL GASTROINTESTINAL DISORDER

- Rome II criteria are used to diagnose FGID.
- There is no specific treatment for FGID, but reassurance and psychological coping skills are most important.

FURTHER READING

Davis P, Cladis F, Motoyoma E (Eds.). *Smith's Anesthesia for Infants and Children*. 8th ed. Philadelphia, PA: Mosby; 2011:445.
Saps M Functional abdominal pain in children. 2009. Available at http://www2.luriechildrens.org/ce/online/article.aspx?articleID=229.

5. ANSWER: B

Abdominal pain can be from somatic or visceral sources. Visceral pain is usually vague and diffuse. In contrast, somatic pain from the abdominal wall is usually well localized. Carnett's sign is positive when abdominal wall pain is exacerbated by tensing the abdominal muscles. The anterior cutaneous branch of the intercostal nerve can become entrapped when entering into the rectus sheath muscle, resulting in anterior cutaneous nerve entrapment. Treatment includes rectus sheath blocks using ultrasound guidance and sometimes surgical release.

KEY FACT: VISCERAL VERSUS SOMATIC ABDOMINAL PAIN

- Carnett's sign is used to diagnose anterior cutaneous nerve entrapment as the cause of abdominal wall pain.

FURTHER READING

Davis P, Cladis F, Motoyoma E (Eds.). *Smith's Anesthesia for Infants and Children*. 8th ed. Philadelphia, PA: Mosby; 2011:445.

6. ANSWER: A

Water-soluble drugs have a small volume of distribution roughly equal to the intravascular volume. Body composition changes during growth and development. Total body water content in full-term newborns is 75% of body weight, and in preterm newborns it is 80–85% of body weight. This decreases to 60% at 5 months of age. Neonates and infants have a larger volume of distribution for water-soluble drugs compared to adults because of the higher total body water content.

Lipophilic drugs that distribute into tissues have a larger volume of distribution. Body composition changes during growth and development. Body fat increases with age from 3% in preterm newborns to 12% in full-term newborns and 30% at 12 months. In toddlers, body fat decreases to adult levels of 18% once they are walking. Neonates and infants have a smaller volume of distribution for lipophilic drugs compared to adults because of their smaller fat content.

KEY FACTS: PHYSIOLOGY AND DEVELOPMENT—VOLUME OF DISTRIBUTION

- Neonates and infants have a larger volume of distribution for water-soluble drugs.
- Neonates and infants have a smaller volume of distribution for lipophilic drugs.
- Total body water content decreases with age.
- Total body fat increases with age until 12 months of age.

FURTHER READING

Davis P, Cladis F, Motoyoma E (Eds.). *Smith's Anesthesia for Infants and Children*. 8th ed. Philadelphia, PA: Mosby; 2011:179–182.

7. ANSWER: A

Neonates and infants have thinner skin, greater perfusion and hydration, as well as a larger surface area-to-volume ratio, resulting in a greater transdermal bioavailability. Intramuscular bioavailability is greater in neonates and infants because of a large number of skeletal muscle capillaries.

Rectally administered drugs undergo first-pass metabolism. Because neonates and infants have immature hepatic metabolism, their rectal bioavailability is greater.

KEY FACT: ABSORPTION— BIOAVAILABILITY

- Intramuscular, transdermal, and rectal bioavailability are greatest in neonates and infants.

FURTHER READING

Davis P, Cladis F, Motoyoma E (Eds.). *Smith's Anesthesia for Infants and Children*. 8th ed. Philadelphia, PA: Mosby; 2011:183–184.

8. ANSWER: B

Ketamine is a dissociative anesthetic that is frequently used for sedation because most reflexes are preserved. Respiration and blood pressure are usually well maintained. Undesirable side effects, such as acute increases in pulmonary artery pressure in infants with congenital heart disease, hallucinations, bad dreams, and exacerbated excitement of the awakening phase of anesthesia, may occur. Generalized extensor spasm and opisthotonos have occurred in infants.

Infants have a reduced metabolism and decreased renal excretion of ketamine, resulting in reduced clearance and prolonged elimination half-life.

Ketamine can be administered orally as a premedication or analgesic adjuvant, but it has a bitter taste that children may not tolerate.

KEY FACTS: ABSORPTION— BIOAVAILABILITY

- Infants with congenital heart disease may have increases in pulmonary artery pressure when given ketamine.
- Ketamine is associated with extensor spasms and opisthotonos in infants.

FURTHER READING

Davis P, Cladis F, Motoyoma E (Eds.). *Smith's Anesthesia for Infants and Children*. 8th ed. Philadelphia, PA: Mosby; 2011:205–206.

9. ANSWER: D

Epidural fat acts as a reservoir for local anesthetics. Because there is less epidural fat in neonates and infants, the peak plasma concentrations occur earlier in this age group compared to older children and adults, who have biphasic absorption of local anesthetics because of the epidural fat.

Neonates and infants also have a higher cardiac output that increases uptake from the epidural space. This results in a higher peak plasma concentration and a shorter duration of action.

Lung extraction for amide local anesthetics is high. Infants with right-to-left cardiac shunts may be at greater risk of toxicity. Amide local anesthetics are metabolized by the liver and bound by plasma proteins. Neonates and infants have immature metabolism, reduced liver blood flow, as well as decreased plasma proteins. This results in higher levels of free drugs and may cause toxicity.

KEY FACTS: PHARMACOLOGY— LOCAL ANESTHETICS

- Neonates and infants have quicker onset and higher peak plasma concentrations of epidural-administered local anesthetics.
- Infants with right-to-left cardiac shunts may be at greater risk of toxicity.
- Neonates and infants have immature metabolism, reduced liver blood flow, as well as decreased plasma protein, leading to increased free drug.

FURTHER READING

Davis P, Cladis F, Motoyoma E (Eds.). *Smith's Anesthesia for Infants and Children*. 8th ed. Philadelphia, PA: Mosby; 2011:235–238, 440–441.

10. ANSWER: E

Parental interactions may encourage or limit activities in their children. Activities are reinforced by emotional or behavioral responses from the parents. In answer choices A and B, the parents are having catastrophizing thoughts about their child's pain. Catastrophizing thoughts in parents lead to more pain, distress, and disability in the child. Optimism leads to lower pain scores. Both the parents' and the child's cognitive processing are important. Higher pain scores are found in patients who have less optimism or reactive temperaments (fear, anger, and frustration). Catastrophizing increases fear and anxiety, leading to avoidance of painful behaviors and physical inactivity.

Reinforcing the child to use positive coping strategies such as distraction is an appropriate response.

KEY FACTS: PAIN PERCEPTION—CATASTROPHIZING

- Catastrophizing in parents or the patient leads to more pain, distress, and disability.

- Catastrophizing increases fear and anxiety, leading to avoidance of painful behaviors and physical inactivity.

FURTHER READING

McGrath PJ, Stevens BJ, Walker SM, et al. (Eds.). *Oxford Textbook of Paediatric Pain*. Cambridge, UK: Oxford University Press; 2014:10.

11. ANSWER: A

Perception of pain varies by developmental level. Infants as young as 6 months will become fearful and actively avoid anticipated needle punctures if previously exposed. Infants will develop sleep and eating disturbances as well as difficulties with separation from parents.

Toddlers regard their skin as "self" and are preoccupied with wounds. The smallest scrape can be extremely distressful. Common words to describe pain are "owie," "booboo," and "hurt." Fear and anxiety from health care providers as well as unintelligible speech make communication with the child challenging. Parents and caregivers frequently rely on clues of decreased play, fussiness, and loss of appetite to notice that something is wrong.

Preschoolers are in the preoperational thinking stage described by Piaget. Their thinking is egocentric, concrete, and perceptually dominated. They live in a magical world in which reality and fantasy are intertwined. It is important to ensure that they do not believe that their bad behaviors caused their pain.

Elementary-aged children are able to better express and describe their pains. They understand internal cues related to pain such as nausea means they are sick. However, they lack external cues such as the bad sushi eaten last night as the cause of the nausea. At approximately 11 years of age, the affective component of pain starts to develop. These children may continue to believe their bad behavior is the reason for their pain. In this stage, boys are learning to model differences between sexes and will try to be more stoic.

Teenagers can think abstractly and can think about the future. This may lead to worry about recurrence of pain, disease, and disability. They understand how pain works and that pain is protective. They have also learned maladaptive responses to pain and may ignore it or have amplification.

KEY FACTS: PAIN PERCEPTION— DEVELOPMENTAL LEVELS

- Infants do feel and react to painful stimuli.
- Toddlers are preoccupied with wounds.
- Preschoolers have magical thinking and may believe their behavior caused their pain.

- Elementary-aged children at approximately age 11 years start to understand the affective component of pain.
- Teenagers can think abstractly about pain and understand how pain works.

FURTHER READING

Kuttner L. *A Child in Pain: What Health Professionals Can Do to Help.* Bancyfelin, UK: Crown House; 2010:113–119.

Schechter N, Berde C, Yaster M. *Pain in Infants, Children and Adolescents.* 2nd ed. Philadelphia, PA: Lippincott Williams & Wilkins; 2003:132–139.

12. ANSWER: D

Appropriate acetaminophen dosing is 10–15 mg/kg IV/PO q4hr prn. Maximum daily dose from all routes of administration is 70 mg/kg/day for full-term infants, 60 mg/kg/day for preterm infants, and 90 mg/kg/day up to a maximum of 4 g/day for older children and adults. Rectal absorption is variable and has a slower onset time except in newborns and infants. Rectal dosing requires higher doses of 20–40 mg/kg.

Acetaminophen is a centrally acting COX-3 inhibitor that produces analgesia. Acetaminophen is metabolized in the liver by conjugation (primary), sulfation (most important for neonates), and oxidation. Oxidation leads to *N*-acetyl-*p*-benzoquinone imine metabolite, which is hepatotoxic.

Clearance is reduced in neonates and infants. The elimination half-life in infants is approximately 3.5 hours, whereas in adults it is approximately 2 hours. The half-life in premature infants at 28–30 weeks of gestation is 11 hours, and that in premature infants at 32–36 weeks of gestation is 4.8 hours. There have been reports of hepatotoxicity in infants. The dosing interval for premature infants may need to be increased.

KEY FACTS: PHARMACOLOGY— ACETAMINOPHEN

- Maximum dose of acetaminophen
  - Preterm: 60 mg/kg/day
  - Term: 70 mg/kg/day
  - Older children/adults: 90 mg/kg/day
- Elimination is delayed in premature infants, and the dosing interval may need to be increased.

FURTHER READING

Davis P, Cladis F, Motoyoma E (Eds.). *Smith's Anesthesia for Infants and Children.* 8th ed. Philadelphia, PA: Mosby; 2011:258–260, 424–426.

13. ANSWER: D

Elimination half-life of morphine in older children and adults is 3 or 4 hours. Newborns less than 1 week old have an elimination half-life twice as long as that of adults. Clearance is also decreased in newborns. The longer elimination half-life and decreased clearance may explain the increased respiratory depression found in newborns. Premature infants (<37 weeks of gestation) who are younger than 52–60 weeks post conception age or full-term infants younger than 2 months old who receive opioids should be in a monitored setting.

KEY FACTS: PHARMACOLOGY— MORPHINE

- The elimination half-life of morphine in newborns is twice that of older children and adults.
- Clearance is also reduced in newborns.
- Premature infants younger than 52–60 weeks post conception age and full-term infants younger than 2 months old who receive opioids should be in a monitored setting.

FURTHER READING

Davis P, Cladis F, Motoyoma E (Eds.). *Smith's Anesthesia for Infants and Children.* 8th ed. Philadelphia, PA: Mosby; 2011:258–260, 427–430.

14. ANSWER: E

Methadone is a lipophilic, opium-derived alkaloid and exists in a racemic mixture. The D-isomer antagonizes the NMDA receptor, whereas the L-isomer is an opioid receptor agonist. The NMDA properties are thought to help with neuropathic pain. None of the other opioids included in the answer choices have NMDA properties.

Methadone can by conveniently administered IV or orally and is the only liquid long-acting opioid available. The $t\frac{1}{2}\beta$ in children averages 19 hours. Oral bioavailability is 80–90%. Methadone is 60–90% protein bound; this may lead to higher levels of free drug concentrations in neonates.

Methadone blocks the delayed rectifier potassium ion channel and may result in QT prolongation and produce torsades de pointes ventricular tachycardia. Hypokalemia and drugs that prolong the QT interval in patients who are receiving methadone should be avoided.

KEY FACTS: PHARMACOLOGY— METHADONE

- Methadone has NMDA properties.
- Methadone is the only liquid long-acting opioid.

- Methadone is highly protein bound, and neonates may have higher levels of free drug concentrations.
- Methadone may prolong QT interval.

FURTHER READING

Benzon H, Raja S, Liu S, et al. (Eds.). *Essentials of Pain Medicine*. 3rd ed. Philadelphia, PA: Saunders; 2011:91–93.
Davis P, Cladis F, Motoyoma E (Eds.). *Smith's Anesthesia for Infants and Children*. 8th ed. Philadelphia, PA: Mosby; 2011:219–220.

15. ANSWER: A

Codeine is metabolized by three different liver pathways: glucuronidation, N-demethylation, and O-demethylation. A total of 5–15% is excreted unchanged in urine. O-demethylation is dependent on the enzyme cytochrome P450 CYP2D6 gene. The CYP2D6 gene is polymorphic, resulting in four phenotypes: poor metabolizers, intermediate metabolizers, extensive metabolizers, and ultrarapid metabolizers. Normally, approximately 10% of codeine is metabolized to morphine in patients.

The polymorphic gene results in unpredictably analgesia and side effects from codeine administration. Poor metabolizers will have little or no analgesic effect (~7% of the US population), whereas the ultrarapid metabolizers are likely to have undesirable side effects (3–5% of the US population). The incidence of ultrarapid metabolizers varies by racial and ethnic groups; for example, it is 1% in European and Chinese populations and up to 29% in Ethiopians. The ultrarapid metabolizers will convert more codeine to morphine, and respiratory depression or arrest may occur.

KEY FACTS: PHARMACOLOGY—CODEINE

- Normally 10% codeine is metabolized to morphine.
- Metabolism of codeine by the CYP2D6 gene varies. Ethiopians and other racial and ethnic groups may be ultrarapid metabolizers, resulting in toxic doses of morphine.

FURTHER READING

Davis P, Cladis F, Motoyoma E (Eds.). *Smith's Anesthesia for Infants and Children*. 8th ed. Philadelphia, PA: Mosby; 2011:222–223, 430.

16. ANSWER: D

In situations in which pain is minimal at rest but significantly increased with activity, a demand-only PCA may be appropriate. Basal and demand as well as demand-only PCA have been shown to be safe and effective in children.

Table 26.2 provides suggested starting doses for opioids based on the size of the patient. The PCA computer allows for different programing options and stores the history of the attempts by the patient so that individual variation can be considered and the computer can be reprogrammed to make the pump more efficient.

Contraindications to PCA include not being physically capable of pushing the button, not understanding how to use it, or not wanting to use it.

KEY FACT: PHARMACOLOGIC TREATMENT OF PAIN—PCA

- Morphine, fentanyl, and Dilaudid PCA can be used in pediatrics with or without a basal infusion.

FURTHER READING

Davis P, Cladis F, Motoyoma E (Eds.). *Smith's Anesthesia for Infants and Children*. 8th ed. Philadelphia, PA: Mosby; 2011:431–432.

17. ANSWER: D

Nalbuphine is a phenanthrene opioid derivative with agonist and antagonist activities. Overall, it has high affinity for the μ receptor but poor efficacy, so that it is useful only for mild pain. The analgesic ceiling dose is between 150 and 300 μg/kg. In 2006, Dalens et al. showed that one dose of 0.1 mg/kg before extubation decreased emergence delirium by 30%.

Table 26.2 **INTRAVENOUS PATIENT-CONTROLLED ANALGESIA DOSING GUIDELINES**

DRUG	CONTINUOUS BASAL INFUSION (RANGE) (μG/KG/HR)	DEMAND DOSE (RANGE) (μG/KG)	LOCKOUT INTERVAL (RANGE) (MINUTES)	NUMBER OF DEMAND DOSES/ HOUR (RANGE)	4-HOUR LIMIT (μG/KG)
Morphine	20 (10–30)	20 (10–30)	8 (6–15)	5 (1–10)	250–400
Fentanyl	0.5 (0.2–1)	0.5 (0.2–1)	15 (6–15)	4 (1–10)	7–10
Dilaudid	4 (2–6)	4 (2–6)	8 (6–15)	5 (1–10)	50–80

Nalbuphine has good bioavailability from intramuscular and subcutaneous injections at approximately 80% but poor bioavailability from oral absorption at 12%. The elimination half-life is shorter in children at 57 minutes compared to adults at 135 minutes.

Nalbuphine can also be used for the treatment of opioid-induced itching at 50 μg/kg/dose.

KEY FACTS: PHARMACOLOGIC TREATMENT OF PAIN—NALBUPHINE

- Nalbuphine's low analgesic ceiling effect makes it useful Dalens for mild pain.
- Nalbuphine is both an agonist and an antagonist.

FURTHER READING

Dales BJ, Pinard AM, Letourneau DR, Albert NT, Truchon RJ. Prevention of Emergence Agitation After Sevoflurane Anesthesia for Pediatric Cerebral Magnetic Resonance Imaging by Small Doses of Ketamine or Nalbuphine Administered Just Before Discontinuing Anesthesia. *Ants Analg.* 2006 Apr;102(4):1056–61.
Davis P, Cladis F, Motoyoma E (Eds.). *Smith's Anesthesia for Infants and Children.* 8th ed. Philadelphia, PA: Mosby; 2011:223, 435.

18. ANSWER: C

Chronic pain in children is frequently managed by noninterventional therapies. Psychological support for improved coping skills is a mainstay of treatment. Cognitive–behavioral therapy (CBT) has the most evidence-based approach for psychological treatment in the pediatric population. The CBT premise is on the relationship of thoughts, feelings, and behaviors being integrated. CBT is a combination of cognitive theory, which emphasizes interpretation of experiences, and behavioral learning theory, which emphasizes shaping of behaviors through reinforcement. Types of CBT include biofeedback, distraction, thought-stopping, guided imagery, hypnosis, cognitive reframing, relaxation, positive self-statements, and desensitization.

Biofeedback is one type of CBT in which patients use computers to learn how to change their own physiologic response. This allows immediate, real-time feedback that enables children to make the mind–body connection, decrease sympathetic tone, increase relaxation, and provide a sense of control over their own bodies. Types of biofeedback include thermal, EMG, heart rate variability, respiration, and skin conductance. Children usually enjoy using computers in their therapy sessions, and there are many age-based applications that can be downloaded to their electronic devices for them to use at home and school.

KEY FACTS: NONPHARMACOLOGIC TREATMENT OF PAIN—CBT

- Chronic pain in children is usually first treated with noninterventional treatments.
- CBT in pediatrics is the most evidence-based psychological therapy to provide benefit.
- Biofeedback is one type of CBT that allows the connection between mind and body to be seen in real time.

FURTHER READING

McGrath PJ, Stevens BJ, Walker SM, et al. (Eds.). *Oxford Textbook of Paediatric Pain.* Cambridge, UK: Oxford University Press; 2014:11.
Palermo T. *Cognitive–Behavioral Therapy for Chronic Pain in Children and Adolescents.* New York, NY: Oxford University Press; 2012:75–91.

19. ANSWER: B

Treatment of chronic pain in children often involves teaching parents how to restructure their previous emotional and behavioral approaches to their child's pain. A psychologist is frequently needed to help teach the parents as well as the child new ways of coping. Many parents believe they are uncaring if they do not ask their child whether he or she is having pain or if they ignore pain-related behaviors. Parents should not stop caring or ignore their children, but they should shift the framework to focus on positive thinking and reinforcements. They should avoid giving attention to verbal and nonverbal pain complaints and instead praise the child for using coping strategies. Parents should not allow fun activities on days when their child has reduced activity from pain. Parents should restructure their statements with hope, more tolerable words, and a positive spin. They should help their child understand that the pain will come to an end and remind him or her of all the body parts that do not hurt.

KEY FACTS: NONPHARMACOLOGIC TREATMENT OF PAIN—COGNITIVE REFRAMING

- Parents and patients frequently need a psychologist to help them improve coping skills.
- Focus attention away from the pain and use positive reinforcement for appropriate coping strategies.

FURTHER READING

Kuttner L. *A Child in Pain: What Health Professionals Can Do to Help.* Bancyfelin, UK: Crown House; 2010:147–182.

Palermo T. *Cognitive–Behavioral Therapy for Chronic Pain in Children and Adolescents*. New York, NY: Oxford University Press; 2012:75–91.

20. ANSWER: B

In normally developing 2-year-old children, self-report may be limited to pointing to various locations of pain on their body and vocalization. However, by 3 years of age, most normally developing children can quantify the intensity of their pain and describe its location as well as the sensory qualities of their pain reliably if provided with the appropriate tools.

KEY FACT: PAIN ASSESSMENT TOOLS

- Self-assessment tools can be useful but are not reliable for use in children younger than age 3 years.

FURTHER READING

McGrath PJ, Stevens BJ, Walker SM, et al. (Eds.). *Oxford Textbook of Paediatric Pain*. Cambridge, UK: Oxford University Press; 2014:370–371.

21. ANSWER E

To reliably self-report pain using the VAS or NRS tool, one must be able to count numbers (to use the NRS) and understand the concept of measuring intensity level. A faces scale requires only the ability to point at a picture that represents how one is feeling with regard to distress or pain. Multiple faces scales have been developed, but the three that are most commonly used in practice and are the best validated are the Faces Pain Scale-Revised, the OUCHER, and the Wong–Baker FACES Pain Rating Scale (Figure 26.1).

KEY FACT: PAIN ASSESSMENT TOOLS

- Faces scales are helpful tools to ascertain pain levels in younger children.

FURTHER READING

McGrath PJ, Stevens BJ, Walker SM, et al. (Eds.). *Oxford Textbook of Paediatric Pain*. Cambridge, UK: Oxford University Press; 2014:372–373.
Wong–Baker FACES Foundation. Wong–Baker FACES Pain Rating Scale. 2015. Available at http://www.WongBakerFACES.org.

22. ANSWER: B

Children with cancer pain consider painful procedures such as venipuncture, intravenous catheter placement, central line placement, lumbar puncture, bone marrow biopsies, and tissue biopsies to be the most difficult aspect of cancer treatment. Although venipuncture is not as invasive and painful as a procedure such as bone marrow biopsy, the frequency and repetition of this procedure utilized during the treatment for cancer can be a major source of distress to pediatric patients.

KEY FACT: CANCER PAIN

- Venipuncture is a major source of distress in pediatric cancer patients due to the high frequency of this procedure in this patient population, even though it is less invasive than other less frequently performed procedures.

FURTHER READING

American Pain Society. *Guideline for the Management of Cancer Pain in Adults and Children*. Chicago, IL: American Pain Society; 2005.

Wong-Baker FACES® Pain Rating Scale

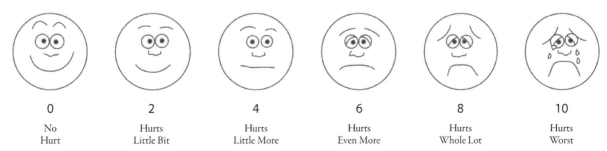

0	2	4	6	8	10
No Hurt	Hurts Little Bit	Hurts Little More	Hurts Even More	Hurts Whole Lot	Hurts Worst

Figure 26.1 Wong–Baker FACES Pain Rating Scale.
SOURCE: Reprinted with permission from the Wong–Baker FACES Foundation. FGID, functional gastrointestinal disorder.

23. ANSWER: B

Many children with cancer develop neuropathic pain following chemotherapy. There are no randomized control trials pertaining to the treatment of neuropathic pain in children. Most of the data are extrapolated from the results of studies on adult patients and from case reports. Opioid medications are the most commonly used agents for the treatment of neuropathic pain in children. TCAs, SNRIs, calcium channel $\alpha_2\delta$ ligands, NMDA antagonists, and membrane stabilizers such as lidocaine patches all have been used as adjuvant agents in children.

KEY FACTS: NEUROPATHIC PAIN IN CHILDREN

- Neuropathic pain commonly develops after chemotherapy.
- Opioids are the most common medications used to treat neuropathic pain in children.

FURTHER READING

McClain BC, Suresh S (Eds.). *Handbook of Pediatric Chronic Pain*. New York, NY: Springer; 2011:200–204.

24. ANSWER: A

Three types of justifications have been proposed to describe the reasons for not adequately treating pain in children and adolescents. A comparative justification is used when a practitioner compares the risks of having unrelieved pain versus the benefits of having adequate pain relief when utilizing a certain treatment. For instance, many practitioners may choose not to utilize opioid medications in children and adolescents out of fear that they will become addicted even if these are the best choice for pain control in a particular patient. However, there are few data confirming that addiction will result with the use of opioids if these medications are prescribed and monitored appropriately in the pediatric population.

A revisionist justification describes the tendency of a caregiver to revise a child's pain complaint based on preconceived beliefs regarding how much pain is acceptable and normal in a given situation. To combat this type of justification, reliable and valid methods of assessing pain in children have been developed.

A pragmatic justification rationalizes that in some circumstances, unrelieved pain can be beneficial in achieving a greater goal. For example, some clinicians believe that eliminating or masking a patient's pain could harm the patient because the ability to monitor the effects of

a treatment or to indicate limits of a certain treatment is removed. When determining whether maintaining a level of pain in a patient is beneficial, one must be certain that (1) the pain will provide useful information for a specific goal, (2) the pain is necessary in achieving that goal, and (3) the pain is maintained at the lowest useful level needed for monitoring purposes. Another example of a pragmatic justification is when a child's pain is not controlled specifically to encourage the development of traits such as courage, self-discipline, or self-sacrifice. Although instilling virtues such as bravery is important in some cultures, prioritizing character development in a child who is suffering from illness or pain is ethically concerning.

KEY FACTS: ETHICS

- A comparative justification is used when a practitioner compares the risks of having unrelieved pain with the benefits of having adequate pain relief when utilizing a certain treatment.

FURTHER READING

McGrath PJ, Stevens BJ, Walker SM, et al. (Eds.). *Oxford Textbook of Paediatric Pain*. Cambridge, UK: Oxford University Press; 2014:661–664.

25. ANSWER: C

Baclofen withdrawal can be a life-threatening situation. Early signs of withdrawal include fever, tachycardia, changes in blood pressure, irritability, increased spasticity, dysphoria, and pruritus. If not identified in the early stages and managed appropriately, the withdrawal can lead to severe hyperthermia, seizures, rhabdomyolysis, disseminated intravascular coagulation, altered mental status, and psychomotor agitation followed by multisystem organ failure and death. If you have any concerns that the patient may be experiencing withdrawal from baclofen, it is important to initiate treatment immediately while ruling out other causes for the patient's symptoms. An X-ray of the spine can be obtained in the emergency room to evaluate the integrity of the catheter and the pump.

KEY FACTS: BACLOFEN WITHDRAWAL

- Early signs of withdrawal include fever, tachycardia, changes in blood pressure, irritability, increased spasticity, dysphoria, and pruritus.
- Withdrawal can lead to severe hyperthermia, seizures, rhabdomyolysis, disseminated intravascular coagulation,

altered mental status, and psychomotor agitation followed by multisystem organ failure and death.

FURTHER READING

Alexander MA, Matthews DJ (Eds.). *Pediatric Rehabilitation: Principles and Practice.* 4th ed. New York, NY: Demos Medical; 2009:181–182.

26. ANSWER: C

Opioid withdrawal can occur in patients who have been administered opioid medication for as few as 7 days. An abrupt cessation of the medication will lead to a decreased concentration of opioid in the blood, which can cause the withdrawal symptoms. Withdrawal can occur within a few days of cessation of the medication. This patient had been receiving opioid medication for pain control for 2 weeks but was not weaned off of the medication after being discharged from the hospital. It is important to develop a plan for weaning patients off opioid medication in order to prevent withdrawal from occurring. Commonly, IV medications are first converted to oral preparations, and the dose is decreased by 10–20% every 24–48 hours.

KEY FACT: OPIOID WITHDRAWAL

- Opioid withdrawal can occur in patients who have been administered opioid medication for as few as 7 days.

FURTHER READING

Galinkin J, Koh JL; Committee on Drugs and Section on Anesthesiology and Pain Medicine. Recognition and management of iatrogenically induced opioid dependence and withdrawal in children. *Pediatrics.* 2014;133:152–155.

27. ANSWER: B

Phantom limb pain is a pain that is experienced in the region of the missing limb following amputation. It can be described as sharp, throbbing, pins and needles, stabbing, tingling, squeezing, and tight. The pain is typically episodic and of short duration. However, a small cohort of children will complain of constant pain. Nonpainful sensations following amputation are reported by 50–100% of children following amputation and in up to 20% in children with congenitally deficient limbs. Children with increased risk of developing painful sensations after amputation are those who have had the limbs surgically removed as opposed to having a congenitally deficient limb, those who are older at the time of amputation, those who had the limb removed due to cancer, those who have had chemotherapy, those who had electrical burns to the limb necessitating the amputation, and those who had pain preoperatively in the affected limb.

KEY FACTS: PHANTOM LIMB PAIN

- Phantom limb pain is a pain that is experienced in the region of the missing limb following amputation and is often described as sharp, throbbing, pins and needles, stabbing, tingling, squeezing, and tight.
- The pain is typically episodic and of short duration.

FURTHER READING

McGrath PJ, Stevens BJ, Walker SM, et al. (Eds.). *Oxford Textbook of Paediatric Pain.* Cambridge, UK: Oxford University Press; 2014:207–208.

28. ANSWER: C

Joint pain is typically the primary presenting complaint in children with chronic inflammatory arthritis. Typically, the pain is associated with other signs, such as swelling and/or pain on movement. There is often limited range of motion in the affected joint(s) as well. Pain at rest is unusual, but it does worsen with inactivity. These patients will complain of pain after prolonged sitting or after sleeping. Pain from arthritis does not usually awaken a patient from sleep, so if this is a complaint, other causes of joint pain should be investigated. There are no laboratory or radiographic studies that can make the diagnosis of juvenile idiopathic arthritis. The diagnosis is typically made clinically.

KEY FACTS: JUVENILE IDIOPATHIC ARTHRITIS

- Joint pain is typically the primary presenting complaint in children with chronic inflammatory arthritis.
- Pain from arthritis does not usually awaken a patient from sleep, so if this is a complaint, other causes of joint pain should be investigated.

FURTHER READING

McGrath PJ, Stevens BJ, Walker SM, et al. (Eds.). *Oxford Textbook of Paediatric Pain.* Cambridge, UK: Oxford University Press; 2014:217–219.

29. ANSWER: E

Complex regional pain syndrome is diagnosed clinically based on the Budapest criteria (Box 26.1), which were validated in 2010 by Harden et al. Often, there is a precipitating injury that leads to the development of this condition, but there are cases that develop without previous injury. The pain is usually out of proportion to the mechanism of injury. In children, the lower limb is most commonly affected, and this is more common in females. Signs and symptoms can resolve only to reappear months to years later. Symptoms can also affect another limb. Children are less likely to suffer long-term disability from this condition compared to adults.

The underlying pathophysiology of complex regional pain syndrome is poorly understood. Possible etiologies include dysfunction in the autonomic nervous system, peripheral small fiber neuropathy, or exaggerated regional inflammation. The endocrine system may also be involved, as well as environmental and behavioral factors.

Box 26.1 THE BUDAPEST CRITERIA

The patient must have continuing pain that is out of proportion to the inciting event.

The patient must report at least one symptom in three of the following four categories:

1. Sensory: Complains of allodynia and/or hyperesthesia
2. Vasomotor: Reports temperature asymmetry and/or skin color changes and/or skin color asymmetry
3. Sudomotor/edema: The presence of edema and/or changes in sweat pattern or asymmetry
4. Motor/trophic: Decreased range of motion and/or motor dysfunction, such as weakness, tremor, or dystonia; trophic changes in the hair, nails, or skin

The patient must display at least one sign at the time of evaluation in two or more of the following categories:

1. Sensory: Evidence of hyperalgesia to pinprick and/or allodynia to light touch, deep somatic pressure, or joint movement
2. Vasomotor: Evidence of temperature asymmetry and/or skin color changes and/or asymmetry
3. Sudomotor/edema: Evidence of edema and/or sweating changes and/or asymmetry
4. Motor/trophic: Evidence of decreased range of motion and/or motor dysfunction including weakness, tremor, or dystonia and/or trophic changes in the hair, nails, or skin

There cannot be any other diagnosis that better explains the patient's signs or symptoms.

KEY FACTS: DIAGNOSIS OF COMPLEX REGIONAL PAIN SYNDROME

- Complex regional pain syndrome is a diagnosis of exclusion.
- The Budapest criteria are used as the standard for diagnosis of this condition.
- In children, this condition is predominant in females.
- The lower limb is more commonly affected.

FURTHER READING

Harden RN, Bruehl S, Perez RS, et al. Validation of proposed diagnostic criteria (the "Budapest criteria") for complex regional pain syndrome. *Pain.* 2010;150(2):268–274.

McGrath PJ, Stevens BJ, Walker SM, et al. (Eds.). *Oxford Textbook of Paediatric Pain.* Cambridge, UK: Oxford University Press; 2014:239–240.

30. ANSWER: D

The diagnostic criteria for headaches was established originally in 1988 and updated in 2004 as the International Classification of Headache Disorders, second edition (ICHD-2), but it was designed for adult headache conditions only. However, modified migraine headache criteria for children have been suggested that have significantly improved diagnostic sensitivity.

Modified migraine diagnostic criteria for children include the following features:

A. At least five attacks fulfilling criteria B–D
B. Headaches lasting 1–72 hours (untreated or unsuccessfully treated)
C. Headache has at least two of the following characteristics
   1. Focal location (unilateral, bifrontal, bitemporal, or biparietal)
   2. Pulsing quality
   3. Moderate or severe pain intensity
   4. Worsening or limiting physical activity
D. Nausea and/or vomiting or two of the following five symptoms
   1. Photophobia
   2. Phonophobia
   3. Difficulty thinking
   4. Lightheadedness
   5. Fatigue
E. Not attributed to another disorder

Based on these criteria, this patient's symptoms are consistent with migraine without aura. However, because her headaches have evolved to occur almost every day, they would be categorized as chronic migraine. These headaches can be successfully treated with migraine-specific pharmacologic agents such as triptans or ergots.

KEY FACTS: MIGRAINE HEADACHES IN CHILDREN

- Modified migraine diagnostic criteria were developed by Hershey et al., which increased the diagnostic sensitivity of children with migraines.

- Migraines and chronic migraines can be treated with triptans or ergots.

FURTHER READING

Hershey AD, Winner P, Kabbouche MA, et al. Use of the ICHD-II criteria in the diagnosis of pediatric migraine. *Headache.* 2005;45:1288–1297.
McClain BC, Suresh S (Eds.). *Handbook of Pediatric Chronic Pain.* New York, NY: Springer; 2011:149–170.

27.

GERIATRIC PAIN

Elizabeth Huntoon

INTRODUCTION

Advances in health care have provided improved longevity and improved daily functioning in many elderly individuals. However, the increase in longevity contributes to the complexity of caring for the elderly pain patient by exposing often multiple comorbidities. Unfortunately, many elderly pain patients are undertreated as a result of inadequate pain assessment, cognitive limitations, or physiologic processes. Therefore, it is imperative to have an awareness and understanding of how the aging process affects the body. The treatment of pain in the elderly includes a variety of pain medications that are commonly used in other age groups but must be approached with caution in older patients due to the differences caused by age-related physiologic changes as well as psychological and socioeconomic differences. The International Association for the Study of Pain (IASP)'s Global Year Against Pain in Older Persons was in 2006. IASP has published a comprehensive review of issues related to pain in the elderly as part of the *Progress in Pain Research and Management* series.

QUESTIONS

1. Which of the following statements is most true regarding the elderly population?

A. The population of adults aged 60 years or older is the fastest growing age group in the United States.
B. The population of adults aged 60 years or older is the fastest growing age group in the world.
C. The percentage of people older than age 60 years experiencing chronic pain is similar to the percentage of patients younger than age 60 years experiencing chronic pain, but these groups differ with regard to the location of the pain problem.
D. Approximately 20% of adults older than age 60 years will experience chronic pain.

2. The elderly pain patient is different from a middle-aged pain patient because of the following generalizations:

A. Middle-aged adults consume more alcohol and thus are at greater risk for developing an addiction to prescription pain medication.
B. Elderly patients consume more prescription drugs than their middle-aged counterparts.
C. Elderly patients with cancer make up the largest proportion of cancer pain visits.
D. Elderly pain patients are more likely to complain of back pain compared to middle-aged pain patients.

3. A 62-year-old female has developed a nontraumatic vertebral compression fracture (VCFx) at T11. Her bone density T score is –1.5. She is otherwise healthy and active. She rates her back pain as a 6 out of 10 on a verbal analogue scale. Which of the following statements is most true?

A. Vertebral compression fractures are a relatively rare occurrence in patients younger than age 75 years; thus, the physician caring for the patient should investigate for possible domestic violence as the cause.
B. Osteoporotic vertebral compression fractures always cause pain.
C. Bracing can be an effective, nonpharmacologic treatment for this patient's back pain.
D. This patient's vertebral compression fracture is not related to osteoporosis because her T score is not within the range for a diagnosis of osteoporosis.

4. An 82-year-old recently widowed female would be expected to be at higher risk for experiencing more pain related to her diagnosis of terminal breast cancer because of the following:

A. She has metastatic disease.
B. She is recently widowed.

C. She has been deemed terminal.

D. B and D.

E. All of the above.

5. All of the following are true of pain and disability in the elderly adult except:

A. Older adults can present atypically with signs and symptoms of a particular disease.

B. An older adult's pain may present as a syndrome of multiple etiologies rather than as a specific disease state.

C. Sensory impairments such as retinal deterioration and hearing loss are independent risk factors for development of disability in the elderly.

D. Neuropsychological decline is not associated with development of persistent pain in the elderly.

6. Which statement is most true regarding a group of community-dwelling older adults?

A. The percentage of elderly patients undertreated for pain increases with age and minority status.

B. Elderly patients with cognitive dysfunction are overtreated with regard to pain medication for osteoarthritis of the spine.

C. Elderly patients without cognitive dysfunction overreport pain compared to elderly patients with cognitive dysfunction.

D. Older adults are more likely to report that they are experiencing pain even though they believe that their pain is a normal part of aging.

7. The Beers criteria are guidelines for safe prescribing in elderly patients. Which of the following statements most closely aligns with the guidelines published in the Beers criteria?

A. All opioids should be avoided in the elderly regardless of their diagnosis.

B. The guidelines do not apply to patients in hospice care.

C. Opioids should be used with caution in patients older than age 55 years.

D. Nortriptyline is safe if used alone without concurrent opioids.

E. Muscle relaxants should be used only at night and at low doses.

8. You are consulted to evaluate an 89-year-old patient with dementia who was recently admitted to the hospital after a fall. She is pleasant and alert but not oriented and is cooperative with your exam. Some of her answers to your questions are nonsensical. Her family members tell you that they think she is in pain. Which of the following will give you the most accurate assessment of this patient's pain?

A. A visual analogue scale because this has been validated for use in the elderly

B. A simple verbal rating scale with the patient indicating if she has "none," "some," or " a lot" of pain

C. The McGill Pain Questionnaire, which can be used if a family member assists the patient in filling out the form

D. The use of behavioral indicators

9. A 79-year-old male with knee osteoarthritis and back pain is brought to your clinic by his son. The patient lives alone, but his son is worried that his father's back and knee pain is becoming problematic for him and interfering with his ability to participate in normal activities of daily living. Which scenario are you likely to encounter in this situation?

A. The patient will deny that his pain is bad enough to warrant a trip to the doctor but will report that he comes in today to please his son.

B. The patient will deny your advice to try pain medication with physical therapy because physical therapy has been shown to be ineffective for treating spinal stenosis and he does not want to become addicted to "pain drugs."

C. The patient is likely to believe that his pain must represent something ominous such as cancer.

D. The patient will overreport his pain as a consequence of personal, societal, or familial expectations.

10. A previously obstinate 80-year-old female with a past history of breast cancer suffered a stroke 1 month ago and is now aphasic. After the stroke, she had some limited mobility and could ambulate with assistance. Prior to her stroke, her oncologist told her she was still in remission. Her breast cancer was successfully treated with cisplatin 5 years ago. During the past 2 weeks, she has started refusing to get out of bed. The nurse on the floor believes that the patient is just being cranky and stubborn. What issue could most likely explain this patient's behavior?

A. She might be experiencing pain caused by her stroke and thus does not want to ambulate.

B. Her refusal to ambulate may be a behavioral issue prompting a psychological evaluation.

C. Her cancer has spread.

D. She might be developing pain from peripheral neuropathy and is not having her pain treated.

11. When assessing the clinical presentation of pain in the elderly patient, which of the following is true?

   A. A healthy elderly patient is more likely to present with typical signs and symptoms of illness or injury, whereas an unhealthy elderly patient is more likely to present atypically.
   B. Pain may be absent or atypical in acute infections.
   C. Older adults are less vulnerable to developing persistent pain after an acute injury.
   D. When present, acute neuropathic pain in an elderly patient presents as a typical pattern in the lower extremities and atypically in the upper extremities.

12. Which of the following is most consistent with age?

   A. Increased renal and hepatic function
   B. Sarcopenia
   C. Increased myelinated and decreased unmyelinated nerve fibers
   D. Increased bone density

13. A 70-year-old insulin-dependent diabetic patient was complaining of back pain; a thorough investigation revealed lumbar spinal stenosis. His primary care doctor placed him on hydrocodone 5/325 mg, four to six times per day. The patient was also advised by his orthopedic surgeon to take 1000 mg acetaminophen three or four times a day and gabapentin 600 mg QID for his knee pain. This patient is at highest risk for all of the following except:

   A. Renal failure since the diabetes may have injured his kidneys, resulting in a buildup of toxic metabolites
   B. Hepatic damage from the hydrocodone that exceeds the recommended dose for the elderly
   C. Fracture because the dose of gabapentin that he is on can cause dizziness and falls
   D. Hepatic damage from the acetaminophen that exceeds the recommended dose

14. Which of the following statements is most true?

   A. Innervation of skeletal muscle decreases as the body ages.
   B. Muscle mass decreases in relation to body weight by approximately 30–50% in men and 10–20% in women.
   C. Muscle mass decreases as a result of loss of type 1 fast-twitch muscle fibers.
   D. Exercise will prevent the decline of muscle mass.

15. A decline in renal function in a healthy elderly patient is most likely to be directly associated with which of the following?

   A. Sarcopenia in the large, weight-bearing muscles of the lower extremities due to increased risk of dehydration
   B. An increased risk of falling following the initiation of gabapentin therapy for peripheral neuropathy
   C. A decreased risk of opioid addiction due to the increased renal clearance of these medications
   D. Gender because elderly males are twice as likely to experience a decline in renal function compared to age-matched females

16. The physiologic differences between a healthy 85-year-old male and an 85-year-old male with diabetes, cardiovascular disease, and arthritis can contribute to the frailty of the patient with multiple medical problems. Aging in either patient can result in which of the following situations?

   A. The rate of an orally administered medication's absorption is inversely related to aging.
   B. Reduced glomerular filtration rates and renal blood flow raise the risk of side effects.
   C. The elderly have higher concentrations of body fat, and this contributes to accumulation of hydrophilic agents.
   D. There is an increase in serum protein concentration in the elderly, and this can cause decreased bioavailability for the highly protein-bound drugs.

17. Which of the following is most true regarding the effects of aging among patients of similar chronological age?

   A. Twin studies show that genetics accounts for 25% and environmental factors account for 50% of the variation in longevity among twins.
   B. Aging is characterized by progressive, unpredictable changes in the renal, hematopoetic, and neurologic systems.
   C. The gastrointestinal tract is unaffected by the aging process.
   D. Persons of the same chronological age will have similar molecular changes related to the aging process in their functional capacity, renal function, and immunologic function.

18. The cognitive function in elderly patients may play a significant role in treatment outcomes. Of the following statements, which is most true for healthy, community-dwelling elderly patients?

   A. The ability to recognize familiar objects and faces remains stable over a lifetime, but skills, ability, and knowledge will decrease past the seventh decade of life.

B. Executive function is well preserved in the elderly as long as they remain healthy.
C. Problem-solving and reasoning skills increase with age, but attention span and processing speed for new information decrease with age.
D. Time-limited testing of cognitive skills begins to decline after the age of 50 years.

19. A 72-year-old female with diet-controlled diabetes presents with right-sided thorax pain of 2 months' duration. She takes a multivitamin regularly and occasionally uses acetaminophen, but otherwise she does not take any prescribed medications. The pain in her thorax is located in the T8 dermatome on the right, in the same location where she had a rash with blisters 2 months previously. She tells you that the rash came on suddenly without much pain. As the blisters healed, the area became more painful. She shares with you that her twin brother had a similar rash that resolved after a few weeks and he is fine now. She did not visit her doctor when the rash was present, so she was not sure if she had herpes zoster. Which of the following best explains her predicament?

A. As a fraternal twin, her female gender makes it more likely she has increased pain; if she had been a male twin, then her pain would have been the same as that of her brother.
B. There is a reasonable chance that the pain will resolve in the next few months because her brother's rash has already resolved and was not painful.
C. Usually, males have more severe onset of herpes zoster but are less likely to go on to develop postherpetic neuralgia.
D. Her age, gender, and diabetes make her more likely to develop postherpetic neuralgia.

20. A 65-year-old female presents to your office with complaints of unilateral leg pain. The pain seems localized to the area around the groin and knee. In addition to leg pain, she complains of leg weakness. On exam, you note that she is 5 feet tall and weighs 280 pounds; she has an antalgic gait favoring the right and a normal neurologic exam with the exception of weakness in the hip flexor muscle group on the right. There is no varus or valgus malalignment of the knees in standing position. There is crepitance around the knee with passive range of motion, and hip range of motion is limited in internal rotation.

Which of the following statements is most likely true?

A. Absence of valgus deformity weighs against a diagnosis of knee osteoarthritis.
B. She may have an L3 lumbar radiculopathy.
C. Radiography likely reveals narrowing of the medial knee joint space.
D. Radiography likely reveals degenerative changes of the hip joint.

ANSWERS

1. ANSWER: B

The world population reached 7.3 billion as of mid-2015, with 12% of that number being age 60 years or older. globally, life expectancy at birth is projected to rise from 70 years in 2010–2015 to 77 years in 2045–2050 and 83 years in 2095–2100.

In 2015, there were 901 million people aged 60 years or older, in the world. This population is growing at a rate of 3.26% per year, making this the fastest growing age group. It has been estimated that up to 50% of community-dwelling elderly adults suffer from chronic pain.

KEY POINT

- The population aged 60 years or older is growing at a rate of 3.26% per year, making this the fastest growing segment of the world's population.

FURTHER READING

Hughs J, Dodds C. Principles of chronic pain therapy in elderly patients. In: Wilson P, Watson P, Haythornthwaite J, et al. (Eds.), *Clinical Pain Management: Chronic Pain*. 2nd ed. London: Hodder & Stoughton; 2008:641–642.

United Nations Department of Economic and Social Affairs, Population Division. World population prospects: The 2015 revision, key findings and advance tables. 2015. Available at https://esa.un.org/unpd/wpp/publications/files/key_findings_wpp_2015.pdf.

2. ANSWER: B

A recent study found that prescription drug use has increased in older adults during the past 20 years. Elderly patients make up the largest proportion of cancer patients; however, they are not the largest proportion to visit pain centers/clinics, and many are undertreated with respect to their pain. The reasons for this undertreatment are multifactorial, with risk factors for higher levels of pain being institutionalization, being widowed, or termed terminal and having impaired mental or physical functioning. Most visits for back pain involve middle-aged patients, particularly working-age adults, rather than the elderly, although there is a significant percentage of elderly reporting back pain.

FURTHER READING

Arnstein P, Herr K. Pain in the older person. In: Fishman S, Ballantyne J, Rathmell J (Eds.), *Bonica's Management of Pain*. 4th ed. Philadelphia, PA: Lippincott Williams & Wilkins; 2010:782–785.

Charlesworth CJ, Smit E, Lee DS, et al. Polypharmacy among adults aged 65 years and older in the United States: 1988–2010. *J Gerontol A Biol Sci Med Sci*. 2015;70A:989–995.

3. ANSWER: C

Many osteoporotic VCFx are painless; however, these types of fractures are a relatively common cause of back pain in the elderly. It is estimated that 75 million people in the United States are affected by osteoporosis, with the majority of this group being elderly postmenopausal women. An estimated one-third of women older than age 65 years will be diagnosed with a vertebral fracture, and one in three women and one in six men will experience a hip fracture by the age of 80 years. The risk of osteoporosis increases with age. Osteoporosis is considered if a patient's T score is–2.5 or less; however, the patient may still suffer from a vertebral compression fracture even if the T score is greater than –2.5. Bracing is an effective nonpharmacologic treatment strategy for many patients with VCFx.

FURTHER READING

Clark G, Kortebein P, Siebens H. Aging and rehabilitation. In: Frontera W (Ed.), *Delisa's Physical Medicine & Rehabilitation: Principles and Practice*. 5th ed. Philadelphia, PA: Lippincott Williams & Wilkins; 2010:1560–1561.

4. ANSWER: D

Cancer can present in different ways in different populations and age groups. Older adults comprise the largest proportion of cancer patients, and risk factors for higher levels of pain in institutionalized elderly include being widowed, deemed terminal, or having dementia. Impaired physical functioning is also considered a risk factor for having higher levels of pain; however, impaired physical functioning may be a consequence of having intense pain. Metastatic disease does not always present with increased pain.

FURTHER READING

Arnstein P, Herr K. Pain in the older person. In: Fishman S, Ballantyne J, Rathmell J (Eds.), *Bonica's Management of Pain*. 4th ed. Philadelphia, PA: Lippincott Williams & Wilkins; 2010:784–785.

5. ANSWER: D

Older patients will commonly present with signs and symptoms that are not typical for a particular problem or disease, and often their pain will appear as a syndrome with many factors or possible etiologies. Sensory impairments do render the elderly at increased risk for developing disability. Neuropsychological decline in this group of patients is associated with the development of persistent pain; postherpetic neuralgia is one common medical problem in which this has been well studied.

FURTHER READING

Arnstein P, Herr K. Pain in the older person. In: Fishman S, Ballantyne J, Rathmell J (Eds.), *Bonica's Management of Pain*. 4th ed. Philadelphia, PA: Lippincott Williams & Wilkins; 2010:783–784.

6. ANSWER: A

The percentage of elderly patients undertreated for pain increases with both age and minority status. Approximately 25–59% of community-dwelling older adults have pain that interferes with normal function. Cognitively impaired elderly patients are rarely overtreated for pain; Rather, they are more likely to be undertreated. Patients who are cognitively intact will often underreport pain as a consequence of personal, societal, or familial expectations. Older adults may be less likely to report pain when they believe that their pain is considered normal and a natural part of the aging process.

KEY POINT

- Pain is a common problem for older persons, with more than 50% of community-dwelling elderly and 80% of nursing home residents reporting pain.

FURTHER READING

American Geriatrics Society. AGS Panel on Persistent Pain in Older Persons. Clinical practice guidelines: The management of persistent pain in older persons. *J Am Geriatr Soc.* 2002;50(6 Suppl):S205–S224.

7. ANSWER: B

The Beers criteria are guidelines for safe prescribing in elderly patients. They were updated in 2015 by the American Geriatrics Society (AGS). The interdisciplinary expert panel added two major components to the prior edition: (1) a nonexhaustive list of drugs that require dose adjustments based on renal function and (2) a nonexhaustive list of drug–drug interactions.

The new Beers criteria are not applicable to elderly patients in hospice or palliative care. The criteria are intended for use in all ambulatory, acute, and institutionalized settings of care for populations aged 65 years or older in the United States. Both nortriptyline and muscle relaxants in general are listed as potentially inappropriate medications for older adults. The strength of recommendation within the Beers criteria is "strong" to avoid both these categories of medications. Most muscle relaxants are poorly tolerated by the elderly because of potential anticholinergic side effects and sedation, potentially resulting in falls. Antidepressants can cause orthostatic hypotension, sedation, or anticholinergic side effects.

FURTHER READING

The American Geriatrics Society 2015 Beers Criteria Update Expert Panel. American Geriatrics Society 2015 updated Beers criteria for potentially inappropriate medication use in older adults. *J Am Geriatr Soc.* 2015;63(11):2227–2246.

8. ANSWER: D

Pain assessment in the elderly is as important as in any other age group; however, there can be limitations on how the assessment tools are used and interpreted. Cognitive impairment can interfere with accurate assessment of pain if one relies on self-report pain scales such as visual analogue scales (VAS), verbal rating scales (VRS), or numerical rating scales (NRS). AGS recommends the use of behavioral indicators such as facial expressions, vocalizations, body movements, changes in interpersonal interactions, changes in activity patterns, and mental status changes to assess pain in cognitively impaired individuals. Overall, the use of VRS or NRS is considered preferable to use of a VAS pain scale for the cognitively intact elderly because comparison studies suggest that increasing age is associated with a higher frequency of incomplete or nonscoreable responses on a VAS even in cognitively intact older adults. Furthermore, the McGill Pain Questionnaire long form may be inappropriate for use in the elderly because they may have difficulty completing the form due to its complexity and length/time requirement, rendering the results inaccurate.

KEY POINT

- Pain assessment often is more difficult in certain older populations, such as those with dementia or those who are noncommunicative, and one must rely on nonverbal signs of pain (e.g., grimacing, guarding, agitation, and frown eyebrows) or behavioral changes such as decreased appetite, increased moodiness, or disorientation.

FURTHER READING

Arnstein P, Herr K. Pain in the older person. In: Fishman S, Ballantyne J, Rathmell J (Eds.), *Bonica's Management of Pain*. 4th ed. Philadelphia, PA: Lippincott Williams & Wilkins; 2010:783–784.

Jaramillo CA. The geriatric patient. In: Cifu D (Ed.), *Braddom's Physical Medicine & Rehabilitation*. 5th ed. Philadelphia, PA: Elsevier; 2016:655–656.

9. ANSWER: A

Part of the challenge in adequately treating an elderly patient is the underreporting of pain. Older adults may be less likely to state when they are experiencing pain due to possible beliefs that pain is a normal part of aging or that if they do admit that there is pain, their independence may be challenged. Many have fears about addiction to pain medications and the cognitive impairments that can sometimes result from taking these medications. Family concern is appropriate if the ability to perform activities of daily living is becoming compromised. Physical therapy is actually helpful for managing pain in many patients with musculoskeletal pain.

FURTHER READING

American Geriatrics Society. AGS Panel on Persistent Pain in Older Persons: Management of persistent pain in older persons *J Am Geriatr Soc*. 2002;50:S205–S224.

Arnstein P, Herr K. Pain in the older person In: Fishman S, Ballantyne J, Rathmell J (Eds.), *Bonica's Management of Pain*. 4th ed. Philadelphia, PA: Lippincott Williams & Wilkins; 2010:783–785.

10. ANSWER: D

It is unlikely that the stroke is causing any extra pain at this point because she was ambulating with assistance for a few weeks after the stroke and before this recent change. Behavioral changes can occur after strokes and should be evaluated, but a higher priority would be to rule out any physiologic or physical causes of her behavior change before attributing this change to her premorbid "crankiness. " It is possible that her cancer has spread (and should be investigated), but a more likely possible explanation at this juncture is that the cisplatin has caused a peripheral neuropathy, making ambulation painful for this patient.

KEY POINTS

• More than one clinical diagnosis typically contributes to chronic pain in older adults.

• The elderly can present with multiple comorbidities that can adversely affect accurate diagnosis and treatment outcome.

FURTHER READING

Vargo M, Riutta J, Franklin D. Rehabilitation for patients with cancer diagnoses. In: Frontera W (Ed.), *Delisa's Physical Medicine & Rehabilitation: Principles and Practice*. 5th ed. Philadelphia, PA: Lippincott Williams & Wilkins; 2010:1162–1163.

11. ANSWER: B

Both healthy and unhealthy elderly pain patients may present with a variety of signs and symptoms that are atypical for both acute and chronic pain. The seemingly discrepant symptoms can delay diagnosis, which could prove deadly in this often frail population; these symptoms include a lack of fever with an infection, lack of typical referred pain pattern, or an atypical referred pain pattern in acute myocardial infarctions. Vague signs such as confusion or restlessness in a dementia patient could easily be mistaken for behavioral problems rather than signs of infection or a nontraumatic vertebral compression fracture. Both acute and chronic pain can present with increased confusion, agitation, and fatigue, although these changes are more likely to be seen in the acute setting.

FURTHER READING

Arnstein P, and Herr K. Pain in the Older Person In: Fishman S, Ballantyne J, Rathmell J. eds. *Bonica's Management of Pain* 4th ed. Philadelphia, PA: Lippincott Williams & Wilkins; 2010: 783–785.

Clark G, Kortebein P, Siebens H. Aging and rehabilitation. In: Frontera W (Ed.), *Delisa's Physical Medicine & Rehabilitation: Principles and Practice*. 5th ed. Philadelphia, PA: Lippincott Williams & Wilkins; 2010:1560–1561.

12. ANSWER: B

Sarcopenia is the loss of muscle tissue as a natural part of the aging process.

Other physiologic changes associated with aging include the progressive loss of bone density, muscle cell atrophy, and loss of myelinated and unmyelinated nerve fibers with increases in the number of damaged nerve fibers. Decreased renal and hepatic function along with loss of hearing and vision changes such as macular degeneration, diabetic retinopathy, glaucoma, and cataract formation can affect the way an elderly patient presents and responds to treatment.

- Aging is associated with progressive physiologic changes that influence susceptibility to many diseases and pain states.

of skeletal muscle decreases in patients older than age 50 years, and the number of motor units decreases with a compensatory increase in motor unit size, which contributes to early fatigability of the muscle fibers.

FURTHER READING

Camacho-Soto A, Sowa G, Weiner D. Geriatric pain. In: Benzon H, Raja S, Liu S, et al. (Eds.), *Essentials of Pain Medicine*. 3rd ed. Philadelphia, PA: Saunders; 2011:409–411.

FURTHER READING

Degens H. Age-related skeletal muscle dysfunction: Causes and mechanisms. *J Musculoskelet Neuronal Interact*. 2007;7:246–252.
Ryall JG, Schertzer JD, Lynch GS. Cellular and molecular mechanisms underlying age-related skeletal muscle wasting and weakness. *Biogerontology*. 2008;9(4):213–228.

13. ANSWER: B

The treatment of pain in the elderly includes a variety of pain medications that are commonly used in other age groups but must be approached with caution in older patients. Acetaminophen, nonsteroidal anti-inflammatory drugs (NSAIDs), opioids, and adjuvants are the mainstay of pharmacotherapy; however, prescribing for the older patient presents unique challenges. Due to changes that occur in the human body as people age, alterations in renal and hepatic function affect the clearance and metabolism of medications; sarcopenia and atrophy result in decreased muscle mass and can affect the way topical agents are absorbed. Analgesics that are affected by aging-associated decline in renal function include codeine; duloxetine; gabapentin; meperidine; pregabalin; propoxyphene; salicylate; tramadol; and the opioids morphine, oxycodone, hydromorphone, fentanyl, and methadone.

FURTHER READING

Barber JB, Gibson S. Treatment of chronic non-malignant pain in the elderly: Safety considerations. *Drug Saf*. 2009;32(6):457–474.
Charlesworth CJ, Smit E, Lee DS, et al. Polypharmacy among adults aged 65 years and older in the United States: 1988–2010. *J Gerontol A Biol Sci Med Sci*. 2015;70A:989–995.

14. ANSWER: A

Muscle mass decreases in the elderly by approximately 30–50% in both men and women. The type 1 slow-twitch fibers are less affected by age compared to fast-twitch type 2 fibers; muscle quality and mass decrease with infiltration of fat and connective tissue. The loss of muscle contributes to age-related insulin resistance, changes in body composition, and changes in volumes of distribution for water-soluble drugs.

Lower extremity strength is lost at a faster rate than upper extremity strength, and exercise will slow the rate of decline but will not prevent loss of muscle mass. Innervation

15. ANSWER: B

One of the side effects of gabapentin is dizziness, which increases the risk of falling in elderly patients even if the starting dose has been adjusted downward to account for the decreased renal function. The most recent Beers criteria suggest that anticonvulsants be avoided in the elderly unless safer alternatives are not available.

Sarcopenia is not directly related to a decline in renal function, and although there may be a decreased risk of opioid addiction in the elderly, this decreased risk is not related to an increased or decreased renal clearance. Decreased renal function occurs in both males and females at approximately the same rate.

FURTHER READING

The American Geriatrics Society 2015 Beers Criteria Update Expert Panel. American Geriatrics Society 2015 updated Beers criteria for potentially inappropriate medication use in older adults. *J Am Geriatr Soc*. 2015;63(11):1–20.

16. ANSWER: B

The rate of medication absorption is not significantly influenced by aging, except for absorption through the rectal route, but there is an age-related selective decline in gut function overall. The risk of side effects increases in patients with reduced glomerular filtration and renal blood flow due in part to the accumulation of active and toxic metabolites. The elderly do have higher concentrations of body fat, and this would contribute to the accumulation of lipophilic, not hydrophilic, agents. The aging process also causes a decline in the serum protein concentrations, which can increase the bioavailability of drugs that are highly protein-bound, such as NSAIDs. This causes an increased free serum concentration of the active analgesic.

Arnstein P, Herr K. Pain in the older person. In: Fishman S, Ballantyne J, Rathmell J (Eds.), *Bonica's Management of Pain.* 4th ed. Philadelphia, PA: Lippincott Williams & Wilkins; 2010:785–787.
Camacho-Soto A, Sowa G, Weiner D. Geriatric pain. In: Benzon H, Raja S, Liu S, et al. (Eds.), *Essentials of Pain Medicine.* 3rd ed. Philadelphia, PA: Saunders; 2011:409–410.

17. ANSWER: A

Aging is characterized by progressive predictable changes in all the physiologic systems of the human body, including the gastrointestinal tract, which can be seen as thinning of the epithelial lining of the oral mucosa, decreased gastric acid production, hypertrophy of the skeletal muscles in the upper third of the esophagus, and loss of esophageal muscle compliance. Genetics and environmental factors significantly influence the way a person ages; a Danish twin study found that genetics accounted for 25% and environmental factors accounted for 50% of the variation in longevity between twins. The process of aging, although predictable, is not a homogenous process, and organs in the same person age at different rates influenced by genetics and other factors. Because aging is significantly affected by environmental factors, persons of the same chronological age may have vastly different physiological responses to the aging process.

Fulp SR, Dalton CB, Castell JA, et al. Aging-related alterations in human upper esophageal sphincter function. *Am J Gastroenterol.* 1990;85:1569–1572.
Soenen S, Rayner CK, Jones KL, et al. The ageing gastrointestinal tract. *Curr Opin Clin Nutr Metab Care.* 2016;19(1):12–18.
vB Hjelmborg J, Iachine I, Skytthe A, et al. Genetic influence on human lifespan and longevity. *Hum Genet.* 2006;119:312–321.

18. ANSWER: A

Certain performances on cognitive testing are well preserved with aging, such as the ability to recognize familiar faces and objects. Well-practiced, familiar skills and abilities such as vocabulary remain intact for a while but will begin to decrease after the age of 70 years. Executive function, which is critical for independent living, declines as a natural part of aging, with the most dramatic decrease in executive functioning occurring after the age of 70 years. Problem-solving and reasoning skills about unfamiliar things show a steady decline after the age of 30 years. Attention span and processing speed for new information decrease with the aging process, which may lead to decreased testing performance on cognitive testing, particularly when the testing is time limited.

Tam HM, Lam CL, Huang H, et al. Age-related difference in relationships between cognitive processing speed and general cognitive status. *Appl Neuropsychol Adult.* 2015;22(2):94–99.
Wilson RS, Beckett LA, Barnes LL, et al. Individual differences in rates of change in cognitive abilities of older persons. *Psychol Aging.* 2002;17(2):179–193.

19. ANSWER: D

Diabetes and gender are both likely to be the main risk factors for this patient, but not the fact that she is a fraternal twin with her brother because genetics is not proven to play a significant role in the development of postherpetic neuralgia (PHN). This patient does not have a history of a prodrome, and her rash was not painful in the beginning; both of these factors weigh in her favor for not developing PHN.

Common risk factors for developing PHN include the presence of a prodrome (suggesting earlier and possibly more extensive involvement in the sensory ganglion), gender (females > males), severity of acute pain, and greater vesicle severity suggesting more extensive involvement of the epidermal nerves. An estimated 10–25% of patients with herpes zoster will develop PHN. Approximately 20% of patients older than age 50 years will continue to have pain 6–12 months after the onset of the rash. The elderly are more susceptible to the development of PHN that is refractory to usual treatment regimens. Other risk factors for developing PHN include the presence of polyneuropathy and ophthalmic distribution of the rash.

Thakur R, Kent J, Dworkin R. Herpes zoster and postherpetic neuralgia. In: Fishman S, Ballantyne J, Rathmell J (Eds.), *Bonica's Management of Pain.* 4th ed. Philadelphia, PA: Lippincott Williams & Wilkins; 2010:348–349.

20. ANSWER: D

Osteoarthritis (OA) is an age-related condition found in a significant percentage of elderly patients, in whom it is an important cause of disability. It is the most common form of arthritis in the world. Radiographic evidence of OA is present in nearly all patients older than age 75 years, but estimates suggest that only approximately 20% of patients will have significant symptoms. Weight-bearing and frequently used joints are most often affected; obesity predisposes the knees to OA; and age, genetics, and trauma are all known risk factors.

The presence of a valgus deformity in the standing position is suggestive of medial knee joint degenerative changes, but the absence of this deformity does not rule out the diagnosis of OA. An upper lumbar level radiculopathy is an option and should be included in the differential; however, in light of the presenting symptoms and physical exam findings, radiography of the hip will potentially show degenerative changes. Hip OA symptoms can present as groin pain or lateral hip or buttock pain that will often radiate down the thigh. Internal rotation limitations are found on hip ranging, and weakness of the hip flexors is common and usually related to pain rather than true neurologic weakness.

FURTHER READING

Baqai T, Jawad A, Kidd B. Chronic joint pain. In: Wilson P, Watson P, Haythornthwaite J, et al. (Eds.), *Clinical Pain Management: Chronic Pain*. 2nd ed. London: Hodder & Stoughton; 2008:525–531.

Gardner G. Joint pain. In: Fishman S, Ballantyne J, Rathmell J (Eds.), *Bonica's Management of Pain*. 4th ed. Philadelphia, PA: Lippincott Williams & Wilkins; 2010:434–436.

Miro J, Paredes S, Rull M, et al. Pain in older adults: A prevalence study in the Mediterranean region of Catalonia. *Eur J Pain*. 2007;11:83–92.

28.

PAIN RELIEF IN AREAS OF DEPRIVATION AND CONFLICT

John Corey and Kelly McQueen

INTRODUCTION

This chapter addresses pain relief in areas of deprivation and conflict. There is variability in the causes of pain worldwide, including HIV/AIDS, torture-related pain and suffering, and war-related injuries. There is also great variability in the availability of adequate pain treatment worldwide due to limitations of education, training, knowledge of pain and its treatment, beliefs and communication about pain, and the inadequacy of access to drugs and palliative care in many countries. Research reflects the importance of extending pain care worldwide and addressing ethical and political issues surrounding pain care.

QUESTIONS

1. The idea of pain treatment being a universal right is declared by what international organization?

A. United Nations
B. International Association for the Study of Pain (IASP)
C. World Health Organization (WHO)
D. All of the above

2. According to the Global Burden of Disease 2010 study, what individual condition ranked highest in terms of years lived with disability (YLD)?

A. Depression
B. Low back pain
C. Neck pain
D. Cancer

3. The World Health Organization defines disability-adjusted life years (DALYs) as the sum of what components?

A. Number of deaths (N) and standard life expectancy at death (L)
B. Years of life lost (YLL) and number of prevalent cases (P)
C. Years lost to disability (YLD) and YLL
D. Incidence (I) and average duration until resolution or death

4. According to a publication by Human Rights Watch on the global state of pain treatment as part of palliative care, what area of the world has the lowest access to opioid medications for those dying with advanced cancer and HIV?

A. Middle East
B. Asia
C. The Americas
D. Sub-Sahara Africa

5. Pain is secondary in prevalence to what symptom in global ambulatory HIV/AIDs patients?

A. Fever
B. Weight loss
C. Diarrhea
D. Cough

6. Survivors of torture often develop symptoms of major depression, generalized anxiety, traumatic stress, and what kind of descriptive pain?

A. Neuropathic
B. Visceral
C. Musculoskeletal
D. Central

7. Which of the following is not defined by Human Rights Watch as a barrier to the use of opioids for palliative care?

A. Lack of availability of policies that promote palliative care and pain treatment
B. Insufficient number of health care workers
C. Insufficient training for health care workers concerning opioid use in palliation
D. Lack of drug availability

8. Regarding limb amputation for patients of disasters or humanitarian emergencies, which of the following statements is true concerning the consensus statement of the 2011 Humanitarian Action Summit Surgical Working Group?

A. Amputations should proceed immediately to prevent infection.
B. Ketamine reduces the risk of developing phantom limb pain.
C. Limb amputation surgery in field hospital settings must never proceed in the absence of effective anesthesia and analgesia.
D. Total intravenous anesthesia (TIVA) has little utility in this setting.

9. What condition is considered to be a hidden and neglected epidemic in low- and middle-income countries (LMICs) according to WHO?

A. Trauma
B. Malaria
C. HIV/AIDS
D. Asthma

10. Which is not a barrier to delivery of effective acute and chronic pain care in LMICs?

A. Poor road networks
B. Insufficient public transportation
C. Sufficient access to analgesic medications
D. Poorly trained health care personnel

11. What model has WHO urged countries to adopt to assist with palliative care?

A. Hospital-based palliative care service
B. Free-standing pain clinic
C. Mobile team of pain physicians
D. Visiting nurse or health worker under the supervision of a physician

12. Kerala, India, used what kind of model to develop cost-effective and sustainable long-term and palliative care?

A. A regional community-based palliative care model
B. An inpatient palliative care hospital
C. A regional pain clinic
D. A nurse-run long-term and palliative care center

13. In LMICs, what important role can anesthesia providers play in reducing chronic pain after traumatic injuries?

A. Provide general anesthesia
B. Provide effective perioperative pain control
C. Use of succinylcholine
D. Intravenous access

14. As we struggle to increase pain care in LMICs, what is an important concept to keep in mind related to opioid medications?

A. There are few side effects from long-term use of opioids.
B. Chronic pain is not the result of an opioid deficit.
C. Opioids for pain are always appropriate.
D. There is no ceiling associated with opioid use.

15. What arguments contribute to the idea of pain being treated as an individual disease in terms of public health policy as opposed to the symptom of another disease process?

A. Failure to do so has led to the neglect of this condition in the world of public health.
B. The staggering prevalence of pain affecting more than 10–20% of the world's population.
C. The combination of persistent pain and psychological comorbidities produces significant disability throughout the world.
D. All of the above.

16. Cultural experiences with pain, both for patients and for health care providers, vary widely and greatly impact the diagnosis and treatment options for patients within their home country. These experiences may include:

A. Religion
B. Myth
C. Fear
D. Superstition
E. All of the above

17. Access to narcotics as one modality for pain treatment is severely limited in most LMICs primarily due to what factor?

A. Expense
B. Government regulation
C. Black markets
D. WHO does not include them on the essential medicine list

18. What percentage of total global disability (YLD) is caused by musculoskeletal (MSK) conditions?

A. 21%
B. 35%
C. 11%
D. Has not been measured

19. The following disparity of trained providers contributes to limited ability to diagnose and treat pain:

A. In LMICs, there are fewer than one physician per 10,000 population.
B. In LMICs, health care is often provided by traditional healers and technicians.
C. In most LMICs, there are only one or two experts trained in pain management within the entire country.
D. The treatment of pain is significantly limited by both available treatment modalities and the opportunity for diagnosis.
E. All of the above.

20. With musculoskeletal and psychological distress causing such a large percentage of global YLD, what therapy has been advocated as one of the most comprehensively successful?

A. Chronic opioid therapy
B. Epidural steroids
C. Cognitive–behavioral therapy
D. Lumbar and cervical traction

ANSWERS

1. ANSWER: D

The United Nations *Universal Declaration of Human Rights* was adopted on December 10, 1948. This document was largely the result of World War II, with the international community vowing to never again allow atrocities such as those of that conflict to happen again. Eleanor Roosevelt chaired the drafting committee, and overall, the drafters skillfully represented ideas consistent with both Eastern and Western philosophies of governance: Western liberal societies such as the United States, Great Britain, and France were represented, as were China and the Soviet Union. Although not specific to pain treatment, Article 25 states that "everyone has a right to a standard of living adequate for the health and well-being of himself and his family."

IASP launched a global day against pain in 2004. The emphasis of the meeting was to promote and reinforce that pain relief should be a human right. This meeting was cosponsored by WHO. In 2006, a convening summit by IASP with the same mission was held in Montreal, Canada. More than 260 pain specialist from 62 countries attended this summit, at which *The Declaration of Montreal* was accepted. The declaration highlights findings that pain management is inadequate in most of the world and that there is poor knowledge and treatment of chronic pain with a significant amount of stigma associated with it. This is followed by three articles stating that all people should have access to pain management without discrimination and also should be provided information and access to pursue appropriate assessment and treatment by appropriately trained providers.

FURTHER READING

Brennan F, Carr DB, Cousins M. Pain management: A fundamental human right. *Anesth Analg.* 2007;105(1):205–221.

International Association for the Study of Pain website. http://www.iasppain.org/Advocacy/Content.aspx?ItemNumber=1821&navItemNumber=582.

United Nations website. http://www.un.org/en/documents/udhr/index.shtml#a25.

2. ANSWER: B

Analysis of the Global Burden of Disease 2010 study showed that of 291 condition studied, low back pain ranked highest in terms of disability (YLD). In terms of DALYs, low back pain ranked sixth. Neck pain ranked fourth highest in terms of YLD and 21st for DALYs.

Although osteoarthritis, rheumatoid arthritis, and gout were significant contributors to the global disability burden, "other musculoskeletal disorders" ranked sixth highest for YLD. Unfortunately, the number of people experiencing MSK conditions in LMICs is likely to increase substantially. Age is one of the most common risk factors for MSK conditions. The ratio of old to young will continue to increase throughout the world. Compared to high-income countries, LMICs have inherently higher risk because work demands of subsistence communities such as collection of water and farming activities can increase the risk of low back pain and knee pain. The negative impact of incapacitation due to low back pain is significant in rural, poor areas, where decreased work and decreased ability to collect essential materials such as clean water and to harvest crops can have a profound impact on the entire family.

FURTHER READING

Hoy DG, Smith E, Cross M, et al. Reflecting on the global burden of musculoskeletal conditions: Lessons learnt from the Global Burden of Disease 2010 study and the next steps forward. *Ann Rheum Dis.* 2015;74(1):4–7.

3. ANSWER: C

One DALY can be thought of as one lost year of "healthy" life. The sum of these DALYs across the population, or the burden of disease, can be thought of as a measurement of the gap between current health status and an ideal health situation in which the entire population lives to an advanced age, free of disease and disability. DALYs for a specific condition are the sum of YLL due to early mortality and the YLD. The YLL represents the number of deaths multiplied by the standard life expectancy at the age at which death occurs. The basic formula for YLL (without yet including other social preferences) is the following for a given cause, age, and sex: $YLL = N \times L$, where N is the number of deaths, and L is the standard life expectancy (in years) at age of death. YLD is calculated as the number of incident cases in that period (I) multiplied by the average duration of the disease (L) and a weight factor (DW; 0 = perfect health, 1 = dead). Thus, the formula is $YLD = I \times L \times DW$.

FURTHER READING

Murray CJ, Vos T, Lozano R, et al. Disability-adjusted life years (DALYs) for 291 diseases and injuries in 21 regions, 1990–2010: A systematic analysis for the Global Burden of Disease Study 2010. *Lancet* 2013;380(9859):2197–2223.

World Health Organization website. http://www.who.int/en.

4. ANSWER: D

Sub-Saharan Africa has the lowest consumption of opioid analgesics worldwide. It is speculated that even if countries in sub-Saharan Africa used opioid analgesics exclusively to treat pain in patients with terminal cancer and HIV, fewer than 10% of these patients could receive adequate pain treatment. As a result, a very conservative estimate is that at least 1.2 million people in sub-Saharan Africa die from cancer or HIV/AIDS without adequate pain treatment each year. Clearly, a challenging economic environment and poor health care infrastructure undoubtedly are major reasons for this situation; findings suggest that government failure to take reasonable, low-cost steps to improve availability of opioid analgesics is a significant contributing factor in many countries.

Although access is poorest in sub-Sahara Africa, the absolute number of people dying without any treatment of pain is highest in Asia due to the world's two most populous countries, India and China. Respectively, these countries can treat just 12% and 53% of their terminal cancer patients, resulting in at least 1.7 million terminal cancer and HIV/AIDS patients untreated.

In the Americas, there is wide variability, with Canada and the United States having good access and some of the countries in Central America having the poorest access. In general, the large countries (Columbia, Brazil, Argentina, and Chile) have some availability based on surveys.

The Middle East also shows a large range, with Israel and Iran having the best access, and Pakistan, Iraq, and Djibouti having the poorest access.

FURTHER READING

Human Rights Watch. Global state of pain treatment: Access to palliative care as a human right. June 2, 2011. Available at https://www.hrw.org.

5. ANSWER: A

Pain is second only to fever as the most common symptom in ambulatory persons with HIV/AIDS. It often presents as a combination of nociceptive pain associated with inflammation (including autoimmune responses), infection (e.g., syphilis or tuberculosis), or neoplasia (lymphoma or sarcoma), as well as neuropathic pain from direct viral infection, secondary pathogens, or neurotoxic side effects from therapy. Prevalence can be up to 60–70% for more advanced AIDS. Similar to cancer, pain associated with HIV/AIDS tends to increase in severity as the disease progresses.

Common pain syndromes by prevalence include abdominal pain (26%), peripheral neuropathy (25%), throat pain (20%), and HIV-related headaches (17%). More than half of the presenting pain complaints are neuropathic in nature. The painful neuropathies can be classified according to HIV stage. The acute or seroconversion phase is associated with mononeuritis, brachial plexopathy, and acute demyelinating polyneuropathy (Guillain–Barré syndrome); the latent phase (CD4 > 500/mm^3) with Guillain–Barré syndrome and chronic inflammatory demyelinating polyneuropathy; the transition phase (CD4 200–500 /mm^3) with herpes zoster and mononeuritis multiplex; and the late phase (<200 /mm^3) with predominant sensory polyneuropathy, autonomic neuropathy, cytomegalovirus polyradiculopathy, severe mononeuritis multiplex, mononeuropathies associated with meningitis, and nucleoside toxicity.

FURTHER READING

Carr DB. Pain in HIV/AIDS: A major global healthcare problem. Accessed at http://www.iasp-pain.org/files/Content/ContentFolders/GlobalYearAgainstPain2/20042005RighttoPainRelief/paininhivaids.pdf.

O-Nei WM, Sherrard S. Pain in human immunodeficiency virus disease: A review. *Pain.* 1993;54:3–14.

Singer EJ, Zorilla C, Fahy-Chandon B, et al. Painful symptoms reported by ambulatory HIV-infected men in a longitudinal study. *Pain.* 1993;54:15–19.

6. ANSWER: C

Pain in the musculoskeletal system is the dominant physical symptom in the chronic phase. The pain tends to be widespread or regional muscle and joint pain, pain related to the spine and pelvic girdle, and neurological complaints. Visceral pain, headaches, and neuropathic pain are also prevalent. Many symptoms can be correlated with the type of torture the victim suffered (e.g., brachial plexus lesions after suspension by the upper extremities). However, the dominant feature is musculoskeletal pain that shares features similar to other widespread pain conditions.

Torture aims to destroy the victim as a human being through the systematic infliction of severe pain, brutalization, and psychological suffering. Not surprisingly, there is a high degree of post-traumatic stress disorder (PTSD). Symptoms of PTSD and chronic pain share some characteristics, particularly anxiety and attentional bias toward somatic cues, as well as avoidance of provoking cues. Ultimately, the psychological and physiologic trauma set the stage for symptoms consistent with central sensitization. These syndromes share common characteristic similar to the constellation of symptoms found in many torture survivors: regional or generalized musculoskeletal pain, often associated with poor sleep, fatigue, sensory disturbances, headache, and visceral symptoms. Diagnosis in other settings would be chronic widespread pain, fibromyalgia, and chronic fatigue syndrome.

FURTHER READING

International Association for the Study of Pain. *Pain Clin Updates.* October 2007;15(7).
Williams ACC, Amris K. Pain from torture. *PAIN.* 2007;133(1):5–8.

7. ANSWER: B

A survey study by Human Rights Watch found that lack of availability of policies that promote palliative care and pain treatment, training for health care workers, and drug availability are all defined as barriers to effective palliative care for those dying of cancer and HIV/AIDS. Of these, one of the major obstacles is training for health care workers.

Key informants from 16 countries surveyed told Human Rights Watch that although some health care workers feared potential legal repercussions when using opioid medications, the larger problem was that there was a reluctance to use opioid medications because of exaggerated fears that they would cause dependence syndrome or respiratory distress in patients. Education in pain management was available to undergraduate medical students in only 5 of the 40 countries surveyed. In Ethiopia, Tanzania, Cameroon, Guatemala, Iran, Jordan, and China, no postgraduate training in palliative care is available.

Manufacture, import and export, distribution, prescription, and dispensation can only occur with government authorization and are overseen by a body created by the Single Convention—the International Narcotics Control Board. Because many countries respond to this regulation by enacting drug control laws that make it difficult for doctors to prescribe medications and for patients to receive them, their cost escalates, unnecessarily limiting their use. In reality, these medications can be produced at very low cost.

FURTHER READING

Human Rights Watch. Global state of pain treatment: Access to palliative care as a human right. June 2, 2011. Available at https://www.hrw.org.
World Health Organization. *Cancer Pain Relief: A Guide to Opioid Availability.* 2nd ed. Geneva, Switzerland: World Health Organization; 1996.

8. ANSWER: C

Best practices for delivery of humane and competent anesthesia and analgesia must be provided even in difficult settings. Lessons learned from prior disasters, including the 2010 earthquake in Haiti, have revealed that delaying definitive surgery may sometimes be the wisest decision, especially when the patient can be stabilized and provided with antibiotics to prevent infection. Often, in the first days and weeks post crisis, anesthesia medications and monitoring equipment may be scarce. If surgery must proceed, resuscitation is a priority, and appropriate anesthesia and pain management must be available.

TIVA via portable, battery-operated infusion pumps may be a cost-effective, safe, and practical anesthesia delivery system for amnesia and hypnosis in austere settings. Regional anesthesia techniques, including central neuraxial and peripheral upper and lower extremity blocks, have clear benefits both intraoperatively and postoperative by superior pain control. Because pain control is a rate-limiting step in the recovery of amputation patients, parenteral ketamine may be a good option for both anesthesia and analgesia after surgery. Ketamine has been shown to reduce severity of chronic phantom limb pain but not the prevalence.

FURTHER READING

Knowlton LM, Gosney JE, Chackungal S, et al. Consensus statements regarding the multidisciplinary care of limb amputation patients in disasters or humanitarian emergencies: Report of the 2011 Humanitarian Action Summit Surgical working group on amputations following disasters or conflict. *Prehospital Disaster Med.* 2011;26(6):438–448.

9. ANSWER: A

Traumatic injuries related to transportation are a neglected epidemic in developing countries causing approximately 5 million deaths each year, roughly equal to the number of deaths from HIV/AIDs, malaria, and tuberculosis combined. When including nontransport injuries, the number increases by approximately 2 million additional deaths annually. There are no definitive data on the number of people who survive with some form of permanent disability for every injury-related death, but estimates are between 10 and 50 times more. More than 90% of injury deaths occur in LMICs, where preventive efforts are often nonexistent.

Although data on burden, epidemiology, effectiveness, and cost-effectiveness of many diseases and interventions in LMICs are available, information for injuries and their management is lacking. Clearly, this has area of mortality and morbidity has not been given the status of many other "high-visibility" conditions, such as communicable disease and nutrition. There is evidence that relatively small investments in prevention can have major impacts in outcome.

FURTHER READING

Gosselin RA, Spiegel DA, Coughlin R, et al. Injuries: The neglected burden in developing countries. *Bull World Health Organization.* 2009;87(4):246–246a.

Murray CJ, Vos T, Lozano R, et al. Disability-adjusted life-years (DALYs) for 291 diseases and injuries in 21 regions, 1990–2010: A systematic analysis for the Global Burden of Disease Study 2010. *Lancet* 2013;380(9859):2197–2223.

10. ANSWER: C

Infrastructure can be a major barrier to effective health care delivery in LMICs. The populations tend to be rural subsistence farmers and are connected by poor road networks with nonexistent public transport. Frequently, health care is delivered by a network of small clinics (some without a doctor) serving massive populations of patients over wide geographical areas. Better facilities and services may be available in larger metropolitan areas, but the cost makes access prohibitive.

Often, provision of anesthesia and analgesia is viewed as a low priority in comparison with the treatment of diseases such as malaria, tuberculosis, and HIV/AIDs. In many places, opioid analgesia is unavailable intraoperatively and postoperatively. A survey of anesthesia officers in Uganda showed that only 45% always had either pethidine or morphine available, whereas 21% never had these drugs available. A study of postoperative pain in Nigeria showed that two-thirds of patients complained of moderate to unbearable pain 24 hours postoperatively. In a rural hospital in sub-Saharan Africa, it is not uncommon for two nursing staff to look after a ward of 50 patients. Lack of training may lead to unreasonable fear of side effects or addiction, which propagates a culture of non-intervention.

FURTHER READING

Faponle AF, Soyannwo OA, Ajayi IO. Postoperative pain therapy: A survey of prescribing patterns and adequacy of analgesia in Ibadan, Nigeria. *Central African J Med*. 2001;47(3):70–74.
Size M, Soyannwo OA, Justins DM. Pain management in developing countries. *Anaesthesia*. 2007;62(Suppl 1):38–43.

11. ANSWER: D

WHO has emphasized that palliative care is particularly important in developing countries, in which the burden of HIV/AIDS is greatest; treatment is not universally available; and many patients with cancer seek medical attention only when the disease is in an advanced stage, beyond cure but causing severe pain. Although palliative care providers may offer inpatient services at hospices or hospitals, their focus is frequently on home-based care for people who are terminally ill or have life-limiting conditions, thus reaching people who otherwise might not have any access to health care services, including pain management. WHO has urged countries with limited resources to focus on developing home-based palliative care services, which can be provided by a visiting nurse or community health worker under the supervision of a doctor, making them very cost-effective.

FURTHER READING

World Health Organization. National cancer control programs: Policies and managerial guidelines. 2002; pp 85–87. Available at http://www.who.int/cancer/media/en/408.pdf. Accessed August 6, 2010.

12. ANSWER: A

The Neighborhood Network in Palliative Care (NNPC) in Kerala, India, is a successful program that involves volunteers at various levels. In the program, people who can spare at least 2 hours per week to care for the sick in their area are enrolled in structured training (16 hours of interactive theory in addition to 4 days of clinical practice under supervision, with an evaluation at the end). On successful completion of this "entry point" training, the volunteers are encouraged to form into groups of 10–15 people per community. Each group then works to identify the problems of the chronically ill in their area and to organize appropriate interventions. These NNPC groups are supported by trained doctors and nurses. The NNPC groups work closely with existing palliative care facilities in their area or, if necessary, create such facilities themselves. Volunteers from these groups make regular home visits to follow up with the patients seen by the palliative care team. Volunteers also identify patients in need of care and address a variety of nonmedical concerns, including financial problems, organizing programs to create awareness in the community, and raising funds for palliative care activities.

FURTHER READING

Kumar S. Kerala, India: A regional community-based palliative care model. *J Pain Symptom Manage*. 2007;33:623–627.
World Health Organization. Cancer control: Palliative care. Available at http://www.who.int/cancer/publications/cancer_control_palliative/en. Accessed November 13, 2015.

13. ANSWER: B

In many LMICs, accidents, especially from road traffic, account for one-third of the disease burden in adult males between 15 and 44 years of age. For those who survive, disability due to chronic pain is a significant problem, and these men are traditionally the primary wage earners for their families.

Because opioid analgesics may be scarce in these settings, other analgesics, such as NSAIDS and ketamine, and regional anesthesia techniques are particularly important. Peripheral nerve blocks have many advantages in operating rooms in which electricity, oxygen delivery, ventilators, monitoring, staffing, and recovery room care are often inadequate or unavailable.

Many groups are focused on increasing awareness, resources, and access for better delivery of perioperative pain care. In 2010, the African Society of Regional Anesthesia was founded to promote education and practice in regional anesthesia on the African continent. The World Federation of Societies of Anesthesiologists has published guidelines pertaining to the management of acute pain in developing countries and has provided educational materials in these areas. Health Volunteers Overseas includes pain management in its anesthesia curriculum in many of the countries to which it sends its volunteers.

FURTHER READING

Warfield CA. Pain management in developing countries. ASA Newsletter. June 2012;76(6).

14. ANSWER: B

The Global Burden of Disease (GBD) study reports low back pain is now the leading cause of years lost to disability worldwide. In fact, 8 of the top 12 disabling conditions globally (low back and neck pain, migraine, arthritis, other musculoskeletal conditions, depression, anxiety, and drug use disorder) are all chronic pain conditions or psychological conditions strongly associated with persistent pain.

Appropriate global access to essential pain medicines, including opioids, for acute and cancer pain is a necessary and worthy goal in LMICs. However, lessons should be learned from opioid use in wealthy countries, especially the United States. Widespread prescriptions of opioids and benzodiazepines to treat chronic pain and anxiety/insomnia have paralleled unprecedented increases in mortality from accidental overdose. In conjunction, there is a lack of demonstrable increases in quality of life and physical function.

In a 2007 review in the journal *Anesthesia and Analgesia*, the authors argued that part of the deficient pain management for worldwide pain care is due to "opiophobia and opioignorance." The associated editorial by White and Kehlet expressed caution for this perspective due to a lack of scientific evidence of benefit and contrary evidence of harm for using opioids for "maintenance" analgesia therapy in patients with chronic noncancer pain.

FURTHER READING

Brennan F, Carr DB, Cousins M. Pain management: A fundamental human right. *Anesth Analg*. 2007;105(1):205–221.
Jackson T, Stabile VS, McQueen KK. The global burden of chronic pain. ASA Newsletter. 2014;78(6).
White PF, Kehlet H. Improving pain management: Are we jumping from the frying pan into the fire? *Anesth Analg*. 2007;105(1):10–12.

15. ANSWER: D

The high prevalence and incidence of global chronic pain, its substantial and growing comorbidities, and its linkage with social and economic determinants collectively provide justification for regarding pain as a public health priority. There are positive public policy consequences in turn. It implies immediately that the global focus on access to essential medicines such as opioids is insufficient as a primary policy strategy. A public health focus requires stakeholders to be aware of multiple potential causes (e.g., traffic and work safety and access to primary care). Chronic pain, as well as most diseases on the planet, are strongly determined by the social and economic conditions in which people work and live. No matter how important essential medicines are to treating chronic pain, a public health model recommends that significant global attention and resources be shifted to the macrosocial determinants that most powerfully shape the patterns of chronic pain, associated comorbid diseases, and the distribution of both. This shift in policy from the micro-level focus on the provision of health care services to a macro-level approach addressing the structural determinants of health dovetails with a number of practices and reports urging the same kind of health policy shift, including but not limited to the those of WHO, the Marmot Review, and the Commission to Build a Healthier America.

FURTHER READING

Goldberg DS, McGee SJ. Pain as a global public health priority. *BMC Public Health*. 2011;11(1):770.
University of Wisconsin School of Medicine and Public Health. Improving global opioid availability for pain & palliative care: A guide to a pilot evaluation of national policy. 2013. Available at http://www.painpolicy.wisc.edu/sites/www.painpolicy.wisc.edu/files/Global%20evaluation%202013.pdf.

16. ANSWER: E

One of the major obstacles in delivery of appropriate palliative and pain care is a lack of appropriate training. Without this training, many continue to practice based on cultural norms that often include perspectives based on myth, superstition, and religion. Based on surveys, in LMICs many providers also still have an unwarranted fear of addiction and respiratory depression, even in the palliative setting. These fears supersede concerns over legal ramifications.

To overcome these obstacles, WHO has recommended that countries provide training on palliative care to health care workers. Under the right to health, countries are obliged to ensure that health care workers at least receive training in the basics of palliative care. Given that almost all doctors will encounter patients in need of palliative care and pain treatment, instruction in these disciplines should be a standard part of undergraduate medical curriculum and postgraduate training in medical disciplines that routinely deal with patients who require palliative care.

FURTHER READING

Human Rights Watch. Global state of pain treatment: Access to palliative care as a human right. June 2, 2011. Available at https://www.hrw.org.
Soyannwo O. Obstacles to pain Management in low-resource settings. In: Kopf A, Patel NB (Eds.), *Guide to Pain Management in Low-Resource Settings*. Seattle, WA: International Association for the Study of Pain; 2010.

17. ANSWER: B

Barriers can be classified into three categories: lack of health policies in support of palliative care development, lack of relevant training for health care workers, and poor availability of essential palliative care drugs. Within the latter category, there are a number of different common barriers, including the failure of states to put in place functioning drug supply systems, the existence of unnecessarily restrictive drug control regulations and practices, fear among health care workers of legal sanctions for legitimate prescribing of opioid medications, and the unnecessarily high cost of pain medications.

The 1961 Single Convention on Narcotic Drugs lays out three minimum criteria that countries must observe in developing national regulations regarding the handling of opioids:

1. Individuals must be authorized to dispense opioids by their professional license to practice, or be specially licensed to do so.
2. Movement of opioids may occur only between institutions or individuals so authorized under national law.
3. A medical prescription is required before opioids may be dispensed to a patient.

Governments may, under the Convention, impose additional requirements if deemed necessary, such as requiring that all prescriptions be written on official forms provided by the government or authorized professional associations. The additional restrictions that many countries have imposed have resulted in diminished or no availability.

FURTHER READING

Human Rights Watch. Global state of pain treatment: Access to palliative care as a human right. June 2, 2011. Available at https://www.hrw.org.
Human Rights Watch. "Please do not make us suffer any more": Access to pain treatment as a human right. 2009. Available at https://www.hrw.org.

18. ANSWER: A

The GBD 2010 study is the most comprehensive effort to date for estimating the global burden of MSK conditions. Taking almost 6 years to complete, the GBD 2010 study estimated for the first time the burden for all MSK conditions, which include osteoarthritis, rheumatoid arthritis, gout, low back pain, neck pain, and all other MSK disorders captured in a group titled "other MSK disorders."

The increasing number of people affected by MSK conditions in LMICs is of great concern because the impact is likely to be extreme and compound other forms of disadvantage, especially because these patients are usually in the most productive years of their life. Although WHO has been measuring and monitoring the prevalence of chronic disease risk factors in developing countries through its STEPwise surveillance program for heart disease, stroke, chronic lung disease, cancer, and diabetes, no such effort has been made to include MSK, despite it being a major cause of global disability.

FURTHER READING

Hoy DG, Smith E, Cross M, et al. Reflecting on the global burden of musculoskeletal conditions: Lessons learnt from the Global Burden of Disease 2010 study and the next steps forward. *Ann Rheum Dis.* 2015;74(1):4–7.

19. ANSWER: E

In LMICs, there is a paucity of trained health care providers, especially physicians but also nurses and others trained in specialty areas of care. A majority of the population in developing countries seek medical attention only when they are seriously ill and often only after consulting traditional healers in their community. Concurrent with this reality is that even clinical officers and general physicians have limited abilities beyond physical examination to diagnose disease in general, and especially complex pain syndromes. Acute and chronic pain often go undertreated or untreated even when anticipated (injury or following surgery) due to limited access to narcotics and other pain medicines, and few or no advanced pain treatments are available. Although WHO recommends availability of narcotics, NSAIDS, and even antiepileptics for the treatment of pain, some countries opt not to invest in WHO recommended medications or frequently restrict the prescription of these medications. Furthermore, health care systems in LMICs frequently refuse to pay for outpatient pain medicines, and even the least expensive available narcotics and NSAIDS are frequently too expensive for the average patient to afford.

FURTHER READING

Africa Health Workforce Observatory. Country monitoring. Available at http://www.hrh-observatory.afro.who.int/en/country-monitoring.html.
World Health Organization. Essential medicines. Available at http://www.who.int/topics/essential_medicines/en.
World Health Organization. The world health report 2006: Working together for health. Available at http://www.who.int/whr/2006/en.

20. ANSWER: C

Although chronic musculoskeletal pain (i.e., back and neck pain and osteoarthritis) and associated psychological comorbidities are a major problem, current treatments are quite limited in their ability to relieve chronic pain. Systematic reviews of 34 commonly used treatments for this disorder have revealed that the vast majority (85%) reduce average pain levels by less than 20%. Also, iatrogenic morbidity in the treatment of chronic pain can be best exemplified by the overprescribing of opioids in wealthy countries that has resulted in a concomitant increase in overdose, death, and addiction treatment. However, cognitive–behavioral therapy has continued to show promise. In fact, reviews of randomized controlled trials of treatments aimed at the self-management of chronic pain have repeatedly concluded that approaches that use cognitive–behavioral therapy methods are most effective.

Acceptance that chronic, disabling pain is a chronic condition for which there is no simple solution has been even slower to achieve than recognition of its existence, with many health systems still supporting ineffective short-term treatments over more appropriate longer-term options.

Despite the difficulties, there is increasing agreement that a chronic care approach may provide a more comprehensive solution for all. Explicit within a chronic care approach is the imperative for those with the condition to play a major role in managing it.

FURTHER READING

International Association for the Study of Pain. Expanding patients' access to help in managing their chronic pain. *Pain Clin Update*. 2015;23(1).

INDEX

References to tables, figures, and boxes are indicated by an italic *t*, *f*, or *b* respectively, following the page number

International Commission on Non-
Ionizing Radiation Protection
(ICNIRP), 201
International normalized ratio (INR), 113
Interneurons, 108
PAG and, 3
Interstitial cystitis (IC), 280
Carnett's sign and, 358
comorbidities with, 276
CPP and, 276
diagnostic test for, 276
gender and, 66
irritable bowel syndrome and, 276, 281
stellate ganglion block and, 76
vulvodynia and, 274
Interval variables, 24t
Intervertebral discs, 256, 265
Intervertebral foramen, 245, 248, 251f
Intervertebral space, cervicobrachialgia
and, 247
Intra-articular hip injection, ultrasound
guide for, 257
Intrathecal opioids, 132–33, 138–40
for C-section, 285, 288
for left-sided abdominal pain, 3
Introspection, 48–49
Investigator bias, 12
Iontophoresis, 173, 177
IPG. See Implantable pulse generator
IRBs. See Institutional review boards
Iritis, 164
Irritable bowel syndrome
gender and, 64
IC and, 276, 281
vulvodynia and, 274
Ischiofemoral impingement, 83
MRI for, 74
Isokinetic exercise, 182, 182t
Isolation, gender and, 64
Isometheptene (Midrin), for migraine
headache, 308
Isometric exercise, 182, 182t
for CRPS, 350
Isoniazid, 327, 335
Isotonic exercise, 182, 182t
ITBS. See Iliotibial band syndrome

Janis reports, 29
Jewett brace, 180
JIA. See Juvenile idiopathic arthritis
Joint of Luschka, 246, 248
J sign, 163, 168
Julien, N., 265
Jumping to conclusions, 46, 55–56
Justice, 31–32, 39, 42
Juvenile idiopathic arthritis (JIA),
360–61, 371

Kappa opioid agonists, 93
Kappa opioid receptor, 88
Kaptchuk, T. J., 17
Kenalog. See Triamcinolone
Kerala, India, 385, 390
Ketamine, 216, 223, 229
for CRPS, 349, 350, 353, 354
in LMICs, 391
for neuropathic pain, 332, 343
in pediatrics, 358, 364
Ketorolac (Toradol), 106, 117, 123
Klumpke's palsy, 187
Knee
areflexia of, ventilatory support for, 328
flexion, 75
OA of, 164, 169, 377
activities of daily living and, 375
shoe modifications for, 174, 181

Korszun, A., 324
Kyphoplasty, 239

Labia majora, 276
Labia minora, 276
Labor pain, 283–84
acupuncture for, 286, 295
anxiety and, 285, 290
first-stage, 283, 288, 290–91
oxytocin and, 290
PCA for, 296
second stage, 284, 291
epidural analgesia for, 289
pelvic pain with, 284, 291
Lachman test, 163, 168
Lacrimal neuralgia, 316
Lamina II (substantia gelatinosa), 3–4
Lamivudine, 327, 335
Lamotrigine, 120, 126
SJS and, 121, 330, 339
Lamotrigine and, 121
LANSS. See Leeds Assessment of
Neuropathic Symptoms and Signs
Laparoscopic presacral neurectomy, 282
Laparoscopic uterine nerve ablation
(LUNA), 282
Laparoscopy, for CPP, 275, 279
Làsegue's sign, 257, 264
Laser-evoked potentials, 176, 188
LAST. See Local anesthetic systemic
toxicity syndrome
Late first stage labor, 284
Lateral epicondylitis, 169, 174, 182
Lateral femoral cutaneous nerve (LFCN),
82, 217, 336–37
Lateral plantar allodynia, 258
Lateral spinothalamic tract, cordotomies
to, 8–9
Latissimus dorsi, 269
Learning theory, 46
Leeds Assessment of Neuropathic
Symptoms and Signs (LANSS),
329, 339t
Leptomeningeal metastatic
disease, 227–28
Leukemia, 105–6, 228
Leukopenia, risperidone overdose
and, 121
Levator ani syndrome, hypertonic pelvic
floor dysfunction and, 278, 280
Levels of evidence, 12, 16
Levetiracetam, 120
Levorphanol, 121
LFCN. See Lateral femoral
cutaneous nerve
Lhermitte's sign, 245
Libido reduction, methadone and, 103
Lidocaine, 28–29, 120, 122, 125, 343
for medial branch nerve block, 303
for neuropathic pain in pediatrics, 360
Lifetime prevalence, 35
of low back pain, 29, 30, 36–37
Ligamentum flavum, 79, 87
hypertrophy, 256
Light work, 202, 206
Limb amputation, 385
Limbic system, neuropathic pain and,
327, 332
Lipophilia, opioids and, 133
Lipophilic drugs, 364
Lissauer's tract, 6
Literature review and evidence, for pain,
12–27, 21t–22t
LMICs. See Low- and middle-income
countries
Local anesthetics, 140

for cancer pain, 231
for cervical radicular pain, 250
for neuropathic pain, 328
in pediatrics, 358, 364–65
in pregnancy, 285, 293–94
Local anesthetic systemic toxicity
syndrome (LAST), 145, 154
Localized external beam radiotherapy,
231, 241
Loewenberg-Weisband, Y, 289
Longus colli, stellate ganglion block and, 76
Low- and middle-income countries
(LMICs)
chronic pain syndrome in, 385, 391
narcotics in, 386
opioids in, 385
trauma in, 390–91
Low back pain, 143, 164, 256–72
activities of daily living and, 375
BRPs for, 205
cause of, 165
celiac plexus block and, 275, 278
corticosteroids for, 258
from degenerative disc disease, 172, 190
disability from, 206
EMG for, 175
flag system for, 202, 206, 258
from FM, 257
hydrocodone for, 45
lifetime prevalence of, 29, 30, 36–37
MRI for, 74, 258
PACE sign with, 74
physical functioning measurement
for, 13
rehabilitation for, 261
risk factors for, 202
SCS for, 260
SI and, 282
therapeutic heat for, 173, 177
X-ray for, 72, 73f, 258, 260
YLD and, 384
zygapophyseal joints and, 260
Low-energy laser, 173
Low-frequency probes, 81
Lumbar facet
injection, spinal stenosis and, 78
synovial cysts, 262
Lumbar plexopathy, 143
Lumbar plexus, 217, 224–25
injury, 332
Lumbar puncture, 303–4, 307
for orofacial pain, 316
Lumbar spinal stenosis, 87
in elderly, 376
Lumbar sympathetic block, 75–76, 76f,
84, 147, 150f
for CRPS, 349, 350, 354
in pediatrics, 359
Lumbar sympathetic chains, 159–60
Lumbar traction, 174, 178–79, 268
Lumbosacral plexus, 235
LUNA. See Laparoscopic uterine nerve
ablation
Lung cancer, 228, 229, 232
Lyme disease, orofacial pain and, 316
Lymphoma, 228
depression and, 232, 243

MACE. See Major adverse cardiac event
Magnesium, 122–23
as NMDA antagonist, 129
Magnetic resonance imaging (MRI), 68,
71, 75, 75f. See also Functional
magnetic resonance imaging
for cervical radicular pain, 246,
247, 253

for CRPS, 349
for CTS, 340, 341
for disc herniation, 259
for discogenic pain, 260
for end-stage colon cancer, 145
for headache, 300–301
for ischiofemoral impingement, 74
for low back pain, 74, 258
for neuropathic pain, 330, 331
for pars interarticularis, 270
for PDPH, 285, 311
for radiculopathy, 258–59
for spine pain, 78, 78f, 84
Magnets, 200–201
Maigne's syndrome, 264, 266
Maintenance, in transtheoretical model of
behavioral change, 59–60
Major adverse cardiac event (MACE), 161
Malingering, 45, 53, 260
in pediatrics, 357
Mandibular branch, of trigeminal nerve
block of, 316, 322
postherpetic neuralgia and, 328
Mandibular foramen, 316
Mandibular nerve, 315, 325
Marijuana, 193, 200
Masculinity, 64, 67
Massage therapy, 174, 179
Mastication muscles, 323
Maternal Opioid Treatment Human
Experimental Research
(MOTHER), 91, 98
Matrix metalloproteinase 7 (MMP-7), 267
Maxillary branches, of trigeminal nerve
block of, 316, 322
postherpetic neuralgia and, 328
Maximal medical improvement (MMI),
205, 213–14
McGill Pain Questionnaire (MPQ), 13,
45, 53, 205, 212
for elderly, 375, 379
McKenzie method, 182–83
McMurray sign, 163, 168
MD Anderson Symptom Inventory
(MDASI), 235
Mechanical diagnosis and treatment
(MDT), 182–83
Mechanonociceptors, 1, 5
Medial branch nerve, 80
block, 147, 151–52, 160
false positives with, 152b
for headache, 303
lidocaine for, 303
Medial spinothalamic tract, ablation of, 9
Median innervated muscles, 187
Median nerve mononeuropathy,
duloxetine and, 105
Medicare
CAM and, 195–96
hospice care and, 227, 234
Medication overuse headache (MOH),
301, 306
Meditation, 44
Medium work, 202, 206
Meloxicam, 118
coronary artery disease and, 107
for neuropathic pain, 328
for rheumatoid arthritis, 106
Memantine, for neuropathic pain,
332, 343
Membrane stabilizers, for CRPS, 350, 354
Memorial Symptom Assessment Scale
(MSAS), 228
Meningitis, 307
epidural analgesia and, 284
Meningococcal meningitis, 307

Taylor brace, 180
TCAs. *See* Tricyclic antidepressants
Tegretol. *See* Carbamazepine
Temazepam, 95
Temporal arteritis, 301
Temporomandibular joint (TMJ)
    disorder, 165, 317, 322–23, 324
    gender and, 66
Tender points (TPs), 195
TENS. *See* Transcutaneous electrical
    nerve stimulation
Tension myalgia, hypertonic pelvic floor
    dysfunction and, 278
Tension-type headaches, 36
    migraine headache from, 304, 311
    in pediatrics, 361
    as primary headache, 313
    VAS for, 301
Teres major, 162
Teres minor, 162
Termination, 44
Testicular cancer, 229
Testosterone
    opioids and, 110
    for transsexuals, 67
Tetracaine, 122
Tetrahydrocannabinol (THC), 95–96
Thalamotomy, 345
Thalamus, 165, 170, 332
Thalidomide, 236
THC. *See* Tetrahydrocannabinol
Therapeutic heat, for low back pain,
    173, 177
Therapeutic ultrasound, in physical
    therapy, 173, 177
Thermal neuritis, 144
Thermal radiofrequency, 261, 271–72
Thigh numbness, 147–48
Thiopental, in pediatrics, 358
Thiothixene, 120
Third-generation psychotherapeutic
    treatment, 44
Third occipital headache, 303, 310
Third-order neurons, 2
Thompson test, 175
Thoracic splanchnic nerve neurolysis, 231
Thoracolumbar junction, 264
Three-phase bone scintigraphy, for CRPS,
    349, 353–54
Tibial nerve, total hip arthroplasty
    and, 176
Tinel's sign, for neuropathic pain, 331
Tipranavir, 327, 335
Tissue pain, 215–26
Tizanidine, 121
TLSO, 180
TMJ. *See* Temporomandibular joint
TN. *See* Trigeminal neuralgia
TNF. *See* Tumor necrosis factor
Topiramate
    for migraine headache, 106, 116–17,
        305, 308
    oral contraceptives and, 313
    in pregnancy, 312
Toradol. *See* Ketorolac
Torsades de pointes, methadone and, 111
Torture, 384, 388
Total hip arthroplasty, 74, 121, 176
    persistent post-surgical pain from, 217
TPs. *See* Tender points
Tramadol
    CYP and, 113
    for DPN, 339
    methadone and, 104
    mu opioid receptor and, 120

for neuropathic pain, 104, 328
    NMDA antagonist and, 112
    for orofacial pain, 318
    pharmacologic actions of, 104
    for PHN, 329
    WHO and, 229, 237–38
Transaminase, acetaminophen and, 104
Transcutaneous electrical nerve
    stimulation (TENS), 3, 9, 131,
    134, 173, 177, 216
    GABA and, 222
    for OA, 163
Transition "end zone" pain, spinal cord
    injury and, 245
Transsexuals, testosterone for, 67
Transtheoretical model of behavioral
    change, 44, 48, 50, 59–60
Transversus abdominis plane block
        (TAP), 75–76, 76*f*, 84–85, 330
    for C-section, 76, 283, 288
Trauma
    in LMICs, 385, 389, 390–91
    from surgery, 217, 224
Traumatic brain injury, 174–75
Trendelenburg gait, 183
Triamcinolone (Kenalog), 120
    hydrocortisone and, 122
Tricyclic antidepressants (TCAs), 115
    in animal research, 41, 114
    for CPP, 277, 282
    for CRPS, 352, 353
    cyclobenzaprine and, 127
    CYP and, 128
    for DPN, 339
    for neuropathic pain, 10, 333, 344, 356
        in pediatrics, 360
    for PHN, 105, 337
    for pressure pain, 31
    side effects of, 105
    for type 2 diabetes mellitus, 3
Trigeminal ganglion block, 316
Trigeminal nerve, 325
    block, 316, 322
    PHN and, 328, 337
Trigeminal neuralgia (TN), 105–6, 116,
        316, 319, 325, 344–45
    CBT for, 58
    glycerol for, 159
    headache from, 305
    microvascular decompression and,
        133, 142
    TENS for, 177
Trigeminocervical nucleus, 309
Trigger points (TrPs), 195
    headaches and, 301
    injections of, for CRPS, 350
    for myofascial pain syndrome, 249, 324
Trileptal. *See* Oxcarbazepine
Triple-blinded study, 14
Triptans
    for migraine headache, 308, 312
    MOH from, 301, 306
Triptan sensations, 311–12
    sumatriptan and, 304
TrPs. *See* Trigger points
True negatives, 27
True positives, 27
Tuberculosis, neuropathic pain
    with, 327–28
Tumor necrosis factor (TNF), 263, 267
    antagonists
        CRPS and, 353
        for musculoskeletal pain, 163
        for RA, 167
    CRPS and, 349

Turk, D. C., 20
Turner, L., 22
Tuskegee study, 32
TXA$_2$, 118
Type 2 diabetes mellitus, 106
    lower extremity pain with, 3
    neuropathic pain with, 328
Type I error, 24
Type II error, 24

Ultrasound guide
    for injections, 73–74
    for interscalene block, 72–73, 81–82
    for intra-articular hip injection, 257
    for piriformis injection, 72, 74
    for stellate ganglion block, 76, 77*f*, 145
Uncovertebral joints, 245, 248, 248f
United Nations, 384, 387
*Universal Declaration of Human
    Rights*, 387
Urgent catheter dye study, 70, 70*f*
Urinary incontinence
    hypertonic pelvic floor dysfunction
        and, 275, 278
    stellate ganglion block and, 76
Urine drug screens
    cannabinoids in, 89, 95–96
    false positives with, 96
    heroin in, 92
    opioids in, 95
Urothelial ulcers, 281
Uterine cancer, 75
    depression and, 232

Vaginismus, hypertonic pelvic floor
    dysfunction and, 278
Valacyclovir, 328
Valproic acid (Depakote), 302
    for neuropathic pain, 328
    SJS and, 330, 339
Variables, 24, 24*t*
VAS. *See* Visual analogue scale
Vasoactive inhibitory peptide (VIP),
    328, 336
VCFx. *See* Vertebral compression
    fracture
Venipuncture, in pediatrics, 360, 369
Venlafaxine
    for brachial plexus neuralgia, 331
    neuropathic pain and, 104
Ventilatory support, for areflexia of
    knee, 328
Ventral posterolateral nucleus
    (VPN), 8
Ventral tegmental area, addiction and, 88
Verbal rating scale (VRS), 52
    for elderly, 375, 379
Vertebral compression fracture (VCFx)
    in elderly, 374, 378
    X-ray for, 80
Vertebroplasty/kyphoplasty, 71, 80
Very heavy work, 202, 206
Vinca alkaloids, 228
Vincristine-induced neuropathy, 31
VIP. *See* Vasoactive inhibitory peptide
Visceral nociceptors, 5
Visceral pain, 233, 241, 242*t*, 244
Visceral tegmental area (VTA), addiction
    and, 93, 93*f*
Viscous distention model, 31
Visual analogue scale (VAS), 13, 14, 22,
    22*b*, 52–53, 215
    for cancer pain, 230, 235
    for elderly, 375, 379
    for headache, 300–301

for migraine headache, 300
    in pediatrics, 360, 369
    for tension-type headaches, 301
Vitamin B$_6$, 328
Vitamin B$_{12}$, 328
    deficiency, 316
Vitamin D, 190, 194–95
Vitamin E, 328
Vitamin K, 199
Volunteer bias, 19
VPN. *See* Ventral posterolateral nucleus
VRS. *See* Verbal rating scale
VTA. *See* Visceral tegmental area
Vulnerable populations, 14–15, 32
Vulvodynia, 274
    hypertonic pelvic floor dysfunction
        and, 275, 278

Waddell, Gordon, 207
Wallerian degeneration, 328, 334, 336
WDR. *See* Wide dynamic range neurons
West Haven-Yale Multidimensional Pain
    Inventory (WHYMPI), 45, 53
Whiplash injury
    EBP for, 304
    orofacial pain and, 316
Whipple procedure, 231, 241
WHO. *See* World Health Organization
WHYMPI. *See* West Haven-Yale
    Multidimensional Pain Inventory
Wide dynamic range neurons (WDR), 2, 6
    central sensitization and, 7
    first-order neurons and, 7
    Rexed lamina and, 10
    second-degree burns and, 2
    wind-up and, 9
Wide-spread pain index (WPI), 264
Wilcoxon rank-sum test, 14
Wind-up, central sensitization and, 9
Wong-Baker FACES Pain
    Scale, 45, 53
    in pediatrics, 369, 369*f*
Work rehabilitation, 202–14
World Health Organization (WHO),
    238–39, 384, 385, 387, 390, 392
    tramadol and, 229, 237–38
WPI. *See* Wide-spread pain index

Xenon, 121
X-ray
    for low back pain, 72, 73*f*, 258, 260
    for pars interarticularis, 270
    for vertebral compression fracture, 80

Yale-Brown Obsessive-Compulsive Scale,
    28, 33–34
Years lived with disability (YLD),
    384, 387
    for musculoskeletal pain, 386
Yeoman's test, 266
Yergason's test, for neuropathic
    pain, 330
YLD. *See* Years lived with disability

Zalcitabine, for HIV, 335
Ziconotide (Prialt), 105, 121, 126, 132,
    137, 156
    calcium channels and, 116
    for CRPS, 350, 354
    for multiple sclerosis, 145
Zidovudine, for HIV, 335
Zygaphyseal cyst, 256
Zygaphyseal joints, 270, 310
    low back pain and, 260
Zyprexa, 230, 238